Recovery after Stroke

One-third of people after stroke, having survived the first few weeks, return home with significant residual disability and can, therefore, benefit from an active, multidisciplinary rehabilitation program. This is a comprehensive guide to rehabilitation after stroke in which leading international authorities set out the basic neuroscientific principles that underlie brain recovery, including chapters on neural plasticity and neural imaging, and describe appropriate rehabilitation strategies for the many different functional problems that can arise after stroke. These include movement disorders, sensory loss, dysphagia and dysarthria, problems with continence and sexual difficulties, and cognitive disorders. Also covered are measurement of disability and quality of life, assistive technology, and vocational rehabilitation.

It is, therefore, an essential handbook and reference for all members of the multidisciplinary stroke rehabilitation team, including medical personnel, therapists, clinical neuropsychologists, and rehabilitation nurses.

Michael P. Barnes is head of the Academic Unit of Neurological Rehabilitation at the University of Newcastle upon Type, UK, and current President of the World Federation for Neurorehabilitation. His previous books include *Upper Motor Neurone Syndrome and Spasticity: Clinical Management and Neurophysiology*, Cambridge University Press, 2001.

Bruce H. Dobkin is Professor of Neurology at the University of California Los Angeles, and directs the UCLA Neurological Rehabilitation and Research Program. He has written extensively in the field.

Julien Bogousslavsky is Professor and Chair in the Department of Neurology and Professor of Cerebrovascular Disease, University of Lausanne, Switzerland, and current President of the International Stroke Society. He has edited several books on stroke including *Stroke Syndromes*, Cambridge University Press, 2001.

Recovery after Stroke

Edited by

Michael P. Barnes

Professor of Neurological Rehabilitation, Hunters Moor Regional Neurological Rehabilitation Centre, Newcastle upon Tyne, UK

Bruce H. Dobkin

Professor of Neurology, University of California Los Angeles, USA

Julien Bogousslavsky

Professor and Chair, Department of Neurology, University of Lausanne, Switzerland

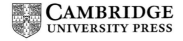
CAMBRIDGE
UNIVERSITY PRESS

CAMBRIDGE UNIVERSITY PRESS
Cambridge, New York, Melbourne, Madrid, Cape Town, Singapore, São Paulo

CAMBRIDGE UNIVERSITY PRESS
The Edinburgh Building, Cambridge, CB2 2RU, UK

Published in the United States of America by Cambridge University Press, NewYork

http://www.cambridge.org
Information on the title: www.cambridge.org/978052182236X

First published 2005

Printed in the United Kingdom at the University Press, Cambridge

A catalog record for this book is available from the British Library

Library of Congress Cataloging in Publication data

ISBN-13 978-0-521-82236-X hardback
ISBN-10 0-521-82236-X hardback

Medical disclaimer
Every effort has been made in preparing this book to provide accurate and up-to-date information which is
in accord with accepted standards and practice at the time of publication. Although case histories are drawn
from usual cases, every effort has been made to disguise the identities of the individuals involved.
Nevertheless, the authors, editors and publishers can make no warranties that the information contained
herein is totally free from error, not least because clinical standards are constantly changing through research
and regulation. The authors, editors and publishers therefore disclaim all liability for direct or consequential
damages resulting from the use of material contained in this book. Readers are strongly advised to pay careful
attention to information provided by the manufacturer of any drugs or equipment that they plan to use.

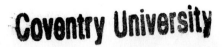

Contents

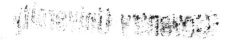

Contributors

Gillian Baer
Department of Physiotherapy, Queen
Margaret University College, Duke St,
Edinburgh EH6 8HF, UK

Michael P. Barnes
Hunters Moor Regional Neurorehabilitation
Centre, Hunters Rd, Newcastle-upon-Tyne
NE2 4NR, UK

Claudio Bassetti
Department of Neurology, University
Hospital of Zurich, Frauenklinikstrasse 26,
CH-8091 Zurich, Switzerland

Daniel C. Bezerra
Department of Neurology, Centre
Hospitalier Universitaire Vaudois, 1011
Lausanne, Switzerland

Claire Bindschaedler
Division de Neuropsychologie, Centre
Hospitalier Universitaire Vaudois, Rue du
Bugnon, CH-1011 Lausanne, Switzerland

Julien Bogousslavsky
Department of Neurology, Centre
Hospitalier Universitaire Vaudois, 1011
Lausanne, Switzerland

Adolfo M. Bronstein
Academic Dept of Neurootology, Faculty of
Medicine, Imperial College, Charing Cross
Hospital, Fulham Palace Rd, London,
W6 8RF, UK

Thomas S. Carmichael
Department of Neurology, Reed Neurologic
Research Center, 710 Westwood Plaza, Los
Angeles, CA 90095, USA

Antonio Carota
Clinique de Rééducation, University
Hospital Geneva, Av. de Berau-Sejour 26,
Ch-1211 Geneva 14, Switzerland

Barbara J. Chandler
Hunters Moor Regional Neurorehabilitation
Centre, Newcastle upon Tyne NE2 4NR, UK

Stephanie Clarke
Division de Neuropsychologie, Centre
Hospitalier Universitaire Vaudois, Rue du
Bugnon, CH-1011 Lausanne, Switzerland

Gabriel R. de Freitas
Rua Mario Pedermeiras 55 206-I, Rio de
Janeiro, RJ, CEP, 2261–060, Brazil

Karin Diserens
Department of Neurology, University of
Lausanne and Centre Hospitalier
Universitaire Vaudois, Rue du Bugnon, 1011
Lausanne, Switzerland

Bruce H. Dobkin
Department of Neurology, Reed Neurologic
Research Center, 710 Westwood Plaza, Los
Angeles, CA 90095, USA

Susan E. Fasoli
77 Massachusetts Ave, Bldg 3–147,
Cambridge, MA 02139, USA

Joseph Ghika
Service de Neurologie, Centre Hospitalier
Universitaire Vaudois, Rue du Bugnon,
CH-1011 Lausanne, Switzerland

Angus Graham
Brain Injury Rehabilitation Unit, Frenchay
Hospital, Bristol B516, UK

Vladimir Hachinski
London Health Sciences Centre, University
Campus, 339 Windermere Rd, London, ON
N6A 5A5, Canada

Dirk Hermann
Department of Neurology, University
Hospital of Zurich, Frauenklinikstrasse 26,
CH-8091 Zurich, Switzerland

Neville Hogan
Newman Laboratory for Biomechanics,
Room 3–146, Massachusetts Institute
of Technology, Cambridge, MA 02139,
USA

Barbro B. Johansson
Division for Experimental Brain
Research, Wallenberg Neuroscience
Center, BMC A13, SE-2211 84 Lund,
Sweden

Hermano I. Krebs
77 Massachusetts Ave, Bldg 3–137,
Cambridge, MA 02139, USA

Gert Kwakkel
Department of Physical Therapy, VU
Medical Centre/Institute for Rehabilitation,
PO Box 7057, De Boelelaan 1117, 1007 MB
Amsterdam, the Netherlands

B. Laurent
Saint-Etienne Center for Pain, Department
of Neurology, Hôpital de Bellevue, 42055
Saint-Etienne, Cedex 02, France

Jeri A. Logemann
Northwestern University, 2299 North
Campus Drive, Evanston, IL 60208–3580,
USA

Ashish Macaden
Hunters Moor Regional,
Neurorehabilitation Centre, Hunters Rd,
Newcastle upon Tyne, NE2 4NR, UK

Alexandre B. Maulaz
Department of Neurology, Centre
Hospitalier Universitaire Vaudois, 1011
Lausanne, Switzerland

José Merino
University of Florida Health Sciences
Center, 580 West 8th St, Tower 1, 9th Floor,
Jacksonville, FL 32209–6511, USA

Marjorie Nicholas
MGH Institute of Health Professions,
Charleston Navy Yard, 36 First Avenue,
Boston, MA 02129, USA

Donal O'Kelly
Different Strokes, 9 Canon Harnett Court,
Wolverton Mill, Milton Keynes, MK12 5NF,
UK

Dominique A. Perennou
Service de Rééducation Neurologique,

Centre Hospitalier-Universitaire de
Rééducation, 23 rue Gaffarel, 21034 Dijon
Cedex, France

R. Peyron
Saint-Etienne Center for Pain, Department
of Neurology, Hôpital de Bellevue, 42055
Saint-Etienne, Cedex 02, France

Radek Ptak
Clinique de Rééducation, University
Hospital Geneva, Av. de Beau-Sejour 26,
Ch-1211 Geneva 14, Switzerland

Michel Rijntjes
Department of Neurology
Universitätsklinikum Hamburg-Eppendorf,
UKE, Martinstraβe 52, 20246 Hamburg,
Germany

Brandon R. Rohrer
Sandia National Laboratories, MS 1010,
PO Box 5800, Albuquerque, NM 87185, USA

Gerhard Rothacher
Kliniken Schmieder Gailingen, Auf dem
Berg, 78262 Gailingen, Germany

Armin Schnider
Clinique de Rééducation, University
Hospital Geneva, Av. de Beau-Sejour 26,
CH-1211 Geneva 14, Switzerland

Rudiger J. Seitz
Department of Neurology, University
Hospital Düsseldorf, Moorenstrasse 5,
D-40225 Düsseldorf, Germany

Fabienne Staub
Department of Neurology, University of
Lausanne, Rue du Bugnon 26, 1011
Lausanne, Switzerland

Joel Stein
Spaulding Rehabilitation Hospital, 125
Nashua St, Boston, MA 02114, USA

Frederike M. J. van Wijck
Department of Physiotherapy, Queen
Margaret University College, Duke St,
Edinburgh EH6 8HF, UK

Bruce T. Volpe
The Burke Medical Research Institute, 785
Mamaroneck Ave, White Plains, NY 10605,
USA

Philippe Vuadens
Clinique Romande de Réeadaptation, Av
Grand-Champsec, CH-1951 Sion,
Switzerland

Cornelius Weiller
Department of Neurology
Universitätsklinikum Hamburg-Eppendorf,
UKE, Martinstraβe 52, 20246 Hamburg,
Germany

Sharon Wood-Dauphinee
School of Physical and Occupational
Therapy, McGill University, 3654
Promenade Sir-William-Osler, Montreal,
Quebec H3G 1Y5, Canada

Preface

Stroke is one of the commonest types of disabling neurological disease worldwide. It represents a significant cost, not only in terms of personal and family disability but also in economic cost to the state. In many developed countries, there are now good-quality acute stroke care facilities and also remarkable achievements in stroke prevention, although events will continue to occur, justifying advances in recovery management. There is an increasing understanding of the various etiologies of stroke disease and increasingly effective ways to limit the degree of consequent brain damage. Despite these advances, approximately one-third of those who survive the first few weeks after stroke return home with a significant residual disability. There is increasing evidence that these people can benefit from an active multidisciplinary rehabilitation program. Neurological rehabilitation is an expanding speciality and is increasingly based on sound principles underlying neural recovery and neural plasticity.

Although there are many textbooks that comprehensively cover acute stroke management, there are surprisingly few textbooks that concentrate on recovery and rehabilitation after stroke. We hope that this textbook fills that gap. We have attempted to outline the basic neuroscientific principles that underlie brain recovery. We have then outlined appropriate clinical rehabilitation strategies that can be used to aid recovery of the many different functional problems that can arise after stroke. Each chapter is designed to be of practical help to practitioners in the field. The book is designed for a multidisciplinary audience and we hope it is of value not only to neurologists, rehabilitation physicians/physiatrists, geriatricians, and other medical specialists but will also be of interest and value to senior therapists and nurses working as members of a multidisciplinary stroke rehabilitation team.

It has been a pleasure to write and edit this book and we hope it is of value in this important and developing speciality.

Stroke: background, epidemiology, etiology and avoiding recurrence

Gabriel R. de Freitas

Federal University of Rio de Janeiro, Brazil

Daniel C. Bezerra, Alexandre B. Maulaz and Julien Bogousslavsky

Centre Hospitalier Universitaire Vaudois, Lausanne, Switzerland

Epidemiology

The impact of stroke

In both the developing and developed countries, the burden of stroke is enormous. Stroke was responsible for 1 in every 15 deaths in the USA in 2001 and, on average, every three minutes someone dies from a stroke (American Heart Association, 2004). Stroke is the second leading cause of death worldwide and the third in developed countries (Murray and Lopez, 1997; Sarti *et al.*, 2000). In 2002, there were more than 5.47 million deaths from cerebrovascular disease worldwide (World Health Organization [WHO], 2003a).

However, stroke is more disabling than lethal, with at least 30% of the survivors making a incomplete recovery and a further 20% requiring assistance for activities of daily living (Bonita *et al.*, 1997). Cerebrovascular diseases are the first cause of serious long-term disability in the USA (American Heart Association, 2004) and the second worldwide in individuals more than 60 years of age (WHO, 2003a). In addition, the psychosocial burden of caregiving should be mentioned. The long-term caregivers of people with stroke more frequently complain of restraints in social life, uncertainty about care needs, constant worries, and feelings of heavy responsibility. A lower quality of life, as well as an increased prevalence of depression, was also found among stroke caregivers (Morimoto *et al.*, 2003).

Finally, because stroke is a leading cause of lost years and disability, it has a very high economic cost. Although the cost may vary according to the type (Bergman *et al.*, 1995; Taylor *et al.*, 1996; Payne *et al.*, 2002) (e.g. hemorrhagic vs. ischemic) and severity of stroke (Caro *et al.*, 2000), the mean lifetime cost for ischemic stroke (IS) including inpatient care, rehabilitation and follow-up is expected to be at

Recovery after Stroke, ed. Michael P. Barnes, Bruce H. Dobkin and Julien Bogousslavsky. Published by Cambridge University Press. © Cambridge University Press 2005.

US$ 140, 048, and the estimated direct and indirect cost of stroke in the USA for 2004 is US$ 53.6 billion (Taylor *et al.*, 1996; American Heart Association, 2004).

Secular trends in stroke mortality

The mortality from stroke has been clearly changing over time. In the USA, it is estimated that between 1915 and 1968 stroke mortality has decreased approximately 1.5% per year, probably as a result of improvements in general public health and nutritional status of the citizens (Wolf and D'Agostino, 1998). Between 1950 and 1968, although mortality from coronary heart disease (CHD) increased about 10%, stroke continued to decrease (National Institutes of Health [NIH], 2002) and there is evidence that it is still declining (Howard *et al.*, 2001). Nevertheless, since the population is aging, the actual number of deaths is rising; consequently, even though the death rate fell approximately 3.4% between 1991 and 2001, the actual number of deaths rose 7.7% in the USA (American Heart Association, 2004).

In most of the other developed countries, mortality rates have also fallen since the early 1990s, especially in Japan and Western Europe (Sarti *et al.*, 2000; Feigin *et al.*, 2003; Truelsen *et al.*, 2003). In the WHO MONICA (Multinational Monitoring of Trends and Determinants in Cardiovascular Disease) project (2003b), the average stroke mortality in Turku-Loimaa, Finland fell from 82 per 100 000 in 1983–1985 to 60 per 100 000 in 1990–1992 (Tuomilehto *et al.*, 1996) (Fig. 1.1). Conversely, the mortality from countries in Eastern Europe has increased in recent years (Truelsen

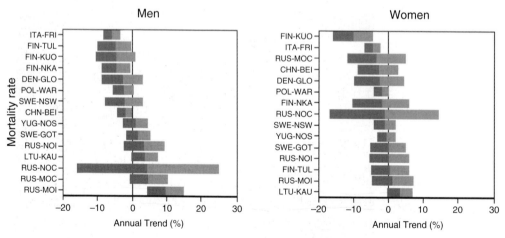

Fig. 1.1   Mortality trends in the MONICA project (WHO, 2003b). Horizontal bars in the mortality rate show the 95% confidence intervals around the estimated annual trend. Note that stroke mortality has lowered in countries from Western Europe, China and Poland whereas the opposite has happened to countries in most of the populations studied in Eastern Europe. ITA, Italy; FIN, Finland; DEN, Denmark; POL, Poland; SWE, Sweden; CHN, China; YUG, Yugoslavia; RUS, Russia; LTU, Lithuania.

et al., 2003; WHO, 2003a). Data from the WHO indicate that in Russia between 1985 and 1994 mortality rates increased by 2.19% per year for men aged 35–74 years (Sarti *et al.*, 2000).

There are few studies concerning mortality trends in developing countries making it, difficulty to draw conclusions. Except for some places such as Mauritius (which has not shown an evident variation in time), in most countries mortality rates have also been declining (Sarti *et al.*, 2000; de Padua Mansur *et al.*, 2003), especially for the population aged 35–74 years.

The determinants of stroke mortality: incidence and case-fatality

Stroke mortality is a function of the incidence (new cases per year) and the case-fatality (proportion of those who die). It varies widely in different regions of the world (Fig. 1.2) and depends on factors such as local environmental, cultural, socioeconomic and genetic variables. Incidence can only be drawn from population-based stroke studies. Most of the studies capable of providing such information show that incidence of stroke declined during the 1970s and 1980s, but between the 1980s and 1990s this decline slowed, reaching a plateau or even increasing in some populations, such as in Söderhamn, Sweden or in Auckland, New Zealand (Bonita *et al.*, 1993; Feigin *et al.*, 1995, 2003; Brown *et al.*, 1996; Numminen *et al.*, 1996; Morikawa *et al.*, 2000; Pessah-Rasmussen *et al.*, 2003; Terént, 2003). Nonetheless, there are other populations, such as in Turku, Finland

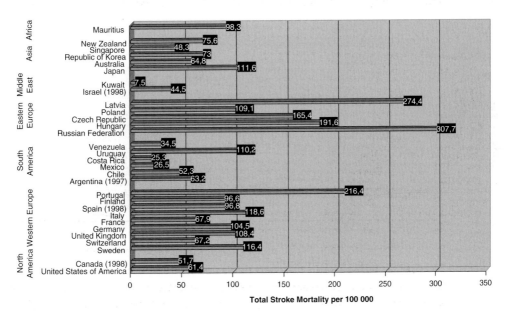

Fig. 1.2   Stroke mortality worldwide. Note the wide variation and the higher rates in countries located in Eastern Europe and Portugal. Data are from 1999 unless otherwise specified. (From WHO, 2003c.)

or in Perth, Australia, that have continued to show a decline (Jamrozik *et al.*, 1999; Immonen-Raiha *et al.*, 2003; Kubo *et al.*, 2003; Sivenius *et al.*, 2004).

Since there are many studies that report a plateau in the incidence levels of stroke over recent years, it seems that the decline in stroke mortality is mainly a consequence of lowering case-fatality rather than a lowering of the incidence rate (Asplund *et al.*, 1998; Asplund, 2001; Sarti *et al.*, 2003; Truelsen *et al.*, 2003).

There are plausible explanations for the reduction in case-fatality. The first is better acute stroke care. Although there are no new specific treatments for stroke that would lead to a clear difference in case-fatality since the early 1990s, the management of medical complications could have improved. The second possibility is a decline in stroke severity. In fact, there are many studies that indicate a reduction in the cases of intracerebral haemorrhage (ICH), a subtype of stroke with high case-fatality (Lawlor *et al.*, 2002; Kubo *et al.*, 2003; Terént, 2003), and an increase in milder strokes. In Sweden, for example, between 1975 and 2001, the incidence of ICH decreased by approximately two-thirds, whereas the incidence of milder strokes almost doubled (Terént, 2003). In Portland, USA (Barker and Mullooly, 1997), stroke severity declined between 1967 and 1985, with a reduction in the rates of people in coma or wheelchair bound. Finally, the development of newer methods for the diagnosis of stroke (such as computed tomography and magnetic resonance) have allowed easier diagnosis of strokes that are mild in nature, with minimal neurological deficits. In Rochester, USA, for example, the incidence of stroke has increased but stroke severity has decreased coincidently with the advent of computed tomography (Broderick, 1993).

Etiology

Although primary prevention interventions are outwith the scope of this chapter (Bronner *et al.*, 1995; de Freitas and Bogousslavsky, 2001), results of randomized controlled trials are reported here, since they provide the best data on clinical epidemiology. The demonstration that specific modification of a presumed risk factor in one group reduces the incidence of stroke compared with the other similar (randomized) group, which had no intervention, is one of the best ways for establishing a causal relationship.

Risk factors

Classically, stroke can be divided into IS (accounting for about 80%) and hemorrhagic stroke (20%). IS is further broadly subdivided into lacunar infarction (small artery disease), large artery disease and cardioembolic stroke; hemorrhagic stroke could be subdivided into ICH and subarachnoid haemorrhage (SAH). The

Table 1.1 Stroke risk factors

Non-modifiable	Modifiable	Emerging
Age	Hypertension	Fibrinogen
Gender	Diabetes mellitus	Hyperhomocysteine
Race	Hypercholesterolemia	Inflammation/infection
Heredity	Cigarette smoking	
	Alcohol abuse	
	Diet	
	Oral contraceptive	
	Atrial fibrillation	

classification of stroke into several types and further subtypes is of great importance. The incidence of morbidity, mortality, and recurrence of hemorrhage and
infarction in the various types/subtypes is entirely different, as are their physio-
pathology and natural history (de Freitas and Bogousslavsky, 2003).

About two-thirds of stroke patients have well known risk factors for stroke. Risk
factors can be divided into modifiable and non-modifiable, and new potential risk
factors are also being studied (Table 1.1) (Sacco, 1995). Risk factors may also be
specific for one stroke type or subtype.

Age

In all studies of stroke, there is a clear increase in the incidence and prevalence with
age. The main reasons for this are reduction of incidence and case-fatality of stroke
in the younger population; the longer time for effect of environmental risk factors;
and higher prevalence of risk factors with age, such as atrial fibrillation, hypertension, diabetes, and CHD (Stolk et al., 1997; Wattigney et al., 2003).

Race and ethnic origin

Although the definitions of ethnicity are controversial (Shriver, 1997; Fustinoni
and Biller, 2000; Saposnik et al., 2003), there is an important variation in mortality
among the different racial and ethnic groups studied.

In USA and Europe, the death rates from cerebrovascular disease among black
people are consistently higher than other groups (Broderick et al., 1998; Qureshi
et al., 1999; Rosamond et al., 1999; Stewart et al., 1999; Longstreth et al., 2001;
Wolfe et al., 2002; Centers for Disease Control and Prevention [CDC], 2003). In
the USA, between 1991 and 1998, the decline in mortality rate was about 2.0% per
year in Asian and Pacific Islanders, followed by Hispanics and black people (1.4%),
Alaskan Natives (1.1%) and white people (0.8%) (CDC, 2003). Possible reasons for
these higher mortality rates in black people are a more stressful socioeconomic

lifestyle and less access to medical therapy, reflected in a lower probability of receiving secondary prevention therapy (Kaplan and Keil, 1993; Giles *et al.*, 1995; Gorelick, 1998; Cabrera *et al.*, 2001; Christian *et al.*, 2003). In addition, black people have higher predisposition and incidence of hypertension and diabetes mellitus compared with white people (Burt *et al.*, 1995a, b; Giles *et al.*, 1995; Baker *et al.*, 1998; Hajat *et al.*, 2001; Gupta *et al.*, 2003). Finally, there seem to be differences in IS subtypes, with black people showing a higher risk for lacunar infarction and large-artery intracranial occlusive disease, whereas white people may be more prone to cerebral embolism, transient ischemic attack (Gorelick *et al.*, 1998), and extracranial atherosclerotic disease (Gupta *et al.*, 2003). Asians have the highest frequency of hemorrhagic stroke, compared with other groups (CDC, 2003).

Family history

In a recent review of the most important studies about the relationship between stroke and family history (Floeβmann *et al.*, 2004), there seemed to be a small genetic contribution to stroke, based on twin studies, with monozygotic twins being 1.6 times more likely to be concordant for stroke compared with dizygotic twins. Moreover, the genetic factors seemed to be more linked to stroke in younger people, particularly those less than 70 years.

This genetic predisposition could be, in part, a reflection of the fact that many risk factors for cardiovascular diseases may have genetic influences, such as hypertension (Oparil *et al.*, 2003), diabetes (Florez *et al.*, 2003), hypercholesterolemia (Snieder *et al.*, 1999), CHD (Hirashiki *et al.*, 2003), carotid stenosis (Fox *et al.*, 2003), and obesity (Damcott *et al.*, 2003). In addition, some genetic mutations, such as factor V Leiden, prothrombin G20210A, methylenetetrahydrofolate reductase C677T, and the genotypes of angiotensin-converting enzyme (ACE) I/D and apolipoprotein allele e4, have been shown to augment the risk of stroke particularly in the presence of hypertension, diabetes mellitus, smoking, and drinking (Szolnoki *et al.*, 2003).

Recently, it was found that the gene encoding phosphodiesterase 4D was associated with IS and that it was not correlated with known risk factors (Gretarsdottir *et al.*, 2003).

Hypertension

Hypertension is the most prevalent and modifiable risk factor for stroke and is associated with IS, ICH, and SAH (Teunissen *et al.*, 1996; Eastern Stroke and Coronary Heart Disease Collaborative Research Group, 1998). It is difficult to determine a relative risk for hypertension, since it interacts with other risk factors, such as age and atrial fibrillation (Whisnant, 1997). In addition, the relative risk is dependent on blood pressure. For example, in a meta-analysis, the relative risk of stroke for people in the highest quintile of diastolic blood pressure was up to 10-fold

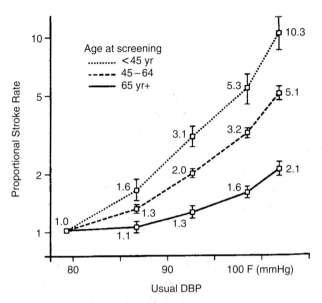

Fig. 1.3   Proportional stroke risk by age and usual diastolic blood pressure (DBP). (Data from Prospective Studies Collaboration, 1995.)

higher than for those in the lowest quintile (Prospective Studies Collaboration, 1995) Fig. 1.3).

Antihypertensive therapy substantially reduces the risk of stroke. A meta-analysis of 14 randomized trials showed that a significant reduction of 42% (95% confidence interval [CI], 33–55) in stroke in treated patients resulted from only a 5–6 mmHg reduction in diastolic blood pressure (Collins et al., 1990).

Although there is no longer uncertainty about whether hypertension should be treated, many questions have only recently been answered. In the early 1990s, there was a reluctance to reduce high blood pressure in the elderly (Wolf, 1993).The Swedish Trial in Old Patients with Hypertension showed that antihypertensive treatment in people aged 70–84 years was safe and conferred a 45% reduction (95% CI, 14–67) in risk of stroke compared with placebo (Dahlöf et al., 1991). Although this trial excluded persons with isolated systolic hypertension (systolic blood pressure >160 mmHg and diastolic blood pressure <90 mmHg), a common condition in the elderly, this issue was addressed in another trial, the Systolic Hypertension in the Elderly Program, which showed that management of isolated systolic hypertension in persons older than 60 years reduced the total incidence of stroke by 36% (95% CI, 18–50) (SHEP Cooperative Research Group, 1991). These results were supported by the Systolic Hypertension in Europe trial, which achieved a 42% (95% CI, 17%–60) reduction in the risk of stroke in people older than 60 years with isolated systolic hypertension (Staessen et al., 1997).

The two main issues at present are to what extent blood pressure should be lowered and which medical regimen should be chosen (Cutler, 1999). It has been argued that mortality increases at a certain level of reduction of blood pressure, resulting in the so-called J curve. However, the J curve has never been confirmed for mortality from stroke and whether it exists in CHD is a matter of controversy (Fletcher and Bulpitt, 1992). The Hypertension Optimal Treatment Study demonstrated the benefits of lowering systolic and diastolic pressures, respectively, to 140 and 85 mmHg, or lower (Hansson *et al.*, 1998). Efforts to lower blood pressure further (to 120 mmHg systolic and 70 mmHg diastolic) appeared to give little further benefit but did not result in any additional risk. Moreover, in the Heart Outcomes Prevention Evaluation Study (Yusuf *et al.*, 2000a), further blood pressure reduction in patients at high risk for cardiovascular events using ramipril, an ACE inhibitor, was associated with a significant 32% (95% CI, 16%–44) reduction in the rate of stroke.

It has been questioned whether newer antihypertensive agents (ACE inhibitors and calcium channel blockers [calcium antagonists]) give the same benefits as conventional treatment (diuretics and beta-blockers). According to recent guidelines (Chobanian *et al.*, 2003), there is similar cardiovascular protection from lowering blood pressure with ACE inhibitors, angiotensin-receptor blockers, and calcium antagonists as with thiazide-type diuretics and beta-blockers.

Diabetes mellitus and glucose intolerance

Diabetes is a well-established, independent risk factor for IS, but not for hemorrhagic stroke. In the Honolulu Heart Program, the age-adjusted incidence rate of IS in diabetics was more than two-fold higher than in subjects in the low–normal category of glucose tolerance (adjusted relative risk [RR], 2.45; 95% CI, 1.73–3.47) (Burchfiel *et al.*, 1995). In contrast, the incidence of hemorrhagic stroke did not differ between the groups. However, it is not clear whether strict control of blood glucose is effective. In fact, in patients with type 2 diabetes, intensive sulphonylurea and/or insulin therapy ameliorated microvascular complications but not macrovascular complications, such as stroke (UK Prospective Diabetes Study Group, 1998). Similarly, although intensive insulin therapy (given either by an external pump or by three or more daily injections) in patients with type 1 diabetes delayed the onset of microvascular complications, the reduction of macrovascular complications was not significant (Diabetes Control and Complications Trial Research Group, 1993, 1995).

Asymptomatic hyperglycemia was also considered to be an independent risk factor for stroke, but prospective studies yielded inconsistent results (Fuller *et al.*, 1983; Burchfiel *et al.*, 1995; Balkau *et al.*, 1998; Wannamethee *et al.*, 1999). In addition, it remains unclear whether the serum insulin concentration is an independent risk factor for stroke. In the British Regional Heart Study, a J-shaped relationship was seen between serum insulin and risk of stroke, the lowest risk being seen in the second quintile of the distribution (Wannamethee *et al.*, 1999). In the Atherosclerosis Risk in Communities Study, the fasting serum insulin level was weakly associated with IS after adjusting for confounding risk factors (adjusted RR, 1.14; 95% CI, 1.01–1.3), and, again, the association was non-linear (Folsom *et al.*, 1999a).

Obesity

Data linking obesity and stroke are limited. It is not clear whether otherwise healthy mildly or moderately obese persons are at a higher risk of stroke than healthy non-obese people (Kassirer and Angell, 1998). One study reported a lack of relationship between the body mass index and stroke (Folsom *et al.*, 1999a), whereas another demonstrated a relationship but made no adjustment for blood pressure and blood lipids (Sharper *et al.*, 1997). Nevertheless, overall, the evidence suggests that there is an U-shaped relationship between weight and stroke: that is, persons at either extreme of the body mass index are at highest risk (Sharper *et al.*, 1997; Stevens *et al.*, 1998; Wassertheil-Smoller *et al.*, 2000). The RR associated with a greater body mass index declines with age, and, in older people, the risk of death and stroke is similar across a wide range of values (Stevens *et al.*, 1998).

Lipids

Total cholesterol

The relationship between cholesterol levels and CHD is well established, and hypercholesterolemia is one of the most important risk factors for this disease. Although there are strong links between CHD and cerebrovascular diseases, the association between cholesterol levels and stroke is still debated.

In the Framingham Study, a negative relationship was found between high cholesterol levels and stroke in females (Wolf *et al.*, 1983). The Multiple Risk Factor Intervention Trial found that, in men with a diastolic blood pressure $\geq$ 90 mmHg, the risk of ICH was three times higher in those with low–normal cholesterol (<4.24 mmol/l or 160 mg/dl) than in those with higher cholesterol levels (Iso *et al.*, 1989). However, the risk of death from IS increased significantly with increasing serum cholesterol levels. These conclusions were recently reinforced by an overview of Japanese and Chinese studies, which revealed a trend towards an increased risk of hemorrhagic stroke (RR, 1.27; 95% CI, 0.84–1.91) and a reduction in the risk of IS (RR, 0.77; 95% CI, 0.57–1.06) with decreasing cholesterol concentrations (Eastern Stroke and Coronary Heart Disease Collaborative Research Group, 1998). However, the results of this last study did not support the earlier suggestion that the risk of hemorrhagic stroke was higher in patients with both low cholesterol concentrations and high blood pressure. The above results on IS also contrast with those of another meta-analysis of 45 prospective cohorts, which showed no association between total cholesterol and mortality from stroke except, perhaps, in subjects under 45 years (Prospective Studies Collaboration, 1995).

There are many possible explanations for the discrepant results of the above studies. First, some studies included only fatal stroke and the results for less severe stroke may be different. Moreover, stroke subtypes were not identified, and, in studies in which no association between all strokes and cholesterol was found, a positive association with IS linked to large artery disease might be counterbalanced by a negative association with hemorrhagic stroke.

The results of the first three large trials of cholesterol reduction using 3-hydroxy-3-methyl-glutaryl-coenzyme A (HMG-CoA) reductase inhibitors (statins) published in the middle 1990s (WOSCOP [Shepherd *et al.*, 1995], 4S [Scandinavian Simvastatin Survival Study Group, 1994], and CARE [Sacks *et al.*, 1996]) have challenged previous concepts, and we can now divide opinion regarding cholesterol as a risk factor into two eras; pre- and post-statin. Seven meta-analyses, including the above and newer studies, revealed a reduction of about 25% in stroke as a result of statin use (Blaw *et al.*, 1997; Crouse *et al.*, 1997, 1998; Herbert *et al.*, 1997; Bucher *et al.*, 1998; Ross *et al.*, 1999; di Mascio *et al.*, 2000; Corvol *et al.*, 2003).In the setting of primary prevention, the meta-analysis revealed a non-significant 4–20% reduction in stroke (Crouse *et al.*, 1997; Herbert *et al.*, 1997; di Mascio *et al.*, 2000; Corvol *et al.*, 2003). However, none of these analyses included recent large trials, such as the AFCAPS/TexCAPS (Downs *et al.*, 1998), Heart Protection Study (Heart Protection Study Collaborative Group, 2002a), the ALLHAT-LLT trial ALLHAT Officers and Coordinators for the ALLHAT Collaborative Research Group, 2002), and the PROSPER trial (Shepherd *et al.*, 2002), which included 6605, 2629, 8880, and 3239 patients, respectively, without history of vascular disease.

High-density lipoprotein cholesterol, triglycerides, and lipoprotein (a)

The British Regional Heart Study (Wannamethee *et al.*, 2000) and the Copenhagen City Heart Study (Lindenstrom *et al.*, 1994) reported that higher levels of high density lipoprotein (HDL) were associated with a decrease in the risk of stroke, while this inverse relation was not observed in the recent analysis of the Atherosclerosis Risk in the Communities Study (Shahar *et al.*, 2003). In a study that included very old people (older than 85 years), when the relevance of lipids as determinants of cardiovascular disease risk is disputable, low HDL cholesterol, in contrast to high low density lipoprotein (LDL) cholesterol levels, was associated with mortality from stroke (Weverling-Rijnsburger *et al.*, 2003).

There are limited and conflicting data on the association between serum triglycerides (Lindenstrom *et al.*, 1994; Wannamethee *et al.*, 2000; Shahar *et al.*, 2003), lipoprotein (a) (Glader *et al.*, 1999) and stroke.

Interventions aimed to lower serum triglycerides and increase HDL cholesterol produced inconsistent results. The primary prevention trials were negative (may be because of the low stroke numbers) (Corvol *et al.*, 2003). While the recent secondary prevention Benzafibrate Infarction Prevention (BIP) study showed no reduction in stroke rates in men with CHD (BIP Study Group, 2000). The Veterans Affair HDL Intervention Trial showed a 31% reduction of stroke in the same clinical setting (Rubins *et al.*, 2001).

Cigarette smoking

Studies published in the 1980s clearly established cigarette smoking as a powerful risk factor for stroke, especially IS and SAH (Abbott *et al.*, 1986; Bonita *et al.*, 1986; Colditz *et al.*, 1988; Shinton and Beevers, 1989). Although, in the Honolulu Heart Program, an excess of hemorrhagic stroke was seen among smokers, this may have resulted from the inclusion of SAH in this group of patients (Abbott *et al.*, 1986) and it is, therefore, not yet clear whether a relationship exists between ICH and cigarette smoking. The estimated overall RR of IS for cigarette smoking was 1.92 (95% CI, 1.71–2.16), whereas the risk of SAH was 2.93 (95% CI, 2.48–3.46) (Shinton *et al.*, 1989). The mechanism by which smoking causes SAH is not clear, but it may be through an acute rise in blood pressure, which may predispose to arterial rupture. It appears that cigarette smoking provokes IS by more than one mechanism. One mechanism that is irreversible and cumulative is linked to carotid atherosclerosis progression. Indeed, the Atherosclerosis Risk in Communities Study showed that progression of carotid atherosclerosis was higher in current, past, and passive smokers than in non-smokers (Howard *et al.*, 1998). The other, and probably most important, effect of smoking on IS is through short-term effects, which include increased fibrinogen levels and platelet aggregability, elevated hematocrit values, and reduced cerebral blood flow as a result of arterial vasoconstriction (Wannamethee *et al.*, 1995). The importance of these short-term effects is supported by the drastic reduction in stroke (IS and SAH) after ceasing smoking (Abbott *et al.*, 1986; Colditz *et al.*, 1988; Shinton *et al.*, 1989; Kawachi *et al.*, 1993; Wannamethee *et al.*, 1995).

Alcohol consumption

The relationship between alcohol consumption and stroke is complex. In the Honolulu Heart Program, heavy drinkers showed a three-fold higher risk of SAH and ICH than non-drinkers (Donahue *et al.*, 1986). These data are supported by those of a Finnish study, in which both binge drinking (i.e. occasional alcohol intoxication) and regular heavy drinking increased the risk of aneurysmal and non-aneurysmal SAH (Hillbom and Kaste, 1982). The effects of alcohol consumption on IS are still a matter of controversy. In the British Regional Heart Study, lifelong abstainers had an increased risk of stroke, but there was no convincing evidence that light or moderate drinking was beneficial for stroke risk (Wannamethee and Sharper, 1996). However, a protective effect of light or moderate alcohol consumption has been suggested in several recent studies (Thun *et al.*, 1997; Berger *et al.*, 1999; Sacco *et al.*, 1999). A recent case–control study of a multiethnic population suggested that moderate consumption (up to two measures of spirits, two cans of beer, or two glasses of wine per day) is associated with a reduced risk of IS, while heavy alcohol consumption is associated with an increased risk (Sacco *et al.*, 1999). Although it has been suggested that certain types of beverage, particularly red wine, are more protective than others, wine, beer, and spirits had approximately the same effect (Sacco *et al.*, 1999). Similarly, analysis of nearly 450 000 subjects included in the Cancer Prevention Study II showed that mortality from all cardiovascular causes, including stroke, was 30–40% lower in men and women who reported taking at least one drink per day than in non-drinkers (Thun *et al.*, 1997). Furthermore, in the recent analysis of the Physicians' Health Study, there was a significant 23% reduction in the risk of IS (adjusted RR, 0.77; 95% CI, 0.63–0.94) in men who had one, or more, drink a week, the greatest reduction being seen in men who had one to four drinks per week (Berger *et al.*, 1999). There was no significant association between alcohol consumption and hemorrhagic stroke, but heavy drinking was very rare in this population.

A meta-analysis including 35 observational studies (19 cohort studies and 16 case–control studies) reported that, compared with abstainers, alcohol consumption of less than 12 g/day (one drink on US conversion) was associated with a decreased risk of total stroke (RR, 0.83; 95% CI, 0.75–0.91), while alcohol consumption of more than 60 g/day (five drinks/day) was significantly associated with an increase risk of total stroke (RR, 1.64; 95% CI, 1.39–1.93). Although the association of alcohol consumption and the relative risk of IS was J shaped, the relative risk of hemorrhagic stroke increased linearly with increasing alcohol consumption (Reynolds *et al.*, 2003).

Physical activity

The association between physical activity and stroke was first described in a report from the Harvard Alumni Study in 1967, which showed that men who had been athletes in college experienced less than half the risk of fatal stroke than non-athletes (Paffenbarger *et al.*, 1967). However, it was in the 1990s that several large studies (Wannamethee and Sharper, 1992; Abbott *et al.*, 1994; Kiely *et al.*, 1994; Gillum *et al.*, 1996a; Bijnen *et al.*, 1998; Lee and Paffenbarger, 1998, Lee *et al.*, 1999; Ellekjær *et al.*, 2000; Hu *et al.*, 2000), but not all (Evenson *et al.*, 1999), demonstrated that physical activity is inversely related to the risk of stroke. Its protective effects extend to IS, ICH, and SAH. A meta-analysis, including 18 cohort and five case–control studies published from 1966 to 2002, showed that moderate and high levels of physical activity were associated with a reduced risk of total, ischemic, and hemorrhagic stroke (Lee *et al.*, 2003). In the analysis of the cohort studies, highly active individuals had a 25% lower risk of stroke incidence or mortality than did low-active individuals (RR, 0.75; 95% CI, 0.69–0.82), while moderate actively individuals had a 17% lower risk of stroke incidence or mortality than did low-active individuals (RR, 0.83; 95% CI, 0.76–0.89; $P < 0.001$). Slightly stronger results were found for case–control studies (64% and 48%, respectively), but there was no evidence of heterogeneity by study type.

Diet

Information on the relationship between diet and stroke is limited and contradictory.

Fat

Although saturated fat intake is directly related to the incidence of CHD, analysis of fat intake in middle-aged men in the Framingham cohort showed that intake of fat, saturated fat, and monounsaturated fat was inversely associated with IS (Gillman *et al.*, 1997). In addition, in the Nurses' Health Study cohort, women in the lowest quintile of either dietary saturated fat or trans-unsaturated fat, which corresponds to the mean consumption in some populations in Asia, had a 2.5-fold increase in the risk of ICH (Iso *et al.*, 2001a, b). These results are in line with a 14-year prospective study of 4775 Japanese aged 40–69 years, in which an increase risk of ICH was found among people in the lowest quintile of saturated fat intake (Iso *et al.*, 2003). These authors claim that the low consumption of saturated fat helps to explain the high rate of this stroke subtype in Asian countries. A recent analysis of more then 40,000 male US healthcare professionals also failed to find any relation between total fat, specific types of fat, and the risk of ischemic, hemorrhagic or total stroke (He *et al.*, 2003).

Fish and omega-3 fatty acids

The low mortality from CHD in certain populations, such as Eskimos, with a high fish consumption contributed to the hypothesis that omega-3 fatty acids in fish oil may have protective effects against vascular diseases (Bang *et al.*, 1976). Further ecologic studies showing that the Mediterranean diet, which is rich in fish and other sources of omega-3 fatty acids, reduced the risk of cardiovascular diseases also supported this hypothesis (Trichopoulou *et al.*, 2003).

In comparison with the literature about the association of omega-3 fatty acids and CHD, there are relatively few data describing the effects of omega-3 fatty acids on stroke (Kris-Etherton *et al.*, 2002). In addition, cohort studies were inconsistent; in the Zutphen study (Kell *et al.*, 1994), fish consumption was associated with a reduced risk of stroke, while the Physicians' Health Study (Morris *et al.*, 1995) and the Chicago Western Electric Study (Orencia *et al.*, 1996) found no association and NHANES I study (Gillum *et al.*, 1996a, b) found an association restricted to white women. More recent evidence, from the Health Professionals' Follow-up Study and the Nurses' Health Study, which separated IS and hemorrhagic stroke, indicated that higher consumption of fish reduced the risk of IS in men (He *et al.*, 2002) and women (Iso *et al.*, 2001b). The GISSI-Prevention Study, the largest randomized controlled trial to test the efficacy of omega-3 fatty acids for secondary prevention of CHD, found a 15% reduction in the primary end point (death, non-fatal MI, and stroke) in patients with pre-existing CHD given 1 g omega-3 fatty acids compared with controls (GISSI-Prevenzione Investigators, 1999). All the benefit, however, was attributable to the decrease in risk for overall and cardiovascular death and there was no difference in the risk of stroke.

Cations

Since the 1980s, it has been suggested that low levels of potassium are associated with stroke mortality (Khaw and Barrett-Connor, 1987). Although it is well known that potassium intake reduces blood pressure, the apparent effect of potassium was greater than would be expected simply from this relationship. In addition, recent large studies have supported the idea of a protective effect of potassium (Ascherio *et al.*, 1998; Iso *et al.*, 1999; Green *et al.*, 2002), mainly seen in hypertensive men (Ascherio *et al.*, 1998).

Intake of calcium, and magnesium has also been associated with reduced stroke (Abbott *et al.*, 1996; Ascherio *et al.*, 1998; Iso *et al.*, 1999), but further studies are necessary.

Fibers

Dietary fiber may come from different food sources: vegetables, fruits, and cereals. Although some studies reported an inverse association between the incidence of stroke and fibers from all sources, other studies showed that effects of dietary fiber might vary depending on food source (Ascherio *et al.*, 1998). In fact, a recent analysis of the Cardiovascular Health Study, including a cohort of 3588 men and women aged 65 years or older, showed that higher cereal fiber intake, but not fruit or vegetable fruit consumption, was associated with lower risk of total stroke and IS (Mozaffarian *et al.*, 2003).

Nevertheless, data from the Framingham study showed a risk reduction of 0.75 (95% CI, 0.55–1.03) for an increment of three servings of fruits and vegetables per day (Gillman *et al.*, 1995). Moreover, a combined analysis of two cohorts, the Nurses' Health Study and the Health Professionals' Follow-up Study, including 75 596 women and 38 683 men, showed that fruit and vegetable intake was inversely related to the risk of IS after adjusting for potential confounders (Joshipura *et al.*, 1999). People in the highest quintile of fruit and vegetable intake (five to six servings per day) had a relative risk of 0.69 (95% CI, 0.52–0.92) compared with those in the lowest quintile.

Vitamins

It has been claimed that low vitamin levels are associated with stroke (Gey *et al.*, 1993; Voko *et al.*, 2003). Moreover, experimental studies on animals suggest that antioxidant dietary supplementation inhibits the atherogenic process, and randomized controlled trials in humans showed that vitamins diminished the carotid atherosclerotic process (Salonen *et al.*, 2003). Nevertheless, the results of published randomized studies, in contrast to these preclinical and observational studies, are inconsistent (Willet and Stampfer, 2001).

The vitamins that have received most attention in the last few years are beta-carotene, alpha-tocopherol (vitamin E), vitamin C, and folic acid.

The Alpha-tocopherol, Beta-carotene Cancer Prevention Study evaluated the effect of vitamin E and beta-carotene in almost 30 000 Finish male smokers. It was found that vitamin E supplementation increased the incidence of SAH and the risk of fatal hemorrhagic strokes but decreased the incidence of IS (Leppala *et al.*, 2000). However, the results of other large randomized trials of vitamin E, such as the Primary Prevention Project (de Gaetano, 2001), Heart Outcomes Prevention Evaluation (Yusuf *et al.*, 2000b), and Heart Protection Study (Heart Protection Study Collaborative Group, 2002b), including approximately 35 000 high-risk subjects, showed no effect on the incidence of any type of vascular disease.

A meta-analysis of randomized trials of beta-carotene and vitamin E has been published (Vivekananthan *et al.*, 2003). In 138 113 patients randomized to beta-carotene or control treatment, the all-cause mortality in patients treated with beta-carotene was slightly increased compared with controls (RR, 1.07; 95% CI, 1.02–1.11). In the analysis of 81 788 patients for vitamin E, the frequency of all-cause plus cardiovascular mortality and that of stroke did not differ between subjects treated and those not treated with vitamin E (11.3 vs. 11.1, 6.0 vs. 6.0, 3.6 vs. 3.5, respectively).

Another review, for the US Preventive Service Task Force, is consistent with these data and provided extended evidence for vitamin A, C, antioxidant combination and a multivitamin preparation (Morris and Carson, 2003). It was concluded that there was no evidence to support the prescribing of the vitamins above for the prevention of cardiovascular disease and it recommended against the use of beta-carotene (US Preventive Service Task Force, 2003).

Hormones

Oral contraceptives

During the 1970s, the association between oral contraceptives (OC) and IS was established (Stadel, 1981). OC are also associated with SAH (Johnston *et al.*, 1998) and IS secondary to cerebral sinus thrombosis (de Bruijn *et al.*, 1998). Although the doses of estrogen and progestogen used in OC have since been reduced, it is only recently that the relationship between low-dose OC and stroke has received more attention (WHO Collaborative Study of Cardiovascular Disease and Steroid Hormone Contraception, 1996a; Heinemann *et al.*, 1997; Schwartz *et al.*, 1998). The WHO Collaborative Study and the Transnational Case Control study revealed a small increased risk of IS (WHO Collaborative Study of Cardiovascular Disease and Steroid Hormone Contraception, 1996a; Heinemann *et al.*, 1997) and hemorrhagic stroke (WHO Collaborative Study of Cardiovascular Disease and Steroid Hormone Contraception, 1996b), even with low-dose OC. A meta-analysis of SAH and OC showed an increased risk of stroke, which, although higher with high-estrogen OC, was also seen with low-dose OC (adjusted RR, 1.51; 95% CI, 1.18–1.92) (Johnston *et al.*, 1998). In contrast, in a pooled analysis of the Kaiser Permanent Medical Care Program of Northern California and University of Washington studies, the risk of stroke was not increased in current users of low-dose OC (Schwartz *et al.*, 1998). Despite these discrepancies, all studies agree that the risk of stroke in young women is very low and that the risk is small compared with the potential benefits of OC. However, women at high risk of SAH or IS, namely those with unruptured aneurysms, a strong positive family history of SAH (Johnston *et al.*, 1998), or a history of cigarette smoking, hypertension, or migraine, should consider alternative modes of contraception until more data are available (Heinemann *et al.*, 1997; Schwartz *et al.*, 1998).

Postmenopausal hormone-replacement therapy

Postmenopausal hormone replacement therapy (HRT) is a good example of how recommendations may change over time and how different evidence regarding the benefits and risks may emerge from different categories of epidemiological study. Since the 1970s, animal research and many observational studies have suggested that HRT was associated with a lower risk of cardiovascular disease (Grodstein *et al.*, 2000) as well as stroke (Falkeborn *et al.*, 1993; Petitti *et al.*, 1998). Such association was biologically plausible: besides improving endothelial vascular function and reversing postmenopausal increase in fibrinogen, estrogen therapy reduces plasma levels of LDL by 10–14% and increases plasma levels of HDL by 7–8% (Manson and Martin, 2001). However, large cohort studies showed that HRT had no significant effect (Grodstein et al., 1996) or increased stroke risk (Wilsom et al., 1985). For example, in an analysis based on a 16-year follow-up of 59 337 postmenopausal women participating in the Nurses' Health Study, no significant association was found between stroke and either combined hormones (adjusted RR, 1.09; 95% CI, 0.66–1.80) or estrogen alone (adjusted RR, 1.27; 95% CI, 0.95–1.69) (Grodstein et al., 1996). Finally, recent randomized clinical trials to evaluate the effect of HRT on primary (Wassertheil-Smoller et al., 2003) or secondary (Hulley et al., 1998; Viscoli et al., 2001) prevention of cardiovascular disease showed a worrisome increase in the risk for CHD and stroke among women in the HRT group. In the Women's Health Initiative Trial, 16 608 postmenopausal women received 0.625 mg equine estrogens plus 2.5 mg medroxyporgesterone daily or placebo (Wassertheil-Smoller et al., 2003). The trial was stopped prematurely because of an excess of breast cancer in women taking hormones. HRT was also associated with an increased risk of CHD (RR, 1.29; 95% CI, 1.02–1.63) and stroke (RR, 1.41; 95% CI, 1.07–1.49). The increased risk with estrogen plus progestin was linked to IS. The increased risk was unrelated to traditional cardiovascular risk factors (e.g. age, prior history of cardiovascular disease, hormone use, and hypertension). The analysis provided no identification of women at the highest risk of stroke when taking estrogen plus progestin (Wassertheil-Smoller et al., 2003). Although the Women's Health Initiative Trial is the only published trial of HRT in primary prevention of cardiovascular disease, its results are in line with two secondary prevention trials. A recent revision of four randomized clinical trials, including over 20 000 women followed for an average of 4.9 years, found a significant excess incidence of stroke (RR, 1.27; 95% CI, 1.06–1.51) in women randomized to HRT compared with the placebo group (Beral et al., 2002). HRT was also associated with an excess of breast cancer and pulmonary embolism but a deficit of colorectal cancer and hip fractures. Although it was argued that the negative results of HRT could result from adverse effects of medroxyprogesterone acetate, the Women's Estrogen Stroke Trial showed no reduction of stroke in women randomized to take oestrogen alone (1 mg estradiol-17 per day) compared with placebo; in fact, fatal strokes were more common in the estradiol group (Viscoli et al., 2001).

Antithrombotic drugs

A number of studies have shown that aspirin can definitely reduce the recurrence of coronary and cerebral vascular events (Antithrombotic Trialists' Collaboration, 2002). However, its effects in healthy people are not clear.

Two large clinical trials, the Physicians, Health Study (Steering Committee of the Physicians' Health Study Research Group, 1989) and the British Male Doctors

Study (Peto *et al.*, 1988), have addressed the use of aspirin in healthy male doctors. In a non-blind British study that analyzed data from 5139 male physicians randomly allocated to receive or not receive 500 mg aspirin daily, there was no difference in the incidence of myocardial infarction, but disabling strokes were more common in those allocated to aspirin (Peto *et al.*, 1988). Given the limited data regarding which of these strokes were ischemic and which hemorrhagic, the higher incidence of strokes in the aspirin group could result from a higher incidence of hemorrhagic stroke. The Physicians' Health Study, a randomized, double-blind, placebo-controlled trial that analyzed data from 22 071 male physicians who received either 325 mg aspirin or placebo every other day, demonstrated a 44% risk reduction in myocardial infarction and a non-significant increased risk of stroke in the aspirin group (Steering Committee of the Physicians' Health Study Research Group, 1989). In the subgroup with hemorrhagic strokes, aspirin was associated with an increased risk of borderline statistical significance.

Four large trials (the Early Treatment Diabetic Retinopathy Study [ETDRS Investigators, 1992], the Thrombosis Prevention Trial [Medical Research Council's General Practice Research Framework, 1998], the Hypertension Optimal Treatment Study [Hansson *et al.*, 1998], and the Primary Prevention Project [de Gaetano, 2001]) assessed the value of aspirin in the prevention of vascular events in subjects with risk factors but without overt cardiovascular disease. All of them showed a significative reduction or a trend for reduction in the incidence of myocardial infarction with aspirin use, contrasting with a lack of significant effect on stroke

These findings are reinforced by a meta-analysis of trials examining the relationship between aspirin use and stroke in low-risk patients (Hart *et al.*, 2000), which found no significant effect of aspirin on stroke in trials involving subjects with or without risk factors (RR, 1.08; 95% CI, 0.95–1.24) (Fig. 1.4), contrasting sharply with a reduction in myocardial infarction (RR, 0.74; 95% CI, 0.68–0.82) and a protective effect against stroke in patients with established vascular disease. Moreover, long-term use of aspirin increased the risk of hemorrhagic stroke (RR, 1.35; 95% CI, 0.88–2.1). Another meta-analysis, including the most recent data from the Primary Prevent Project trial, showed similar results (Eidelman *et al.*, 2003).

Cardiac disease

Atrial fibrillation

Atrial fibrillation is associated with a high rate of IS. A review reported an average stroke rate of 5% per year in patients included in primary prevention trials, with wide clinically important variation between subpopulations of such patients (0.5–12% per year) (Albers *et al.*, 2001). Oral anticoagulation therapy markedly reduced the risk of stroke in patients with atrial fibrillation. This statement is based

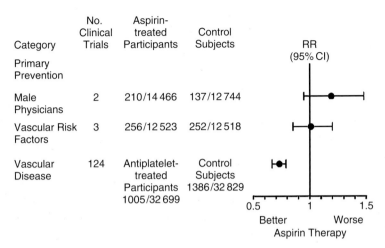

Category	No. Clinical Trials	Aspirin-treated Participants	Control Subjects	RR (95% CI)
Primary Prevention				
Male Physicians	2	210/14 466	137/12 744	
Vascular Risk Factors	3	256/12 523	252/12 518	
Vascular Disease	124	Antiplatelet-treated Participants 1005/32 699	Control Subjects 1386/32 829	

Fig. 1.4   Effect of aspirin therapy and stroke according to the presence of vascular risk factors and clinically manifest vascular disease. RR, relative risk; CI, confidence interval. (Data from Hart *et al.*, 2000.)

on the consistent results of six randomized trials, aggregate analysis of which showed that anticoagulation with the oral vitamin K antagonist warfarin reduced the rate of all stroke (ischemic and hemorrhagic) and of IS by 62% (95% CI, 48%–72), and 65% (95% CI, 48%–72), respectively, compared with untreated patients (Hart *et al.*, 1999). For primary prevention, the absolute risk reduction for all stroke was 2.7% per year and the number needed to treat for one year to prevent one stroke was 37. The rate of intracranial hemorrhage was 0.3% per year with warfarin and 0.1% per year with placebo, although a higher number of intracranial hemorrhages may be found in clinical settings.

Assessment of the optimal intensity of anticoagulation in the European Atrial Fibrillation Study (EAFT Study Group, 1995) showed that therapy resulting in an international normalized ratio (INR) of 2.0–2.9 and 3.0–3.9, respectively, reduced the combined incidence rate for ischemic and hemorrhagic events by 80% and 40%, compared with that with an INR <2.0; > an INR 5.0 resulted in an unacceptable risk of bleeding complications, while an INR<2.0 resulted in no significant reduction in thromboembolic events.

The use of aspirin was assessed in six randomized trials yielding a pooled risk reduction of all stroke of 22% (95% CI, 2%–38), compared with placebo (Hart *et al.*, 1999). The absolute risk reduction was 1.5% year (number needed to treat 67). When the effect of warfarin on stroke was compared with aspirin in five trials, it yielded a 36% (95% CI, 14%–52) and 46% (95% CI, 27%–60) reduction of all stroke and IS, respectively. The absolute risk reduction in all stroke for warfarin compared with aspirin was 0.8 per year (Hart *et al.*, 1999).

Table 1.2 The CHADS$_2$ index for quantifying stroke risk in patients with atrial fibrillation

CHADS$_2$ score [a]	Adjusted stroke rate in the NRAF (95% CI)
0	1.9 (1.2–3.0)
1	2.8 (2.0–3.8)
2	4.0 (3.1–5.1)
3	5.9 (4.6–7.3)
4	8.5 (6.3–11.1)
5	12.5 (8.2–17.5)
6	18.2 (10.5–27.4)

NRAF, National Registry of Atrial Fibrillation; CI, confidence interval.
[a] Calculated by adding 1 point for each of the following conditions: congestive heart failure, hypertension, age at least 75 years, or diabetes mellitus and adding 2 points for having a prior stroke or transient ischemic attack.

As the annual rate of stroke among people with atrial fibrillation has a wide range, risk stratification should separate etiologic subtypes, who should receive different treatments. Consequently, numerous studies have attempted to define clinical criteria that may be used to classify risk as low or high. The best-known risk stratification schemes are those published by the Atrial Fibrillation Investigators, the SPAF investigators, and, more recently, the CHADS$_2$ (Table 1.2) (Gage *et al.*, 2001) and Framingham Heart Study scores (Wang *et al.*, 2003).

Patients with atrial fibrillation and at least one of the risk factors of previous stroke, transient ischemic attack, systemic embolism, over 75 years of age, hypertension, or poor left ventricular function are at high risk of stroke and should be offered anticoagulation therapy (target INR of 2.5: range 2.0–3.0) unless their risk of bleeding is high. Patients with atrial fibrillation and no cardiovascular disease ("lone atrial fibrillation") aged less than 65 years are at such a low risk that they should either be treated with aspirin or not treated. Patients over 65 years without other risk factors may be considered as at moderate risk and therapy could include warfarin or aspirin.

For some patients, aspirin might be preferred to warfarin because of situations that may increase the risk of bleeding, namely increased age (over 80–85 years), poor drug or clinical compliance, uncontrolled hypertension, alcohol excess, liver disease, bleeding lesions (peptic ulcer or previous cerebral hemorrhage), or a tendency to bleeding (including coagulation defects and thrombocytopenia) (Lip and Lowe, 1996).

Carotid artery stenosis

Internal carotid artery atherosclerosis is an important risk factor for IS, being responsible for about 20% of all IS (Bogousslavsky *et al.*, 1988). In the Framingham Study, the prevalence of carotid stenosis of 50% or more in people between 66 and 93 years was low, corresponding to 7% for women and 9% for men (Fine-Edelstein *et al.*, 1984). Risk factors for carotid artery stenosis include older age, cigarette smoking, hypertension, diabetes, obesity, hypercholesterolemia, family history of stroke, and ischemic changes on electrocardiogram (Fine-Edelstein *et al.*, 1984; Bogousslavsky *et al.*, 1985). Carotid stenosis greater than 75% and progressing stenosis are associated with a higher risk of ipsilateral stroke (Chambers and Norris, 1986), which is approximately 1.7 and 5.5% annually (Chambers and Norris, 1986; Bogousslavsky *et al.*, 1986). It should be emphasized that stenosis is not the real problem in every stroke ipsilateral to a carotid stenosis. Indeed, in the North American Study of Carotid Endarterectomy Trial, even after excluding patients with cardioembolic sources, 45% of strokes in patients with asymptomatic stenosis of 60–99% were attributed to lacunes and cardioembolism (Inzitari *et al.*, 2000).

Medical treatment

There is no proved medical treatment for carotid artery stenosis. In a small trial of aspirin in 372 neurologicsally asymptomatic patients with carotid artery stenosis of 50% or more, the annual rate of IS or death of any cause was similar in the placebo and aspirin group (12.3% vs. 11.0%) (Coté *et al.*, 1995). Since randomized controlled trials showed that statins reduced the progression of carotid stenosis (but not the rate of ipsilateral stroke) (Furberg *et al.*, 1994; Salonen *et al.*, 1995; Mercuri *et al.*, 1996), and a trend toward a better efficacy of aspirin was observed in the subgroup of carotid artery stenosis in the Antithrombotic Trialists' Collaboration (Antithrombotic Trialists' Collaboration, 2002), in some centers, aspirin and statin are prescribed to patients with asymptomatic carotid disease.

Endarterectomy

The results of trials assessing endarterectomy (CEA) in asymptomatic patients are still a matter of controversy. The largest of these trials, the Asymptomatic Carotid Atherosclerosis Study, reported that patients with an asymptomatic carotid stenosis greater than 60% had a 53% reduction in the five-year RR of ipsilateral stroke if CEA was performed (Executive Committee for the Asymptomatic Carotid Atherosclerosis Study, 1995). However, the absolute risk reduction was small (5.9% in five years), as was the rate of ipsilateral stroke in the medically treated group (11.0% in five years, or 2.3% annually). Moreover, these results were obtained with a perioperative rate of complications (stroke or death) of only 2.3%, which is difficult to achieve in practice. In addition, in certain subgroups of patients (namely those with contralateral carotid occlusion), the risk of stroke with medical treatment is so low that surgery may be best avoided (Baker *et al.*, 2000).

A meta-analysis of five trials of CEA for asymptomatic carotid stenosis concluded that, although surgery reduced the incidence of ipsilateral stroke, the absolute benefit of CEA was small, as the incidence of stroke in medically treated patients was low (Benavente *et al.*, 1998). The authors suggested that, until high-risk subgroups have been identified, medical management remains the sensible alternative for many patients with asymptomatic carotid stenosis.

Angioplasty

The main problems with carotid angioplasty are that long-term follow-up is not yet available and direct comparison with CEA is scarce. Moreover, recent studies comparing angioplasty with CEA (Naylor *et al.*, 1998; CAVATAS Investigators, 2001) focused mostly on patients with symptomatic stenosis, and it is difficult to extrapolate its results for patients without neurological symptoms. However, in a recent series of 100 patients submitted to carotid angioplasty with stenting (Kastrup *et al.*, 2003), the overall complication rate (any stroke or death) was lower in asymptomatic than in symptomatic patients (0% vs. 8% of stroke and death). It is hoped that the ongoing trials comparing carotid angioplasty with CEA in both symptomatic and asymptomatic patients will help to clarify the optimal indications for each procedure.

Emerging risk factors

Homocysteine

Results from several cross-sectional and case–control studies support an association between elevated homocysteine levels and stroke (Christen *et al.*, 2000). One review showed that results from prospective studies, however, tended to indicate a weak association or a lack of an association (Christen *et al.*, 2000). This suggests that homocysteine may be an acute phase reactant, rather than a risk factor (reverse causality). Recent meta-analysis reappraised the question, including more data, especially from prospective studies. The Homocysteine Studies Collaboration meta-analysis evaluated separately prospective and retrospective studies (Homocysteine Studies Collaboration, 2002). Stronger associations were observed in retrospective studies of homocysteine measured in blood collected after the onset of the disease than in prospective studies among individuals who had no history of cardiovascular disease when blood was collected. Moreover, the association of homocysteine and cardiovascular disease was weaker when adjustment for known cardiovascular risk factors and regression dilution bias were performed. Nevertheless, a 25% lower than normal homocysteine level was associated with a 19% (RR, 0.81; 95% CI, 0.69–0.95) lower stroke risk. Another meta-analysis focusing on prospective studies found that a serum homocysteine increase of 5 μmol/l was associated with an increased risk of stroke (RR, 1.59; 95% CI, 1.29–1.96), after adjusting for known risk factors and adjusting for regression dilution bias (Wald *et al.*, 2002). The same investigators performed a meta-analysis of methylenetetrahydrofolate reductase polymorphism studies and found that people with a common mutation that reduce the activity of the enzyme (and consequently with a moderate [20%] increase in serum homocysteine) showed a higher risk for cardiovascular disease (evaluation of stroke separately was harmed because of few data). This is strong evidence of a causal effect since the presence of a mutation offers a natural experiment in which the population has been "randomly" allocated to one group with higher homocysteine concentrations.

Few randomized controlled trials of treatment with folic acid, vitamin B_6, and B_{12}, and vascular outcomes have been published (Schnyder *et al.*, 2001; Toole *et al.*, 2004). In the Swiss Heart Study, patients assigned to vitamins after percutaneous coronary angioplasty had a lower rate of restenosis and need for revascularization of the target lesion than patients assigned to placebo (Schnyder *et al.*, 2001). The Vitamin Intervention for Stroke Prevention Study randomized patients who sustained a IS to a low or high dosage of B vitamins and found no difference between the two groups for the primary end point, recurrence of IS (Toole *et al.*, 2004). Several primary and secondary prevention trials are testing supplementation with a combination of folic acid and B vitamins in relation to the incidence of cardiovascular disease and will provide important information on this issue (Eikelboom *et al.*, 1999; Hankey *et al.*, 1999).

Fibrinogen and other markers of hemostatic function
Few data are available relating plasma fibrinogen and stroke. A Swedish study (Wilhelmsen *et al.* 1984) and the Edinburgh Artery Study (Smith *et al.*, 1997) showed that, after adjusting for confounding variables, fibrinogen was associated with stroke. However, no such relationship was found in a recent analysis of the Atherosclerosis Risk in Communities cohort (Folsom *et al.*, 1999b).

It has been suggested that high levels of tissue plasminogen activator, fibrin D-dimer (Smith *et al.*, 1997), von Willebrand factor, and factor VIIIc (Folsom *et al.*, 1999a) are associated with IS, but further studies are necessary.

C-reactive protein and other markers of inflammation

C-reactive protein is an acute-phase reactant that markedly increases during an inflammatory response. Not only may it be a marker of systemic inflammation but also may be involved in atherosclerosis. Although there are multiple markers of inflammation, C-reactive protein is the most extensively studied, receiving most focus in momentum.

In a previous case–controlled analysis of the Women's Health Study, including 28 263 women, four markers of inflammation (C-reactive protein, serum amyloid A, interleukin-6, and soluble intercellular adhesion molecule type 1) were found to be independent predictors of future cardiovascular events, the most significant being C-reactive protein (adjusted RR, 1.4; 95% CI, 1.1–1.9) (Ridker *et al.*, 2000). Moreover, a recent prospective study, which extended from the results above, included data from the entire cohort of 27 939 women followed for a mean of eight years for the occurrence of myocardial infarction, IS, coronary revascularization intervention, or death from cardiovascular causes. Measurements of C-reactive protein at baseline were better than LDL cholesterol in predicting cardiovascular events (adjusted RR according to increasing quintiles of CRP, compared with the first quintile: 1.4, 1.6, 2.0, and 2.3), and IS (Ridker *et al.*, 2002). These results are consistent with those of another contemporary analysis, the Cardiovascular Heart Study, which showed that the adjusted hazard ratio for IS in the fourth quartile of baseline C-reactive protein was 1.6 (95% CI, 1.23–2.08) compared with the first quartile (Cao *et al.*, 2003).

Infection

There is growing evidence that chronic infections may be associated with atherosclerosis and, therefore, with cardiovascular diseases (Lindsberg and Grau, 2003). *Chlamydia pneumoniae* is one of the most studied pathogens, but there is no agreement whether serological evidence for *C. pneumoniae* is associated with stroke; this may result from the different methodologies adopted by studies, such as collection of blood for serological analysis before or after the stroke (Glader *et al.*, 1999; Elkind *et al.*, 2000). Final proof of a causal role of infectious mechanisms in stroke pathogenesis is still lacking and will require interventional studies.

Risk factors: future directions

Better identification of individuals at high risk of stroke will be a cornerstone in stroke prevention in the near future. Advances in the genetics of stroke may permit the discovery of "stroke genes" and the molecular determination of individual risk patterns (Auburger, 1998). Surrogate markers of cerebrovascular diseases will allow shorter, less-expensive clinical trials. Novel serum inflammatory markers, such as C-reactive protein, may help to identify asymptomatic subjects at high risk. These new markers may provide a means of recognizing people for whom drugs should be prescribed. Obviously, all these advances will not reduce the burden imposed by stroke if large-population approaches to prevention, aimed at modifying lifestyle factors, are not implemented.

Avoiding recurrence

Secondary prevention is clearly important in the setting of stroke rehabilitation. Stroke recurrence is obviously associated with increased neurological disability and higher mortality (Sacco *et al.*, 1989; Moroney *et al.*, 1998). Those who have already had a stroke are at higher risk of further stroke than the general population (Hardie *et al.*, 2004) Consequently, a stroke rehabilitation team needs to take appropriate precautions to reduce the chances of recurrence.

Obviously many of the risk factors that are associated with the first stroke are also associated with recurrent strokes. Therefore, appropriate action needs to be taken, particularly with regard to hypertension, diabetes mellitus, hypercholesterolemia, cigarette smoking, alcohol intake, diet and, as appropriate, cessation of OC, and appropriate treatment for atrial fibrillation.

The Stroke Council of the American Heart Association (Wolf *et al.*, 1999) has produced clear guidelines for risk reduction after first transient ischemic episode or stroke. These are summarized in Table 1.3. It should be emphasized that this book concentrates on rehabilitation and recovery after stroke. It is not intended as a definitive textbook on all aspects of stroke management. Therefore, it is not appropriate to consider secondary stroke prevention in great detail. However, it is appropriate for a few particular points to be made with regard to reduction of appropriate risk factors after first and subsequent stroke.

Blood pressure

It can clearly be demonstrated that lowering blood pressure is an effective measure to prevent stroke. Each 10 mmHg reduction in systolic blood pressure is associated with a decrease in risk of stroke of 34–36% in people 60–69 years and 25–29% for those in 70–79 years (Lawes *et al.*, 2004). The specific issue of secondary stroke prevention has been investigated in seven randomized studies and analyzed in a recent meta-analysis (Rashid *et al.*, 2003). Trials of beta-blockers (atenolol) have generally been negative although a confounding factor could be that the drugs were administered in the acute phase, which may lead to a worse prognosis (Oliveira-Filho *et al.*, 2003). The Heart Outcomes Prevention Evaluation Study (Yusuf *et al.*, 2000a) indicated effectiveness of ramipril for secondary stroke prevention although the subgroup of individuals with previous cerebrovascular

Table 1.3 Guide to risk reduction for patients with ischemic cerebrovascular disease (patients who have already had their first transient ischemic attack or stroke): specific recommendations for general risk factors

Risk factor	Goal	Recommendations
Hypertension	Systolic blood pressure <140 mmHg and diastolic blood pressure <90 mmHg (systolic blood pressure <135 mmHg and diastolic blood pressure <85 mmHg if target organ damage is present)	Lifestyle modification and antihypertensive medication as appropriate
Smoking	Cessation	Strongly encourage patient and family to stop smoking, provide counselling, nicotine replacement and formal antismoking programs as required
Diabetes mellitus	Glucose <7.0 mmol/l	Diet, oral hypoglycemic drugs and insulin as required
Lipids	Total cholesterol <5.18 mmol/l, triglyceride <2.26 mmol/l, LDL <2.59 mmol/l, HDL <0.91 mmol/l	Start American Heart Association Step II diet (≤30% fat, <7% saturated fat, <200 mg/day cholesterol, and emphasize weight management and physical activity); if target goal not achieved with these measures, add drug therapy (e.g. statins) if LDL >3.37 mmol/l and consider drug therapy if LDL 2.59–3.37 mmol/l
Alcohol	Moderate consumption only (≤2 units/day)	Strongly encourage patient and family to stop excessive drinking and provide formal alcohol cessation program
Physical activity	30–60 minutes of activity at least 3–4 times/week	Moderate exercise (e.g. brisk walking, jogging, cycling, or other aerobic activity); medically supervised programs for high-risk patients (e.g. those with cardiac disease) and appropriately adapted programs for those with neurological disabilities
Weight	≤120% of ideal body weight for height	Diet and exercise

HDL, highdensity lipoproteins; LDL, low density lipoproteins.
From Wolf *et al.*, 1999.

events was rather small. Other studies have indicated the efficacy of diuretics (thiazide or indapamide) in reducing stroke by about 32% (Rashid *et al.*, 2003). The coadministration of indapamide and perindopril in the PROGRESS Trial (PROGRESS Collaborative Group, 2001) led to a reduction in stroke and myocardial infarction, with all vascular events reduced by 40–45%.

The conclusion of these early studies may indicate that appropriate antihypertensive therapy should be given to all people with stroke. At present approach, it seems the combination of perindopril and indapamide is probably the most effective although it is a little too early to state this conclusion too definitively. Since lowering blood pressure in acute stroke is probably detrimental, appropriate therapy should be started in a more stable phase – perhaps around two weeks after the acute event. Consideration also needs to be given to non-pharmacological measures to lower blood pressure, although such measures have not been studied in great detail (Chobanian *et al.*, 2003).

Hypercholesterolemia

As indicated earlier in this chapter, there is a clear relationship between CHD and blood cholesterol concentration. However, the association between blood lipid concentrations and the risk of stroke has been less clear. Most of the statin studies have been conducted in patients with or at high risk of coronary artery disease and there are few high-quality studies that clearly demonstrate the reduction of incidence of stroke with statin usage. However, one recent study does provide some evidence that statin therapy is beneficial for people with previous cerebrovascular disease even if they do not already manifest coronary heart disease (Heart Protection Study Collaborative Group, 2004).

Smoking

There is clear evidence that smoking increases the risk of stroke and that this increase seems to depend on the number of cigarettes smoked per day (Goldstein *et al.*, 2001). However, it is still important to emphasize that smoking cessation is just as important after the first stroke as it is before the first stroke. Smoking cessation reduces the risk of stroke to that of the general population in approximately 2–5 years (Goldstein *et al.*, 2001). There have been few studies on the exact change in risk with reduced smoking in those who have already had a cerebrovascular event; nevertheless, it is firmly recommended that those with stroke, and their partners, reduce and preferably stop smoking after the stroke.

Antithrombotic drugs for secondary stroke prevention

There are considerable data that show the effectiveness of antiplatelet agents to reduce the risk of vascular events, including stroke (see above). In people with a history of stroke or transient ischemic attacks, the absolute risk reduction of new events with antiplatelet therapy is in the order of 36 per 1000 for people treated for two years (Antithrombotic Trialists' Collaboration, 2002).

Among the various antiplatelet agents, aspirin is the most widely studied. In the 11 placebo-controlled randomized trials of aspirin, including more than 10 000 patients with prior transient ischaemic attacks or IS, aspirin reduced the onset of a serious vascular event by 17% (Algra and van Gijn, 1999). The effective dose seems to range between 75–300 mg and there is no evidence that the higher doses are any more effective. Other studies have shown a risk reduction per 1000 patients treated of seven strokes and nine major vascular events when aspirin is administered within 48 hours of the stroke and for at least three weeks after (Antithrombotic Trialists' Collaboration, 2002). The slight problem associated with this therapy is a modest increase (around 2 per 1000) of haemorrhagic strokes. Other agents have been studied for the prevention of stroke recurrence. Until recently, there was very limited evidence that dipyridamole reduced vascular death even when administered with other antiplatelet agents. However, the European Stroke Prevention Study-2 trial showed that dipyridamole plus aspirin was more effective than aspirin alone for secondary prevention in patients with a history of stroke or transient ischemic attacks (Diener *et al.*, 1996). However, the dose of aspirin used in the study was rather low (50 mg per day). A newer and more bio-available preparation is currently being studied and the results of this trial are awaited with interest (de Schryver, 2000).

There have been two large trials of ticlopidine in people with existing cerebrovascular disease (Gent *et al.*, 1989; Hass *et al.*, 1989). The Canadian study (Gent *et al.*, 1989) demonstrated a relative risk reduction of 30.2% (95% CI, 7.5–48.3) for the primary end points (non-fatal stroke, myocardial infarction and vascular death). The Antithrombotic Trialists' Collaboration (2002) found that ticlopidine reduced the odds of vascular events by 10%. This 10% additional decrease in risk was associated with a number of adverse events, such as diarrhea, skin rash, and neutropenia.

There is some limited evidence that clopidogrel is as efficacious or perhaps modestly more efficacious than aspirin (Anonymous 1996). Recently, Ringleb and colleagues (2004) have demonstrated that people with a history of prior symptomatic atherosclerotic disease had a tendency to benefit modestly more from clopidogrel than aspirin (absolute risk reduction, 3.4%, 95% CI, 0.2–7.0; relative risk reduction, 14.9%; $P = 0.045$).

The role of warfarin in secondary prevention of non-cardioembolic stroke has been studied in the WARSS trial (Mohr *et al.*, 2001). The authors found no significant differences between warfarin and aspirin. The primary end point of death or recurrent stroke was reached by 17.8% of the warfarin group and 16% of the aspirin group. There were no significant differences between the treatment

Table 1.4 Cardioembolic sources and embolic risk

High risk	Low/uncertain risk
Atrial fibrillation	Patent foramen ovale
Mechanical valves	Atrial septal aneurysm
Mitral stenosis	Mitral prolapse
Dilated cardiomyopathy	Mitral valve strands
Infective endocarditis	Mitral annulus calcification
Non-infective endocarditis	Calcified aortic stenosis
Left atrial or ventricular thrombus	Akinetic/dyskinetic ventricular wall segment
Atrial myxoma	Subaortic hypertrophic cardiomyopathy
Recent myocardial infarction	
Sick sinus syndrome	

groups in the rate of major haemorrhage. The trial was interpreted as demonstrating that there was no definitive role for anticoagulation therapy in patients with non-cardioembolic ischaemic stroke.

In summary, the present evidence might indicate the following recommendations for secondary prevention of noncardioembolic stroke.

- The first-line agent would be aspirin (75–300 mg per day). It has confirmed efficacy and low cost.
- Clopidogrel could be used for those intolerant of aspirin.
- Coadministration of dipyridamole and aspirin could be considered, although the present authors reserve this combination for those with recurrent stroke despite optimal therapy.
- The current evidence does not support the use of oral anticoagulants for secondary prevention of non-cardioembolic stroke.

Specific situations

Cardioembolic stroke

Strokes caused by cardioembolism are, in general, severe and prone to early recurrence. There is a probability of recurrence of about 22% after two years (Kolominsky-Rabas *et al.*, 2001). Cardiac disorders can be classified according to their potential risk for recurrence (Table 1.4) (Ferro, 2003). A fewer of the more common risks are discussed.

Atrial fibrillation

The risk of stroke is at least five times higher in people with atrial fibrillation than in healthy controls (Wolf *et al.*, 1978). The risk of stroke in atrial fibrillation rises from 1.5% at the age of 50 to 24% at the age of 80 (Wyse *et al.*, 2002). People with atrial fibrillation and transient ischaemic attack or prior stroke should be given anticoagulation treatment. Anticoagulation that results in an INR of 2.0 or greater reduces not only the frequency of stroke but also the severity and risk of death within 30 days (Hylek *et al.*, 2003). Only those people without cerebrovascular risk factors or with contraindications to warfarin should be given aspirin. Aspirin alone has a modest protective effect but only approximately 20% of the protective effect of warfarin (Hart *et al.*, 2000). Despite the preventive potential of continuous oral anticoagulation in people with atrial fibrillation, several studies in the USA and Europe have shown that oral anticoagulation is underused (White *et al.*, 1999).

Patent foramen ovale and atrial septal aneurysm

Patent foramen ovale is present in a third of all patients with stroke who are younger than 55 years of age (Cabanes *et al.*, 1993). Atrial septal aneurysms are detected in 4% of people examined with transesophageal echocardiography (Nater *et al.*, 1992). The risk of stroke, and recurrent stroke, associated with patent foramen ovale and atrial septal aneurysm is controversial. A recent study demonstrated that the risk of recurrent stroke is low (2.3%) amongst patients with patent foramen ovale alone and moderate (15.2%) in those with patent foramen ovale and atrial septal aneurysm, as well as being low (4.2%) in those with neither (Mas *et al.*, 2001). Treatment alternatives are aspirin, warfarin, a combination of antiplatelet drugs, surgical intervention, or closures of the patent foramen ovale. There is no clear consensus in the literature regarding the best preventative treatment in such situations.

Mitral valve prolapse

The recurrent stroke rate in mitral valve prolapse was originally reported to be quite high, at 16% (Jackson *et al.*, 1984). However, more recent cohort and case–controlled studies have cast doubt on the role of uncomplicated mitral valve prolapse in stroke, even in young adults (Orencia *et al.*, 1995; Gilon *et al.*, 1999). Aspirin is generally recommended as an initial secondary preventative agent, and long-term anticoagulation with warfarin should be considered in patients with mitral valve prolapse with mitral regurgitation and large left atria or with recurrent transient ischemic attacks while receiving aspirin therapy (Bonow *et al.*, 1998).

Other situations

Prevention of embolic events in patients with mechanical valvular prosthesis (Turpie *et al.*, 1993) and prevention of serious vascular events in acute myocardial infarction (Hurlen *et al.*, 2002), and probably in congestive heart failure associated with atrial fibrillation (Lip and Gibbs, 2004), are the other evidence-based indications for the use of combined oral anticoagulants and aspirin.

Other rarer causes of stroke

Although it is outwith the scope of this textbook, it is clearly incumbent on the rehabilitation team to make sure that the patient referred for stroke rehabilitation has had the cause of the stroke thoroughly investigated. This is particularly the case, but not exclusively, for younger people. There are obviously a number of conditions that are associated with a higher risk of recurrent stroke and that need specific treatment in their own right. The reader is referred to standard stroke textbooks for detailed discussion of appropriate investigations after a stroke to determine if there are avoidable causes of recurrence.

REFERENCES

Abbott, R. D., Curb, D., Rodriguez, B. L., *et al.* (1996). Effects of dietary calcium and milk consumption on risk of thromboembolic stroke in older middle-aged men: the Honolulu Heart Program. *Stroke* **27**: 813–818.

Abbott, R. D., Rodriguez, B. L., Burchfiel, C. M., and Curb, D. (1994). Physical activity in older middle aged men and reduced risk of stroke: the Honolulu Heart Program. *Am J Epidemiol* **139**: 881–893.

Abbott, R. D., Yin, Y., Reed, D. M., and Yano, K. (1986). Risk of stroke in male cigarette smokers. *N Engl J Med* **315**: 717–720.

Albers, G. W., Dalen, J. E., Laupacis, A., *et al.* (2001). Antithrombotic therapy in atrial fibrillation. *Chest* **119**(Suppl.1): 194S–206S.

Algra, A. and van Gijn, J. (1999). Cumulative meta-analysis of aspirin efficacy after cerebral ischaemia of arterial origin. *J Neurol Neurosurg Psychiatry* **66**: 255.

ALLHAT Officers and Coordinators for the ALLHAT Collaborative Research Group (2002). Major outcomes in moderately hypercholesterolemic, hypertensive patients randomized to pravastatin vs usual care: the Antihipertensive and Lipid-lowering Treatment to Prevent Heart Attack Trial (ALLHAT-LLT). *JAMA* **288**: 2998–3007.

American Heart Association (2004). *Heart Disease and Stroke Statistics.* Dallas, TX: American Heart Association.

Anon. (1996). A randomised, blinded, trial of clopidogrel versus aspirin in patients at risk of ischaemic events (CAPRIE). CAPRIE Steering Committee. *Lancet* **348**: 1329–1339.

Antithrombotic Trialists' Collaboration (2002). Collaborative meta-analysis of randomized trials of antiplatelet therapy for prevention of death, myocardial infarction, and stroke in high risk patients. *BMJ* **324**: 71–86.

Ascherio, A., Rimm, E. B., Hernán, M. A., *et al.* (1998). Intake of potassium, magnesium, calcium, and fiber and risk of stroke among US men. *Circulation* **98**: 1198–1204.

Asplund, K. (2001). The decline in stroke mortality: an ending or a never-ending story? *Stroke* **32**: 2218–2220.

Asplund, K., Stegmayr, B., and Peltonen, M. (1998). From the twentieth to the twenty-first century: a public health perspective on stroke. In *Cerebrovascular Disease: Pathophysiology, Diagnosis and Management*, ed. M. D. Ginsberg and J. Bogousslavsky. Oxford, UK: Blackwell Science, pp. 901–918.

Auburger, G. (1998). New genetic concepts and stroke prevention. *Cerebrovasc Dis* **8**(Suppl. 5): 28–32.

Baker, E. H., Dong, Y. B., Sagnella, G. A., *et al.* (1998). Association of hypertension with T594M mutation in beta subunit of epithelial sodium channels in black people resident in London. *Lancet* **351**: 1388–1392.

Baker, W. H., Howard, V. J., Howard, G., and Toole, J. F., for the ACAS Investigators (2000). Effect of contralateral occlusion on long-term efficacy endarterectomy in the Asymptomatic Carotid Atherosclerosis Study (ACAS). *Stroke* **31**: 2330–2334.

Balkau, B., Shipley, M., Jarret, R. J., *et al.* (1998). High blood glucose concentration is a risk factor for mortality in middle-aged nondiabetic men. 20 year follow-up in the Whitehall Study, the Paris Prospective Study, and the Helsinki Policemen Study. *Diabetes Care* **21**: 360–367.

Bang, H. O., Dyerberg, J., and Hjørne, N. (1976). The composition of food consumed by Greenland Eskimos. *Acta Med Scand* **200**: 69–73.

Barker, W. H. and Mullooly, J. P. (1997). Stroke in a defined elderly population, 1967–1985. A less lethal and disabling but no less common disease. *Stroke* **28**: 284–290.

Benavente, O., Moher, D., and Pham, B. (1998). Carotid endarterectomy for asymptomatic carotid stenosis: a meta-analysis. *BMJ* **317**: 1477–1480.

Beral, V., Banks, E., and Reeves, G. (2002). Evidence from randomised trials on the long-term effects of hormone replacement therapy. *Lancet* **360**: 942–944.

Berger, K., Ajani, U. A., Kase, C. S., *et al.* (1999). Light-to-moderate alcohol consumption and the risk of stroke among US male physicians. *N Engl J Med* **341**: 1557–1564.

Bergman, L., van der Meulen, J. H. P., Limburg, M., *et al.* (1995). Costs of medical care after first-ever stroke in the Netherlands. *Stroke* **26**: 1830–1836.

Bijnen, F. C. H., Caspersen, C. J., Feskens, E. J. M., *et al.* (1998). Physical activity and 10-year mortality from cardiovascular diseases and all causes: the Zutphen Elderly Study. *Arch Intern Med* **158**: 1499–1505.

BIP Study Group (2000). Secondary prevention by raising HDL cholesterol and reducing triglycerides in patients with coronary artery disease: the Benzafibrate Infarction Prevention (BIP) study. *Circulation* **102**: 21–27.

Blaw, G. J., Lagaay, A. M., Smelt, A. H. M., and Westendorp, R. G. J. (1997). Stroke, statins and cholesterol: a meta-analysis of randomized, placebo-controlled, double-blind trials with HMG-CoA reductase inhibitors. *Stroke* **28**: 946–950.

Bogousslavsky, J., Regli, F., and van Melle, G. (1985). Risk factors and concomitants of internal carotid artery occlusion or stenosis: a controlled study of 159 cases. *Arch Neurol* **42**: 864–867.

Bogousslavsky, J., Despland, P.-A., and Regli, F. (1986). Asymptomatic tight stenosis of the internal carotid artery: long term prognosis. *Neurology* **36**: 861–863.

Bogousslavsky, J., van Melle, G., and Regli, F. (1988). The Lausanne Stroke Registry: analysis of 1000 consecutive patients with first stroke. *Stroke* **19**: 1083–1092.

Bonita, R., Scragg, R., Stewart, A., Jackson, R., and Beaglehole, R. (1986). Cigarette smoking and risk of premature stroke in men and women. *BMJ* **293**: 6–8.

Bonita, R., Broad, J. B., and Beaglehole, R. (1993). Changes in stroke incidence and case-fatality in Auckland, New Zealand, 1981–91. *Lancet* **342**: 1470–1473.

Bonita, R., Solomon, N., and Broad, J. B. (1997). Prevalence of stroke and stroke-related disability. Estimates from the Auckland Stroke Studies. *Stroke* **28**: 1898–1902.

Bonow, R. O., Carabello, B., de Leon, A. C., Jr., *et al.* (1998). Guidelines for the management of patients with valvular heart disease: executive summary. A report of the American College of Cardiology/American Heart Association Task Force on Practice Guidelines (Committee on Management of Patients with Valvular Heart Disease). *Circulation* **98**: 1949–1984.

Broderick, J. P. (1993). Stroke trends in Rochester, Minnesota, during 1945 to 1984. *Ann Epidemiol* **3**: 476–479.

Broderick, J., Brott, T., Kothari, R., *et al.* (1998). The Greater Cincinnati/Northern Kentucky Stroke Study preliminary first-ever and total incidence rates of stroke among blacks. *Stroke* **29**: 415–421.

Bronner, L. L., Kanter, D. S., and Manson, J. E. (1995). Primary prevention of stroke. *N Engl J Med* **333**: 1392–1400.

Brown, R. D., Whisnant, J. P., Sicks, J. D., O'Fallon, W. M., and Wiebers, D. O. (1996). Stroke incidence, prevalence, and survival: secular trends in Rochester, Minnesota, through 1989. *Stroke* **27**: 373–380.

Bucher, H. C., Griffith, L. E., and Guyatt, G. H. (1998). Effect of HMG-coA reductase inhibitors on stroke: a meta-analysis of randomized, controlled trials. *Ann Intern Med* **128**: 89–95.

Burchfiel, C. M., Curb, J. D., Rodriguez, B. L., *et al.* (1995). Glucose intolerance and 22-year stroke incidence: the Honolulu Heart Program. *Stroke* **25**: 951–957.

Burt, V. L., Cutler, J. A., Higgins, M., *et al.* (1995a). Trends in the prevalence, awareness, treatment, and control of hypertension in the adult US population: data from the Health Examination Surveys, 1960 to 1991. *Hypertension.* **26**: 60–69.

Burt, V. L., Whelton, P., Roccella, E. J., *et al.* (1995b). Prevalence of hypertension in the US adult population. *Hypertension* **25**: 305–313.

Cabanes, L., Mas, J. L., Cohen, A. *et al.* (1993). Atrial septal aneurysm and patent foramen ovale as risk factors for cryptogenic stroke in patients less than 55 years of age. A study using transesophageal echocardiography. *Stroke* **24**: 1865–1873.

Cabrera, C., Helgesson, O., Wedel, H., *et al.* (2001). Socioeconomic status and mortality in Swedish women: opposing trends for cardiovascular disease and cancer. *Epidemiology* **12**: 532–536.

Cao, J. J., Thach, C., Manolio, T. A., *et al.* (2003). C-reactive protein, carotid intima-media thickness, and incidence of ischemic stroke in the elderly: the Cardiovascular Health Study. *Circulation* **108**: 166–170.

Caro, J. J., Huybrechts, K. F., and Duchesne, I. (2000). Management patterns and costs of acute ischemic stroke: an international study. *Stroke* **31**: 582–590.

CAVATAS Investigators (2001). Endovascular versus surgical treatment in patients with carotid stenosis in the Carotid and Vertebral Artery Transluminal Angioplasty Study (CAVATAS). *Lancet* **357**: 1729–1737.

Centers for Disease Control and Prevention (2003). *The CDC Atlas of Stroke Mortality.* Bethesda, MDi Department of Health and Human Services, Centers for Disease Control and Prevention.

Chambers, B. R. and Norris, J. W. (1986). Outcome in patients with asymptomatic neck bruits. *N Engl J Med* **315**: 860–865.

Chobanian, A. V., Bakris, G. L., Black, H. R., *et al.* (2003). Seventh report of the Joint National Committee on Prevention, Detection, Evaluation, and Treatment of High Blood Pressure. *Hypertension* **42**: 1206–1252.

Christen, W. G., Ajani, U. A., Glynn, R. J., and Hennekens, C. H. (2000). Blood levels of homocysteine and increased risk of cardiovascular disease. *Arch Intern Med* **160**: 422–434.

Christian, J. B., Lapane, K. L., and Toppa, R. S. (2003). Racial disparities in receipt of secondary stroke prevention agents among US nursing home residents. *Stroke* **34**: 2693–2697.

Colditz, G. A., Bonita, R., Stampfer, M. J., *et al.* (1988). Cigarette smoking and risk of stroke in middle-aged women. *N Engl J Med* **318**: 937–941.

Collins, R., Peto, P., MacMahon, S., *et al.* (1990). Blood pressure, stroke, and coronary heart disease, part 2: short-term reductions in blood pressure: overview of randomised drug trials in their epidemiological context. *Lancet* **335**: 827–838.

Corvol, J.-C., Bouzamondo, A., Sirol, M., *et al.* (2003). Differential effects of lipid-lowering therapies on stroke prevention: a meta-analysis of randomized trials. *Arch Int Med* **163**: 669–676.

Côté, R., Battista, R. N., Abrahamowicz, M., *et al.* (1995). Lack of effect of aspirin in asymptomatic patients with carotid bruits and substantial carotid narrowing. *Ann Intern Med* **123**: 649–655.

Crouse, J. R., Byington, R. P., Hoen, H. M., and Furberg, C. D. (1997). Reductase inhibitor monotherapy and stroke prevention. *Arch Intern Med* **157**: 1305–1310.

Crouse, J. R., Byington, R. P., and Furberg, C. D. (1998). HMG-CoA reductase inhibitor therapy and stroke risk reduction: an analysis of clinical trials data. *Atherosclerosis* **138**: 11–24.

Cutler, J. (1999). Which drug for treatment of hypertension? *Lancet* **353**: 604–605.

Dahlöf, B., Lindholm, L. H., Hansson, L., *et al.* (1991). Morbidity and mortality in the Swedish Trial in Old Patients with Hypertension (STOP-Hypertension). *Lancet* **338**: 1281–1285.

Damcott, C. M., Sack, P., and Shuldiner, A. R. (2003). The genetics of obesity. *Endocrinol Metab Clin North Am* **32**: 761–786.

de Bruijn, S. F., Stam, J., Koopman, M. M., and Vandenbroucke, J. P. (1998). Case–control study of risk of cerebral sinus thrombosis in oral contraceptive users and in carriers of hereditary prothrombotic conditions. The Cerebral Venous Sinus Thrombosis Study Group. *BMJ* **316**: 589–592.

de Freitas, G. R. and Bogousslavsky, J. (2001). Primary stroke prevention. *Eur J Neurol* **8**: 1–15. (2003). Classification of stroke. In *Imaging in Stroke*, ed. M. G. Hennerici. London: Remedica, pp. 1–17.

de Gaetano, G. for the Collaborative Group of the Primary Prevention Project (2001). Low-dose aspirin and vitamin E in people at cardiovascular risk: a randomised trial in general practice. *Lancet* **357**: 89–95.

de Padua Mansur, A., de Fatima, M. S., Favarato, D., *et al.* (2003). Stroke and ischemic heart disease mortality trends in Brazil from 1979 to 1996. *Neuroepidemiology* **22**: 179–183.

de Schryver, E. L. (2000). Design of ESPRIT: an international randomized trial for secondary prevention after non-disabling cerebral ischaemia of arterial origin. European/Australian

Stroke Prevention in Reversible Ischaemia Trial (ESPRIT) group. *Cerebrovasc Dis* **10**: 147–150.

Diabetes Control and Complications Trial Research Group (1993). The effect of intensive treatment of diabetes on the development and progression of long-term complications in insulin-dependent diabetes mellitus. *N Engl J Med* **329**: 977–986.

(1995). The effect of intensive diabetes management on macrovascular events and risk factors in the Diabetes Control and Complications Trial. *Am J Cardiol* **75**: 894–903.

di Mascio, R., Marchioli, R., and Tognoni, G. (2000). Cholesterol reduction and stroke occurrence: an overview of randomized clinical trials. *Cerebrovasc Dis* **10**: 85–92.

Diener, H. C., Cunha, L., Forbes, C., *et al.* (1996). European Stroke Prevention Study 2. Dipyridamole and acetylsalicylic acid in the secondary prevention of stroke. *J Neurol Sci* **143**: 1–13.

Donahue, R. P., Abbott, R. D., Dwayne, M. R., and Yano, K. (1986). Alcohol and hemorrhagic stroke: the Honolulu Heart Program. *JAMA* **255**: 2311–2314.

Downs, J. R., Clearfield, M., and Weis, S., for the AFCAPS/TexCAPS Research Group (1998). Primary prevention of acute coronary events in men and woman with average cholesterol levels. *JAMA* **279**: 1615–1622.

EAFT Study Group (1995). Optimal oral anticoagulation therapy with nonrheumatic atrial fibrillation and recent cerebral ischemia. *N Engl J Med* **333**: 5–10.

Eastern Stroke and Coronary Heart Disease Collaborative Research Group (1998). Blood pressure, cholesterol, and stroke in eastern Asia. *Lancet* **352**: 1801–1807.

Eidelman, R. S., Hebert, P. R., Weisman, S. M., Hennekens, C. H. (2003). An update on aspirin in the primary prevention of cardiovascular disease. *Arch Intern Med* **163**: 2006–2010.

Eikelboom, J. W., Lonn, E., Genest, J., Hankey, G., and Yussuf, S. (1999). Homocyst(e)ine and cardiovascular disease: a critical review of epidemiological evidence. *Ann Intern Med* **131**: 363–375.

Elkind, M. S. V., Lin, I. F., Grayston, J. T., and Sacco, R. L. (2000). *Chlamydia pneumoniae* and the risk of first ischemic stroke: the Nothern Manhattan Stroke Study. *Stroke* **31**: 1521–1525.

Ellekjær, H., Holmen, J., Ellekjær, E., and Vatten, L. (2000). Physical activity and stroke mortality in women: ten-year follow-up of the Nord-Trøndelag Health Survey, 1984–1986. *Stroke* **31**: 14–18.

ETDRS Investigators (1992). Aspirin effects on mortality and morbidity in patients with diabetes mellitus: Early Treatment Diabetic Retinopathy Study Report 14. *JAMA* **268**: 1292–1300.

Evenson, K. R., Rosamond, W. D., and Cai, J. for the Atherosclerosis Risk in Communities (ARIC) study investigators (1999). Physical activity and ischemic stroke risk: the Atherosclerosis Risk in Communities Study. *Stroke* **30**: 1333–1339.

Executive Committee for the Asymptomatic Carotid Atherosclerosis Study (ACAS) (1995). Endarterectomy for asymptomatic carotid artery stenosis. *JAMA* **273**: 1421–1428.

Falkeborn, M., Persson, I., Terent, A., *et al.* (1993). Hormone replacement therapy and the risk of stroke: follow-up of a population-based cohort in Sweden. *Arch Intern Med* **153**: 1201–1209.

Feigin, V. L., Wiebers, D. O., Whisnant, J. P., and O'Fallon, W. M. (1995). Stroke incidence and 30-day case-fatality rates in Novosibirsk, Russia, 1982 through 1992. *Stroke* **26**: 924–929.

Feigin, V. L., Lawes, C. M. M., Bennett, D. A. and Anderson, C. S. (2003). Stroke epidemiology: a review of population-based studies of incidence, prevalence, and case-fatality in the late 20th century. *Lancet Neurol* **2**: 43–53.

Ferro, J. M. (2003). Cardioembolic stroke: an update. *Lancet Neurol* **2**: 177–188.

Fine-Edelstein, J. S., Wolf, P. A., O'Leary, D. H., *et al.* (1984). Precursors of extracranial carotid atherosclerosis in the Framingham Study. *Neurology* **44**: 1046–1050.

Fletcher, A. E. and Bulpitt, C. J. (1992). How far should blood pressure be lowered? *N Engl J Med* **326**: 251–254.

Florez, J. C., Hirschhorn, J., and Altshuler, D. (2003). The inherited basis of diabetes mellitus: implications for the genetic analysis of complex traits. *Annu Rev Genom Hum Genet* **4**: 257–291.

Floßmann, E., Schulz, U. G. R., and Rothwell, P. M. (2004). Systematic review of methods and results of studies of the genetic epidemiology of ischemic stroke. *Stroke* **35**: 212–227.

Folsom, A. R., Rasmussen, M. L., Chambless, L. E. for the Atherosclerosis Risk in Communities (ARIC) Study Investigators (1999a). Prospective associations of fasting insulin, body fat distribution, and diabetes with risk of ischemic stroke. *Diabetes Care* **22**: 1077–1083.

Folsom, A. R., Rosamond, W. D., Sahar, E. for the Atherosclerosis Risk in Communities (ARIC) Study Investigators (1999b). Prospective study of markers of hemostatic function with risk of ischemic stroke. *Circulation* **100**: 736–742.

Fox, C. S., Polak, J. F., Chazaro, I., *et al.* (2003). Genetic and environmental contributions to atherosclerosis phenotypes in men and women. Heritability of carotid intima-media thickness in the Framingham Heart Study. *Stroke* **34**: 397–401.

Fuller, J. H., Shipley, M. J., Rose, G., Jarret, R. J., and Keen, H. (1983). Mortality from coronary heart disease and stroke in relation to the degree of glycaemia: the Whitehall study. *BMJ* **287**: 867–870.

Fustinoni, O. and Biller, J. (2000). Ethnicity and stroke. *Stroke* **31**: 1013–1015.

Furberg, C. D., Adams, H. P., Applegate, W. B. for the Asymptomatic Carotid Artery Progression Study (ACAPS) Research Group (1994). Effect of lovastatin on early carotid atherosclerosis and cardiovascular events. *Circulation* **90**: 1679–1687.

Gage, B. F., Waterman, A. D., Shannon, W., *et al.* (2001). Validation of clinical classification schemes for predicting stroke: results from the National Registry of Atrial Fibrillation. *JAMA* **285**: 2864–2870.

Gent, M., Blakely, J. A., Easton, J. D., *et al.* (1989). The Canadian American Ticlopidine Study (CATS) in thromboembolic stroke. *Lancet* **i**: 1215–1220.

Gey, K. F., Stahelin, H. B., and Eichholzer, M. (1993). Poor plasma status of carotene and vitamin C is associated with higher mortality from ischemic heart disease and stroke: Basel Prospective Study. *Clin Invest* **71**: 3–6.

Giles, W. H., Kittner, S. J., Hebel, J. R., Losonczy, K. G., and Sherwin, R. W. (1995). Determinants of black–white differences in the risk of cerebral infarction. *Arch Intern Med.* **155**: 1319–1324.

Gillman, M. W., Cupples, L. A., Gagnon, D., *et al.* (1995). Protective effects of fruits and vegetables on development of stroke in men. *JAMA* **273**: 1113–1117.

Gillum, R. F., Mussolino, M. E., and Ingram, D. D. (1996a). Physical activity and stroke incidence in women and men: the NHANES I Epidemiologic Follow-up Study. *Am J Epidemiol* **143**: 860–869.

Gillum, R. F., Mussolino, M. E., and Madans, J. H. (1996b). The relationship between fish consumption and stroke incidence: the NHANES I epidemiologic follow-up study. *Arch Intern Med* **156**: 537–542.

Gillman, M. W., Cupples, L. A., Millen, B. E., Ellison, R. C., and Wolf, P. A. (1997). Inverse association of dietary fat with development of ischemic stroke in men. *JAMA* **278**: 2145–2150.

Gilon, D., Buonanno, F. S., Joffe, M. M., *et al.* (1999). Lack of evidence of an association between mitral-valve prolapse and stroke in young patients. *N Engl J Med* **341**: 8–13.

GISSI-Prevenzione Investigators (Gruppo Italiano per lo Studio della Sopravvivenza nell'Infarto Miocardico) (1999). Dietary supplementation with *n*-3 polyunsaturated fatty acids and vitamin E after myocardial infarction: results of the GISSI-Prevenzione trial. *Lancet* **354**: 447–455.

Glader, C. A., Stegmayr, B., Boman, J., *et al.* (1999). *Chlamydia pneumoniae* antibodies and high lipoprotein (a) levels do not predict ischemic cerebral infarction: results from a nested case–control study in Northern Sweden. *Stroke* **30**: 2013–2018.

Goldstein, L. B., Adams, R., Becker, K., *et al.* (2001). Primary prevention of ischemic stroke: a statement for healthcare professionals from the Stroke Council of the American Heart Association. *Stroke* **32**: 280–299.

Gorelick, P. (1998). Cerebrovascular disease in African Americans. *Stroke* **29**: 2656–2664.

Green, D. M., Ropper, A. H., Kronmal, R. A., Psaty, B. M., and Burke, G. L. (2002). Serum potassium level and dietary potassium intake as risk factors for stroke. *Neurology* **59**: 314–320.

Gretarsdottir, S., Thorleifsson, G., Reynisdottir, S. T., *et al.* (2003). The gene encoding phosphodiesterase 4D confers risk of ischemic stroke. *Nat Genet* **35**: 131–138.

Grodstein, F. G., Stampfer, M. J., Manson, J. E., *et al.* (1996). Postmenopausal estrogen and progestin replacement use and the risk of cardiovascular disease. *N Engl J Med* **335**: 453–461.

Grodstein, F. G., Manson, J. E., Colditz, G. A., *et al.* (2000). A prospective, observational study of postmenopausal hormone therapy and primary prevention of cardiovascular disease. *Ann Intern Med* **133**: 933–941.

Gupta, V., Nanda, N. C., Yesilbursa, D., *et al.* (2003). Racial differences in thoracic aorta atherosclerosis among ischemic stroke patients. *Stroke* **34**: 408–412.

Hajat, C., Dundas, R., Stewart, J. A., *et al.* (2001). Cerebrovascular risk factors and stroke subtypes. Differences between ethnic groups. *Stroke* **32**: 37–42.

Hankey, G. J. and Eikelboom, J. W. (1999). Homocysteine and vacular disease. *Lancet* **354**: 407–413.

Hansson, L., Zanchetti, A., Carruthers, S. G., *et al.* (1998). Effects of intensive blood-pressure lowering and low-dose aspirin in patients with hypertension: principal results of the Hypertension Optimal Treatment (HOT) randomised trial. *Lancet* **351**: 1755–1762.

Hardie, K., Hankey, G. J., Konrad, J., *et al.* (2004). Ten-year risk of first recurrent stroke and disability after first-ever stroke in the Perth Community Stroke Study. *Stroke* **35**: 731–735.

Hart, R. G., Benavente, O., McBride, R., and Pearce, L. A. (1999). Antithrombotic therapy to prevent stroke in patients with atrial fibrillation: a meta-analysis. *Ann Intern Med* **131**: 492–501.

Hart, R. G., Halperin, J. L., McBride, R., *et al.* (2000). Aspirin for the primary prevention of stroke and other major vascular events: meta-analysis and hypotheses. *Arch Neurol* **57**: 326–332.

Hass, W. K., Easton, J. D., Adams, H. P. Jr., *et al.* (1989). A randomized trial comparing ticlopidine hydrochloride with aspirin for the prevention of stroke in high-risk patients. Ticlopidine Aspirin Stroke Study Group. *N Engl J Med* **321**: 501–507.

He, K., Rimm, E. B., Merchant, A., *et al.* (2002). Fish consumption and risk of stroke in men. *JAMA* **288**: 3130–3136.

He, K., Merchant, A., Rimm, E. B., *et al.* (2003). Dietary fat intake and risk of stroke in male US healthcare professionals: 14 year prospective cohort study. *BMJ* **327**: 777–782.

Heart Protection Study Collaborative Group (2002a). MRC/BHF heart protection study of cholesterol lowering with simvastatin in 20 536 high-risk individuals: a randomized placebo-controlled trial. *Lancet* **360**: 7–22.

(2002b). MRC/BHF heart protection study of antioxidant vitamin supplementation in 20 536 high-risk individuals: a randomised placebo-controlled trial. *Lancet* **360**: 23–33.

(2004). Effects of cholesterol-lowering with simvastatin on stroke and other major vascular events in 20 536 people with cerebrovascular disease or other high-risk conditions. *Lancet* **363**: 757–767.

Heinemann, L. A., Lewis, M. A., Thorogood, M., *et al.* (1997). Case–control study of oral contraceptives and risk of thromboembolic stroke: results from International Study on Oral Contraceptives and Health of Young Women. *BMJ* **315**: 1502–1504.

Herbert, P. R., Gaziano, J. M., Chan, K. S., and Hennekens, C. H. (1997). Cholesterol lowering with statin drugs, risk of stroke, and total mortality. *JAMA* **278**: 313–321.

Hillbom, M. and Kaste, M. (1982). Alcohol intoxication: a risk factor for primary subarachnoid hemorrhage. *Neurology* **32**: 706–711.

Hirashiki, A., Yamada, Y., Murase, Y., *et al.* (2003). Association of gene polymorphisms with coronary artery disease in low- or high-risk subjects defined by conventional risk factors. *J Am Coll Cardiol* **42**: 1429–1437.

Homocysteine Studies Collaboration (2002). Homocysteine and risk of ichemic heart disease and stroke: a meta-analysis. *JAMA* **288**: 2015–2022.

Howard, G., Wagenknecht, L. E., Burke, G. L. for the ARIC Investigators (1998). Cigarette smoking and progression of atherosclerosis: the Atherosclerosis Risk in Communities (ARIC) Study. *JAMA* **279**: 119–125.

Howard, G., Howard, V. J., Katholi, C., Oli, M. K., Huston, S. (2001). Decline in US stroke mortality: an analysis of temporal patterns by sex, race, and geographic region. *Stroke* **32**: 2213–2220.

Hu, F. B., Stampfer, M. J., Colditz, G. A., *et al.* (2000). Physical activity and risk of stroke in women. *JAMA* **283**: 2961–2967.

Hulley, S., Grady, D., Bush, T., *et al.* (1998). Randomized trial of estrogen plus progestin for the secondary prevention of coronary heart disease in postmenopausal women. *JAMA* **280**: 605–613.

Hurlen, M., Abdelnoor, M., Smith, P., *et al.* (2002). Warfarin, aspirin, or both after myocardial infarction. *N Engl J Med* **347**: 969–974.

Hylek, E. M., Go, A. S., Chang, Y., *et al.* (2003). Effect of intensity of oral anticoagulation on stroke severity and mortality in atrial fibrillation. *N Engl J Med* **349**: 1019–1026.

Immonen-Raiha, P., Sarti, C., Tuomilehto, J. *et al.* (2003). Eleven-year trends of stroke in Turku, Finland. *Neuroepidemiology* **22**: 196–203.

Inzitari, D., Eliasziw, M., Gates, P., *et al.* (2000). The causes and risk of stroke in patients with asymptomatic internal-carotid-artery stenosis. *N Engl J Med* **342**: 1693–1700.

Iso, H., Jacobs, D. R., Wentworth, D., Neaton, J. D., and Cohen, J. D. (1989). Serum cholesterol levels and 6-year mortality from stroke in 350 977 men screened for the Multiple Risk Factor Intervention Trial. *N Engl J Med* **320**: 904–910.

Iso, H., Stampfer, M. J., Manson, J. E., *et al.* (1999). Prospective study of calcium, potassium, and magnesium intake and risk of stroke in women. *Stroke* **30**: 1772–1779.

(2001a). Prospective study of fat and protein intake and risk of intraparenchymal hemorrhage in women. *Circulation* **103**: 856–863.

Iso, H., Rexrode, K. M., Stampfer, M. J., *et al.* (2001b). Intake of fish and omega-3 fatty acids and risk of stroke in women. *JAMA* **285**: 304–312.

Iso, H., Sato, S., Kitamura, A., *et al.* (2003). Fat and protein intakes and risk of intraparenchymal hemorrhage among middle-aged Japanese. *Am J Epidemiol* **157**: 32–39.

Jackson, A. C., Boughner, D. R., and Barnett, H. J. (1984). Mitral valve prolapse and cerebral ischemic events in young patients. *Neurology* **34**: 784–787.

Jamrozik, K., Broadhurst, R. J., Lai, N., *et al.* (1999). Trends in the incidence, severity, and short-term outcome of stroke in Perth, Western Australia. *Stroke* **30**: 2105–11.

Johnston, S. C., Colford, J. M., Jr., and Gress, D. R. (1998). Oral contraceptives and the risk of subarachnoid hemorrhage: a meta-analysis. *Neurology* **51**: 411–418.

Joshipura, K. J., Ascherio, A., Manson, J. E., *et al.* (1999). Fruit and vegetable intake in relation to risk of ischemic stroke. *JAMA* **282**: 1233–1239.

Kaplan, G. A. and Keil, J. E. (1993). Socioeconomic factors and cardiovascular disease: a review of the literature. *Circulation* **88**: 1973–1998.

Kassirer, J. P. and Angell, M. (1998). Losing weight – an ill-fated New Year's resolution. *N Engl J Med* **338**: 52–54.

Kastrup, A., Skalej, M., Krapf, H., *et al.* (2003). Early outcome of carotid angioplasty and stenting versus carotid endarterectomy in a single academic center. *Cerebrovasc Dis* **15**: 84–89.

Kawachi, I., Colditz, G. A., Stampfer, M. J., *et al.* (1993). Smoking cessation and decreased risk of stroke in women. *JAMA* **269**: 232–236.

Kell, S. O., Feskens, E. J. M., and Kromhout, D. (1994). Fish consumption and risk of stroke: the Zutphen study. *Stroke* **25**: 328–332.

Khaw, K. T. and Barrett-Connor, E. (1987). Dietary potassium and stroke-associated mortality: a 12-year prospective population study. *N Engl J Med* **316**: 235–240.

Kiely, D. K., Wolf, P. A., Cupples, L. A., Beiser, A. S., and Kannel, W. B. (1994). Physical activity and stroke risk: the Framingham Study. *Am J Epidemiol* **140**: 608–620.

Kolominsky-Rabas, P. L., Weber, M., Gefeller, O., *et al.* (2001). Epidemiology of ischemic stroke subtypes according to TOAST criteria: incidence, recurrence, and long-term survival in ischemic stroke subtypes: a population-based study. *Stroke* **32**: 2735–2740.

Kris-Etherton, P. M., Harris, W. S., and Appel, L. J. for the American Heart Association Nutrition Committee (2002). Fish consumption, fish oil, omega-3 fatty acids, and cardio-vascular disease. *Circulation* **106**: 2747–2757.

Kubo, M., Kiyohara, Y., Kato, I., *et al.* (2003). Trends in the incidence, mortality, and survival rate of cardiovascular disease in a Japanese community: the Hisayama Study. *Stroke* **34**: 2349–2354.

Lawes, C. M., Bennett, D. A., Feigin, V. L., and Rodgers, A. (2004). Blood pressure and stroke: an overview of published reviews. *Stroke* **35**: 1024–1033.

Lawlor, D. A., Smith, G. A., Leon, D. A., Sterne, J. A. C., and Ebrahim, S. (2002). Secular trends in mortality by stroke subtype in the 20th century: a retrospective analysis. *Lancet* **360**: 1818–1823.

Lee, C. D., Folsom, A. R., and Blair, S. N. (2003). Physical activity and stroke risk: a meta-analysis. *Stroke* **34**: 2475–2481.

Lee, I. M. and Paffenbarger, R. S., Jr. (1998). Physical activity and stroke incidence: the Harvard Alumni Health Study. *Stroke* **29**: 2049–2054.

Lee, I. M., Hennekens, C. H., Berger, K., Buring, J. E., and Manson, J. E. (1999). Exercise and risk of stroke in male physicians. *Stroke* **30**: 1–6.

Leppala, J. M., Virtamo, J., Fogelholm, R., *et al.* (2000). Vitamin E and beta carotene supplementation in high risk for stroke: a subgroup analysis of the Alpha-tocopherol, Beta-carotene Cancer Prevention Study. *Arch Neurol* **57**: 1503–1509.

Lindenstrom, E., Boysen, G., and Nyboe, J. (1994). Influence of total cholesterol, high density lipoprotein cholesterol and triglycerides on risk of cerebrovascular disease: the Copenhagen City Heart Study. *BMJ* **309**: 11–15.

Lindsberg, P. J. and Grau, A. J. (2003). Inflammation and infections as risk factors for ischemic stroke. *Stroke* **34**: 2518–2532.

Lip, G. and Gibbs, C. R., (2004). Anticoagulation for heart failure in sinus rhythm. *Cochrane Database of Systematic Reviews*, Issue 1. Oxford: Update Software.

Lip, G. Y. H. and Lowe, G. D. O. (1996). Antithrombotic treatment for atrial fibrillation. *BMJ* **312**: 45–49.

Longstreth, W. T., Bernick, C., Fitzpatrick, A., *et al.* (2001). Frequency and predictors of stroke death in 5888 participants in the Cardiovascular Health Study. *Neurology* **56**: 368–375.

Manson, J. E. and Martin, K. A. (2001). Postmenopausal hormone-replacement therapy. *N Engl J Med* **345**: 34–40.

Mas, J. L., Arquizan, C., Lamy, C., *et al.* (2001). Recurrent cerebrovascular events associated with patent foramen ovale, atrial septal aneurysm, or both. *N Engl J Med* **345**: 1740–1746.

Medical Research Council's General Practice Research Framework (1998). Thrombosis prevention trial: a randomised trial of low-intensity oral anticoagulation with warfarin and low-dose aspirin in the primary prevention of ischaemic heart disease in men at increased risk. *Lancet* **351**: 233–241.

Mercuri, M., Bond, M. G., Sirtori, C. R., *et al.* (1996). Pravastatin reduces carotid intima–media thickness progression in an asymptomatic hypercholesterolemic Mediterranean population: the Carotid Atherosclerosis Italian Ultrasound Study. *Am J Med* **101**: 627–634.

Mohr, J. P., Thompson, J. L., Lazar, R. M., *et al.* (2001). A comparison of warfarin and aspirin for the prevention of recurrent ischemic stroke. *N Engl J Med* **345**: 1444–1451.

Morikawa, Y., Nakagawa, H., Naruse, Y., *et al.* (2000). Trends in stroke incidence and acute case fatality in a Japanese rural area: the Oyabe study. *Stroke* **31**: 1583–1587.

Morimoto, T., Schreiner, A. S., and Asano, H. (2003). Caregiver burden and health-related quality of life among Japanese stroke caregivers. *Age Aging* **32**: 218–223.

Moroney, J., Bagiella, E., Paik, M. C., Sacco, R. L., and Desmond, D. W. (1998). Risk factors for early recurrence after ischemic stroke. The role of stroke syndrome and subtype. *Stroke* **29**: 2118–2124.

Morris, C. D. and Carson, S. (2003). Routine vitamin supplementation to prevent cardiovascular disease: a summary of the evidence for the US Preventive Services Task Force. *Ann Intern Med* **139**: 56–70.

Morris, M. C., Manson, J. E., Rosner, B., *et al.* (1995). Fish consumption and cardiovascular disease in the Physicians' Health Study: a prospective study. *Am J Epidemiol* **142**: 166–175.

Mozaffarian, D., Kumanyika, S. K., Lemaitre, R. N., *et al.* (2003). Cereal, fruit, and vegetable fiber intake and the risk of cardiovascular disease in elderly individuals. *JAMA* **289**: 1659–1666.

Murray, C. J. L. and Lopez, A. D. (1997). Mortality by cause for eight regions of the world: Global Burden of Disease Study. *Lancet* **349**: 1269–1276.

Nater, B. J., Regli, F., Stauffer, J.-C. (1992). Stroke patterns with atrial septal aneurysms. *Cerebrovasc Dis* **2**: 343–346.

Naylor, A. R., Bolia, A., Abbott, R. J., *et al.* (1998). Randomized study of carotid angioplasty and stenting versus carotid endarterectomy: a stopped trial. *J Vasc Surg* **28**: 326–334.

NIH: Morbidity and Mortality (2002). *Chart Book in Cardiovascular, Lung, and Blood Diseases.* Bethesda, MA, National Institutes of Health.

Numminen, H., Kotila, M., Waltimo, O., Aho, K., and Kaste, M. (1996). Declining incidence and mortality rates of stroke in Finland from 1972 to 1991: results of three population-based stroke registers. *Stroke* **27**: 1487–1491.

Oliveira-Filho, J., Silva, S. C., Trabuco, C. C., *et al.* (2003). Detrimental effect of blood pressure reduction in the first 24 hours of acute stroke onset. *Neurology* **61**: 1047–1051.

Oparil, S., Zaman, A., and Calhoun, D. A. (2003). Pathogenesis of hypertension. *Ann Intern Med* **139**: 761–776.

Orencia, A. J., Petty, G. W., Khandheria, B. K., *et al.* (1995). Risk of stroke with mitral valve prolapse in population-based cohort study. *Stroke* **26**: 7–13.

Orencia, A. J., Daviglus, M. L., Dyer, A. R., Shekelle, R. B., and Stamler, J. (1996). Fish consumption and stroke in men: 30-year findings of the Chicago Western Electric Study. *Stroke* **27**: 204–209.

Paffenbarger, R. S., Jr. and Williams, J. L. (1967). Chronic disease in former college students: early precursors of fatal stroke. *Am J Public Health* **57**: 1290–1299.

Payne, K. A., Huybrechts, K. F., Caro, J. J., Craig Green, T. J., and Klittich, W. S. (2002). Long term cost-of-illness in stroke: an international review. *Pharmacoeconomics* **20**: 813–825.

Pessah-Rasmussen, H., Engström, G., Jerntorp, I., Janzon, L. (2003). Increasing stroke incidence and decreasing case fatality, 1989–1998: a study from the Stroke Register in Malmö, Sweden. *Stroke* **34**: 913–918.

Petitti, D. B., Sidney, S., Quesenberry, C. P., Jr., and Bernstein, A. (1998). Ischemic stroke and use of estrogen and estrogen/progestogen as hormone replacement therapy. *Stroke* **29**: 23–28.

Peto, R., Gray, R., Collins, R., *et al.* (1988). Randomised trial of prophylactic daily aspirin in British male doctors. *BMJ* **296**: 313–316.

PROGRESS Collaborative Group (2001). Randomised trial of a perindopril-based blood-pressure-lowering regimen among 6105 individuals with previous stroke or transient ischaemic attack. *Lancet* **358**: 1033–1041.

Prospective Studies Collaboration (1995). Cholesterol, diastolic blood pressure and stroke. 13 000 strokes in 450 000 people in 45 prospective cohorts. *Lancet* **346**: 1647–1653.

Qureshi, A. I., Giles, W. H., and Croft, J. B. (1999). Racial differences in the incidence of intracerebral haemorrhage. Effects of blood pressure and education. *Neurology* **52**: 1617–1621.

Rashid, P., Leonardi-Bee, J., and Bath, P. (2003). Blood pressure reduction and secondary prevention of stroke and other vascular events: a systematic review. *Stroke* **34**: 2741–2748.

Reynolds, K., Lewis, B., Nolen, J. D., *et al.* (2003). Alcohol consumption and risk of stroke: a meta-analysis. *JAMA* **289**: 579–588.

Ridker, P. M., Hennekens, C. H., Buring, J. E., and Rifai, N. (2000). C-reactive protein and other markers of inflammation in the prediction of cardiovascular disease in women. *N Engl J Med* **342**: 836–843.

Ridker, P. M., Rifai, N., Rose, L., Buring, J. E., and Cook, N. R. (2002). Comparison of C-reactive protein and low-density lipoprotein cholesterol levels in the prediction of first cardiovascular events. *N Engl J Med* **347**: 1557–1565.

Ringleb, P. A., Bhatt, D. L., Hirsch, A. T., *et al.* (2004). Benefit of clopidogrel over aspirin is amplified in patients with a history of ischemic events. *Stroke* **35**: 528–532.

Rosamond, W. D., Folsom, A. R., Chambless, L. E. *et al.* (1999). Stroke incidence and survival among middle-aged adults. *Stroke* **30**: 736–743.

Ross, S. D., Allen, I. E., Connelly, J. E., *et al.* (1999). Clinical outcomes in statin treatment trials: a meta-analysis. *Arch Intern Med* **159**: 1793–1802.

Rubins, H. B., Davenport, J., Babikian, V., *et al.* (2001). Reduction in stroke with gemfibrozil in men with coronary heart disease and low HDL cholesterol: the Veterans Affair HDL Intervention Trial (VA-HIT). *Circulation* **103**: 2828–2833.

Sacco, R. L. (1995). Risk factors and outcomes for ischemic stroke. *Neurology* **45**(Suppl. 1): 10–14.

Sacco, R. L., Foulkes, M. A., Mohr, J. P., *et al.* (1989). Determinants of early recurrence of cerebral infarction: the Stroke Data Bank. *Stroke* **20**: 983–989.

Sacco, R. L., Elkind, M., Boden-Albala, B., *et al.* (1999). The protective effect of moderate alcohol consumption on ischemic stroke. *JAMA* **281**: 53–60.

Sacks, F. M., Pfeffer, M. A., Moye, L. A., *et al.* (1996). The effect of pravastatin on coronary events after myocardial infarction in patients with average cholesterol levels. *N Engl J Med* **335**: 1001–1009.

Salonen, R., Nyyssönen, K., Porkkala, E., *et al.* (1995). Kuopio Atherosclerosis Prevention Study (KAPS): a population-based primary prevention trial of the effect of LDL lowering on atherosclerotic progression in carotid and femoral arteries. *Circulation* **92**: 1758–1764.

Salonen, R. M., Nyyssonen, K., and Kaikkonen, J. for the Antioxidant Supplementation in Atherosclerosis Prevention Study (2003). Six-year effect of combined vitamin C and E supplementation on atherosclerotic progression: the Antioxidant Supplementation in Atherosclerosis Prevention (ASAP) Study. *Circulation* **107**: 947–953.

Saposnik, G. and Del Brutto, O. H. for the Iberoamerican Society of Cerebrovascular Diseases (2003). Stroke in South America: a systematic review of incidence, prevalence, and stroke subtypes. *Stroke* **34**: 2103–2108.

Sarti, C., Rastenyte, D., Cepaitis, Z., and Tuomilehto, J. (2000). International trends in mortality from stroke, 1968 to 1994. *Stroke* **31**: 1588–1601.

Sarti, C., Stegmayr, B., Tolonen, H., *et al.* (2003). Are changes in mortality from stroke caused by changes in stroke event rates or case fatality? Results from the WHO MONICA Project. *Stroke* **34**: 1833–1841.

Scandinavian Simvastatin Survival Study Group (1994). Randomised trial of cholesterol lowering in 4444 patients with coronary heart disease: the Scandinavian Simvastatin Survival Study (4S). *Lancet* **344**: 1383–1389.

Schnyder, G., Roffi, M., Pin, R., *et al.* (2001). Decreased rate of coronary restenosis after lowering of plasma homocysteine levels. *N Engl J Med* **345**: 1593–1600.

Schwartz, S. M., Petitti, D. B., Siscovick, D. S., *et al.* (1998). Stroke and use of low-dose oral contraceptives in young women: a pooled analysis of two US studies. *Stroke* **29**: 2277–2284.

Shahar, E., Chambless, L. E., Rosamond, W. D., *et al.* (2003). Plasma lipid profile and incident ischemic stroke: the Atherosclerosis Risk in the Communities (ARIC) study. *Stroke* **34**: 623–631.

Sharper, A. G., Wannammethee, S. G., and Walker, M. (1997). Body weight: implications for the prevention of coronary heart disease, stroke, and diabetes mellitus in a cohort study of middle aged men. *BMJ* **314**: 1311–1317.

SHEP Cooperative Research Group (1991). Prevention of stroke by antihypertensive drug treatment in older persons with isolated systolic hypertension: final results of the Systolic Hypertension in the Elderly Program (SHEP). *JAMA* **265**: 3255–3264.

Shepherd, J., Cobbe, S., Ford, I., *et al.* (1995). Prevention of coronary heart disease with pravastatin in men with hypercholesterolemia. *N Engl J Med* **333**: 1301–1307.

Shepherd, J., Blaw, G. J., Murphy, M. B., *et al.* (2002). Pravastatin in elderly individuals at risk of vascular disease (PROSPER): a randomized controlled trial. *Lancet* **360**: 1623–1630.

Shinton, R. and Beevers, G. (1989). Meta-analysis of relation between cigarette smoking and stroke. *BMJ* **298**: 789–794.

Shriver, M. D. (1997). Ethnic variation as a key to the biology of human disease. *Ann Intern Med* **125**: 401–403.

Sivenius, J., Tuomilehto, J., Immonen-Räihä, P., *et al.* (2004). Continuous 15-year decrease in incidence and mortality of stroke in Finland. The FINSTROKE Study. *Stroke* **35**: 420–425.

Smith, F. B., Lee, A. J., Fowkes, G. R., *et al.* (1997). Hemostatic factors as predictors of ischemic heart disease and stroke in the Edinburgh Artery Study. *Arterioscl or Thromb Vasc Biol* **17**: 3321–3325.

Snieder, H., van Doornen, L. J., and Boomsma, D. I. (1999). Dissecting the genetic architecture of lipids, lipoproteins, and apolipoproteins: lessons from twin studies. *Arterioscler Thromb Vasc Biol* **19**: 2826–2834.

Stadel, B. V. (1981). Oral contraceptives and cardiovascular disease. *N Engl J Med* **305**: 672–677.

Staessen, J. A., Fagard, R., Thijs, L., for the Systolic Hypertension in, Europe (Sys-Eur) Trial Investigators (1997). Randomised double-blind comparison of placebo and active treatment for older patients with isolated systolic hypertension. *Lancet* **350**: 757–764.

Stewart, J. A., Dundas, R., Howard, R. S., Rudd, A. G., and Wolfe, C. D. A. (1999). Ethnic differences in incidence of stroke: prospective study with stroke register. *BMJ* **318**: 967–971.

Steering Committee of the Physicians' Health Study Research Group (1989). Final report of the ongoing physicians health study. *N Engl J Med* **321**: 129–135.

Stevens, J., Cai, J., Pamuk, E. R., *et al.* (1998). The effect of age on the association between body-mass index and mortality. *N Engl J Med* **338**: 1–7.

Stolk, R. P., Pols, H. A., Lamberts, S. W., *et al.* (1997). Diabetes mellitus, impaired glucose tolerance, and hyperinsulinemia in an elderly population. The Rotterdam Study. *Am J Epidemiol* **145**: 24–32.

Szolnoki, Z., Somogyvari, F., Kondacs, A., *et al.* (2003). Evaluation of the modifying effects of unfavorable genotypes on classical clinical risk factors for ischaemic stroke. *J Neurol Neurosurg Psychiatry* **74**: 1615–1620.

Taylor, T. N., Davis, P. H., Torner, J. C., *et al.* (1996). Lifetime costs of stroke in the USA. *Stroke* **27**: 1459–1466.

Terént, A. (2003). Trends in stroke incidence and 10-year survival in Söderhamn, Sweden, 1975–2001. *Stroke* **34**: 1353–1358.

Teunissen, L. L., Rinkel, G. J., Algra, A., and van Gijn, J. (1996). Risk factors for subarachnoid hemorrhage: a systematic review. *Stroke* **27**: 544–549.

Thun, M. J., Peto, R., Lopez, A. D., *et al.* (1997). Alcohol consumption and mortality among middle aged and elderly US adults. *N Engl J Med* **337**: 1705–1714.

Toole, J. F., Malinow, M. R., Chambless, L. E., *et al.* (2004). Lowering homocysteine in patients with ischemic stroke to prevent recurrent stroke, myocardial infarction, and death: the Vitamin Intervention for Stroke Prevention (VISP) randomized controlled trial. *JAMA.* **291**: 565–575.

Trichopoulou, A., Costacou, T., Bamia, C., and Trichopoulos, D. (2003). Adherence to a Mediterranean diet and survival in a Greek population. *N Engl J Med* **348**: 2599–2608.

Truelsen, T., Mähönen, M., Tolonen, H., *et al.* (2003). Trends in stroke and coronary heart disease in the WHO MONICA Project. *Stroke* **34**: 1346–1352.

Tuomilehto, J., Rastenyte, D., Sivenius, J. *et al.* (1996). Ten-year trends in stroke incidence and mortality in the FINMONICA Stroke Study. *Stroke* **27**: 825–832.

Turpie, A. G., Gent, M., Laupacis, A., *et al.* (1993). A comparison of aspirin with placebo in patients treated with warfarin after heart-valve replacement. *N Engl J Med* **329**: 524–529.

UK Prospective Diabetes Study Group (1998). Intensive blood-glucose control with sulphonylureas or insulin compared with conventional treatment and risk complications in patients with type 2 diabetes (UKPDS 33). *Lancet* **352**: 837–853.

US Preventive Service Task Force (2003). Routine vitamin supplementation to prevent cancer and cardiovascular disease: recommendations and rationale. *Ann Intern Med* **139**: 51–55.

Viscoli, C. M., Brass, L. M., Kernan, W. N., *et al.* (2001). A clinical trial of estrogen-replacement therapy after ischemic stroke. *N Engl J Med* **345**: 1243–1249.

Vivekananthan, D. P., Penn, M. S., Sapp, S. K., Hsu, A., and Topol, E. J. (2003). Use of anti-oxidant vitamins for the prevention of cardiovascular disease: meta-analysis of randomised trials. *Lancet* **361**: 2017–2023.

Voko, Z., Hollander, M., Hofman, A., Koudstaal, P. J., and Breteler, M. M. (2003). Dietary antioxidants and the risk of ischemic stroke: the Rotterdam Study. *Neurology* **61**: 1273–1275.

Wald, D. S., Law, M., and Morris, J. K. (2002). Homocysteine and cardiovascular disease: evidence on causality from a meta-analysis. *BMJ* **325**: 1202–1208.

Wang, T. J., Massaro, J. M., Levy, D., *et al.* (2003). A risk score for predicting stroke or death in individuals with new-onset atrial fibrillation in the community: the Framingham Heart Study. *JAMA* **290**: 1049–1056.

Wannamethee, S. G. and Sharper, A. G. (1992). Physical activity and stroke in British middle aged men. *BMJ* **304**: 597–601.

(1996). Patterns of alcohol intake and risk of stroke in middle-aged British men. *Stroke* **27**: 1033–1039.

Wannamethee, S. G., Shaper, A. G., Whincup, P. H., and Walker, M. (1995). Smoking cessation and the risk of stroke in middle-aged men. *JAMA* **274**: 155–160.

Wannamethee, S. G., Perry, I. J., and Shaper, A. G. (1999). Nonfasting serum glucose and insulin concentrations and the risk of stroke. *Stroke* **30**: 1780–1786.

Wannamethee, S. G., Sharper, A. G., and Ebrahim, S. (2000). HDL-cholesterol, total cholesterol, and the risk of stroke in middle-aged British men. *Stroke* **31**: 1882–1888.

Wassertheil-Smoller, S., Fann, C., Allman, R. M., for the SHEP Cooperative Research Group (2000). Relation of low body mass to death and stroke in the Systolic Hypertensive in the Elderly Program. *Arch Intern Med* **160**: 494–500.

Wassertheil-Smoller, S., Hendrix, S. L., Limacher, M., for the WHI Investigators (2003). Effect of estrogen plus progestin on stroke in postmenopausal women: the Women's Health Initiative – a randomized trial. *JAMA* **289**: 2673–2684.

Wattigney, W. A., Mensah, G. A., and Croft, J. B. (2003). Increasing trends in hospitalization for atrial fibrillation in the USA, 1985 through 1999: implications for primary prevention. *Circulation* **108**: 711–716.

Weverling-Rijnsburger, A. W., Jonkers, I. J., van Exel, E., Gussekloo, J., and Westendorp, R. G. (2003). High-density vs. low-density lipoprotein cholesterol as the risk factor for coronary artery disease and stroke in old age. *Arch Intern Med* **163**: 1549–1554.

Whisnant, J. P. (1997). Modeling of risk factors for ischemic stroke. The Willis Lecture. *Stroke* **28**: 1839–1843.

White, R. H., McBurnie, M. A., Manolio, T., *et al.* (1999). Oral anticoagulation in patients with atrial fibrillation: adherence with guidelines in an elderly cohort. *Am J Med* **106**: 165–171.

WHO Collaborative Study of Cardiovascular Disease and Steroid Hormone Contraception (1996a). Ischaemic stroke and combined oral contraceptives: results of an international, multicentre, case–control study. *Lancet* **348**: 498–505.

(1996b). Haemorrhagic stroke, overall stroke risk, and combined oral contraceptives: results of an international, multicentre, case–control study. *Lancet* **348**: 505–510.

WHO (2003a). *The World Health Report 2003*. Geneva: WHO.

(2003b). *MONICA Monograph and Multimedia Sourcebook*. http://www.ktl.fi/monica/.

(2003c). *WHO Mortality Database*. www3.WHO.int/whosis.

Wilhelmsen, L., Svärdsudd, K., Korsan-Bengtsen, K., *et al.* (1984). Fibrinogen as a risk factor for stroke and myocardial infarction. *N Engl J Med* **311**: 501–505.

Willett, W. C. and Stampfer, M. J. (2001). Clinical practice. What vitamins should I be taking, doctor? *N Engl J Med* **345**: 1819–1824.

Wilsom, P. W. F., Garrison, R. J., and Castelli, W. P. (1985). Postmenopausal estrogen use, cigarette smoking, and cardiovascular mortality in women over 50: the Framingham Study. *N Engl J Med* **313**: 1038–1043.

Wolf, P. A. (1993). Lewis A. Conner Lecture. Contributions of epidemiology to the prevention of stroke. *Circulation* **88**: 2471–2478.

Wolf, P. A. and D'Agostino, R. B. (1998). Epidemiology of stroke. In *Stroke: Pathophysiology, Diagnosis and Management*, ed. H. J. M. Barnett, J. P. Mohr, B. M. Stein, and F. M. Yatsu, 3rd edn, New York: Churchill Livingstone, pp. 3–28.

Wolf, P. A., Dawber, T. R., Thomas, H. E., Jr., and Kannel, W. B. (1978). Epidemiologic assessment of chronic atrial fibrillation and risk of stroke: the Framingham study. *Neurology* **28**: 973–977.

Wolf, P. A., Kannel, W. B., and Verter, J. (1983). Current status of risk factors for stroke. *Neurol Clin* **1**: 317–343.

Wolf, P. A., Clagett, G. P., Easton, J. D., *et al.* (1999). Preventing ischemic stroke in patients with prior stroke and transient ischemic attack: a statement for healthcare professionals from the Stroke Council of the American Heart Association. *Stroke* **30**: 1991–1994.

Wolfe, C. D. A., Rudd, A. G., Howard. R, *et al.* (2002). Incidence and case fatality rates of stroke subtypes in a multiethnic population: the South London Stroke Register. *J Neurol Neurosurg Psychiatry* **72**: 211–216.

Wyse, D. G., Waldo, A. L., DiMarco, J. P., *et al.* (2002). A comparison of rate control and rhythm control in patients with atrial fibrillation. *N Engl J Med* **347**: 1825–1833.

Yusuf, S., Sleight, P., Pogue, J., *et al.* (2000a). Effects of an angiotensin-converting-enzyme inhibitor, ramipril, on cardiovascular events in high risk patients. The Heart Outcomes Prevention Evaluation Study Investigators. *N Engl J Med* **342**: 145–153.

Yusuf, S., Dagenais, G., Pogue, J., Bosch, J., and Sleight, P. (2000b). Vitamin E supplementation and cardiovascular events in high-risk patients. The Heart Outcomes Prevention Evaluation Study Investigators. *N Engl J Med* **342**: 154–160.

2

Principles of recovery after stroke

Bruce H. Dobkin and Thomas S. Carmichael

University of California Los Angeles School of Medicine, Los Angeles, CA, USA

Introduction

This chapter introduces concepts about the interacting cascades of ischemia-induced, activity-dependent, and practice- and learning-driven principles that permit gains or prevent gains early and late after stroke. Subsequent chapters will look more specifically at nervous system adaptations and outcomes associated with mechanisms of neuroplasticity and specific biological and training-related interventions. The biological mechanisms and therapeutic applications of training-induced plasticity for motor control and cognitive functions have been more fully reviewed across neurological diseases in other texts (Dobkin, 2003). We illustrate some of these principles by examining gains in the motor control for walking in hemiparetic patients and by describing some of the substrates of biological changes that may contribute to those gains.

Recovery: restitution, substitution, or compensation?

Patients tend to improve over time after an acute stroke, in a general relationship to a few defined impairment groups (Table 2.1). Gains occur in motor impairments, with the largest increases in strength occurring in patients who are not initially paralyzed (Hendricks et al., 2002). Six months after a non-hemorrhagic stroke, approximately half of patients have no significant motor impairment. For motor-related abilities, functional gains tend to follow the level of recovery of selective movement skills. The level of motor control for walking, which perhaps best correlates with manual muscle testing of lower extremity strength, runs in parallel with the level of independence for walking (Jorgensen et al., 1995), but of course it is not the only impairment that can compromise ambulation. Any analysis is limited by how we measure strength and walking skills. Are we measuring selective strength of individual muscle groups? Will the scale use dynamometry or a non-parametric scale such as the British Medical Council scale, with its

Recovery after Stroke, ed. Michael P. Barnes, Bruce H. Dobkin and Julien Bogousslavsky. Published by Cambridge University Press. © Cambridge University Press 2005.

Table 2.1 Recovery of walking by impairment group

Impairment group	Onset (%)	Recovery (%) at month		
		1	3	6
Motor	18	50	75	85
Sensorimotor	10	48	72	72
Motor, hemianopsia	7	28	68	75
Sensorimotor, hemianopsia	3	16	33	38

From: Kaplan–Meier graphs in Patel *et al.*, 2000.

standard five grades? Can we agree that the three-step scale of the Barthel Index or the seven-step scale of the Functional Independence Measure adequately cover the meaning of recovery, or should walking speed over 50 feet (15 m) and walking distance in six minutes, or symmetries of stance and swing times, kinematics, ground reaction forces, and the pattern of muscle activations be included to better ascertain what we mean by recovery? Do assessment procedures reflect changes in the range of adaptive strategies that patients may incorporate over time? Principles of recovery may be subsumed within three general changes within the sensorimotor networks (Dobkin, 2003): restitution, substitution, and compensation.

Restitution

Restitution is relatively independent of external variables such as physical and cognitive stimulation. Restitution includes the biochemical and gene-induced events that take a turn for the better in restoring the functionality of neural tissue, such as reduction of edema, absorption of heme, restoration of ionic currents, and restoration of axonal transport.

Substitution — training brain to make new nerves

Substitution depends on external stimuli such as practice with the affected hemiparetic arm or leg during rehabilitation. The adaptations may depend more heavily on cognitive, visual, and proprioceptive networks that aid learning and drive activity-dependent plasticity. The cognitive networks may include those for conscious control of movement and for attention, motivation, and goal-setting. A shift to greater reliance on a new control strategy may be necessary. Substitution includes the functional adaptations of diminished, but partially restored, neural networks that compensate for components lost or disrupted by the injury. Substitution may proceed through partially spared neural pathways, reorganizational plasticity in cortical representations for movements, changes in activity in components of a motor network, such as central pattern generators for walking, and other biological mechanisms associated with learning and changes in synaptic efficacy. Substitution may add a cost to the mental or physical energy needed to carry out a relearned motor skill. For example, automaticity for walking often suffers. Many patients cannot walk and talk, or otherwise divide their attention, when simply stepping from one place to another. Most patients walk slower to lessen the energy cost of walking with a paretic trunk and leg. Such cognitive and physical costs tend not to be included in functional assessments (Mulder *et al.*, 2002). Some investigators call this the compensatory cost, but we will use the term compensation in a more restricted way.

Compensation —changing goals, help pt, change home

Compensation aims to improve the mismatch between a patient's impaired skills and the demands of the patient or the environment. This approach for rehabilitation is the heart of many interventions for disabilities. Domains of compensation for locomotion may include several aspects.

1. Remediation: increase the time, effort, or amount of training to maintain or regain basic aspects of an affected skill.
2. Behavioral substitution: use a latent skill already in the patient's repertoire or develop a new skill that replaces the defective one. An assistive device such as an ankle–foot orthosis serves as a partial substitute for the biomechanical and physiological control of the ankle and knee.
3. Accommodation: adjust intentions or select new goals. Walking may not be feasible, so training in wheelchair skills becomes more important for daily activities.
4. Assimilation: adjust the expectations of others or modify the environment.

Anatomic nodes for reorganization

The distributed systems for motor control in humans are flexible and adaptable. Functional neuroimaging may reveal changes in the activity of these functional nodes of networks over the process of gains in function (see Chs. 4 and 5). Brain injury from stroke alters the orchestration of the components of this motor learning network, but the system may be driven by restitutive and substitutive biological mechanisms to reconstitute functionally useful upper and lower extremity movements. The most formidable tools for neurological rehabilitation draw upon the activity-dependent plasticity of the sensorimotor regions of the central nervous system (CNS). By placing recent studies of motor control into perspective, the clinician can consider techniques to enhance behavioral outcomes in patients with stroke.

The neurons of the primary motor cortex, M1, dynamically represent multijoint movements and include overlapping representations for the muscles of the lower extremity (Dobkin, 2000a; Graziano *et al.*, 2002), just as nearby regions of M1 do for the control of the fingers, wrist, elbow, and shoulder (Nudo *et al.*, 1996). New physiologic relationships emerge as a consequence of the properties of neurons and their synapses from intrinsic drives during development and then from the drives associated with learning new skills, abilities, and sensory discriminations (Buonomano and Merzenich, 1998). This activity-dependent neuroplasticity is the essence of the CNS's learning machine. Horizontal and vertical corticocortical and intracortical dendritic connections (Donoghue, 1997) allow for rapidly and slowly induced synaptic strengthening or weakening among the cortical ensembles. Neurotransmitters and neuromodulators help to bind these use-dependent integrations.

M1 also contains the giant pyramidal cells of Betz, which account for no more than 50,000 of the several million pyramidal neurons in each precentral gyrus. About 75% supply the leg (Schiebel *et al.*, 1977). The Betz cells appear to be important innervators of the large, antigravity muscles for the back and legs. They phasically inhibit extension and facilitate flexion, which may be especially important for triggering motor activity for walking. Consistent with this tendency, pyramidal tract lesions tend to allow an increase in extension over flexion in the leg.

Movements depend upon multiple regions of the CNS. Only 46% of the axons within the corticospinal tract derive from M1 (Cheney *et al.*, 2000). Other components include portions of S1, as well as axons from the supplementary motor cortex (SMA), and premotor and cingulate motor cortices. Each facilitates aspects of movement. For example, the ventral premotor cortex responds to graspable items by shaping the hand. The corticospinal tract is necessary for altering the amplitude of the H-reflex of the soleus muscle with operant conditioning, suggesting that even stretch reflexes can be modulated by voluntary control (Chen *et al.*, 2002). In addition, frontal and parietal cortices for cognitive and sensory integration are related to motor planning and goals. Goal-oriented movement may be especially important during rehabilitation in order to bind the flexible motor learning capabilities of these regions most effectively.

Subcortical and brainstem regions play important roles for walking and in training-induced plasticity (Dobkin, 1998, 2003). Individual channels of the thalamocortical projections control separate functional units of motor cortex, which, in turn, independently influence the basal ganglia, cerebellum, and other subcortical motor nuclei. These parallel systems may include a partially reiterative capacity to allow some sparing or compensation after a sensorimotor network injury. Midbrain and pontine locomotor regions are important for the initiation of automatic stepping. The cerebellum also plays a major role in locomotion. Purkinje cells are rhythmically active throughout the step cycle (Orlovsky *et al.*, 1999). Neurons of the fastigial and interpositus nuclei burst primarily during the flexor phase of stepping. The cerebellum may contribute more to the ongoing modification of a motor performance than to specific mechanisms of learning a skill (Seidler *et al.*, 2002). Its hemispheres receive inputs from alpha and gamma motor neurons and Ia interneurons, as well as from segmental dorsal root afferents. This input is copied not only to the cerebellum but also to corticomotor neurons and to brainstem locomotor regions. During walking, the neurons of the dorsal spinocerebellar tract in the dorsolateral funiculus of the lumbar cord fire in relation to both Ia and Ib afferent activity (Orlovsky *et al.*, 1999). This activity provides the cerebellum with detailed information about the performance of leg movements. Ventral spinocerebellar neurons project to the cerebellar cortex from the contralateral lateral funiculus and burst during locomotion, reflecting activity in spinal central pattern generators. These spinal oscillating circuits are another flexible and simplifying organization for stepping. In the presence of afferent input, even after spinal transection, cats and rats can be trained on a moving treadmill belt to step with their hindlimbs (Belanger *et al.*, 1996; Edgerton *et al.*, 2001). The training is task specific; practice standing inhibits subsequent treadmill stepping and raises levels of the enzyme glutamic acid decarboxylase (involved in synthesis of the inhibitory gamma-aminobutyric acid [GABA]) and of glycine. Locomotor training reduces inhibitory neurotransmitters toward normal control levels (Tillakaratne *et al.*, 2002).

Training that drives the sensorimotor interactions of residual networks may enable these circuits to regain control of reaching, grasping, and ambulation.

Biological principles

Table 2.2 lists some of the potential biological mechanisms that may lead to spontaneous and activity-dependent gains after a stroke. We examine several mechanisms that may become especially relevant to infarction in human subjects. A more comprehensive view is found in Ch. 3.

Stroke produces substantial changes in neuronal circuits adjacent or connected to the infarct. These changes include dendritic and axonal sprouting and stem cell or neuronal precursor responses. Dendritic spines and sprouts grow with normal learning and both in homologous contralesional and ipsilesional cortex in association with limb use in rodents (Schallert *et al.*, 2000; Bury and Jones, 2002). Axonal sprouting after stroke occurs in both local and long-distance connections and produces novel projection patterns in the brain. The stem cell or neuronal precursor response results in proliferation, migration, and differentiation of new neurons into areas of damage adjacent to the stroke. Through these processes, stroke remodels adjacent brain and creates entirely new systems of connections.

Table 2.2 Potential intrinsic biological mechanisms to lessen impairments and disabilities

---

Plasticity Mechanisms

Network
1. Recovery of neuronal excitability: resolve cell and axon ionic dysequilibrium; reverse edema, resorb blood; reverse transsynaptic diaschisis
2. Activity in partially spared pathways
3. Representational plasticity within neuronal assemblies
4. Recruit a parallel network not ordinarily activitated by a task (e.g. unaffected hemisphere or ipsilesional prefrontal cortex)
5. Engage a subcomponent of a distributed network (e.g. a pattern generator for stepping)
6. Modulation of excitability by neurotransmitters (e.g. serotonin, dopamine)

Pre/Postsynaptic
1. Modulate neuronal intracellular signaling for trophic functions (e.g. neurotrophic factors, protein kinases)
2. Alter synaptic plasticity: modulate basal synaptic transmission; neurotransmitter and peptide modulators alter excitability; denervation hypersensitivity of postsynaptic receptors; regulation of number or types of receptor (e.g., AMPA receptors); activity-dependent unmasking of synaptic connections; experience-dependent learning (e.g. long-term potentiation); dendritic sprouting onto denuded receptors of nearby neurons
3. Axonal and dendritic collateral sprouting from uninjured neurons
4. Axonal regeneration: gene expression for remodeling proteins; modulation by neurotrophic factors; actions of chemoattractants and inhibitors in the milieu
5. Remyelination
6. Reverse conduction block; ion channel changes on axons
7. Neurogenesis

Adapted with permission from B. Dobkin, *The Clinical Science of Neurological Rehabilitation*, Oxford University Press, 2003.

Axonal sprouting

Stroke induces axonal sprouting in local intracortical connections. The best example of this local axonal sprouting is within the rat somatosensory cortex. Focal stroke in the somatosensory cortex produces axonal sprouting in neurons adjacent to the infarct. These neurons are located in areas of partial damage and give rise to substantial and novel intracortical projections within undamaged regions of the somatosensory cortex (Carmichael *et al.*, 2001). In fact, when the connections of the rat somatosensory cortex are compared in stroke and control conditions, stroke induces a wholesale remapping of the adjacent body map. In this remapped area, stroke produces sprouting in a numerically larger pattern of connections than is present in the somatosensory map before the stroke.

Ischemic lesions also induce long-distance axonal sprouting, such as in the callosal connections between cortical hemispheres and in the crossed corticostriatal projection. The neurons that give rise to this long-distance axonal sprouting lie in the hemisphere opposite the lesion, in the corresponding cortical region (the homotypic cortex). From a purely phenomenological perspective, long-distance axonal sprouting after ischemic lesions is a remarkable process for the adult brain. Sprouting axons establish new patterns of connections between hemispheres to peri-infarct cortex and to the striatum below the lesion (Carmichael and Chesselet, 2002). This new projection pattern is formed with areas of partial damage or deafferentation. At the ultrastructural level in the rodent brain, the sprouting in the corticostriatal system after ischemic lesions results in overall preservation in synapses after stroke compared with those in the control (Uryu *et al.*, 2001). The observations of local and long-distance axonal sprouting show that focal cortical ischemia sets off a process that results in partial reinnervation of damaged or deafferented brain regions. Axonal sprouting after a stroke can be followed not only through neuroanatomical mapping, as above, but also through growth cone protein expression. The data show that such axonal sprouting has a time course and pharmacological responsiveness that correlate with functional recovery (Stroemer *et al.*, 1998).

Axonal sprouting after stroke represents a phenotypic change for an adult cortical neuron. Stroke induces normally quiescent cortical neurons to reexpress growth cone proteins, elongate axons, and synapse with new areas in the CNS. Axonal outgrowth and synaptogenesis is a common function of the developing CNS but has been described in only a few areas in the adult CNS, mainly within the hippocampus. In contrast, the axonal sprouting after a stroke occurs simultaneously at multiple, distant sites in the brain and between areas that retain few sprouting-related proteins compared with levels during development. Therefore, ischemic lesions trigger signals that induce profound morphological changes within relatively fixed local and distant cortical networks. Ischemic lesions produce a specific signal that induces axonal sprouting. This was established in a model of differential axonal sprouting after a cortical lesion in the adult rat. As noted, ischemic cortical lesions induce axonal sprouting in projections from the cortical site opposite the lesion to the cortex adjacent to the lesion, and to the striatum below the lesion. In contrast, aspiration lesions that are the same size and in the same location as the ischemic lesions do not induce axonal sprouting (Napieralski *et al.*, 1996; Carmichael and Chesselet, 2002). The aspiration and ischemic cortical lesions share the same degree of tissue damage and axotomy. This means that a signal for axonal sprouting must be specific to focal ischemia and must be distinct from just axotomy.

Ischemic cortical lesions induce a pattern of spontaneous neuronal bursting in peri-lesion cortex and contralateral cortex that serves as a signal for axonal sprouting (Carmichael and Chesselet, 2002). After ischemic lesions, spontaneous bursting of cortical neurons is induced in two distinct patterns in the sites of axonal sprouting. First, in peri-lesion cortex on day one after the lesion, slow field waves and synchronous neuronal bursting occurs with a frequency of 1 Hz. Next in peri-lesion cortex and contralateral homotypic cortex at days two to four after the lesion, a pattern of extracellular field waves and correlated neuronal firing occurs at a slower rate, 0.1–0.4 Hz. This pattern of rhythmic neuronal activity induces axonal sprouting: it is not present in the similarly sized aspiration lesions, which do not induce axonal sprouting, and blockade of this activity pattern prevents post-ischemic axonal sprouting.

The finding of a synchronous electrical activity signal for post-ischemic axonal sprouting has three important implications. First, the pattern of neuronal activity that induces axonal sprouting in experimental animals is identical in location and frequency to that commonly seen in humans after stroke or other brain lesions. In patients, delta activity, maximal at 1 Hz, is often recognized after stroke. This electrical activity may be part of a signal for post-stroke plasticity, or axonal sprouting, in the human brain. Second, the pattern of electrical activity that induces axonal sprouting after ischemic lesions in the adult closely resembles that seen in the developing brain when it is initially sprouting axonal connections. In many different regions in the CNS, spontaneous slow-wave activity and neuronal bursting occur during periods of axonal pathfinding and synaptogenesis (Feller, 1999). In the developing cortex, the frequency and pattern of this bursting activity closely resembles that seen in the adult cortex during post-ischemic axonal sprouting (Napieralski *et al.*, 1996; Carmichael and Chesselet, 2002). This suggests that the adult brain reactivates a developmental electrical rhythm when it engages axonal sprouting programs after ischemia. Third, as noted, axonal sprouting after stroke appears to play a role in functional recovery. Many neuroprotective strategies have, as a byproduct, a direct effect on neuronal activity, such as use of glutamate antagonists, GABA agonists, and sodium channel blockers. Drug interventions may directly impact spontaneous patterns of neuronal activity after stroke. It will be important to ensure that neuroprotective strategies that alter neuronal activity do not reduce infarct size at the cost of limiting the signals that may mediate functional recovery.

Stem cell response

In addition to axonal sprouting, stroke also induces a stem cell or neuronal precursor response. Both global and focal ischemia cause proliferation, neuronal differentiation, and migration of precursor cell populations in the areas of naturally occurring stem cells in the adult brain: the subgranular zone in the hippocampus and the subventricular zone in the cerebral hemisphere. In this stem cell response, the infarct signals these two stem cell zones, and cell proliferation occurs within 7–10 days after stroke (Arvidsson *et al.*, 2002). Stem cells then express glial- and neuronal-specific proteins. Many newly born neurons migrate to areas of damage and further express cytoskeletal- and transmitter-specific markers of the appropriate local neuronal population. This stem cell response occurs within endogenous stem or precursor populations, as opposed to transplanted stem cells, and thus represents a naturally occurring mechanism of cell replacement after stroke. Emerging data suggest that the hypoxic insult in stroke may uniquely activate trophic factor and nitric oxide signaling systems that lead to neurogenesis (Jin *et al.*, 2002). The magnitude of the stem cell response has not been determined. Does the stem cell response after stroke resupply a significant number of neurons adjacent to the stroke? What is a significant number? Unlike axonal sprouting, there has been no correlation between the post-stroke stem cell response and functional outcome. Does the stem cell response produce neurons that establish connections and participate in local brain function? One model of ischemia has demonstrated regenerated neurons that integrate into hippocampal circuits (Nakatomi *et al.*, 2002). In other models of CNS injury, apoptotic cell death in the cortex induces neuronal precursors to migrate to the area of damage, differentiate into neurons, and project to distant brain areas (Magavi *et al.*, 2000).

If the process of neurogenesis *and* reconnection occurs in stroke, it may provide the framework for neural recovery. Behavioral recovery may not require the reconstitution of an entire neural network. The restoration of a small descending input may provide the modulatory tone necessary for central pattern generators to assume a degree of behavioral control (Dobkin, 2000b). Similarly, the reconnection of a small projection between regions in the cerebral hemisphere may be enough to restore a modulatory influence from one region to another that would facilitate the normal function of the damaged region.

To move the field of neural repair toward a more translational setting, animal models that have been used for the study of ischemic cell death will likely need to be altered. Animal models of stroke involve large infarcts compared with those occurring in humans. The two principal models in the stroke field are the intraluminal suture occlusion of the middle cerebral artery and the distal occlusion of the middle cerebral artery through craniotomy. These techniques produce infarction of 10–70% of the forebrain or ipsilateral cortex, sparing a rim of parietal cortex, frontal pole, cingulate cortex, and occipital cortex. Using estimates of human intracranial volume from computed tomography, typical clinical strokes represent 2–4% of intracranial volumes in inpatient neuroprotective studies (Saver *et al.*, 1999) and 0.88–1.2% in outpatient studies (Kissela *et al.*, 2001). The large infarcts in rats and mice are not only less clinically relevant but, in addition, the infarcts spare little cortical tissue to analyze for axonal sprouting and the stem cell response. In addition to a size difference between human and animal models, an important difference in location exists. Animal models of focal stroke produce damage or injury directly within or very closely adjacent to the subventricular zone or sub-granular zone. Stem cell zones are directly involved in the ischemic process and newly born neurons need only migrate a very short distance to the region of damage. Stroke in patients is not often located within or adjacent to these sites. Therefore, it is unclear if a stem cell response will occur in the type and location of infarcts corresponding to human stroke. Finally, animal models of experimental stroke must include a component of reperfusion. Reperfusion occurs in a moderate proportion of human strokes spontaneously and is an outcome measure of fibrinolysis and angioplasty strategies for acute artery thrombosis. Reperfusion also causes a qualitatively different type of cellular injury, notably apoptotic damage (Lipton and Nicotera, 1998). Apoptosis is a potent stimulator of the stem cell response. Therefore, animal models that are relevant to the study of neural repair after stroke ought to mimic human stroke more closely by being smaller, more distant to the germinal zones, and containing a component of reperfusion injury.

Practice and reinforcement

Although some concern about early overuse after cerebral ischemia in rodents has been raised by experimental models (Bland *et al.*, 2000), the degree of use does not have a realistic parallel in the therapy of patients after stroke. Studies in rodents reveal the potential biological effects of such practice. Repetitive, rewarded practice enhances long-term potentiation at many levels of the CNS for memory. Such practice also increases production of neurotransmitters, such as acetylcholine and serotonin, increases synthesis of neurotrophins, such as brain-derived neurotrophic factor and neurotrophin-3, and may lead to the proliferation and greater survival of hippocampal progenitor cells that may be important for new learning and memory (van Praag *et al.*, 1999).

Motor learning is a set of processes for acquiring the capability to produce skilful actions or habitual behaviors via mechanisms of procedural memory. These processes occur within neurons and their synaptic connections and within neural networks, which can be imaged. The representation of goal-directed movements involves discrete regions of the frontal and parietal cortex and striatum. Motor learning occurs as a direct result of experience or practice (i.e. activity-dependent plasticity), which can be affected by problems such as mood, motivation, and fatigue, and by drugs that act on ion fluxes, neurotransmitters, neuromodulators, and gene expression.

One of the most vexing problems for understanding motor control arises from the myriad biomechanical degrees of freedom that must be coordinated by the nervous system to reach and grasp an item, walk, or manage other skills. Task-relevant movement parameters such as force, speed, and direction can vary considerably, for example from one step during walking to the next. Movements are not stereotyped. After a brain injury, the system is perturbed such that fewer options may be available. Substitution or compensation with rehabilitation will have to take into consideration the remaining variability, along with synergies appropriate for a task and task goals. As noted earlier, some systems, such as clinical practice guidelines for stepping, may simplify the necessary computations. Other CNS strategies include the finding that the neural representations of different mechanical contexts, such as the cells in M1 that fire whether a single-joint or multijoint load is required for a movement, provide a basis for how complex motor skills can be learned from simpler ones (Gribble and Scott, 2002). The principle of optimal feedback control has been proposed to account for the noise and variability that alter movements (Todorov and Jordan, 2002). For each motor task, the CNS selects its optimal law of feedback control. This law estimates the state of the CNS and musculoskeletal system (positions, velocities, and forces) based on sensory feedback, efference copy of prior signals, and forward internal models of the limb and somehow computes a movement driven by the goal of the action (Scott, 2002).

Learning a skill, then, fundamentally requires feedback. Particular styles of feedback (Table 2.3) may be better than others when learning to engage substitutive or compensatory mechanisms to improve or reintroduce a skill, depending on the location of the lesion and the residual cerebral substrates for learning. By defining the type of feedback used with a particular patient, the therapist can later switch to another form to determine what works best for learning a skill.

What styles of practice are best for an individual patient? The usual locomotor goal, for example, is to improve performance in the safety and efficiency of the gait pattern, manifested by independence from the need for help from others, improving walking speed, and greater distances walked. Advanced practice includes walking under difficult circumstances, such as on uneven ground or in the community. Styles of practice include the following:

- blocked practice: all practice trials done consecutively
- variable or random practice: practice on one task is interrupted by practice at other tasks, producing contextual interference

Table 2.3 Types of augmented feedback

Concurrent: provide during the movement	Terminal: provide after the movement
Immediate: provide immediately after the relevant action (errorless practice)	Delayed: provide some time after the relevant action
Verbal: spoken or verbalizable form	Non-verbal: non-verbalizable form
Accumulated: feedback represents a compilation of past performance	Distinct: feedback addresses each separate performance
Knowledge of results: verbal or verbalizable postmovement information about the outcome of a movement (correct/incorrect, short/long)	Knowledge of performance: verbal or verbalizable postmovement information about the nature of the pattern of movement (videotape replay, kinematics, forces)

- massed practice: continuous or with little rest
- distributed practice: more rest compared to practice time
- mental rehearsal: imagine doing a task
- virtual reality: practice in a virtual environment.

Constant practice will likely enhance performance when exact reproduction of the skilled movement and its parameters (speed of movement or distance reached or stride taken) are specified. Variable blocked practice aids learning the same motor program and variable random practice enhances learning different programs. Rehabilitation training on a random schedule, rather than with continuous repetition, is generally more effective for long-term retention of functional, skilled movements. Motor learning may not, however, be as evident within a treatment session during acquisition of the skill. Retention will be more apparent in later sessions when the therapist looks for whether the skill can be recalled and replicated. Reinforcement by knowledge of results or of performance may be phased out over the time of practice by going from 100% feedback to 50% to 25% and then no feedback. Learned skills using any of these practice and reinforcement paradigms may not generalize to another setting or to a related set of skills that are not specifically practiced.

Studies in healthy and hemiparetic subjects suggest that task-oriented or task-specific practice is best for skills learning, especially when performed within a massed or contextual interference paradigm. Most studies of constraint-induced movement therapy involve upper extremity tasks (van der Lee *et al.*, 1999; Liepert *et al.*, 2000) and massed practice of a variety of movement skills. The unaffected limb is restricted, permitting massed practice. Shaping, in which a partial movement is acquired for a particular skill before the whole limb movement can be performed, has been recommended by Taub (Taub and Wolf, 1997; Taub *et al.*, 2002), but the evidence for the practice of part of a task over whole task actions, even if assisted by the therapist, is unproven.

Rehabilitation approaches often emphasize compensatory strategies for impairments and disabilities. Patients are trained to make a greater effort to employ a defective skill, substitute a latent skill, learn a new way to accomplish a goal or alter the environment to make a task easier for them, or change their expectations about performing a particular task. Most compensatory approaches require learning and gains may be reflected in experience-dependent plasticity.

The optimal duration and intensity of training is uncertain for human rehabilitation strategies. More intensive, task-oriented practice seems to enhance learning and performance (Kwakkel *et al.*, 1999; Walker *et al.*, 1999). Most patients, however, receive no more than a few months of formal inpatient and outpatient retraining. *Intensive rehabilitation* often amounts to less than 20 hours of engagement in physical, occupational, or speech therapy. Each therapist works at many tasks for two to four weeks of inpatient care and two to four months of outpatient care. This modest amount of practice may be far less than what is needed to, say, regain the ability to walk at a speed that permits community activities or to improve word-finding skills (Nugent *et al.*, 1994; Kwakkel *et al.*, 1997; Dobkin, 1999; Pulvermuller *et al.*, 2001).

Task-oriented practice for walking

The brief review of functional anatomy related to walking suggests that ensembles in M1 and other components of the motor system will encode sensorimotor contingencies as a task is learned. Changes occur in the temporal patterns of firing, in firing rates, and for more correlated firing. The CNS makes flexible associations with sensory stimuli for motor learning. Rehabilitation interventions have been designed around these experience-dependent neural systems.

Task-oriented practice, as opposed to more traditional physical therapies such as the Bobath technique, encourages strategies for walking rather than strategies that reflect concern primarily for spasticity, standing balance, and trunk control, which may take precedence over the action of walking. The techniques of practice, styles of reinforcement for learning, and strengthening and conditioning exercises are components of a task-oriented approach.

Task-oriented therapy for walking with practice at high intensity can be carried out with body-weight-supported treadmill training (BWSTT) in patients who walk cannot walk or who walk with a poor pattern or very slowly (Hesse *et al.*, 1995b; Wernig *et al.*, 1995; Visintin *et al.*, 1998; Sullivan *et al.*, 2002), as well as by a variety of locomotor tasks in patients who have at least fair ability to ambulate

(Dean *et al.*, 2000). Stepping is encouraged over the practice of standing balance as a prerequisite for walking.

BWSTT allows subjects to stand erect without excessive knee flexion so that the therapists can use manual and verbal cures to optimize the kinematics, kinetics, and temporal features of the gait cycle. The subject wears a climbing harness attached to an overhead lift, which preferably allows some vertical displacement during walking. Up to 40% of the subject's body weight is lifted, depending on the need. The therapists aim to allow greater weight bearing and faster treadmill speeds as subjects progress. Treadmill training engrains greater symmetries of the stand and swing phases of gait (Hassid *et al.*, 1997; Hesse *et al.*, 1999). Training at faster speeds, from 1.8 to 2.5 mph (2.9–4.0 km/h), appears to offer the most useful signals recognized by the spinal cord in subjects with complete and incomplete spinal cord injuries and for patients with hemiparetic stroke. Overground training rarely reaches speeds greater than 1 mph (1.6 km/h) in hemiparetic subjects, so treadmill training with or without body weight support allows practice at more normal walking speeds (2.5–3.5 mph [4.0–5.6 km/h]). This training at faster walking speeds equates to more steps per session and to neural accommodations to stepping that are more like the rhythmic sensory input associated with walking in healthy subjects. Faster overground walking velocities accompanies training at faster training speeds (Pohl *et al.*, 2002; Sullivan *et al.*, 2002).

Quasi-experimental trials in patients with stroke (Hesse *et al.*, 1995a) reveal functional ambulatory gains in non-walkers who receive the treadmill training, even at rather slow treadmill walking speeds. Randomized trials of patients with stroke tend not to show gains compared with more conventional treatments with bracing (Kosak and Reding, 2000) or a motor relearning program (Nilsson *et al.*, 2002), perhaps because the treadmill training speeds were generally less than 1 mph (1.6 km/h). A large randomized clinical of subjects who were, on average, two months after their stroke found that patients who received BWSTT walked significantly, if modestly, better than those given treadmill training without body weight support. (Visintin *et al.*, 1998).Treadmill training in patients with chronic hemiparetic stroke may also have a task-specific effect on increasing strength (Smith *et al.*, 1999) in muscles used for walking and on improving endurance (Macko *et al.*, 2001) for walking.

Training-induced plasticity in M1S1 for the lower extremity and SMA were found in patients with hemiparetic stroke who had repeated bouts of 12 sessions of BWSTT (Sullivan *et al.*, 2001). The changes were, in part, related to the location of the infarction. In general, diffuse bilateral activations occurred when subjects dorsiflexed the affected foot during a functional magnetic resonance imaging study before training. After training, the activations became more localized to the contralateral M1S1 and SMA, associated with an increase in the amplitude of the electromyograph trace from the tibialis anterior muscle and overground walking speeds that increased 20%–40%. Another bout of 12 sessions in these rather functional subjects led to further lateralization of the activation and a less-diffuse activation, with higher intensity within M1S1. Walking speed continued to increase into the range of normal and the amplitude of the ankle dorsiflexor muscle rose yet more, consistent with improving activity-dependent motor control. These findings suggest that functional imaging may be used as a physiologic marker for the efficacy of a rehabilitation intervention (Dobkin et al., 2004; Dobkin and Sullivan, 2001). They also reveal close parallels between changes in representational activity after stroke during the practice of an upper extremity task (Carey et al., 2002).

Biomechanical assists (Hesse et al., 2001) and robotic devices (Colombo et al., 2000) may enable similar or greater gains in walking performance and motor relearning, but no trials have yet been completed. Locomotor training with BWSTT has also been combined with functional electrical stimulation in patients with hemiparesis (Hesse et al., 1995b; Daly et al., 2001).

Strengthening and conditioning

Muscle weakness following a stroke is primarily caused by a decrement or loss of spinal motoneuron drive by the cortex and brainstem. Fewer motor units are recruited and firing rates are diminished. Atrophy and fiber type changes in muscle and alterations in connective tissue have also been described, especially in patients with chronic paresis (Ryan et al., 2002). Consequently, resistance exercises may be prescribed for selective muscle strengthening, which can increase the force output across a joint. Weakness associated with a pathophysiological disturbance of muscle itself, however, such as the failure of contractile muscle force production, is not the primary cause of paresis from an upper motor neuron lesion (Landau and Sahrmann, 2002).

Gains in strength that increase motor recovery may derive from a variety of mechanisms, practice of motor skills may increase sensorimotor representations and drives from cortical and subcortical levels onto the spinal motor pools, leading to greater recruitment or firing rates of these pools (Yue and Cole, 1992; Rahnganathan et al., 2001; Dobkin, 2004). Muscle force output is proportional to muscle fiber volume. Selective muscle strengthening through concentric, eccentric, or isometric exercises may reverse any disuse atrophy and paresis, which often occurs in proximal muscle groups in disabled persons who are relatively less physically active. Walking itself, even with treadmill exercise, may or may not increase the strength of most leg muscles, since only about 20% of the maximal force of the knee extensors, for example, is required for walking, at least in normal subjects. Illness or joint pain, however, may lessen muscle force output through underuse and may cause a decline in conditioning, leading to greater impairment and disability. A fitness program that includes selective strengthening, especially of shoulder, hip, and knee muscle groups, can reverse this set back. Many patients with hemiparetic stroke have a low exercise capacity at one to six months after a stroke (MacKay-Lyons and Makrides, 2002). Even the frail elderly and chronic victims of stroke can be trained to improve their strength and level of conditioning (Teixeira-Salmela *et al.*, 1999; Dean *et al.* 2000; Macko *et al.*, 2001). Strengthening and conditioning activities may also lessen fatigability for activities of daily living and for repetitive use of muscle groups. At least one well-designed clinical trial revealed the efficacy of a home program that included strengthening exercises after stroke (Duncan *et al.*, 1998). Therefore, a pulse of therapy aimed at improving strength and fitness through resistance exercises or to increase selective motor control for skills the patient wants to reacquire, even after some intercurrent medical or emotional problem diminished that skill, may allow the hemiparetic person to become more independent.

Summary

To improve motor performance, practice should engage the patient's interests and needs, aim to increase selective movements for skills, optimize sensory feedback, take into consideration potential biological mechanisms of plasticity, and improve strength and endurance for an activity when necessary. This approach to training may lead to synaptic and morphological changes associated with activity-dependent plasticity within cortical, subcortical, and spinal levels of the neuroaxis. In turn, substitutive and compensatory forms of improvements in practiced skills will be elicited.

REFERENCES

Arvidsson, A., Collin, T., Kirik, D., et al. (2002). Neuronal replacement from endogenous precursors in the adult brain after stroke. *Nat Med* **8**: 963–970.

Belanger, M., Drew, T., Provencher, J., and Rossignol, S., et al. (1996). A comparison of treadmill locomotion in adult cats before and after spinal transection. *J Neurophysiol* **76**: 471–491.

Bland, S., Schallert, T., Strong, R., Aronowski, J., and Grotta, J., et al. (2000). Early exclusive use of the affected forelimb after moderate transient focal ischemia in rats. *Stroke* **31**: 1144–1152.

Buonomano, D. and Merzenich, M. (1998). Cortical plasticity: from synapses to maps. *Annu Rev Neurosci* **21**: 149–186.

Bury, S. and Jones, T. (2002). Unilateral sensorimotor cortex lesions in adult rats facilitate motor skill learning with the "unaffected" forelimb and training-induced dendritic structural plasticity in the motor cortex. *J Neurosci* **22**: 8597–8606.

Carey, J., Kimberley, T., Lewis, S., *et al.* (2002). Analysis of fMRI and finger tracking training in subjects with chronic stroke. *Brain* **125**: 773–788.

Carmichael, S. and Chesselet, M.-F. (2002). Synchronous neuronal activity is a signal for axonal sprouting after cortical lesions in the adult rat. *J Neurosci* **22**: 6062–6070.

Carmichael, S., Wei, L., Rovainen, C. *et al.* (2001). New patterns of intracortical projections after focal cortical stroke. *Neurobiol Dis* **8**: 910–922.

Chen, X., Carp, J., Wolpaw, J., *et al.* (2002). Corticospinal tract transection prevents operantly conditioned H-reflex increase in rats. *Exp Brain Res* **144**: 88–94.

Cheney, P., Hill-Karrer, J., Belhaj-Saif, A. *et al.* (2000). Cortical motor areas and their properties: implications for neuroprosthetics. *Prog Brain Res* **128**: 135–160.

Colombo, G., Joerg, M., Schreier, R., *et al.* (2000). Treadmill training of paraplegic patients using a robotic orthosis. *J Rehab Res Develop* **37**: 693–700.

Daly, J., Kollar, K., Debogorski, A., *et al.* (2001). Performance of an intramuscular electrode during functional neuromuscular stimulation for gait training post stroke. *J Rehabil Res Develop* **38**: 513–526.

Dean, C., Richards, C., Malouin, F., *et al.* (2000). Task-related circuit training improves performance of locomotor tasks in chronic stroke: a randomized, controlled pilot trial. *Arch Phys Med Rehabil* **81**: 409–417.

Dobkin, B. (1998). Driving cognitive and motor gains with rehabilitation after brain and spinal cord injury. *Curr Opin Neurol* **11**: 639–641.

(1999). Overview of treadmill locomotor training with partial body weight support: a neurophysiologically sound approach whose time has come for randomized clinical trials. *Neurorehabil Neural Repair* **13**: 157–165.

(2000a). Spinal and supraspinal plasticity after incomplete spinal cord injury: correlations between functional magnetic resonance imaging and engaged locomotor networks. *Prog Brain Res* **128**: 99–111.

(2000b). Functional rewiring of brain and spinal cord after injury: the three R's of neural repair and neurological rehabilitation. *Curr Opin Neurol* **13**: 655–659.

(2003). *The Clinical Science of Neurological Rehabilitation.* New York: Oxford University Press.

(2004). Strategies for stroke rehabilitation. *Lancet Neurol* **3**: 528–536.

Dobkin, B. H. and Sullivan, K. (2001). Sensorimotor cortex plasticity and locomotor and motor control gains induced by body weight-supported treadmill training after stroke. *Neurorehab Neural Repair* **15**: 258.

Dobkin, B. H., Firestine, A., West, M., *et al.* (2004). Ankle dorsiflexion as an fMRI paradigm to assay motor control for walking during rehabilitation. *Neuroimage* **23**: 370–381.

Donoghue, J. (1997). Limits of reorganization in cortical circuits. *Cereb Cortex* **7**: 97–99.

Duncan, P., Richards, L., Wallace, D., *et al.* (1998). A randomized, controlled pilot study of a home-based exercise program for individuals with mild and moderate stroke. *Stroke* **29**: 2055–2060.

Edgerton, V., de Leon, R., Harkema, S. *et al.* (2001). Retraining the injured spinal cord. *J Physiol* **533**: 15–22.

Feller, M. (1999). Spontaneous correlated activity in developing neural circuits. *Neuron* **22**: 653–656.

Graziano, M., Taylor, C., Moore, T., *et al.* (2002). Complex movements evoked by microstimulation of precentral cortex. *Neuron* **34**: 841–851.

Gribble, P. and Scott, S. (2002). Overlap of internal models in motor cortex for mechanical loads during reaching. *Nature* **417**: 938–941.

Hassid, E., Rose, D., Commisarow, J., *et al.* (1997). Improved gait symmetry in hemiparetic patients during body weight-supported treadmill stepping. *J Neurol Rehabil* **11**: 21–26.

Hendricks, H., van Limbeek, J., Guerts, A., *et al.* (2002). Motor recovery after stroke: a systematic review. *Arch Phys Med Rehabil* **83**: 1629–1637.

Hesse, S., Bertelt, C., Jahnke, M., *et al.* (1995a). Treadmill training with partial body weight support compared with physiotherapy in nonambulatory hemiparetic patients. *Stroke* **26**: 976–981.

Hesse, S., Malezic, M., Bertelt, C., *et al.* (1995b). Restoration of gait by combined treadmill training and multichannel electrical stimulation in nonambulatory hemiparetic patients. *Scand J Rehab Med* **27**: 199–203.

Hesse, S., Konrad, M., Uhlenbrock, D., *et al.* (1999). Treadmill walking with partial body weight support versus floor walking in hemiparetic subjects. *Arch Phys Med Rehabil* **80**: 421–427.

Hesse, S., Werner, C., Uhlenbrock, D., *et al.* (2001). An electromechanical gait trainer for restoration of gait in hemiparetic stroke patients. *Neurorehabil Neural Repair* **15**: 39–50.

Jin, K., Zhu, Y., Sun, Y., *et al.* (2002). Vascular endothelial growth factor (VEGF) stimulates neurogenesis in vitro and in vivo. *Proc Natl Acad Sci USA* **99**: 11946–11950.

Jorgensen, H., Nakayama, H., Raaschou, H., *et al.* (1995). Recovery of walking function in stroke patients: the Copenhagen Stroke Study. *Arch Phys Med Rehabil* **76**: 27–32.

Kissela, B., Broderick, J., Woo, D., *et al.* (2001). Greater Cincinnati/Northern Kentucky Stroke Study: volume of first-ever ischemic stroke among blacks in a population-based study. *Stroke* **32**: 1285–1290.

Kosak, M. and Reding, M. (2000). Comparison of partial body weight-supported treadmill gait training versus aggressive bracing assisted walking post stroke. *Neurorehabil Neural Repair* **14**: 13–19.

Kwakkel, G., Wagenaar, R., Koelman, T., *et al.* (1997). Effects of intensity of rehabilitation after stroke: a research synthesis. *Stroke* **28**: 1550–56.

Kwakkel, G., Wagenaar, R., Twisk, J., *et al.* (1999). Intensity of leg and arm training after primary middle cerebral artery stroke: a randomised trial. *Lancet* **354**: 191–196.

Landau, W., and Sahrmann, S. (2002). Preservation of directly stimulated muscle strength in hemiplegia due to stroke. *Arch Neurol* **59**: 1453–1460.

Liepert, J., Bauder, H., Miltner, W., *et al.* (2000). Treatment-induced cortical reorganization after stroke in humans. *Stroke* **31**: 1210–1216.

Lipton, S. and Nicotera, P. (1998). Excitotoxicity, free radicals, necrosis, and apoptosis. *Neuroscientist* **4**: 345–352.

MacKay-Lyons, M. and Makrides, L. (2002). Exercise capacity early after stroke. *Arch Phys Med Rehabil* **83**: 1697–1702.

Macko, R., Smith, G., Dobrovolny, C., *et al.* (2001). Treadmill training improves fitness reserve in chronic stroke patients. *Arch Phys Med Rehabil* **82**: 879–884.

Magavi, S., Leavitt, B., Macklis, J., *et al.* (2000). Induction of neurogenesis in the neocortex of adult mice. *Nature* **405**: 951–955.

Mulder, T., Zijlstra, W., Guerts, A., *et al.* (2002). Assessment of motor recovery and decline. *Gait Posture* **16**: 198–210.

Nakatomi, H., Kuriu, T., Okabe, S., *et al.* (2002). Regeneration of hippocampal neurons after ischemic brain injury by recruitment of endogenous neural progenitors. *Cell* **110**: 429–441.

Napieralski, J., Butler, A., Chesselet, M.-F., *et al.* (1996). Anatomical and functional evidence for lesion-specific sprouting of corticostriatal input in the adult rat. *J Comp Neurol* **373**: 484–497.

Nilsson, L., Carlsson, J., Danielsson, A., *et al.* (2002). Walking training of patients with hemiparesis at an early stage after stroke: a comparison of walking training on a treadmill with body weight support and walking training on the ground. *Clin Rehabil* **15**: 515–527.

Nudo, R., Milliken, G., Jenkins, W., *et al.* (1996). Use-dependent alterations of movement representations in primary motor cortex of adult squirrel monkeys. *J Neurosci* **16**: 785–807.

Nugent, J., Schurr, K., Adams, R., *et al.* (1994). A dose–response relationship between amount of weight-bearing exercise and walking outcome following cerebrovascular accident. *Arch Phys Med Rehabil* **75**: 399–402.

Orlovsky, G., Deliagina, T., Grillner, S., *et al.* (1999). *Neuronal Control of Locomotion: From Mollusc to Man*. Oxford: Oxford University Press.

Patel, A., Duncan, P., Lai, S., *et al.* (2000). The relation between impairments and functional outcomes post-stroke. *Arch Phys Med Rehabil* **81**: 1357–63.

Pohl, M., Mehrholz, J., Ritschel, C., *et al.* (2002). Speed-dependent treadmill training in ambulatory hemiparetic stroke patients. *Stroke* **33**: 553–558.

Pulvermuller, F., Neininger, B., Elbert, T., *et al.* (2001). Constraint-induced therapy of chronic aphasia after stroke. *Stroke* **32**: 1621–1626.

Rahnganathan, V., Siemionow, V., Sahgal, V., *et al.* (2001). Increasing muscle strength by training the central nervous system without physical exercise. *Soc For Neurosci Abstr* **27**: 168.17.

Ryan, A., Dobrovolny, L., Smith, G., *et al.* (2002). Hemiparetic muscle atrophy and increased intramuscular fat in stroke patients. *Arch Phys Med Rehabil* **83**: 1703–1707.

Saver, J., Johnston, K., Homer, D., *et al.* (1999). Infarct volume as a surrogate or auxiliary outcome measure in ischemic stroke clinical trials. *Stroke* **30**: 293–298.

Schallert, T., Fleming, S., Leasure, J., *et al.* (2000). CNS plasticity and assessment of forelimb sensorimotor outcome in unilateral rat models of stroke, cortical ablation, parkinsonism and spinal cord injury. *Neuropharmacology* **39**: 777–787.

Schiebel, M., Tomiyasu, U., Schiebel, A., *et al.* (1977). The aging human Betz cell. *Exp Neurol* **56**: 598–609.

Scott, S. (2002). Optimal strategies for movement: success with variability. *Nat Neurosci* **5**: 1110–1111.

Seidler, R., Purushotham, A., Kim, S.-G., *et al.* (2002). Cerebellum activation associated with performance change but not motor learning. *Science* **296**: 2043–2046.

Smith, G., Silver, K., Goldberg, A., *et al.* (1999). "Task-oriented" exercise improves hamstring strength and spastic reflexes in chronic stroke patients. *Stroke* **30**: 2112–2118.

Stroemer, R., Kent, T., Hulsebosch, C., *et al.* (1998). Enhanced neocortical neural sprouting, synaptogenesis and behavioral recovery with D-amphetamine therapy after neocortical infarction in rats. *Stroke* **29**: 2381–2395.

Sullivan, K., Dobkin, B., Tavachol, M., *et al.* (2001). *Post-stroke Cortical Plasticity Induced by Step Training*. San Diego, CA: Society for Neuroscience.

Sullivan, K., Knowlton, B., Dobkin, B., *et al.* (2002). Step training with body weight support: effect of treadmill speed and practice paradigms on post-stroke locomotor recovery. *Arch Phys Med Rehabil* **83**: 683–691.

Taub, E. and Wolf, S. (1997). Constraint induced movement techniques to facilitate upper extremity use in stroke patients. *Top Stroke Rehabil* **3**: 38–61.

Taub, E., Uswatte, G., Elbert, T., *et al.* (2002). New treatments in neurorehabiltation founded on basic research. *Nat Rev Neurosci* **3**: 228–236.

Teixeira-Salmela, L., Olney, S., Nadeau, S., *et al.* (1999). Muscle strengthening and physical conditioning to reduce impairment and disability in chronic stroke survivors. *Arch Phys Med Rehabil* **80**: 1211–1218.

Tillakaratne, N., de Leon, R., Hoang, T., *et al.* (2002). Use-dependent modulation of inhibitory capacity in the feline lumbar spinal cord. *J Neurosci* **22**: 3130–3143.

Todorov, E. and Jordan, M. (2002). Optimal feedback control as a theory of motor coordination. *Nat Neurosci* **5**: 1226–1235.

Uryu, K., MacKenzie, L., Chesselet, M.-F., *et al.* (2001). Ultrastructural evidence for differential axonal sprouting in the striatum after thermocoagulatory and aspiration lesions of the cerebral cortex in adult rats. *Neuroscience* **105**: 307–316.

van der Lee, J., Wagenaar, R., Lankhorst, G., *et al.* (1999). Forced use of the upper extremity in chronic stroke patients: results from a single-blind randomized clinical trial. *Stroke* **30**: 2369–2375.

van Praag, H., Kempermann, G., Gage, F., *et al.* (1999). Running increases cell proliferation and neurogenesis in the adult mouse dentate gyrus. *Nat Neurosci* **2**: 266–270.

Visintin, M., Barbeau, H., Korner-Bitensky, N., *et al.* (1998). A new approach to retrain gait in stroke patients through body weight support and treadmill stimulation. *Stroke* **29**: 1122–1128.

Walker, M., Gladman, J., Lincoln, N., *et al.* (1999). Occupational therapy for stroke patients not admitted to hospital: a randomised controlled trial. *Lancet* **354**: 278–280.

Wernig, A., Muller, S., Nanassy, A., *et al.* (1995). Laufband therapy based on "Rules of Spinal Locomotion" is effective in spinal cord injured persons. *Eur J Neurosci* **7**: 823–829.

Yue, G. and Cole, K. (1992). Strength increases from the motor program: comparison of training with maximal voluntary and imagined muscle contractions. *J Neurophysiol* **67**: 1114–1123.

3

Regenerative ability in the central nervous system

Barbro B. Johansson

Wallenberg Neuroscience Center, Lund, Sweden

Introduction

Functional improvement after permanent brain lesions results from changes in the remaining non-affected parts of the brain. The mechanisms involved may vary with post-ischemic time and the type and location of the lesion and can take the form of improved connectivity within individual neurons, modification of cortical representation areas, cortical maps, as well as non-synaptic transmission (Jenkins and Merzenich, 1987; Bach-y-Rita, 1990; Johansson and Grabowski, 1994; Nudo et al., 1996; Buonomano and Merzenich, 1998; Xerri et al., 1998; Nudo, 1999; Johansson, 2000; Hallett, 2001; Hickmott and Merzenich, 2002; Chen et al., 2002a; Keyvani and Schallert, 2002; Frost et al., 2003) There is also increasing evidence that astrocytes take an active part in brain plasticity, not only by their metabolic role and as producers of trophic factors but specifically by playing an active part in neural signaling and in synaptic plasticity (Jones and Greenough, 1996; Chvatal and Sykova, 2000; Araque et al., 2001; Ullian et al., 2001; Mazzanti and Haydon, 2003).

An important question is to what extent post-ischemic events can influence lesion-induced plasticity and improve functional restoration. That neuronal cortical connections can be remodeled was suggested half a century ago (Hebb, 1947). The effect of an activity-stimulating environment on brain function, biochemistry, and morphology has been well documented in the healthy as well as the lesioned brain (Bennett et al., 1964; Rosenzweig, 1966; Volkmar and Greenough, 1972; Will and Kelche, 1992; Kolb, 1995). Housing rats in an enriched environment (i.e. large cages allowing various types of activity) but not including forced training improved outcome after focal brain infarcts induced by proximal or distal ligation of the middle cerebral artery (MCA), even when the transfer to an enriched environment was delayed for 15 days after the arterial occlusion (Ohlsson and Johansson, 1995; Johansson, 1996). This chapter deals, first, with how post-ischemic housing conditions can influence functional outcome, gene expression, neuronal morphology,

Recovery after Stroke, ed. Michael P. Barnes, Bruce H. Dobkin and Julien Bogousslavsky. Published by Cambridge University Press. © Cambridge University Press 2005.

and interact with specific interventions in rats. Second, the current evidence that blocking neurite inhibitory factors may be a future therapy to promote axonal outgrowth is examined. Finally, current research on endogenous and exogenous neuronal replacement therapy is described and the relevance of animal studies for clinical stroke rehabilitation will be briefly discussed from a personal perspective.

Post-ischemic gene expression

Ischemia is a strong inducer of gene expression in the brain. Electrophysiological and morphometric alterations after brain lesions occur with different time courses, ranging from minutes or hours to weeks and months; changes these are likely to be associated with activation of various genes at different post-ischemic times. Many genes are induced within minutes after permanent or transient MCA occlusion, often returning to normal levels within the first 24 hours after the lesion (Kinouchi *et al.*, 1994; Akins *et al.*, 1996).

Early changes

In permanent ischemia, early changes probably mainly reflect cell damage and have little relevance to the recovery potential. Also, after transient ischemia, there is so far no evidence that early events after reperfusion predict reversibility of the ischemic injury (Hara *et al.*, 2001). A comparison of the genomic responses 24 hours after permanent occlusion of the MCA, intracerebral haemorrhage, kainate seizures, hypoglycemia and hypoxia in rats was obtained using oligonucleotide microarrays for 8000 transcripts. Brain ischemia regulated more genes than any other condition, with 415 genes upregulated and 158 downregulated. Half of the genes expressed after ischemia, haemorrhage, and hypoglycemia were unique for each condition (Tang *et al.*, 2002). A significant component of the ischemic responses involved immuno-process-related genes likely to represent responses to dying neurons, glia, and blood vessels. A DNA microarray analysis of cortical gene expression for more than 9000 genes three hours following a two-hour occlusion of the MCA likewise showed a number of up- and downregulated genes (Schmidt-Kastner *et al.*, 2002). A complicating factor in interpretation of these data is that many activated genes are not translated to proteins in the injured brain (Hossmann, 1994).

Late changes

Less is known about late post-ischemic events. The expression patterns of 1176 genes were analyzed 10 days after a photothrombotic lesion using DNA macroarrays, which showed a complex pattern with upregulation of several genes in both hemispheres and downregulation of other genes in the ipsilateral neighboring areas

(Keyvani *et al.*, 2002). A clinically relevant question is to what extent gene changes after ischemia can be modified by interventions. Considering the well-known role of brain-derived neurotrophic factor (BDNF) in brain plasticity in intact animals, the hypothesis that housing rats in an enriched environment after ischemic challenge could lead to an enhanced BDNF gene expression was tested. Contrary to the hypothesis, a second marked increase in BDNF gene expression observed during days 2–12 in rats housed in standard environment was prevented in rats in enriched housing; gene expression was significantly downregulated in rats housed in the enriched environment (Zhao *et al.*, 2000). Significant differences occurred between rats in standard and enriched environments; values below baseline were observed in the peri-infarct region, the contralateral cortex, and the hippocampus 2 to12 days after induction of ischemia in the latter group. The BDNF protein levels 12 days after the MCA occlusion likewise showed a significant reduction in the peri-infarct area but not in the contralateral hemisphere (Zhao *et al.*, 2001). A similar dampening of post-ischemic gene expression in rats housed in enriched environment was seen for mRNA of nerve growth factor-induced clone A (NGFI-A). With this gene, however, a late increase was observed in the group in the enriched environment 30 days after the lesion (Dahlqvist *et al.*, 1999).

Cortical networks adjacent to a focal brain infarct are hyperexcitable because of an imbalance between excitatory and inhibitory synaptic function: increased N-methyl-D-aspartate (NMDA) receptor-mediated excitation and reduced gamma-aminobutyric acid (GABA)ergic inhibition (Qu *et al.*, 1998). Hyperexcitability has been recorded also in the contralateral hemisphere one week after an MCA occlusion (Reinecke *et al.*, 1999). A widespread and long-lasting alteration in GABAÂ receptor subtypes has been noted in rats studied 1, 7, and 30 days after photochemically induced cortical infarcts (Redecker *et al.*, 2002). Both detrimental and beneficial plasticity-promoting roles for lesion-induced hyperexcitability have been proposed (Buchkremer-Ratzmann *et al.*, 1996). One possible interpretation of the BDNF mRNA data would be that early post-ischemic dampening of the peri-infarct neuronal hyperactivity activity might be beneficial. Interactions between trophic factors and growth inhibitory factors, also shown to be increased in the post-ischemic phase (Yugushi *et al.*, 1997), have to be considered.

Considering the recent data from techniques allowing investigation of thousands of genes in the same animal, it is evident that the situation is very complex and that pattern of genes rather than isolated genes has to be considered. Furthermore, many genes display posttranscriptional modifications resulting in different isoforms of the corresponding proteins with different functional properties, and mRNA can be differentially translated and the activity of proteins regulated by posttranslational processes such as phosphorylation and glycosylation.

Growth factors, transmitters, and hormones

Growth factors, transmitters, and hormones are clearly involved in many plasticity processes. Considering the many complex events that occur in post-ischemic brain, it is likely that the efficacy of a drug would vary with the post-ischemic time, size and type of lesion, and would interact with other therapeutic interventions. Depending on the time of administration, drugs may either enhance or retard recovery (Kolb *et al.*, 2001). The beneficial effect of a stimulating environment is likely to be related to release and combined action of various endogenous substances, including catecholamines, glutamate, and hormones. Selegeline, an irreversible monoamine oxidase B inhibitor, which alone had no beneficial effect after focal cerebral ischemia, was shown to reduce behavioral and cognitive deficits in rats when combined with housing the animals in an enriched environment (Puurunen *et al.*, 2001). Amphetamine, which in other experimental studies has been shown to improve outcome, had no additional effect in rats housed in enriched environments (Johansson *et al.*, 1997). So far, data on pharmacology and functional outcome are mainly experimental. Except when relevant for the specific issues discussed in this review, the reader is referred to some reviews on the topic (Goldstein, 1998; Johansson, 1998; Abe, 2000; Goldstein, 2000; Keyvani and Schallert, 2002).

Environmental effects on neuronal morphology and dendritic spines

It has long been known that environmental stimulation can influence dendritic branching and spines (Volkmar and Greenough, 1972; Globus *et al.*, 1973). Dendritic spines are the primary postsynaptic targets of excitatory glutaminergic synapses in the mature brain and have been proposed as primary sites of synaptic plasticity (Eilers and Konnerth, 1997; Harris, 1999). The dendritic tree is covered with a variety of excitable synaptic channels operating on different time scales and with activity-dependent sensitivity, enabling a sophisticated neuronal plastic capability (Svoboda *et al.*, 1997). Housing rats in an enriched environment for three weeks significantly increased the number of dendritic spines in pyramidal neurons in cortical layers II/III and V/ VI in intact rats (Fig. 3.1; Johansson and Belichenko, 2001). A marked upregulation of the immediate early gene *arc*, a gene labeling dendrites, has been observed in the same regions after exposure of rats to an enriched environment for one hour daily for three weeks (Pinaud *et al.*, 2001). Postischemic enriched housing after cortical infarcts significantly increased the number of spines in the contralateral hemisphere in layers II–III (Fig 3.2): that is, neurons with extensive horizontal intercortical connections are shown to be important in brain plasticity (Johansson and Belichenko, 2002). It has also been

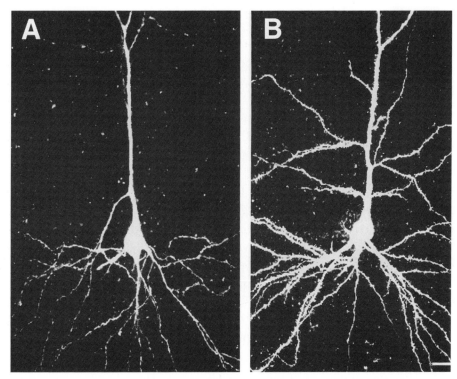

Fig. 3.1.   A pyramidal neuron in cortical layer III in male spontaneously hypertensive rat aged 4 months housed in a standard environment (A) or an enriched environment (B) for 3 weeks. The standard environment was three rats in each cage; in the enriched environment, eight rats were housed in larger cages with opportunities for various activities. (From Johansson and Belichenko (2001) by permission, Springer Verlag.)

reported that skilled reach training combined with enriched environment increases the performance and the dendritic growth in rats compared with training alone (Biernaskie and Corbett, 2001). Nerve growth factor (NGF) treatment prevented dendritic atrophy in the area surrounding the lesion and promoted functional recovery after a devasculariation cortical injury (Kolb *et al.*, 1997), and blockade of basic fibroblast growth factor (bFGF) retarded recovery from motor cortex injury in rats (Rowntree and Kolb, 1997).

Enhancing axonal outgrowth

Myelin in the central nervous system (CNS) strongly inhibited neurite outgrowth after brain lesions (Schwab, 1990; Chen *et al.*, 2000). Three myelin proteins, Nogo, myelin-associated glycoprotein, and oligodendrocyte–myelin glycoprotein inhibit

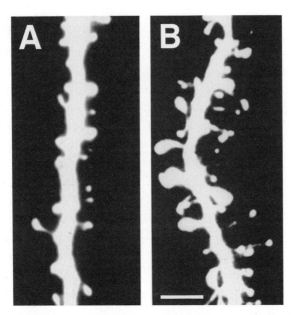

Fig. 3.2.   Spines on a dendrite from a pyramidal neuron in layer III contralateral to a cortical infarct
induced three weeks earlier by a distal ligation of the middle cerebral artery.

regeneration of axons after CNS injury. They share a common receptor, and
blockade of this receptor promoted CNS repair and functional recovery
(Watkins and Barres, 2002). Intrathecal administration of a Nogo receptor antagonist peptide to rats with midthoracic spinal cord hemisection resulted in
significant axon grow of the corticospinal tract and improved functional recovery
(GrandPre and Strittmatter, 2002). Intracerebral injection of the monoclonal
antibody IN-1 in adult rats directly following a MCA occlusion enhanced functional recovery on a forelimb-reaching task. Ten weeks after the lesion, new
corticorubral connections from the opposite, unlesioned hemisphere could be
demonstrated (Papadopolos *et al.*, 2002). Continuous intraventricular infusion of
an anti-Nogo-A antibody for two weeks, starting 24 hours after photothrombotic
cortical injury in normotensive rats or after MCA occlusion in spontaneously
hypertensive rats, significantly increased midline crossing of corticospinal fibers
originating in the unlesioned sensorimotor cortex, with a significant correlation
between the number of crossing fibers and forepaw function (Wiessner *et al.*,
2003). The purine nucleoside inosine, a naturally occurring metabolite, has likewise been shown to induce axonal rewiring and promote behavioral outcome
when infused continuously into the cisterna magna or into the lateral ventricle on
the undamaged side after a partial MCA occlusion (Chen *et al.*, 2002b). The drug
stimulated neurons on the undamaged side of the brain to extend new projections

to denervated areas of the midbrain and spinal cord, and the anatomical changes were paralleled by improved performance on several behavioral measures. The number of crossing corticorubral fibers was low in normal control animals and increased significantly after stroke, even in animals treated with saline alone, but with a further two- to three-fold increase after inosine infusion. Therefore, it seems that lesion alone, and inosine to a larger extent, can overcome at least some of the molecular signals that normally inhibit axonal growth. Subcutaneously administered inosine has earlier been shown to stimulate axonal growth in the rat corticospinal tract after injury (Benowitz *et al.*, 1999).

These two promising approaches to stimulate axonal growth implicate plasticity from the intact hemisphere as a mechanism for recovery in the rat. The role of the contralateral hemisphere for functionally improvement in stroke patients is a controversial issue, and this role may differ with type and location of the lesion. To what extent blockade of Nogo-A or administration of inosine can influence axonal growth in the lesioned hemisphere, where imaging studies have indicated substantial reorganization in patients with good functional outcome (Fridman *et al.*, 2004), has so far not been reported.

Transplantation of fetal tissue, neural and non-neural progenitor cells

A primary role of neurological rehabilitation is to optimize the function of the remaining intact tissue. Another currently discussed question is whether tissue substitution is possible after brain lesions. That transplanted fetal neocortical tissue to cortical cavities can survive was shown by Sharp *et al.* (1987). In adult rats, fetal neocortical dissociated tissue transplanted to the infracted area one to nine weeks after an infarct survived and received afferent connections from ipsilateral and contralateral cortex, the thalamus and several other host brain subcortical nuclei (Grabowski *et al.*, 1992). Grafting to the necrotic tissue during the first five postoperative days was less successful. Sensory stimulation of the rat vibrissae enhanced the metabolic activity in grafts, indicating that the host-to-graft connections could be functionally relevant (Grabowski *et al.*, 1993). Using fetal tissue blocks, rather than dissociated tissue, parts of the grafts developed a morphology reminiscent of normal neocortex and, in addition to afferent connections from the host, the grafts send sparse efferent connections into the host brain (Sørensen *et al.*, 1996). However, functional improvement was only observed when grafting was combined with housing in an enriched environment. When grafting was performed one, but not three, weeks after the ischemic event, the ipsilateral thalamic atrophy was significantly reduced, an effect that most likely resulted from trophic influences of the graft on the surrounding tissue (Mattsson *et al.*, 1997). It has been shown more recently that enriched environment can stimulate branching of fibers from the host after their entry into the graft (Zeng et al., 2000). The significant influence of environment and experience on neural grafts is in agreement with studies on other experimental models, reviewed by Döbrössy and Dunnett (2001).

Ethical considerations combined with restricted availability of fetal tissue has led to the search for alternatives, including immortalized human and murine cell lines, neural embryonic or adult progenitor cells (Savitz et al., 2002). Stem cells are defined by their ability to both self-renew and to differentiate to produce mature progeny cells (Wagern and Weissman, 2004). It is often difficult to draw a sharp line between stem cells and progenitors.

A study on an immortalized stem cell line grafted to either side or infused into the right ventricle two to three weeks after a transient occlusion of the right MCA indicated that the effect can be related to the site of the graft, which was thought to indicate that the cells were utilized in repair processes on both the lesioned and contralateral side (Modo et al., 2002). Searching for valid control grafts, dead stem cells were grafted into the sites previously used for active grafts. Unexpectedly, spatial learning was substantially impaired and the lesion volume was increased by 55% with ipsilateral dead cell grafts, indicating the potential hazards in the use of dead cells for sham grafts (Modo et al., 2003).

Methods have been developed to enable in vivo studies of migration of transplanted cells. Undifferentiated murine embryonic stem cells, labeled by a lipofection procedure with a magnetic resonance imaging (MRI) contrast agent, were injected in the contralateral intact hemisphere two weeks after MCA occlusion for one hour. The movement of the cells was traced by high-resolution MRI at 78 μm isotropic spatial resolution. During the following three weeks, the cells migrated from the injection sites in the hemisphere opposite to the lesion over the corpus callosum into the border zone of the damaged brain tissue, where a large fraction of the cells differentiated into neurons (Hoehn et al., 2002). However, when the same cells, which originated from mice, were transplanted to mice, they did not migrate to the lesion but produced highly malignant teratocarcinomas (Trapp et al., 2002; Erdö et al., 2003). Macroscopically visible tumors were observed as early as one week following transplantation of as few as 500 cells. The study documents a difference in malignant transformation of stem cells following homologous and xenotransplantation, and it raises serious concerns about safety, suggesting that testing human stem cells in animal models may not be sufficient to established safety for patients.

In another in vivo MRI study of cell migration, cells from the subventricular zone were isolated from young adult rats, cultured in the presence of bFGF for eight days, labeled by ferromagnetic particles, and injected into the cisterna magna 48 hours after an embolic right MCA occlusion. Transplanted cells selectively migrated towards the ischemic parenchyma at a mean speed of 65 ± 15 μm/h.

The cells appeared integrated into the microenvironment with well-formed axo-synaptic junctions, and rats with transplanted cells performed significantly better than controls without transplanted cells in some behavioral tests (Zhang *et al.*, 2003). A third technique is to prelabel neural stem cells with the bimodal contrast agent Gadelinium-Rhodamine Dextran, detectable by both MRI and subsequent histological analyses (Modo *et al.*, 2004).

Another strategy has been to use non-neural progenitor cells. (Anderson *et al.*, 2001). A number of non-neural stem cells have been claimed to be able to trans-differentiate into neurons and to influence functional outcome in experimental stroke models. Whether mammalian stem cells are in fact pluripotent and capable of differentiation across tissue lineage boundaries is controversial (Raff, 2003; Wagers and Weissman, 2004). Other or additional mechanisms including cell fusion have been proposed and shown to occur although to a limited and maybe not clinically relevant extent. At the current stage I think it is fair to say that trans-differentiation of other cells into neurons has so far not been verified in a way that satisfies most researchers in the field. This should be kept in mind when reading the claims made in some of the studies discussed below. Although the claims of stem cell plasticity may have been exaggerated, functional improvement may be obtained by non-neural cells through various mechanisms discussed below (Li *et al.*, 2002). Adult rat and human bone marrow stromal (non-hematopoietic) cells have been claimed to differentiate into neurons in vitro (Woodbury *et al.*, 2000). In experimental studies on mice and rats, the majority of bone marrow-derived cells develop into endothelial cells (Hess *et al.*, 2002), and even with bone marrow stroma-derived cells, the proportion of cells that develop into neurons is low. Nevertheless, functional improvement was obtained, and neurological benefit could derive from increase of growth factors in the ischemic tissue, from reduction of apoptosis in the penumbral zone, and from proliferation of endogenous cells in the subventricular zone (Li *et al.*, 2002). Administration of granulocyte colony-stimulating factor and stem cell factor expand and modulate circulating bone marrow stem cells and enhance their capacity to acquire neuronal characteristics in the brain (Corti *et al.*, 2002).

Human umbilical cord blood contains many immature progenitor cells and has been reported to reduce behavior deficits in the rat after MCA occlusion with a better effect when given intravenously 24 hours after the insult rather than a week later (Chen *et al.*, 2001).

Lesion-induced proliferation of endogenous progenitor cells

The subventricular zone and the subgranular zone of the dentate gyrus contain neural stem cells or progenitor cells that continuously give rise to new neurons in the adult brain, including that of humans (Eriksson *et al.*, 1998; Gage, 2000). Small numbers of progenitor cells are thought to be present in other brain areas, including the cerebral cortex in rodents, and cortical neurogenesis has been induced by bFGF in intact rodents (Palmer *et al.*, 1999). Whether neurogenesis occurs in the adult primate neocortex is highly controversial. It has been reported in one study (Gould *et al.*, 1999) but questioned by other researchers (Nowakowski and Hayes, 2000; Rakic, 2002).

The progenitor cell proliferation in subventicular zone and hippocampus can be stimulated by exogenous factors including trophic factors, hormones, physical activity, drugs, brain trauma, and ischemic lesions, including focal brain ischemia (Jin *et al.*, 2001; Arvidsson *et al.*, 2001; Zhang et al., 2001; Komitova *et al.*, 2002; Parent *et al.*, 2002). An ischemic brain lesion apparently induces some so far unknown chemotactic signals that attract endogenous and exogenous immature cells. Proliferating cells from the subventricular zone migrated to the striatum after large striatocortical lesions induced by a transient MCA occlusion. A small number of the cells developed into medium-sized striatal neurons (Arvidsson *et al.*, 2002; Parent *et al.*, 2002). Although cortical lesion-induced neurogenesis has been reported to occur in the same experimental model (Jiang *et al.*, 2001), neither of these studies, nor a study after MCA embolization (Zhang *et al.*, 2001), have been able to confirm this observation.

A stimulating environment enhances the survival of newly formed neurons in the hippocampus of intact rats and mice (Kemperman *et al.*, 1997; Nilsson *et al.*, 1999), even in old mice, where the cellular plasticity occurs together with significant improvements of learning parameters and exploratory behavior (Kemperman *et al.*, 2002). The combined effect of cortical ischemia and environmental stimulation has been studied in 6-month-old spontaneously hypertensive rats with selective cortical infarcts. Bromodeoxyuridine, which labels dividing cells, was given daily during the first week after infarct. Five weeks later, a five- to six-fold ipsilateral increase in labeled cells compared with sham operated rats was seen in all rats, and about 80% of the new cells were neurons. Although there was no difference in newly formed neurons between the groups housed in standard or enriched environments a highly significant difference was observed in the number of new astrocytes. In rats housed in standard environment, few new astrocytes were formed, resulting in a many-fold increase in the neuron-to-glia ratio, a ratio that was normalized in rats housed in enriched environment (Komitova *et al.*, 2002). It seems likely that the low number of astrocytes in the group housed in standard conditions is insufficient to support the newly formed neurons whatever their function. Most studies on brain plasticity have concentrated on neurons. As mentioned in at the beginning of this chapter, there is increasing evidence that astrocytes play an active part in neural signaling and in synaptic plasticity (Araque *et al.*, 2001; Ullian and Sapperstein, 2001; Mazzanti and

Haydon, 2003). Furthermore, a subtype of astrocytes in the subventricular zone and in the subgranular zone in the dentate gyrus has been proposed to function as precursors in neurogenesis in these regions (Doetsch *et al.*, 1999; Seri *et al.*, 2001).

Do new neurons integrate into synaptic circuitry in the adult mammalian brain?

Evidence that newborn neurons integrate into synaptic circuitry in the olfactory bulb and hippocampus in adult intact mice has only recently been obtained (Carlen *et al.*, 2002; van Praag *et al.*, 2002). A model of selective apoptotic damage to pyramidal neurons in adult mice has been used to show that endogenous neural precursors can be induced to differentiate into mature neurons in adult mammalian neocortex. Retrograde labeling from thalamus demonstrated that new neurons formed long-distance corticothalamic connections (Magavi *et al.*, 2000). In the same model of targeted apoptosis, mature astrocytes transform into transitional radial glia that support directed migration of transplanted immature neurons (Leavitt *et al.*, 1999), and late-stage immature neocortical neurons could reconstruct interhemispheric connections and form synaptic contacts within adult mouse cortex (Fricker-Gates *et al.*, 2002). It is an elegant model of great interest for degenerative disorders but is less relevant for cortical infarcts with large tissue loss.

Transient global ischemia that selectively damages hippocampal CA I neurons is a strong stimulant for neurogenesis in the hippocampus (Liu *et al.*, 2000). Intraventricular infusion of FGF-2 and epidermal growth factor (EGF) for four days following a transient global ischemia has been shown to markedly increase regeneration of hippocampal pyramidal neurons. Based on electrophysiological evidence that the neurons were integrated into the existing brain circuitry, it was proposed that the new cells contributed to the amelioration of neurological deficits observed in the treated rats (Nakatomi *et al.*, 2002).

Apart from these studies on selective neuronal damage, there is little evidence for endogenous or exogenous cellular integration. Local contacts, including synapses, do not necessarily mean integration. Whether any integration will be possible and be clinically relevant for brain lesions with a substantial loss of brain tissue, such as infarcts, is indeed an open question. To reinstate sophisticated neocortical networks that have developed during many years would be a formidable task. However, transplanted cells or tissue can have effect as producers of growth factors or transmitters and could optimize the function of the surrounding tissue, as suggested by studies on fetal neocortical transplantation and on non-neural stem cell administration to rodents.

Currently there is no evidence that the endogenous neurogenesis induced by focal brain ischemic is of any relevance for functional outcome. Whether administration of growth-promoting factors that stimulate neurogenesis in intact animals such as

EGF (Craig *et al.*, 1996), FGF (Palmer *et al.*, 1999), and erythropoietin (Shingo *et al.*, 2001) can enhance proliferation, migration, and differentiation of progenitor cells, and if so whether or not such measures influence functional recovery, remains to be shown. Lesioned and intact brain may differ, as recently shown in a study on global ischemia when brain-derived neurotrophic factor suppressed rather than increased lesion-induced neurogenesis (Larsson *et al.*, 2002). It is evident that many questions remain to be answered in this very active field of research. The reason for the apparent diminished capacity for adult neurogenesis in monkeys compared with rodents is not known, and the genes and factors that inhibit neurogenesis in most of the adult brain have not been identified.

How relevant are experimental studies for clinical stroke rehabilitation?

A number of experimental focal brain lesion models have been used as experimental stroke models, including transient or permanent vascular occlusions, cortical ablation, electrolytic, excitotoxic, and photothrombotic models. The time course of lesion progression, influence on the surrounding tissue, and regenerative capability are likely to differ and could influence the efficacy of interventions. Thus grafting after a cortical infarct gives better host-to-graft connectivity than grafting to a cortical aspiration lesion (Zeng *et al.*, 2000). Photothrombotic lesions are associated with an immediate breakdown of the blood–brain barrier and rapid edema development different from the edema patterns seen after arterial ligations or embolization, and after cortical ablation lesions the surrounding tissue is not exposed to the same environment as in the vascular models, factors that are likely to influence plasticity events in the surrounding tissue (Gonzales and Kolb, 2003). We do not know what influence such factors might have on the restoration processes in the brain. One important difference between rodents and humans is that the human brain has a much larger proportion of white matter. The commonly used model of a two-hour transient MCA intraluminal occlusion reduces protein synthesis also in areas outside the MCA territory, including ipsilateral thalamus, hypothalamus, hippocampus, and substantia nigra; it has been suggested that this model should be referred to as an internal carotid artery occlusion and not as an MCA occlusion (Kanemitsu *et al.*, 2002). In a comparison between a two-hour suture occlusion and permanent diathermy occlusion of MCA, axonal degeneration and oligodendrocyte damage was much more severe in the former. The different distribution of axonal pathology in the two models was not a reflection of differences in the size of the neuronal perikarya pathology but rather a consequence of occlusion of additional vessels (McCulloch *et al.*, 2002). Pharmacological interventions may well differ with the models used. Stroke is, after all, a clinical term, and in animal experiments it would be much preferred that authors described clearly in their abstracts what was done rather than using the diffuse term experimental stroke. If well defined, results obtained with different models may help to answer some relevant questions. Another problem is the lack of information on age and gender. Having said this, there is no doubt that we have learnt much from animal studies. However, many research protocols could be improved to enable better comparison between different research groups and between animals and humans.

The animal data referred to in this review demonstrate that postischemic housing in an enriched environmental influences outcome after focal brain ischemia. Concerning the relevance for human stroke patients, two arguments can be raised. One is that standard laboratory housing is a deprived environment not comparable to normal human life; therefore, the result obtained in animal studies may not be relevant for patients. This is a valid argument, which, however, leads to the conclusion that a stimulating environment should be the base in all animal recovery studies to which specific rehabilitative interventions can be added. An opposite argument would be that some elderly stroke patients might have lived a rather isolated life before stroke onset, also a valid argument considering that half of the first-ever stroke patients in Sweden are 75 years or older. In any case, the transfer from home to hospital after an acute stroke involves for most patient a drastic change in environment that justifies any attempts to optimize the hospital and rehabilitation environment.

Summary

The patient's own attitude, activity, and social interaction influence functional outcome and quality of life after stroke (Johansson et al., 1992; Johansson, 2003). Individuals have different capabilities to handle crisis, including diseases. Expectation plays a significant role in all treatments and may even have lesion-specific effects (Petrovic et al., 2002; de la Fuente-Fernandez and Stoessl, 2002; Mayberg et al., 2002). Previous brain lesions may limit later plasticity processes, as indicated from a study indicating that penetrating head injury in young adulthood exacerbated cognitive decline in later years (Corkin, 1989). However, experimental evidence that post-ischemic environmental enrichment can significantly improve functional outcome, influence gene expression, increase dendritic branching and the number of dendritic spines, and modify lesion-induced stem cell differentiation, as well as interact with drug treatment, transplantation and skill training, emphasizes the importance of general stimulation and activation in stroke rehabilitation, clearly in addition and not as a substitute to the specific interventions required. Promising new therapeutic approaches are being developed in animals, but the time windows for the various interventions and the molecular mechanisms for cell proliferation, migration, and differentiation need to be explored.

REFERENCES

Abe, K. (2000). Therpeutic potential of neurotrohic factors and neural stem cells against ischemic injury. *J Cereb Blood Flow Metab* **21**: 1393–1418.

Akins, P. T., Liu, P. K., and Hsu, C. Y. (1996). Immediate early gene expression in response to cerebral ischemia. Friend or foe? *Stroke* **27**: 1682–1687.

Anderson, D. J., Gage, F. H., and Weissman, I. L. (2001). Can stem cells cross lineage boundaries? *Nat Med* **7**: 393–395.

Araque, A., Carmignoto, G., and Haydon, P. G. (2001). Dynamic signaling between astrocytes and neurons. *Annu Rev Physiol* **63**: 795–813.

Arvidsson, A., Kokaia, Z., and Lindvall, O. (2001). N-Methyl-D-aspartate receptor-mediated increase of neuorogenesis in adult rat dentate gyrus following stroke. *Eur J Neurosci* **14**: 10–18.

Arvidsson, A., Collin, T., Kirik, D., Kokaia, Z., and Lindvall, O. (2002). Neuronal replacement from endogenous precursors in the adult brain after stroke. *Nat Med* **8**: 963–970.

Bach-y-Rita, P. (1990). Receptor plasticity and volume transmission in the brain: emerging concepts with relevance to neurologic rehabilitation. *J Neurol Rehab* **4**: 121–128.

Bennett, E. L., Diamond, M. C., Krech, D., and Rosenzweig, M. R. (1964). Chemical and anatomical plasticity of brain. *Science* **146**: 610–619.

Benowitz, L. I., Goldberg, D. E., Madsen, J. R., Soni, D., and Irwin, N. (1999). Inosine stimulates extensive axon collateral growth in the rat corticospinal tract after injury. *Proc Natl Acad Sci USA* **96**: 13486–13490.

Biernaskie, J. and Corbett, D. (2001). Enriched rehabilitative training promotes improved forelimb motor function and enhanced dendritic growth after focal ischemic injury. *J Neurosci* **21**: 5272–5278.

Björklund, A. and Lindvall, O. (2000). Cell replacement therapies for central nervous system disorders. *Nat Neurosci* **3**: 537–544.

Buchkremer-Ratzmann, I., August, M., Hagemann, G., and Witte, O. W. (1996). Electrophysiological transcortical diaschisis after cortical photothrombosis in rat brain. *Stroke* **27**: 1105–1119.

Buonomano, D. V. and Merzenich, M. M. (1998). Cortical plasticity: from synapses to maps. *Annu Rev Neurosci* **21**: 149–186.

Carlen, M., Cassidy, R. M., Brismar, H., *et al.* (2002). Functional integration of adult-born neurons. *Curr Biol* **12**: 606–608.

Chen, J., Sanberg, P. R., Li, Y., *et al.* (2001). Intravenous administration of human umbilical cord blood reduces behavioral deficits after stroke in rats. *Stroke* **32**: 2682–2688.

Chen, M. S., Huber, A. B., van der Haar, M. E., *et al.* (2000). Nogo-A is a myelin-associated neurite outgrowth inhibitor and an antigen for monoclonal antibody IN-1. *Nature* **403**: 369–370.

Chen, P., Goldberg, D. E., Kolb, B., Lanser, M., and Benowitz, L. I. (2002b). Inosine induces axonal rewiring and improves behavioral outcome after stroke. *Proc Natl Acad Sci USA* **99**: 9031–9036.

Chen, R., Cohen, L. G., and Hallett, M. (2002a). Nervous system reorganization following injury. *Neuroscience* **11**: 761–773.

Chen, Y. and Swanson, R. A. (2003). Astrocytes and brain injury. *J Cereb Blood Flow Metab* **23**: 137–149.

Chvatal, A. and Sykova, E. (2000). Glial influence on neuronal signaling. *Prog Brain Res* **125**: 199–216.

Corkin, S., Rosen, T. J., Sullivan, E. V., and Clegg, R. A. (1989).Penetrating head injury in young adulthood exacerbates cognitive decline in later years. *J Neurosci* **9**: 3876–3883.

Corti, S., Locatelli, F., Strazzer, S., *et al.* (2002). Modulated generation of neuronal cells from bone marrow by expansion and mobilization of circulating stem cells with *in vivo* cytokine treatment. *Exp Neurol* **177**: 443–452.

Craig, C. G., Tropepe, T., Morshead, C. M., *et al.* (1996). *In vivo* growth factor expansion of endogenous subependymal neuroal precursor cell populations in the adult mouse brain. *J Neurosci* **16**: 2649–2658.

Dahlqvist, P., Zhao, L., Johansson, I.-M., *et al.* (1999). Environmental enrichment alters NGFI-A and glucocorticoid receptor mRNA expression after MCA occlusion in rats. *Neuroscience* **93**: 527–535.

Dahlqvist, P., Rönnbäck, A., Risedal, A., *et al.* (2003). Effects of postischemic environment on transcription factor and serotonin receptor expression after permanent focal cortical ischemia in rats. *Neuroscience* **119**: 643–652.

de la Fuente-Fernandez, R. and Stoessl, A. J. (2002). The placebo effect in Parkinson's disease. *Trands Neurosci* **159**: 728–737.

Doetsch, F., Caillé, I., Lim, D. A., García-Verdugo, J., and Alvarez-Buylla, A. (1999). Subventrical zone astrocytes are neural stem cells in the adult mammalian brain. *Cell* **97**: 703–716.

Döbrössy, M. D. and Dunnett, S. B. (2001). The influence of environment and experience on neural grafts. *Nat Neurosci* **2**: 871–879.

Eilers, J. and Konnerth, A. (1997). Dendritic signal integration. *Curr Opin Neurobiol* **7**: 385–390.

Erdö, F., Bührle, C., Blunk, J., *et al.* (2003). Host-dependent outcome of embryonic stem cell implantation in experimental stroke. *J Cereb Blood Flow Metab* **23**: 780–785.

Eriksson, P. S., Perfilieva, E., Björk-Eriksson, T., *et al.* (1998). Neurogenesis in the adult human hippocampus. *Nat Med* **4**: 1313–1317.

Fricker-Gates, R. A., Shin, J. J., Tai, C. C., Catapano, L. A., and Macklis, J. D. (2002). Late-stage immature neocortical neurons reconstruct interhemispheric connections and form synaptic contacts with increased efficiency in adult mouse cortex undergoing targeted neurodegeneration. *J Neurosci* **22**: 4045–4056.

Fridman, E. A., Hanakawa, T., Chung, M., Hummel, F., Leiguarda, R. C., and Cohen, L. G. (2004). Reorganisation of the human ipsilesional premotor cortex after stroke. *Brain* **127**: 747–758.

Frost, S. B., Barbay, S., Friel, K. M., Plautz, E. J., and Nudo, R. J. (2003). Reorganisation of remote cortical regions after ischemic brain injury: a potential substrate for stroke recovery. *Neurophysiology* **89**: 3205–3214.

Gage, F. H. (2000). Mammalian neural stem cells. *Science* **287**: 1433–1438.

Globus, A., Rosenzweig, M. R., Bennett, E. L., and Diamond, M. C. (1973). Effect of differential experience on dendritic spines counts in rat cerebral cortex. *J Comp Physiol Psychol* **82**: 175–181.

Goldstein, L. B. (1998). *Restorative Neurology: Advances in Pharmacotherapy for Recovery after Stroke*. Armonk, NY: Futura.

 (2000). Rehabilitation and recovery after stroke. Current treatment options. *Neurology* **2**: 319–328.

Gonzalez, C. L. and Kolb, B. (2003). A comparison of different models of stroke on behaviour and brain morphology. *Eur J Neurosci* **18**: 1950–1962.

Gould, E., Reeves, A. J., Graziano, M. S., and Gross, C. G. (1999). Neurogenesis in the neocortex of adult primates. *Science* **286**: 548–552,

Grabowski, M., Brundin, P., and Johansson, B. B. (1992). Fetal neocortical grafts implanted in adult hypertensive rats with cortical infarcts following a middle cerebral artery occlusion. Ingrowth of afferent fibers from the host brain. *Exp Neurol* **116**: 105–121.

(1993). Functional integration of cortical grafts placed in brain infarcts of rats. *Ann Neurol* **34**: 362–368.

Grabowski, M., Sørensen, J. C., Mattsson, B., Zimmer, J., and Johansson, B. B. (1995). Influence of an enriched environment and cortical grafting on functional outcome in brain infarcts of adult rats. *Exp Neurol* **133**: 96–102.

Grandpre, T. and Strittmatter, S. M. (2002). Nono-66 receptor antogonist peptide promotes axonal regeneration. *Nature* **417**: 547–551.

Hallett, M. (2001). Plasticity of the human motor cortex and recovery from stroke. *Brain Res Brain Res Rev* **36**: 169–174.

Hara, T., Mies, G., Hata, R., and Hossmann, K. A. (2001). Gene expressions after thrombolytic treatment of middle cerebral artery clot embolism in mice. *Stroke* **32**: 1912–1919,

Harris, K. M. (1999). Structure, development, and plasticity of dendritic spines. *Curr Opin Neurobiol* **9**: 343–348.

Hebb, D. O. (1947). The effect of early experience on problem solving at maturity. *Am Psychol* **2**: 737–745.

Hess, D. C., Hill, W. D., Martin-Studdard, A., *et al.* (2002). Bone marrow as a source of endothelial cells and NeuN-expressing cells after stroke. *Stroke* **33**: 1362–1368.

Hickmott, P. W. and Merzenich, M. M. (2002). Local circuit properties underlying cortical reorganization. *J Neurophysiol* **88**: 1288–1301.

Hoehn, M., Kustermann, E., Blunk, J., *et al.* (2002). Monitoring of implanted stem cell migration in vivo: a highly resolved in vivo magnetic resonance imaging investigation of experimental stroke in rat. *Proc Natl Acad Sci USA* **99**: 16267–16272.

Hossmann, K. A. (1994). Viability thresholds and the penumbra of focal ischemia. *Ann Neurol* **36**: 557–565.

Jenkins, W. M. and Merzenich, M. M. (1987). Reorganization of neocortical representations after brain injury: a neurophysiological model of the bases of recovery from stroke. *Progr Brain Res* **71**: 249–266.

Jiang, W., Gu, W., Brännström, T., Rosqvist, R., and Wester, P. (2001). Cortical neurogenesis in adult rats after transient middle cerebral artery occlusion. *Stroke* **32**: 1201–1207.

Jin, K., Minami, M., Lan, J. Q., *et al.* (2001). Neurogenesis in dentate subganular zone and rostral subventricular zone after focal cerebral ischemia in the rat. *Proc Natl Acad Sci USA* **98**: 4710–4715.

Johansson, B. B. (1996). Functional outcome in rats transferred to an enriched environment 15 days after focal brain ischemia. *Stroke* **27**: 324–326.

(1998). Neurotrophic factors and transplants. In *Restorative Neurology: Advances in Pharmacotherapy for Recovery after Stroke*, ch. 6, ed. L. B. Goldstrein., Armonk, NY: Futura.

(2000). Brain plasticity and stroke rehabilitation. The Willis Lecture. *Stroke* **31**: 223–231.

(2003). Environmental influence on recovery after brain lesions: experimental and clinical data. *J Rehabil Med Suppl.* **41**: 11–16.

Johansson, B. B. and Belichenko, P. V. (2001) Environmental influence on neuronal and dendritic spine plasticity after permanent focal brain ischemia. In *Maturation Phenomenon in Cerebral Ischemia IV*, ed. U. Ito Bazan, N. G., Marcheselli, V. L., Kuroiwa, T., and I. Klatzo. Berlin: Springer Verlag, pp. 77–83.

(2002). Neuronal plasticity and dendritic spines: effect of environmental enrichment on intact and postischemic rat brain. *J Cereb Blood Flow Metab* **22**: 89–96.

Johansson, B. B. and Grabowski, M. (1994). Functional recovery after brain infarction. Plasticity and neural transplantation. *Brain Pathol* **4**: 85–95.

Johansson, B. B. and Ohlsson, A.-L. (1996). Environment, social interaction and physical activity as determinants of functional outcome after cerebral infarction in the rat. *Exp Neurol* **139**: 322–327.

Johansson, B. B., Jadbäck, G., Norrving, B., and Widner, H. (1992). Evaluation of long-term functional status in first-ever stroke patients in a defined population. *Scand J Rehab Med Suppl* **26**: 103–114.

Johansson, B. B., Mattsson, B., and Ohlsson, A.-L. (1997). Functional outcome after brain infarction: effect of enriched environment and amphetamine. In *Maturation Phenomenon in Cerebral Ischemia II*, ed. U. Ito, T. Kirino, T. Kuroiwa, and I. Klatzo. Heidelberg: Springer, pp. 159–167.

Jones, T. A. and Greenough, W. T. (1996). Ultrastructural evidence for increased contact between astrocytes and synapses in rats reared in a complex environment. *Neurobiol Learn Mem* **65**: 48–56.

Kanemitsu, H., Nakagomi, T., Tamura, A., *et al.* (2002). Differences in the extent of primary ischemic damage between middle cerebral artery coagulation and intraluminal occlusion models. *J Cereb Blood Flow Metab* **22**: 1196–1204.

Kempermann, G., Kuhn, H. G., and Gage, F. H. (1997). More hippocampal neurons in adult mice living in an enriched environment. *Nature* **386**: 493–495.

Kempermann, G., Gast, D., and Gage, F. H. (2002). Neuroplasticity in old age: sustained fivefold induction of hippocampal neurogenesis by long-term environmental enrichment. *Ann Neurol* **52**: 133–4.

Keyvani, K. and Schallert, T. (2002). Plasticity-associated molecular and structural events in the injured brain. *J Neuropath Exp Neurol* **61**: 831–840.

Keyvani, K., Witte, O. W., and Paulus, W. (2002). Gene expression profiling in peri-lesional and contralateral areas after ischemia in rat brain. *J Cereb Blood Flow Metab* **22**: 153–160.

Kinouchi, H., Sharp, F. R., Chan, P. H., *et al.* (1994). Induction of c-Fos, junB, c-Jun, and hsp70 mRNA in cortex, thalamus, basal ganglia, and hippocampus following middle cerebral artery occlusion. *J Cereb Blood Flow Metab* **14**: 808–817.

Kolb, B. (1995). *Brain Plasticity and Behavior*, Hillsdale, NJ: Lawrence Erlboum.

Kolb, B., Cote, S., Ribeiro de Silva, A., and Cuello, A. C. (1997). Nerve growth factor prevents dendritic atrophy and promotes recovery of function after cortical injury. *Neuroscience* **76**: 1139–1151.

Kolb, B., Brown, R., Witt-Lajeunesse, A., and Gibb, R. (2001). Neural compensations after lesion of the cerebral cortex. *Neural Plast* **8**: 1–16.

Komitova, M., Perfilieva, E., Mattsson, B., Eriksson, P. S., and Johansson, B. B. (2002). Effects of cortical ischemia and post-ischemic environmental enrichment on hippocampal cell genesis and differentiation in the adult rat. *J Cereb Blood Flow Metab* **22**: 852–860.

Kondziolka, D., Wechsler, L., and Achim, C. (2002). Neural transplantation for stroke. *J Clin Neurosci* **9**: 225–230.

Larsson, E., Mandel, R. J., Klein, R. L., *et al.* (2002). Suppression of insult-induced neurogenesis in adult rat brain by brain-derived neurotrophic factor. *Exp Neurol* **177**: 1–7.

Leavitt, B. R., Hernit-Grant, C. S., and Macklis, J. D. (1999). Mature astrocytes transform into transitional radial glia whihin adult mouse neocortex that supports directed migration of transplanted immature neurons. *Exp Neurol* **157**: 43–47.

Li, Y., Chen, J., Chen, X. G., *et al.* (2002). Human marrow stromal cell therapy for stroke in rat. *Neurology* **59**: 514–523.

Liu, J., Bernabeu, R., Aigang, L., and Sharp, F. R. (2000). Neurogenesis and gliogenesis in the post-ischemic brain. *Neuroscientist* **6**: 362–370.

Magavi, S. S., Leavitt, B. R., and Macklis, J. D. (2000). Induction of neurogenesis in the neocortex of adult mice. *Nature* **405**: 951–955.

Mattsson, B., Sørensen, J. C., Zimmer, J., and Johansson, B. B. (1997). Neural grafting to experimental neocortical infarcts improves behavioral outcome and reduces thalamic atrophy in rats housed in an enriched but not in standard environments. *Stroke* **28**: 1225–1232.

Mayberg, H. S., Silva, J. A., Brannan, S. K., *et al.* (2002). The functional neuroanatomy of the placebo effect. *Am J Psychiatry* **159**: 728–737.

Mazzanti, M. and Haydon, P. G. (2003). Astrocytes selectively enhance N-type calcium current in hippocampal neurons. *Glia* **41**: 128–136.

McCulloch, J., Komajti, K., Valeriani, V., and Dewar, D. (2002). Beyond neuroprotection: the protection of axons and oligodendrocytes in cerebral ischemia. In *The 22nd Princeton Conference: Cerebrovascular Disease*, ed. P. H. Chan. Cambridge: Cambridge University Press, pp. 404–415.

Modo, M., Stroemer, R. P., Tang, E., Patel, S., and Hodges, H. (2002). Effects of implantation site of stem cell grafts on behavioral recovery from stroke damage. *Stroke* **33**: 2270–2278. (2003). Effects of implantation site of dead stem cells in rats with stroke damage. *NeuroReport* **24**: 39–42.

Modo, M., Mellodew, K., Cash, D. *et al.* (2004). Mapping transplanted stem cell migration after a stroke: a serial, in vivo magnetic resonance imaging study. *Neuroimage* **21**: 311–317.

Nakatomi, H., Kuriu, T., Okabe, S., *et al.* (2002). Regeneration of hippocampal pyramidal neurons after ischemic brain injury by recruitment of endogenous neural progenitors. *Cell* **110**: 429–441.

Nilsson, M., Perfilieva, E., Johansson, U., Orwar, O., and Eriksson, P. S. (1999). Enriched environment increases neurogenesis in the adult rat dentate gyrus and improves spatial memory. *J Neurobiol* **39**: 569–578.

Nowakowski, R. S. and Hayes, N. L. (2000). New neurons: extraordinary evidence or extra-ordinary conclusion? *Science* **288**: 771.

Nudo, R. J. (1999). Recovery after damage to motor cortical areas. *Curr Opin Neurobiol* **9**: 740–747.

Nudo, R. J., Wise, B. M., SiFuentes, F., and Milliken, G. W. (1996). Neural substrates for the effect of rehabilitative training on motor recovery after ischemic infarct. *Science* **272**: 1791–1794.

Ohlsson, A.-L. and Johansson, B. B. (1995). Environment influences functional outcome of cerebral infarction in rats. *Stroke* **26**: 644–649.

Palmer, T. D., Markakis, E. A., Willhoite, A. R., Safar, F., and Gage, F. H. (1999). Fibroblast growth factor-2 activates a latent neurogenic program in neural stem cells from diverse regions of the adult CNS. *J Neurosci* **19**: 8487–8497.

Papadopoulos, C. M., Tsai, S. Y., Alsbiei, T., *et al.* (2002). Functional recovery and neuroanatomical plasticity following middle cerebral artery occlusion and IN-1 antibody treatment in the adult rat. *Ann Neurol* **51**: 433–441.

Parent, J. M., Vexler, Z. S., Gong, C., Derugin, N., and Ferriero, D. M. (2002). Rat forebrain neurogenesis and striatal neuron replacement after focal stroke. *Ann Neurol* **52**: 802–813.

Petrovic, P., Kalso, E., Petersson, K. M., and Ingvar, M. (2002). Placebo and opioid analgesia: imaging a shared neuronal network. *Science* **295**: 1737–1740.

Pinaud, R., Penner, M. R., Robertson, H. A., and Currie, R. W. (2001). Upregulation of the immediate early gene arc in the brains of rats exposed to environmental enrichment: implications for molecular plasticity. *Brain Res Mol Brain Res* **91**: 50–56.

Plautz, E. J., Millikan, G. W., and Nudo, R. J. (2000). Effect of repetitive motor training on movement prepresentations in adult squirrel monkeys: role of use versus learning. *Neurobiol Learn Mem* **74**: 27–55.

Puurunen, K., Jolkkonen, J., Sieviö, J., Haapalinna, A., and Sivenius, J. (2001). Selegiline combined with enriched-environment housing attenuates spatial learning deficits following focal cerebral ischemia in rats. *Exp Neurol* **167**: 348–355.

Qu, M., Mittmann, T., Luhmann, H. J., and Schleicher, A. (1998). Long-term changes of ionotropic glutamate and GABA receptors after unilateral permanent focal cerebral ischemia in the mouse brain. *Neuroscience* **85**: 29–43.

Raff, M. (2003). Adult stem cell plasticity: fact or artifact. Ann Rev Cell Dev Biol **19**: 1–22.

Rakic, P. (2002). Neurogenesis in adult primate neocortex: an evaluation of the evidence. *Nat Neurosci* **3**: 65–71.

Redecker, C., Wang, W., Fritschy, J. B., and Witte, O. W. (2002). Widespread and long-lasting alterations in GABA(A)-receptor sybtypes after focal cortical infarcts in rats: mediation by NMDA-dependent processes. *J Cereb Blood Flow Metab* **22**: 1463–1475.

Reinecke, S., Lutzenburg, M., Hagemann, G., *et al.* (1999). Electrophysiological transcortical diaschisis after middle cerebral artery occlusion (MCAO) in rats. *Neurosci Lett* **261**: 85–88.

Risedal, A., Mattsson, B., Dahlqvist, P., *et al.* (2002). Environmental influences on functional outcome after a cortical infarct in the rat. *Brain Res Bull* **58**: 315–321.

Rosenzweig, M. R. (1966). Environmental complexity, cerebral change, and behavior. *Am Psychol* **21**: 321–332.

Rowntree, H. and Kolb, B. (1997). Blockade of basic fibroblast growth factor retards recovery from motor cortex injury in rats. *Eur J Neurosci* **9**: 2432–2442.

Savitz, S. I., Rosenbaum, D. M., Dinsmore, J. H., Wechsler, L. R., and Caplan, L. R. (2002). Cell transplantation for stroke. *Ann Neurol* **52**: 266–275.

Schmidt-Kastner, R., Zhang, B., Belayev, L., *et al.* (2002). DNA microarray analysis of cortical gene expression during early recirculation after focal brain ischemia in rat. *Mol Brain Res* **108**: 81–93

Schwab, M. E. (1990). Myelin-associated inhibitors of neurite growth and regeneration in the CNS. *Trends Neurosci* **13**: 452–456.

Seri, B., Carcia-Verdugo, J. M., McEwen, B., and Alvarez-Buylla, A. (2001). Astrocytes give rise to new neurons in the adult mammalian hippocampus. *J Neurosci* **21**: 71153–7160.

Sharp, F. R., Gonzalez, M. F., and Sagar, S. M. (1987). Fetal frontal cortex transplanted to injured motor/sensory cortex of adult rats. II: VIP-, somatostatin, and NPY-immunoreactive neurons. *J Neurosci* **7**: 3002–3015.

Shingo, T., Sorokan, S. T., Shimazaki, T., and Weiss, S. (2001). Erythropoietin regulates the in vitro and in vivo production of neuronal progenitors by mammalian forebrain neural stem cells. *J Neurosci* **21**: 9733–9743.

Sørensen, J.-C., Grabowski, M., Zimmer, J., and Johansson, B. B. (1996). Fetal neocortical tissue blocks implanted in brain infarcts of adult rats interconnect with the host brain. *Exp Neurol* **138**: 227–235.

Svoboda, K., Dent, W., Kleinfeld, D., and Tank, D. (1997). In vivo dendritic calcium dynamics in neocortical pyramidal neurons. *Nature* **385**: 161–165.

Tang, Y., Lu, A., Aronow, B. J., Wagner, K. R., and Sharp, F. R. (2002). Genomic responses of the brain to ischemic stroke, intracerebral haemorrhage, kainate seizures, hypoglycemia, and hypoxia. *Eur J Neurosci* **15**: 1937–5002.

Trapp, T., Erdö, F., Bührle, J., *et al.* (2002). Stem cells for the treatment of stroke: malignant transformation of homologous transplants. *Acta Neuropathol* **1004**: 527

Ullian, E. M., Sapperstein, S. K., Christopherson, K. S., and Barres, B. A. (2001). Control of synapse number by glia. *Science* **291**: 657–661.

van Praag, H., Schinder, A. F., Christie, B. R., *et al.* (2002). Functional neurogenesis in the adult hippocampus. *Nature* **415**: 1030–1034.

Volkmar, F. R. and Greenough, W. T. (1972). Rearing complexity affects branching of dendrites in the visual cortex of the rat. *Science* **176**: 1445–1447.

Wagers, A. J. and Weissman, I. L. (2004). Plasticity of adult stem cells. *Cell* **116**: 639–648.

Watkins, T. A. and Barres, B. A.(2002). Nerve generation: regrowth stumped by shared receptor. *Curr Biol* **12**: R654–656.

Wiessner, C., Bareyre, F. M., Allegrini, P. R., *et al.* (2003). Anti-Nogo-A antibody infusion 24 hours after experimental stroke improved behavioral outcome and corticospinal plasticity in normotensive and spontaneously hypertensive rats. *J Cereb Blood Flow Metab* **23**: 154–165.

Will, B. and Kelche, C. (1992). Environmental approaches to recovery of function from brain damage: a review of animal studies (1981–1991). In *Recovery from Brain Damage,* ed. F. D. Rose and D. A. Johnson. New York: Plenum, pp. 79–103.

Woodbury, D., Schwarz, E. J., Prockop, D. J., and Black, I. B. (2000). Adult rat and human bone marrow stromal cells differentiate into neurons. *J Neurosci Res* **61**: 364–370.

Xerri, C., Merzenich, M. M., Peterson, B. E., and Jenkins, W. M. (1998). Plasticity of primary somatosensory cortex paralleling sensorimotor skill recovery from stroke in adult monkeys. *J Neurophysiol* **79**: 2119–2148.

Yuguchi, T., Kohmura, E., Sakaki, T., *et al.* (1997). Expression of growth inhibitory factor mRNA after focal ischemia in rat brain. *J Cereb Blood Flow Metab* **17**: 745–752.

Zeng, J., Mattsson, B., Schulz, M., Johansson, B. B., and Sørensen, J. C. (2000). Expression of Zink-positive cells and terminals in fetal neocortical homografts to adult rat depends on lesion type and rearing conditions. *Exp Neurol* **164**: 176–183.

Zhang, G. Z., Chopp, M., Goussev, A., *et al.* (2001). Cerebral microvascular obstruction by fibrus is associated with upregulation of PAI-1 acutely after onset of focal embolic ischemia in rats. *J Neurosci* **19**: 10898–10907.

Zhang, Z. G., Jiang, Q., Zhang, R., *et al.* (2003). Magnetic resonance imaging and neurosphere therapy of stroke in rat. *Ann Neurol* **53**: 259–263.

Zhao, L. R., Mattsson, B., and Johansson, B. B. (2000). Environmental influence on brain-derived neurotrophic factor messenger RNA expression after middle cerebral artery occlusion in spontaneously hypertensive rats. *Neuroscience* **97**: 177–184.

Zhao, L. R., Rosedl, A., Wojcik, A., *et al.* (2001). Enriched environment influences brain-derived neurotrophic factor levels in rat forebrain after focal stroke. *Neurosci Lett* **305**: 169–172.

4

Cerebral reorganization after sensorimotor stroke

Rüdiger J. Seitz

University Hospital Düsseldorf, Düsseldorf, Germany

Introduction

Stroke can interfere with every single capacity of the human brain. Many patients experience transient deficits that disappear within 24 hours (Hennerici *et al.*, 1988) or suffer from slight or moderate hemiparesis that regresses completely within a couple of days (Donnan *et al.*, 1991; Duncan *et al.*, 1992). Of the patients with severe completed stroke, approximately 50% recover from hemiparesis (Heinemann *et al.*, 1987; Gresham *et al.*, 1998). In most of these patients, recovery takes place within the first four weeks after infarction, usually starting with shoulder and synergistic arm–hand movements (Donnan *et al.*, 1991; Duncan *et al.*, 1992; Katrak *et al.*, 1998). In subcortical infarctions, functional restoration may be slower, continuing over several years (Fries *et al.*, 1993; Manto *et al.*, 1995). This suggests that a variety of mechanisms may be involved in the restoration of motor functions after brain infarction. Also, clinically undetected white matter changes and the prevalence of silent stroke lesions in patients presenting with the symptoms of acute stroke affect the cognitive and attention state of patients and their capacity to recover (Kase *et al.*, 1989; Sultzer *et al.*, 1995; van Zagten *et al.*, 1996). Therefore, the challenging aspect in each stroke patient is the question to what degree he or she will recover. To monitor recovery, the importance of an adequate assessment of the functional deficit and of the disability level of daily activities has increasingly been recognized (Duncan *et al.*, 2000), since correlation with the tissue perfusion state, the recruitment of peri-lesional and remote areas during functional activation, and changes of cortical excitability, as assessed with transcranial magnetic stimulation (TMS), will provide the basis for an evaluation of the recovery mechanisms and of the efficacy of new therapeutic interventions that have been or will be introduced into clinical use.

Neurological recovery is thought to be the behavioral equivalent to post-lesional cerebral reorganization. However, recovery may be differentiated into spontaneous recovery occurring early after stroke and induced recovery occurring later as

Recovery after Stroke, ed. Michael P. Barnes, Bruce H. Dobkin and Julien Bogousslavsky. Published by Cambridge University Press. © Cambridge University Press 2005.

a result of dedicated physiotherapeutic approaches. Since most of the recovery takes place early after stroke, a major question regarding the underlying mechanisms is how far the restitution of tissue function is mediated by reorganization of the residual neural network. Today's non-invasive investigation techniques provide the means to explore the living human brain for processes related to normal behavior and cerebral reorganization. Neuroimaging with positron emission tomography (PET) and functional magnetic resonance imaging (fMRI) allows investigators to map the cerebral structures that participate in the execution of an experimental task or in producing a certain function. Specifically, PET and fMRI have been employed for studying normal brain function, including brain plasticity related to normal learning (see Toga and Mazziotta, 2000). More recently, PET and fMRI have also been used to study the reorganization of functional representations in relation to recovery from human brain diseases, including ischemic stroke. Similar to other disease conditions, such as psychosis, it is important to study stroke patients with tasks they can perform (Price and Friston, 1999), since the activation patterns are heavily influenced both by the disease-related brain damage and the secondary behavioral changes, which may obscure the task-specific activation patterns. In addition, TMS has recently been advanced as a technique to probe the mechanisms and the specificity of cortical activation areas as demonstrated with functional imaging (Jahanshahi and Rothwell, 2000). Originally, TMS provided a means to study the human corticospinal motor output system and changes in the maps of cortical excitability related to training in healthy volunteers and to abnormalities from brain diseases such as stroke. More recently, however, paired-pulse TMS has provided a means to analyze the disease-related changes of cortical excitability that may underlie abnormal brain activation as in recovery after stroke. In addition, "artificial reversible brain lesions" can be introduced with repetitive TMS, which allows investigators to probe the specific role of a cortical area for a given behavioral task (Jahanshahi and Rothwell, 2000).

The pioneering work of Merzenich and colleagues (see Merzenich and Sameshima, 2000) demonstrated that reorganization can take place in the adult nervous system. In classical experiments, the overuse or disuse of particular inputs was shown to lead to an increase or decrease, respectively, of the corresponding cortical representations. The pivotal question for restorative neurology of whether such plasticity also operates after cortical damage was answered by specific ablation experiments. For example, destruction of areas 1, 2 and 3 in the hand area of primary somatosensory cortex of the monkey (SI) has been shown to lead to an immediate unresponsiveness of the hand representation in SII, the second somatosensory cortex, a functionally related but distinct cooperative area (Pons *et al.*, 1988). Twenty-four hours later, the formally unresponsive hand area was occupied by a foot representation. Further, Nudo *et al.* (1996) observed that the cortical finger representations adjacent to partly damaged finger representations became enlarged in monkeys during rehabilitative treatment, while they remained unchanged in monkeys not subjected to such treatment. In experiments of this type, evidence was provided showing that reorganization occurs in the adult nervous system both adjacent to focal brain damage, leading to plastic changes of the representation within the affected system, as well as remote from the lesion in related systems (Witte *et al.*, 2000).

This chapter on cerebral reorganization after sensorimotor stroke will focus on representational plasticity, reorganization of neural networks beyond the peri-lesional area, and strategies for rehabilitative interventions as investigated in humans with fMRI and TMS.

Representational plasticity

Representational plasticity refers to reorganization of a cortical representation within a given functional brain system. It has been assumed that the changes of cortical representation occur by a Hebbian strengthening of neuronal synapses, enabling improved performance. Since it was shown by functional imaging that motor learning induced an enlargement of the cortical activation area (Schlaug *et al.*, 1994; Karni *et al.*, 1995) and by TMS that cortical excitability increased upon task acquisition (Pascual-Leone *et al.*, 1994, 1995), it should be possible to study representational plasticity in the human brain in diseases such as stroke.

Functional imaging

In patients with a transient functional impairment, as in a transient ischemic attack, recovery may result from restitution of tissue function after short-lasting ischemia or from reorganization adjacent to a small brain lesion within the remaining functional network. These mechanisms can now be studied in humans with MRI techniques such as perfusion imaging (PI) and diffusion-weighted imaging (DWI). Interruption of circulation by cerebral artery occlusion induces immediate changes in cerebral electrical activity, with a perinfarct depolarization resulting in repeated episodes of metabolic stress, growth of the infarction from 4 to 24 hours post-occlusion, and characteristic lesion patterns (Heiss *et al.*, 1992; Mohr *et al.*, 1993; Hossmann *et al.*, 1994; Lee *et al.*, 2000; Li *et al.*, 2000). Clinically, a middle cerebral artery (MCA) occlusion becomes manifest by con-tralateral hemiplegia within 60 seconds (Brunberg *et al.*, 1992). During ischemia, the thresholds for selective neuronal and tissue necrosis are a function of regional cerebral blood flow (rCBF) reduction (Hossmann, 1994). As evident from PI and DWI, during stroke evolution the hypoperfused area is typically larger than the

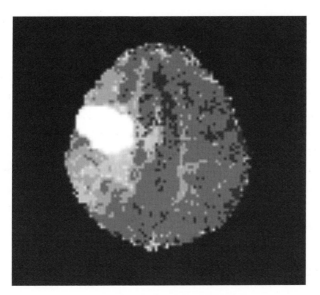

Fig. 4.1   The mismatch between images obtained with perfusion imaging (PI) and diffusion-weighted imaging (DWI) within five hours after stroke onset. The circumscribed stroke lesion shown in the DWI map (white) is superimposed onto the time-to-peak PI map, which indicates a critically delayed arrival of the intravenous gadolinium bolus in the brain (bright gray). Right in the image corresponds to left in the patient.

lession detected by DWI, resulting in a prominent PI–DWI mismatch (Lovblad *et al.*, 1997; Rordorf *et al.*, 1998; Tong *et al.*, 1998; Neumann-Haefelin *et al.*, 1999; Wittsack *et al.*, 2002). This is illustrated in Fig. 4.1. Accordingly, recovery may well be the consequence of reperfusion. Large areas of the brain may become functional again with a restricted functional deficit that is identified as a DWI lesion. Usually, recanalization of the occluded cerebral artery leads to partial restoration of perfusion within 24 hours (Hakim *et al.*, 1987; Heiss *et al.*, 1997). Moreover, good leptomeningeal collaterals and early recanalization of MCA occlusion, in particular during thrombolytic therapy, critically increase the chances of functional restitution with favorable clinical outcome (Ringelstein *et al.*, 1992; Toni *et al.*, 1997, 1998). This view is supported by functional imaging (Heiss *et al.*, 1998a; Kidwell *et al.*, 2000) and monitoring with MRI and transcranial Doppler sonography (Alexandrov *et al.*, 2000, 2001). Therefore, recovery of function in brain infarction is critically determined by the spatial extent and duration of severe ischemia. While hemiplegia and depression of rCBF produced by temporary carotid artery balloon occlusion have been shown to normalize completely with 15 minutes (Brunberg *et al.*, 1992), hyperglycemia adds to brain damage even in early reperfusion after thrombolysis (Els *et al.*, 2002; Parsons *et al.*, 2002). Consequently, tissue recovery seems to be a relatively fast process. In

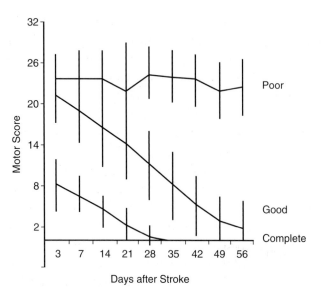

Fig. 4.2   Post-stroke recovery irrespective of cortical and subcortical lesion location. Less-severely affected patients recover within 30 days (complete recovery). Severely affected patients may show negligible recovery (recovery) or recover with a similar temporal dynamic (good recovery). (Data from Binkofski *et al.*, 2001a.)

contrast, recovery through representational plasticity has a far longer time course, typically lasting for weeks. As shown in Fig. 4.2, the protracted recovery from hemiparesis follows the same time course in patients who are affected by both slight and severe strokes, suggesting that similar processes may underlie their functional restitution.

In human stroke, the area of compromised perfusion is considerably larger than the manifest ischemic brain lesion (Fig. 4.1). Therefore, hypothesized reorganiza- tion processes at the border of the manifest ischemic brain lesion will take place in brain tissue that was critically compromised in terms of blood supply but remained structurally intact. Notably, persisting metabolic abnormalities beyond the necrotic core of brain infarction, but within the affected perfusion area, are probably the result of selective ischemic nerve cell damage in the presence of viable glia (Heiss *et al.*, 1992; Weiller *et al.*, 1990; Seitz *et al.*, 1994). This implies that a chronic structural brain lesion as evident in computed tomographic and MRI studies reflects only a portion of the total amount of brain tissue affected in the acute stage of brain infarction. MRI-based in vivo morphometry has shown that profound atrophy of peri-lesional brain tissue develops secondary to ischemic brain infarction (Ritzl *et al.*, 2004; Kraemer, 2004). Consequently, the neuronal loss after transient ischemia significantly exceeds the area of a DWI-detected abnormality (Li *et al.*, 2000). Since lesion volume alone is not sufficient to determine the degree of recovery, lesion location within the affected hemisphere and location in the right versus left hemisphere are important determinants for post-stroke recovery (DiPiero *et al.*, 1992; Sunderland *et al.*, 1994; Pedersen *et al.*, 1998; Chen *et al.*, 2000; Binkofski *et al.*, 2001a). This point is well illustrated by the famous case described by Foerster (1936). This patient underwent ablation of motor cortex for intractable focal epilepsy and later, at autopsy, showed complete unilateral pyramidal tract degeneration. He had regained the capacity to lift his arm straight over his head and to hold a pen. However, his fractionated finger movements remained severely handicapped. Similar evidence for the important role of the pyramidal tract for motor recovery was obtained from morphometric measurements, which revealed a good correlation of neurological impairment and extent of pyramidal tract damage, as well as from MR diffusion tensor imaging (Warabi *et al.*, 1990; Fukui *et al.*, 1994; Binkofski *et al.*, 1996; Werring *et al.*, 1998).

Functional imaging studies in patients who had recovered from their first hemiparetic stroke involving the internal capsule and the basal ganglia consistently showed enlarged areas of activation in the cortical areas in the affected cerebral hemisphere during movement activity of the affected hand (Chollet *et al.*, 1991; Weiller *et al.*, 1992; Marshall *et al.*, 2000). The magnitude of the rCBF increase in the partially damaged motor cortex was as high as that normally detected and so was not a function of the cortical decrease in rCBF at rest and probably corresponded to the normal motor evoked potential (MEP) in the affected hand (Weder and Seitz, 1994; Weder *et al.*, 1994). Therefore, there are good reasons to believe that the motor cortex of the affected hemisphere was actively involved in task performance in these patients who had recovered from subcortical stroke.

In contrast, after recovery from hemiparetic stroke in the MCA territory with predominant involvement of the cortex in the pericentral area, there was a lack of activation in motor cortex and SI, although the corticospinal tract and the afferent somatosensory tract were largely functional as assessed by evoked potential and metabolic studies (DiPiero *et al.*, 1992; Seitz *et al.*, 1998). No rCBF changes related to finger movements of the affected hand were observed in sensorimotor cortex adjacent to the stroke lesion using PET in the chronic phase. Also, fMRI showed only minute activation of areas related to sensorimotor activity just adjacent to the lesion (Fig. 4.3). While these activation areas were still present in the acute phase after focal ischemia, they were far less prominent and markedly displaced in the subacute stage after stroke. Similarly, diminished rCBF increases following sensorimotor stimulation have been reported after transient ischemic attacks and subcortical stroke (Powers *et al.*, 1988; Weder and Seitz, 1994). Possibly, these observations corresponded to the reported uncoupling of rCBF (no response) and regional cerebral glucose metabolism (persistent response),

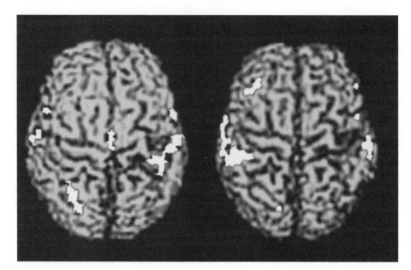

Fig. 4.3   Activation pattern in left sensorimotor infarction is shown during tactile exploration of a complex geometrical object after a first ischemic stroke with the affected hand in the acute (left) and subacute stage (right) as obtained with functional magnetic resonance imaging. Note the prominent peri-lesional activation in the initial scan and the lateral displacement of the reduced postcentral activation in the follow-up scan. Simultaneously, the activation in the homologue area in the contralesional hemisphere and in left premotor and right prefrontal cortex were increased. (Further details in Binkofski and Seitz, 2004.)

which has been explained by an ischemia-induced inhibition of the neuronal nitric oxide synthetase (Cholet *et al.*, 1997). In contrast, subjects with brain tumors in the precentral gyrus had a peri-lesional hand representation (Seitz *et al.*, 1995; Wunderlich *et al.*, 1998) with lateral displacement of the region of activation areas. A systematic posterior shift of the activation after recovery from stroke has been observed in other studies (Pineiro *et al.*, 2001; Carey *et al.*, 2002). Interestingly, activations related to sensorimotor activity occurred in somatosensory cortex after motor cortex infarction, and activation in motor cortex occurred after infarction of somatosensory cortex (Cramer *et al.*, 2001). Apart from their divergence concerning the direction of functional displacement, these data suggest local reorganization of the cortical representation through employment of the plastic capacity of the underlying peri-lesional neural machinery (Seitz and Azari, 1999). Event-related fMRI was used to investigate the time course of activation in motor cortex after a right subcortical stroke (Newton *et al.*, 2002). The major observation was that the hemodynamic response was delayed, particularly in the right motor cortex during activity of the paretic contralateral left hand (Fig. 4.4). In contrast, the hemodynamic response was well timed in the left motor cortex, as it was in both hemispheres in healthy subjects. One may speculate that this

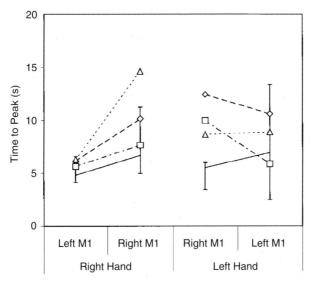

Fig. 4.4   Retarded hemodynamic response in right motor cortex during left-hand activity in three patients (broken lines) after right striatocapsular infarction. Note that during activity with the non-affected right hand, the hemodynamic response in the left motor cortex was as well timed as in young healthy subjects (continuous line is median value with bar indicating range). In healthy subjects, the ipsilateral motor response was slightly delayed and far less time locked than in the motor cortex contralateral to the acting arm. (From Newton *et al.* (2002) with permission.)

impairment of hemodynamics in the patients resulted from changes in the supplying artery, abnormalities of hemodynamic signaling, or from both augmenting the hemodynamic–electrical decoupling.

Transcranial magnetic stimulation

One of the most important factors influencing motor recovery appears to be the integrity of the pyramidal motor output system (see above). Physiological evidence of the importance of the pyramidal output system for motor recovery in humans has been obtained from TMS, which showed that, in the acute stage and also two months after stroke, absence of MEPs and somatosensory evoked potentials was related to poor motor recovery after stroke (Macdonell *et al.*, 1989; Dominkus *et al.*, 1990; Heald *et al.*, 1993; Stephan *et al.*, 1995a). Conversely, it was shown that the reduction of corticospinal tract affection during the first four weeks after stroke was related in a quantitative manner to the increase of MEP amplitudes and clinical motor recovery (Binkofski *et al.*, 1996). It should be emphasized, however, that cerebral infarction results in changes of the motor threshold of the MEPs. A severely enhanced threshold was shown to predict poor motor recovery as early as 24 hours after stroke (Nardone and Tezzon, 2002). Also,

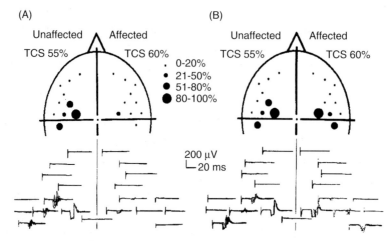

Fig. 4.5   Reoccurrence of motor evoked potentials after recovery from hemispheric middle cerebral artery infarction. Recovery was associated with a symmetrical map without anomalous additional activation sites. (A) Measurement performed in the subacute stage (after day 30); (B) Follow-up measurement after an additional eight weeks of rehabilitative training. (From Traversa *et al.* (1997) with permission.)

a prolonged silent period may lead to the clinical symptom of paresis (Classen *et al.*, 1997). Upon recovery, the MEPs reoccurred first in the proximal muscles and later in the distal hand muscles, approaching normal values of amplitude and central conduction times in parallel to the clinical pattern of recovery (Colebatch and Gandevia, 1989). Notably, the patterns and cerebral locations of the most effective stimulation sites of MEPs in patients who have recovered from cortical infarction upon rehabilitative training were not distinguishable from those in patients who had recovered from subcortical cortical infarction (Traversa *et al.*, 1997) (Fig. 4.5). These findings show that, both in subcortical and cortical brain infarctions, motor cortex-regained functionality after stroke accounted for clinical recovery.

These findings support the notion that beyond the structural lesion there is a peri-lesional zone that is functionally abnormal soon after focal brain damage. Indeed, there is plenty of evidence from experimental studies showing that the peri-lesional zone after focal ischemia is grossly abnormal. This does not simply refer to the concept of penumbra, which has been defined as tissue at risk to undergo ischemic tissue damage during the first minutes and hours after the insult. Rather, the peri-lesional zone accommodates persistent and severe changes in tissue function in a surprisingly large area surrounding a lesion (Witte *et al.*, 2000). In the photothrombosis model in the rat, small focal cortical lesions led to peri-lesional changes that could be monitored by electrophysiological, anatomical, and audioradiographic methods. Specifically, it was found that the stimulation threshold increased while simultaneously the intracortical inhibition decreased, leading to distinctly altered spontaneous activity and stimulus response characteristics within the affected hemisphere (Witte *et al.*, 2000). In close accordance, receptor studies revealed a diversified pattern of altered gamma-aminobutyric acid (GABA) receptor expression, which initially resembled the juvenile expression pattern (Schiene *et al.*, 1996; Hagemann *et al.*, 1998). In addition, glutamate receptor densities increased. These changes persisted over many weeks. The implications of these prolonged changes for functional restoration and the cooperation of the peri-lesional region with the remaining network is as yet unknown.

Owing to the multifold effects on cortex initiated by ischemia, both enhanced inhibition and disinhibition have been shown to develop in a spatially distinct manner and with a defined time course (Witte *et al.*, 2000). In humans, enhanced inhibition, shown by TMS studies, occurred after extensive ischemia of premotor or parietal cortex in addition to motor cortex, resulting in hemiparesis (Classen *et al.*, 1997; Hauptmann *et al.*, 1997; Nardone and Tezzon, 2002). This inhibition regressed in parallel with clinical recovery. Similarly, experimental studies in rats showed that cortical ischemia impaired synaptic transmission, while the direct wave of MEPs and the early potential of somatosensory evoked potentials promptly recovered, suggesting functional efferent and afferent tracts (Bolay and Dalkara, 1998). Conversely, disinhibition occurred after circumscribed infarction within motor cortex, demonstrated by a shortened silent period after TMS (Schnitzler and Benecke, 1994; von Giesen *et al.*, 1994). This disinhibition may provide a path for post-lesional reorganization. Indeed, in such patients, paired TMS revealed disinhibition of the residual cerebral cortex, which was associated with clinical recovery (Liepert *et al.*, 2000; Butefisch *et al.*, 2004).

Unfortunately, the peri-lesional area cannot be visualized by MRI methods even at high field strengths (7 Tesla) and when peri-lesional electrophysiological, audioradiographic, and metabolic patterns are grossly abnormal (Schroeter and Hoehn, 2000). Rather, decreased labeling of the $GABA_B$ receptor by PET imaging indicates irreversibly damaged brain tissue (Sette *et al.*, 1993; Hatazawa *et al.*, 1995; Hayashida *et al.*, 1996; Takahashi *et al.*, 1997; Heiss *et al.*, 1998b). Therefore, the excitability changes shown with TMS to characterize the peri-lesional changes in humans suggest profound physiological alterations that are elusive to modern neuroimaging.

Reorganization of neural networks

Functional imaging

There is clinical evidence showing that the motor system in the contralesional hemisphere plays an important role for deficit compensation in postischemic reorganization (Fisher, 1992). Chollet *et al.* (1991) were the first to show contrale-sional motor cortex activation in brain lesions acquired in adulthood, using PET; this was replicated by Cao *et al.* (1998) using fMRI. One aspect of this contrale-sional activation was that those patients who exhibited significant rCBF increases in motor cortex contralateral to the cerebral infarction had associated movements of the non-affected hand (Weiller *et al.*, 1993). This corresponded to electromyo-graphic findings in healthy subjects, in whom effort, force, and activity with the non-dominant hand were accompanied by increased muscle activity in the homologous muscles contralateral to the moving hand (Durwen and Herzog, 1989, 1992). Notably, the associated rCBF increases in the motor cortex of the non-affected hemisphere occurred in those patients with limited recovery (Weder *et al.*, 1994; Weiller *et al.*, 1993). Nevertheless, fMRI showed that the ipsilateral activation did not occur in a strictly homoguous location compared with the contralateral motor cortical representation but in different locations along the contralesional motor cortex (Cramer *et al.*, 1999). One may argue that recovery was brought about by recruitment of ipsilateral corticospinal projections (Benecke *et al.*, 1991; Farmer *et al.*, 1991; Carr *et al.*, 1993; Lewine *et al.*, 1994). Usually, this leads to initial recovery of proximal movements compared with the later recovery of distal movements (Colebatch and Gandevia, 1989; Lemon *et al.*, 1996). Conversely, there is an ipsilateral impairment of forearm function in the acute stage after stroke (Jones *et al.*, 1989). Similarly, active and passive sensorimotor tasks were reported to show a largely bilateral activation pattern as recovery progressed (Calautti *et al.*, 2001a; Nelles *et al.*, 2001). Remarkably, more sym-metric activations were associated with greater white matter loss and a worse clinical outcome (Rossini *et al.*, 1998a; Reddy *et al.*, 2002).

The situation is different in congenital hemispheric brain lesions involving the pre- and postcentral gyrus. In these patients, motor function in the contralateral hand may be remarkable and even allows for independent finger movements (Muller *et al.*, 1991). Sabatini *et al.* (1994) reported a patient presenting 19 years after a large porencephalic lesion in the area of the right MCA, in whom rCBF increases were confined to the motor cortex of the non-affected hemisphere during finger movements of either hand. Electrophysiological support for such findings was obtained in patients with congenital hemiplegic palsy and hemi-spherectomy, showing unmasking of ipsilateral corticospinal motor projections that are usually not excitable in healthy people (Benecke *et al.*, 1991; Farmer *et al.*, 1991; Carr *et al.*, 1993). It should be stressed, however, that these observations were obtained many years after birth and hemispherectomy, respectively. One can, therefore, postulate that in these patients the cortical reorganization mediating recovery of motor functions had occurred very early in life and had sufficient time to develop. For comparison, with respect to the limited post-lesional changes in

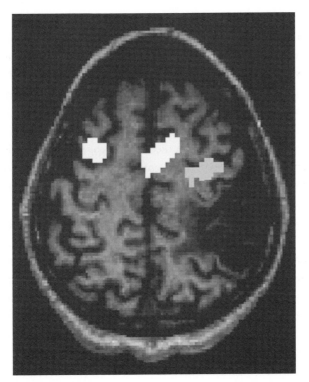

Fig. 4.6   Abnormal activations in patients who have recovered from their first brain infarction involving the middle cerebral artery territory as demonstrated with positron emission tomography. The patients had activations of bilateral premotor cortex and of the supplementary motor area. The white shaded activations in the supplementary motor area and contralesional premotor cortex constituted a network that was relevant for higher motor control in the patients and healthy subjects. (From Seitz *et al.*, 1998.)

adult rats compared with neonatal lesions (Kossut *et al.*, 1988), it appears likely that the capacity for cerebral reorganization of the focally damaged brain, as for instance after stroke, may be less extensive.

Individual and group data analysis in patients recovering from stroke demonstrated that, in addition to motor cortex activation, rCBF increases related to sensorimotor activity of the affected limb occurred in premotor and frontomesial cortical areas of both cerebral hemispheres (Weiller *et al.*, 1993; Weder *et al.*, 1994; Honda *et al.*, 1997). This is illustrated in Fig. 4.6. These findings suggested involvement of bihemispheric cortical areas related to sensorimotor activity during motor restitution. Analysis of imaging data in individual patients revealed large differences of the activation patterns that could be caused by differences in individual lesion location and extent, differences in performance, or, possibly, interindividual functional variability (Weiller *et al.*, 1993; Weder *et al.*, 1994; Cramer *et al.*,

1997). Group data from patients with fairly homogeneous infarct types and lesions, however, provided more consistent data concerning post-lesional activation patterns. The dorsal premotor cortex in the affected hemisphere was more active after prolonged recovery than early after stroke (Calautti et al., 2001b). This area seemed to coincide with a premotor cortical area being more active in elderly than in young subjects during sensorimotor activity (Calautti et al., 2001c). In contrast, in single-movement tasks involving only one digit rather than multiple fingers, the premotor cortex did not become engaged (Carey et al., 2001). Nevertheless, the contralateral premotor cortex is of particular importance for control of temporally or sequentially complex finger movements, as evident in learning, motor adaptation, and post-stroke recovery (Deecke, 1990; Seitz et al., 1999; Stephan et al., 2002). Recently, in patients who had recovered from stroke, inhibition of the contralesional premotor cortex was associated with an impairment of motor performance (Johansen-Berg, 2002). Furthermore, stroke patients who had involvement of premotor cortex exhibited an additional motor deficit that was associated with poorer outcomes (Miyai et al., 1999; Freund and Hummelsheim, 1985). Consequently, evidence is accumulating that points to the important role of the dorsal premotor cortex for recovery after hemiparetic stroke.

In contrast to patients with cortical MCA infarctions, there was relatively little activation in the frontomesial cortex including the supplementary motor area (SMA) in patients who had recovered from striatocapsular infarction (Weder et al., 1994; Dettmers et al., 1997). Activation of the SMA probably corresponded to the initiative role of this area in movement control (Jahanshahi et al., 1995; MacKinnon et al., 1996). From longitudinal studies on recovery from hemispheric stroke, it became apparent that activity of the SMA was enhanced early after stroke but declined as learning proceeded (Carey et al., 2001, 2002). The lack of SMA activation in the striatocapsular infarctions probably resulted from damage to the corticospinal projection from the SMA to the basal ganglia by the infarct. These patients appeared to activate, instead, the contralesional premotor cortex (Weder et al., 1994) underscoring the impact of lesion location for the activation pattern related to sensorimotor recovery.

In this connection, it is noteworthy that a combined activation of the SMA and parietal cortex was shown to be related to the exertion of force (Dettmers et al., 1995). It is reasonable to assume that parietal activation reflects reorganization of the sensorimotor system to meet the task demands of the sensorimotor activation paradigm. In accordance with this interpretation, a contralesional activation of the anterior parietal cortex after stroke was reported in relation to both active somatosensory object discrimination and passive arm movements (Seitz et al., 1998; Nelles et al., 1999). Further, kinematic evidence showed that patients with parietal cortex lesions retained abnormal finger movements when required to explore macrogeometric objects after recovery from hemiparesis (Binkofski *et al.*, 2001b). Therefore, the rCBF increases in the contralesional parietal cortical regions during somatosensory discrimination of macrogeometric objects (Seitz *et al.*, 1998) were probably related to deficit compensation. Notably, they occurred in an area that in normal subjects seems to participate in voluntarily controlled forelimb movement (Seitz *et al.*, 1997; Binkofski *et al.*, 1999). In addition, there was abnormal prefrontal cortex activation, suggesting enhanced cognitive control for a task that is relatively difficult for patients after stroke compared with healthy subjects (Seitz *et al.*, 1998; Calautti *et al.*, 2001b). Continued training with passive arm movements enhanced the bilateral activation of the cortex along the intraparietal sulcus and premotor cortex even further (Nelles *et al.*, 2001). Since the parietal region subserves sensorimotor integration and is heavily interwoven with executive functions mediated in the frontal motor cortical areas, these data emphasize the importance of the non-affected hemisphere for post-stroke recovery of sensorimotor functions.

Recovery from hemiplegia may also be connected with activation of other parts of the sensorimotor circuitry. Similar to activation of the lower premotor cortical areas in recovery from aphasia (Knopman *et al.*, 1984; Karbe *et al.*, 1995; Weiller *et al.*, 1995), there was inferior frontal cortex activation ipsilateral to the moving hand during execution of fast and sequential finger movements with the recovered hand (Weiller *et al.*, 1993; Seitz *et al.*, 1998). Since this area was activated in healthy subjects during learning of finger movement sequences (Jenkins *et al.*, 1994; Schlaug *et al.*, 1994) but not after skill acquisition (Seitz and Roland, 1992), it represents a key area for establishing a motor program. Probably, this function is mediated by the property of this area to relate perception of gestures to body movements (Bonda *et al.*, 1995; Parsons *et al.*, 1995; Decety *et al.*, 1997; Binkofski *et al.*, 2000).

More recently, relation of the dynamics of the cerebral activation maps with the course of motor recovery has been studied. Complex modulations of activity that were determined by the lesion were found. For example, areas showing progressively increasing or sustained activity were located in contralesional prefrontal and premotor cortex as well as in the contralesional cerebellum (Calautti *et al.*, 2001a; Feydy *et al.*, 2002; Fraser *et al.*, 2002; Small *et al.*, 2002). Conversely, areas in the contralesional hemisphere were reported to become progressively less engaged when motor cortex was spared (Feydy *et al.*, 2002). However, patients with poor recovery showed far less cortical and cerebellar activation (Carey *et al.*, 2002; Small *et al.*, 2002). These last observations are of particular relevance, since they emphasize that the cerebellar route participates critically in motor recovery, supporting earlier observations (Azari *et al.*, 1996). Further, patients with poor recovery did not seem to activate the motor system endogenously, which contrasts with motor imagery in healthy subjects (Stephan *et al.*, 1995b; Decety *et al.*, 1997; Binkofski *et al.*, 2000; Lafleur *et al.*, 2002). Nevertheless, the changes in patients who recovered well reflected more or less the pattern in recovery brought about by dedicated physiotherapy. Initial studies using constraint-induced movement therapy or bilateral movement training basically seemed to replicate the activation patterns during spontaneous recovery (Levy *et al.*, 2001; Staines *et al.*, 2001; Carey *et al.*, 2002).

Apart from recovery mediated within the original sensorimotor domain, shifts in the strategy of task performance have to be considered. These included the resumption of abnormal movement patterns (Friel and Nudo, 1998) as well as abnormal movement guidance. For example, monkeys with focal ischemic lesions in motor cortex visually inspected their hand when retrieving objects with the affected hand (Nudo *et al.*, 2000). In humans, it was observed that patients who had recovered from ischemic stroke differed significantly from healthy controls by the recruitment of a predominantly contralesional network, involving visual cortical areas, prefrontal cortex, thalamus, hippocampus, and cerebellum, during the blindfolded performance of sequential finger movements (Seitz *et al.*, 1999). Greater expression of this cortical–subcortical network correlated with a more severe sensorimotor deficit in the acute stage after stroke, reflecting its greater role for post-stroke recovery. Thus, a visuomotor brain system appeared to compensate a sensorimotor deficit in patients who had recovered from hemiparetic stroke. This observation corresponded to animal models of focal brain lesions and to the developing human visual and auditory systems (Clark and Delay, 1991; Cohen *et al.*, 1997; Neville and Bavelier, 1998; Sadato *et al.*, 1998), suggesting that post-lesional reorganization involves a network usually not active in sensorimotor activity.

In addition, it was shown that the lesion-affected and the recovery-related network in stroke patients shared the same structures in the contralesional thalamus and bilateral visual association areas (Seitz *et al.*, 1999). Therefore, these sharing structures accommodated simultaneously passive lesion effects and active recovery-related changes in locations remote to the site of the brain infarction. This observation corresponded to the original conception of diaschisis as a restorative mechanism in functional recovery. That is, recovery was mediated by areas that had regained activity after initial inhibition by a distant brain lesion (von Monakow, 1914). Thus, post-lesional reorganization was not only effective in the peri-lesional vicinity but appeared as a task-related rewiring of intrinsic cerebral networks (Seitz and Azari, 1999). Similar conclusions have also been proposed for psychologically impaired patients (Price and Friston, 1999). As evidenced by activation studies in patients who had recovered from hemiplegic stroke, such

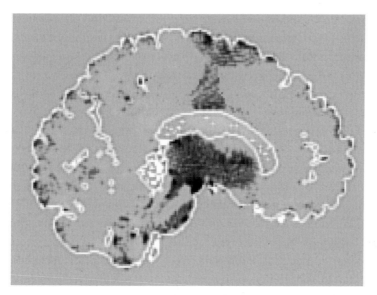

Fig. 4.7   Brain atrophy as shown by voxel-guided morphometry after first hemispheric brain infarction. In this sagittal image, the cortical lesion is shown as well as the affected areas in the corpus callosum, the ipsilesional thalamus, and the pons. Outlined are the inner and outer cerebral surface of the patient. (Further details in Kraemer (2004).)

unused, but functionally related, pathways may take on back-up or facilatatory functions (Chollet *et al.*, 1991; Ringelstein *et al.*, 1992; Weiller *et al.*, 1993; Weder *et al.*, 1994). Even in patients with congenital or developmental brain diseases, these pathways may become engaged as alternative neural routes (Benecke *et al.*, 1991; Farmer *et al.*, 1991; Carr *et al.*, 1993; Sabatini *et al.*, 1994). From a phenomenological point of view, these patients show a temporary loss of function caused by the brain damage with reappearance of the transiently compromised function after some time. Likewise, disturbances of complex motor behavior such as neglect and limb kinetic apraxia also tend to disappear with time (Freund and Hummelsheim, 1985; Heilman *et al.*, 1985). As yet, however, it is unclear how long this period of disturbed function lasts.

The network action for stroke recovery is surprising in view of the widespread atrophy of the brain secondary to brain infarction (Ritzl *et al.*, 2004; Kraemer, 2004). As illustrated in Fig. 4.7, voxel-guided morphometry is able to detect brain atrophy beyond the infarct lesion that involves remote brain structures in the contralesional cerebral hemisphere, the thalamus, and the contralesional cerebellum. Notably, the atrophy in the corpus callosum would suggest that these atrophic changes may result from nerve fiber degeneration and ensuing denervation. Accordingly, these secondary structural changes follow the same patterns as the abnormal remote activations observed in stroke recovery. Therefore, there is an apparent discrepancy between the beneficial role of the connected areas for post-stroke recovery and their liability to secondary tissue shrinkage. If, however, both paths follow identical routes, they may indicate the limits of possible recovery, particularly in recurring brain lesions.

Transcranial magnetic stimulation

The rCBF increases in relation to sensorimotor activity of the affected hand in the contralesional motor cortex were in accordance with the presence of ipsilateral MEPs in such patients (Turton *et al.*, 1996; Netz *et al.*, 1997). It may be argued that they reflected an unmasking of ipsilateral corticospinal projections in relation to heightened effort and action with the affected hand (Durwen and Herzog, 1989, 1992). It has been known for many years that associated finger movements can occur in hemiparesis (Zülch and Müller, 1969). Typically, their onset is significantly shorter than those evoked by intense effort of the normal hand (Hopf *et al.*, 1974). It is possible that these movements are mediated by exposure of the zone in the motor cortex that has been shown in the monkey to be involved in bilateral hand movements (Aizawa *et al.*, 1990). Recently, an area in left motor cortex was found from which ipsilateral MEPs could be elicited (Caramia *et al.*, 2000). Others argue that the ipsilateral MEPs originate from hyperexcitable premotor cortex in stroke patients (Alagona *et al.*, 2001). Nevertheless, the persistence of ipsilateral MEPs after stroke was related to poor recovery (Fig. 4.8), which would be compatible with cortical hyperactivity related to movement of the affected hand.

To elucidate the mechanisms possibly mediating the abnormal activity in motor cortex of the unaffected hemisphere, studies with paired-pulse TMS were performed. It was found that enhanced excitability occurred in the homotopic motor cortex of the non-affected hemisphere after ischemic infarction of the primary motor output system (Butefisch *et al.*, 2003; Shimizu *et al.*, 2002). These remote changes were found to result from a shift in the balance between excitatory and inhibitory activity towards an increase of excitatory activity for higher stimulus intensities (Fig. 4.9). Specifically, the similarity of motor threshold, mean test MEP, and recruitment curves in patients and age-matched controls indicated that the excitability of the cortical motor neurons of the non-affected motor cortex had not changed in the patients (see also Liepert *et al.*, 2000). Rather, cortical interneurons seemed to be affected by pair-pulse TMS at a short interstimulus interval of two milliseconds. Since the increase in paired-pulse excitability was not accompanied by an increase in cortical motor neuron or spinal motor neuron excitability, this would support a cortical site for the enhanced cortical excitability (Kujirai *et al.*, 1993; Ziemann *et al.*, 1996a; Nakamura *et al.*, 1997; Di Lazzaro *et al.*, 1998). Indeed, there is evidence that the inhibitory effect of the conditioning pulse at short interstimulus intervals was mediated by GABAergic interneurons in the

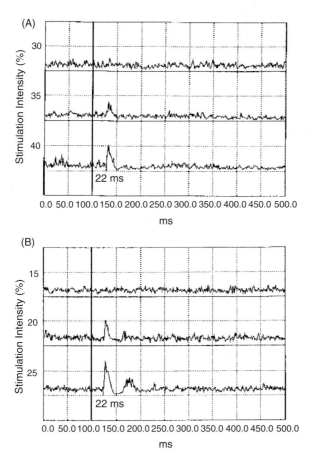

Fig. 4.8   Recording of ipsilateral motor evoked potentials after stroke in a patient with incomplete recovery and persisting associated movements of the non-affected hand. Surface electromyography of the affected (A) and non-affected (B) thenar muscle (relative units) during stimulation of the non-affected hemisphere. Note the identical latency of the potentials that built up upon higher stimulation intensity of the non-affected hemisphere. (Data from Netz *et al.* (1997) with permission.)

vicinity of the tested corticospinal neurons (Ziemann *et al.*, 1996b; Ashby *et al.*, 1999). Further, the relative independence of the absolute conditioning stimulus intensities necessary to elicit inhibition from the threshold of the motor cortical neurons supported the concept that intracortical inhibition and motor threshold were governed by different mechanisms (Ziemann 1996a; Chen *et al.*, 1998). These data are corroborated by paired stimulation experiments in rats after focal cortical lesions, which showed enhanced cortical excitability in both cerebral hemispheres after the lesion (Buchkremer-Ratzmann *et al.*, 1996). Simultaneously, however, these evoked potentials in rats were reduced, supporting the concept of different

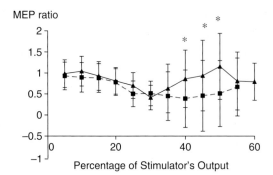

Fig. 4.9   Altered excitability after brain infarction in the contralesional motor cortex. Shown is the intracortical inhibition and excitation as tested by paired-pulse transcranial magnetic stimulation (TMS) at interstimulus interval of 2 ms for different intensities of subthreshold conditioning TMS in patients (▲) and healthy volunteers (■). The conditioning TMS intensity is expressed as a percentage of the stimulator's output. The amplitude of motor evoked potentials (MEP) elicited by the succeeding, conditioned suprathreshold TMS is expressed as a ratio of the mean MEP amplitude evoked by five single test pulses. $P < 0.01$ for modulation of the MEPs between patients and controls. (Further details in Butefisch *et al.*, 2003.)

mechanisms governing the inhibitory and excitatory balance in cortex (Buchkremer-Ratzmann *et al.*, 1996).

Consecutive observations during the course of recovery indicated that stroke patients with good motor recovery showed a persisting disinhibition in the affected hemisphere and a normalization in the non-affected hempishere. In contrast, patients with poor recovery had a persisting disinhibition in both hemispheres of at least at 30 days after stroke (Manganotti, Patuzzo *et al.*, 2002). Four months after stroke, however, intracortical inhibition had normalized in the unaffected hemisphere in patients with persisting hand palsy both after cortical and subcortical stroke (Shimizu *et al.*, 2002; Butefisch *et al.*, 2003). Thus, intracortical disinhibition in the non-affected contralesional hemisphere seemed to accompany clinical progress but vanished when recovery ceased. Since this modulation of cortical excitability was not controlled by transcallosal inhibition (Shimizu *et al.*, 2002), the mechanism for the abnormal recruitment of ipsilateral MEPs in patients with poor motor recovery remains unclear as yet.

Strategies for rehabilitative interventions

It appears from Fig. 4.2 that both patients with a slight stroke-induced deficit and those who are severely impaired initially may recover well and early. The differences in the capacity for functional restoration among stroke patients make it likely that, apart from the cortical motor output system, sensory feedback provided by the use of a partly compromised limb may play a major role for reshaping the remaining circuits. This is best illustrated by the inability of patients with deafferentation to learn new movements patterns. The situation in a paralysed limb may be similar, because the lack of active limb movement precludes motor-related feedback (Rothwell *et al.*, 1982). Evidence from combined clinical and electrophysiological studies support this view, since the presence of somatosensory evoked potentials indicated good recovery (Feys *et al.*, 2000). Furthermore, illusory arm movements in healthy subjects have been reported to activate beyond motor areas, also the somatosensory cortex (Naito *et al.*, 1999). It may, therefore, be assumed that the absence of residual function over a critical time span after stroke prevents functional restitution. Conversely, animal experiments show an enlargement of the somatosensory representations during skill recovery after focal lesions of the primary somatosensory cortex (Xerri *et al.*, 1998). Further, monkeys with deafferentation that did not use the affected limb for weeks after injury failed to recover (Taub *et al.*, 1999). The hypothesis that a critical minimum of residual executive capacity is a prerequisite for tuning recovery holds promise for new approaches in rehabilitative strategies (Wolf *et al.*, 1989; Taub *et al.*, 1994). In fact, from these observations, it was considered that the animals learned to avoid using the affected limb because of discomfort, stress, and frustration when doing so, but rather used the intact arm. This concept of "learned non-use" laid the ground for therapy studies in human stroke. Based on this concept, constraints were imposed on the unaffected limb by keeping it in a cast, which forced the patient to use the minimal residual functions of the affected arm for daily purposes. This so-called constrained-induced therapy has now been shown to be successful even when applied in the chronic state to severely affected patients (Liepert *et al.*, 1998; Taub *et al.*, 1999). Consequently, there is good evidence to support the view that reafferent somatosensory information from the partly compromised limb is critically required for tuning the remaining network into function, which is also evident from scanning passive movements (Nelles *et al.*, 1999). These data are corroborated further by the observation that there is a posterior shift of the sensorimotor area in patients with sensorimotor strokes (Rossini *et al.*, 1998b; Pineiro *et al.*, 2001). However, feedback can even be provided by the visual domain. For example, visual neglect compromises recovery from hemiparesis (Kalra *et al.*, 1997; Paolucci *et al.*, 1998). Neuroimaging data suggest that patients who have recovered from hemiparesis employ the visual system in relation to the execution of finger movements (Seitz *et al.*, 1999).

Epidemiological studies have shown that early physiotherapy and patient mobilization after stroke is beneficial (Jorgensen *et al.*, 2000). It is unclear at present how these data obtained in humans can be reconciled with observations in animal experiments showing that training during the first days aggravates post-ischemic brain lesions (Kozlowski *et al.*, 1996; Risedal *et al.*, 1999). In the early chronic phase, the intensity of repetitive training has been shown to facilitate motor recovery (Butefisch *et al.*, 1995; Hesse *et al.*, 1995; Hummelsheim *et al.*, 1995; Kwakkel *et al.*, 1999). Even rhythmic movement facilitation as well as robot training appeared to be beneficial for motor recovery (Aisen *et al.*, 1997; Thaut *et al.*, 1997; Volpe *et al.*, 1999). Repetitive training and voluntary contraction of affected muscles facilitate motor cortical activity, as shown by TMS (Hauptmann and Hummelsheim, 1996; Aisen *et al.*, 1997). These data agreed with evidence from animal experiments that showed an enlargement of the motor cortical representation in monkeys subjected to rehabilitative training after experimental stroke in the motor cortex (Nudo *et al.*, 1996). Furthermore, it was shown by functional neuroimaging that the supplementary motor area that plays a prominent role in movement initiation is activated in patients who have recovered from hemiparetic infarction in the MCA (Fig. 4.6; Azari *et al.*, 1996; Seitz *et al.*, 1998; Carey *et al.*, 2001). These data underline the importance of a voluntary contribution by the patient for successful therapy rather than just passive training approaches.

It is important to realize that stroke patients retain subtle motor and cognitive deficits even after excellent clinical recovery (Mori *et al.*, 1994; Platz *et al.*, 1994; Weder and Seitz, 1994). Such deficits may be augmented by changes related to a vascular encephalopathy (Heiss *et al.*, 1993; Schmidt *et al.*, 1995). Nevertheless, it is conceivable that recovering patients select an alternative strategy to compensate for their neurological deficit, as was shown in monkeys (Friel and Nudo, 1998). A simple approach is that patients employ more extended finger movements for object manipulation than they usually would (Binkofski *et al.*, 2001b). In contrast to the hand representation in motor cortex (Sato and Tanji, 1989; Schieber and Hibbard, 1993; Sanes *et al.*, 1995), there is no overlapping somatotopy of digit representation in the somatosensory cortex (Sutherling, Levesque *et al.*, 1992). Consequently, because of the exaggerated finger movements, a spatially enhanced input is likely to be processed in an abnormally large portion of the sensorimotor cortex in these patients. Similarly, there is evidence suggesting that patients with hemianopia can learn to perform enlarged saccadic eye movements to compensate for their visual field defect (Zihl and von Cramon, 1985; Pommerenke and Markowitsch, 1989). Likewise, hemiparetic patients may engage muscles for moving a paretic limb that are usually only used for auxillary actions or are reserved for high levels of exertion. This compensatory behavior is most prominent in patients with dystrophic muscle diseases, for instance while they are standing up or lifting a limb (Dubowitz, 1978) but it probably also holds for brain lesions. Lastly, patients with Parkinson's disease sometimes employ sensory cues to initiate locomotion (Marsden, 1982; Schneider *et al.*, 1987; Montgomery *et al.*, 1991). Clearly, these altered actions rely on abnormal sensorimotor or visuomotor information processing and are most likely to produce abnormal cortical activation patterns, as recorded with neuroimaging, and possibly altered cortical excitability, as measured with TMS.

How can these residual deficits be improved? How do patients learn to use their affected limb in a normal manner again? One possible approach is to employ bilateral arm movements and to apply a number of motor tasks for training. Both ways have proved successful in improving recovery (Mudie and Matyas, 2000; Staines *et al.*, 2001; Cauraugh and Kim, 2002). These approaches make use of the transmodal transfer of learning or of skill generalization, which are considered to be prominent modes for learning (Seitz and Matyas, 2002). In addition, focusing attention by eliminating efferent and afferent flow from the adjacent proximal body part was shown to improve post-stroke recovery (Muellbacher *et al.*, 2002). Botulinum toxin reduces spasticity and may lessen some impairments (Brashear *et al.*, 2002). This intervention may provide more residual function and consequently greater improvement by diminishing spasticity. Sensory-driven recovery using rapid TMS is based on a similar hypothesis and has been shown to enhance recovery and the corresponding fMRI signal (Fraser *et al.*, 2002). Common to all these approaches is that they underline the reorganization of the sensorimotor cortex of the affected hemisphere as a major contributor to recovery.

Summary and perspectives

Hemiparesis after stroke represents a good model for studying cerebral reorganization. In addition, the sensorimotor system is suitable for exploring the modulating actions of neurotransmitters and pharmaceuticals. There is evidence from animal experiments of the importance of the widely projecting adrenergic and cholinergic neurons for brain function (Moore, 1982; Mesulam *et al.*, 1983; McCormick, 1992). These neurons become retrogradely affected by the ischemic tissue lesion and their damage has been linked to the occurrence of diaschisis (Boyeson *et al.*, 1994). Likewise, adrenergic mediators have been shown to promote sensorimotor recovery in animals, while adrenoceptor blockers and related drugs are found to impair it (Feeney and Hovda, 1983). A single dose of fluoxetine improved motor skill and enhanced motor cortex activation during a one-week training period in the subacute stage after lacunar brain infarction in humans but reduced cerebellar activations (Pariente *et al.*, 2001). Therefore, functional recovery mediated by cerebral reorganization may be enhanced by drug action.

REFERENCES

Aisen, M. L., Krebs, H. I., Hogan, N., McDowell, F., and Volpe, B. T. (1997). The effect of robot-assisted therapy and rehabilitative training on motor recovery following stroke. *Arch Neurol* **54**: 443–446.

Aizawa, H., Mushiake, H., Inase, M., and Tanji, J. (1990). An output zone of the monkey primary motor cortex specialized for bilateral hand movement. *Exp Brain Res* **82**: 219–221.

Alagona, G., Delvaux, V., Gerard, P., *et al.* (2001). Ipsilateral motor responses to focal transcranial magnetic stimulation in healthy subjects and acute-stroke patients. *Stroke* **32**: 1304–1309.

Alexandrov, A. V., Demchuk, A. M., Felberg, R. A., *et al.* (2000). High rate of complete recanalization and dramatic clinical recovery during tPA infusion when continuously monitored with 2-MHz transcranial doppler monitoring. *Stroke* **31**: 610–614.

Alexandrov, A. V., Burgin, W. S., Demchuk, A. M., El Mitwalli, A., and Grotta, J. C. (2001). Speed of intracranial clot lysis with intravenous tissue plasminogen activator therapy: sonographic classification and short-term improvement. *Circulation* **103**: 2897–2902.

Ashby, C. R. Jr., Rohatgi, R., Ngosuwan, J., *et al.* (1999). Implication of the GABA(B) receptor in gamma vinyl-GABA's inhibition of cocaine-induced increases in nucleus accumbens dopamine. *Synapse* **31**: 151–153.

Azari, N. P., Binkofski, F., Pettigrew, K. D., Freund, H.‑J., and Seitz, R. J. (1996). Enhanced regional cerebral metabolic interactions in thalamic circuitry predicts motor recovery in hemiparetic stroke. *Hum Brain Mapp* **4**: 240–253.

Benecke, R., Meyer, B. U., and Freund, H. J. (1991). Reorganization of descending motor pathways in patients after hemispherectomy and severe hemispheric lesions demonstrated by magnetic brain stimulation. *Exp Brain Res* **83**: 419–426.

Binkofski, F. and Seitz, R. J. (2004). Modulation of the BOLD-response in early recovery from sensorimotor stroke. *Neurology* **63**: 1223–1229.

Binkofski, F., Seitz, R. J., Arnold, S., *et al.* (1996). Thalamic metbolism and corticospinal tract integrity determine motor recovery in stroke. *Ann Neurol* **39**: 460–470.

Binkofski, F., Buccino, G., Posse, S., *et al.* (1999). A frontoparietal circuit for object manipulation in man: evidence from an fMRI-study. *Eur J Neurosci* **11**: 3276–3286.

Binkofski, F., Amunts, K., Stephan, K. M., *et al.* (2000). Broca's area subserves imagery of motion: a combined cytoarchitectonic and MRI study. *Hum Brain Mapp* **11**: 273–285.

Binkofski, F., Seitz, R. J., Hackländer, T., *et al.* (2001a). The recovery of motor functions following hemiparetic stroke: a clinical and MR-morphometric study. *Cerebrovasc Dis* **11**: 273–281.

Binkofski, F., Kunesch, E., Dohle, C., Seitz, R. J., and Freund, H.‑J. (2001b). Tactile apraxia: unimodal apractic disorder of tactile object exploration associated with parietal lobe lesions. *Brain* **124**: 132–144.

Bolay, H. and Dalkara, T. (1998). Mechanisms of motor dysfunction after transient MCA occlusion: persistent transmission failure in cortical synapses is a major determinant. *Stroke* **29**: 1988–1993.

Bonda, E., Petrides, M., Frey, S., and Evans, A. (1995). Neural correlates of mental transformations of the body-in-space. *Proc Natl Acad Sci* USA **92**: 11180–11184.

Boyeson, M. G., Jones, J. L., and Harmon, R. L. (1994). Sparing of motor function after cortical injury. A new perspective on underlying mechanisms. *Arch Neurol* **51**: 405–414.

Brashear, A., Gordon, M. F., Elovic, E., *et al.* (2002). Intramuscular injection of botulinum toxin for the treatment of wrist and finger spasticity after a stroke. *N Engl J Med* **347**: 395–400.

Brunberg, J. A., Frey, K. A., Horton, J. A., and Kuhl, D. E. (1992). Crossed cerebellar diaschisis: occurrence and resolution demonstrated with PET during carotid temporary balloon occlusion. *Am J Neuroradiol* **13**: 58–61.

Buchkremer-Ratzmann, I., August, M., Hagemann, G., and Witte, O. W. (1996). Electrophysiological transcortical diaschisis after cortical photothrombosis in rat brain. *Stroke* **27**: 1105–1109.

Butefisch, C., Hummelsheim, H., Denzler, P., and Mauritz, K. H. (1995). Repetitive training of isolated movements improves the outcome of motor rehabilitation of the centrally paretic hand. *J Neurol Sci* **130**: 59–68.

Butefisch, C. M., Netz, J., Wessling, M., Seitz, R. J., and Homberg, V. (2003). Remote changes in cortical excitability after stroke. *Brain* **126**: 470–481.

Calautti, C., Leroy, F., Guincestre, J. Y., Marie, R. M., and Baron, J. C. (2001a). Sequential activation brain mapping after subcortical stroke: changes in hemispheric balance and recovery. *NeuroReport* **12**: 3883–3886.

Calautti, C., Leroy, F., Guincestre, J. Y., and Baron, J. C. (2001b). Dynamics of motor network overactivation after striatocapsular stroke: a longitudinal PET study using a fixed-performance paradigm. *Stroke* **32**: 2534–2542.

Calautti, C., Serrati, C., and Baron, J. C. (2001c). Effects of age on brain activation during auditory-cued thumb-to-index opposition: a positron emission tomography study. *Stroke* **32**: 139–146.

Cao, Y., D'Olhaberriague, L., Vikingstad, E. M., Levine, S. R., and Welch, K. M. (1998). Pilot study of functional MRI to assess cerebral activation of motor function after post-stroke hemiparesis. *Stroke* **29**: 112–122.

Caramia, M. D., Palmieri, M. G., Giacomini, P., *et al.* (2000). Ipsilateral activation of the unaffected motor cortex in patients with hemiparetic stroke. *Clin Neurophysiol* **111**: 1990–1996.

Carey, L. M., Abbott, D. F., Egan, G. F., *et al.* (2001). Evolution of brain activation with good and poor motor recovery after stroke. *Neuroimage* **13**: 5774.

Carey, J. R., Kimberley, T. J., Lewis, S. M., *et al.* (2002). Analysis of fMRI and finger tracking training in subjects with chronic stroke. *Brain* **125**: 773–788.

Carr, L. J., Harrison, L. M., Evans, A. L., and Stephens, J. A. (1993). Patterns of central motor reorganization in hemiplegic cerebral palsy. *Brain* **116**: 1223–1247.

Cauraugh, J. H. and Kim, S. (2002). Two coupled motor recovery protocols are better than one: electromyogram-triggered neuromuscular stimulation and bilateral movements. *Stroke* **33**: 1589–1594.

Chen, R., Tam, A., Butefisch, C., *et al.* (1998). Intracortical inhibition and facilitation in different representations of the human motor cortex. *J Neurophysiol* **80**: 2870–2881.

Chen, C. L., Tang, F. T., Chen, H. C., Chung, C. Y., and Wong, M. K. (2000). Brain lesion size and location: effects on motor recovery and functional outcome in stroke patients. *Arch Phys Med Rehabil* **81**: 447–452.

Cholet, N., Seylaz, J., Lacombe, P., and Bonvento, G. (1997). Local uncoupling of the cerebrovascular and metabolic responses to somatosensory stimulation after neuronal nitric oxide synthase inhibition. *J Cereb Blood Flow Metab* **17**: 1191–1201.

Chollet, F., DiPiero, V., Wise, R. J., *et al.* (1991). The functional anatomy of motor recovery after stroke in humans: a study with positron emission tomography. *Ann Neurol* **29**: 63–71.

Clark, R. E. and Delay, E. R. (1991). Reduction of lesion-induced deficits in visual reversal learning following cross-modal training. *Restor Neurol Neurosci* **3**: 247–255.

Classen, J., Schnitzler, A., Binkofski, F., *et al.* (1997). The motor syndrome associated with exaggerated inhibition within the primary motor cortex of patients with hemiparetic. *Brain* **120**: 605–619.

Cohen, L. G., Celnik, P., Pascual-Leone, A., *et al.* (1997). Functional relevance of cross-modal plasticity in blind humans. *Nature* **389**: 180–183.

Colebatch, J. G. and Gandevia, S. C. (1989). The distribution of muscular weakness in upper motor neuron lesions affecting the arm. *Brain* **112**: 749–763.

Cramer, S. C., Nelles, G., Benson, R. R., *et al.* (1997). A functional MRI study of subjects recovered from hemiparetic stroke. *Stroke* **28**: 2518–2527.

Cramer, S. C., Finklestein, S. P., Schaechter, J. D., Bush, G., and Rosen, B. R. (1999). Activation of distinct motor cortex regions during ipsilateral and contralateral finger movements. *J Neurophysiol* **81**: 383–387.

Cramer, S. C., Nelles, G., Schaechter, J. D., *et al.* (2001). A functional MRI study of three motor tasks in the evaluation of stroke recovery. *Neurorehabil Neural Repair* **15**: 1–8.

Decety, J., Grezes, J., Costes, N., *et al.* (1997). Brain activity during observation of actions. Influence of action content and subject's strategy. *Brain* **120**: 1763–1777.

Deecke, L., (1990). Electrophysiological correlates of movement initiation. *Rev Neurol* **146**: 612–619

Dettmers, C., Fink, G. R., Lemon, R. N., *et al.* (1995). Relation between cerebral activity and force in the motor areas of the human brain. *J Neurophysiol* **74**: 802–815.

Dettmers, C., Stephan, K. M., Lemon, R. N., and Frackowiak, R. S. J. (1997). Reorganization of the executive motor system after stroke. *Cerebrovasc Dis* **7**: 187–200.

Di Lazzaro, V., Restuccia, D., Oliviero, A., *et al.* (1998). Magnetic transcranial stimulation at intensities below active motor threshold activates intracortical inhibitory circuits. *Exp Brain Res* **119**: 265–268.

DiPiero, V., Chollet, F. M., MacCarthy, P., Lenzi, G. L., and Frackowiak, R. S. (1992). Motor recovery after acute ischaemic stroke: a metabolic study. *J Neurol Neurosurg Psychiatry* **55**: 990–996.

Dominkus, M., Grisold, W., and Jelinek, V. (1990). Transcranial electrical motor evoked potentials as a prognostic indicator for motor recovery in stroke patients. *J Neurol Neurosurg Psychiatry* **53**: 745–748.

Donnan, G. A., Bladin, P. F., Berkovic, S. F., Longley, W. A., and Saling, M. M. (1991). The stroke syndrome of striatocapsular infarction. *Brain* **114**: 51–70.

Dubowitz, V. (1978) *Muscle Disorders in Childhood*. London: Saunders.

Duncan, P. W., Goldstein, L. B., Matchar, D., Divine, G. W., and Feussner, J. (1992). Measurement of motor recovery after stroke. Outcome assessment and sample size requirements. *Stroke* **23**: 1084–1089.

Duncan, P. W., Lai, S. M., and Keighley, J. (2000). Defining post-stroke recovery: implications for design and interpretation of drug trials. *Neuropharmacology* **39**: 835–841.

Durwen, H. F. and Herzog, A. G. (1989). Electromyographic investigation of mirror movements in normal adults. Variation of frequency with side of movements, handedness, and dominance. *Brain Dysfunct* **2**: 84–92.

(1992). Electromyographic investigation of mirror movements in normal adults. Variation of frequency with site, effort and repetition of movements. *Brain Dysfunct* **5**: 310–318.

Els, T., Klisch, J., Orszagh, M., *et al.* (2002). Hyperglycemia in patients with focal cerebral ischemia after intravenous thrombolysis: influence on clinical outcome and infarct size. *Cerebrovasc Dis* **13**: 89–94.

Farmer, S. F., Harrison, L. M., Ingram, D. A., and Stephens, J. A. (1991). Plasticity of central motor pathways in children with hemiplegic cerebral palsy. *Neurology* **41**: 1505–1510.

Feeney, D. M. and Hovda, D. A. (1983). Amphetamine and apomorphine restore tactile placing after motor cortex injury in the cat. *Psychopharmacology* **79**: 67–71

Feydy, A., Carlier, R., Roby-Brami, A., *et al.*, (2002). Longitudinal study of motor recovery after stroke: recruitment and focusing of brain activation. *Stroke* **33**: 1610–1617.

Feys, H., Van Hees, J., Bruyninckx, F., Mercelis, R., and De Weerdt, W. (2000). Value of somatosensory and motor evoked potentials in predicting arm recovery after a stroke. *J Neurol Neurosurg Psychiatry* **68**: 323–331.

Fisher, C. M. (1992). Concerning the mechanism of recovery in stroke hemiplegia. *Can J Neurol Sci* **19**: 57–63.

Foerster, O. (1936). Motorische Felder und Bahnen. In *Allgemeine Neurologie*, ed. O. Bumke, O. Foerster. Berlin: Julius Springer Verlag, pp. 1–357.

Fraser, C., Power, M., Hamdy, S., *et al.* (2002). Driving plasticity in human adult motor cortex is associated with improved motor function after brain injury. *Neuron* **34**: 831–840.

Freund, H. J. and Hummelsheim, H. (1985). Lesions of premotor cortex in man. *Brain* **108**: 697–733.

Friel, K. M. and Nudo, R. J. (1998). Recovery of motor function after focal cortical injury in primates: compensatory movement patterns used during rehabilitative training. *Somatosens Mot Res* **15**: 173–189.

Fries, W., Danek, A., Scheidtmann, K., and Hamburger, C. (1993). Motor recovery following capsular stroke. Role of descending pathways from multiple motor areas. *Brain* **116**: 369–382.

Fukui, K., Iguchi, I., Kito, A., Watanabe, Y., and Sugita, K. (1994). Extent of pontine pyramidal tract Wallerian degeneration and outcome after supratentorial hemorrhagic stroke. *Stroke* **25**: 1207–1210.

Gresham, G. E., Kelly-Hayes, M., Wolf, P. A., *et al.* (1998). Survival and functional status 20 or more years after first stroke: the Framingham Study. *Stroke* **29**: 793–797.

Hagemann, G., Redecker, C., Neumann-Haefelin, T., Freund, H. J., and Witte, O. W. (1998). Increased long-term potentiation in the surround of experimentally induced focal cortical infarction. *Ann Neurol* **44**: 255–258.

Hakim, A. M., Pokrupa, R. P., Villanueva, J., *et al.* (1987). The effect of spontaneous reperfusion on metabolic function in early human cerebral infarcts. *Ann Neurol* **21**: 279–289.

Hatazawa, J., Satoh, T., Shimosegawa, E., *et al.* (1995). Evaluation of cerebral infarction with iodine 123-iomazenil SPECT. *J Nucl Med* **36**: 2154–2161.

Hauptmann, B. and Hummelsheim, H. (1996). Facilitation of motor evoked potentials in hand extensor muscles of stroke patients: correlation to the level of voluntary contraction. *Electroencephalogr Clin Neurophysiol* **101**: 387–394.

Hauptmann, B., Skrotzki, A., and Hummelsheim, H. (1997). Facilitation of motor evoked potentials after repetitive voluntary hand movements depends on the type of motor activity. *Electroencephalogr Clin Neurophysiol* **105**: 357–364.

Hayashida, K., Hirose, Y., Tanaka, Y., *et al.* (1996). Reduction of ^{123}I-iomazenil uptake in haemodynamically and metabolically impaired brain areas in patients with cerebrovascular disease. *Nucl Med Commun* **17**: 701–705.

Heald, A., Bates, D., Cartlidge, N. E., French, J. M., and Miller, S. (1993). Longitudinal study of central motor conduction time following stroke. 2. Central motor conduction measured within 72 h after stroke as a predictor of functional outcome at 12 months. *Brain* **116**: 1371–1385.

Heilman, K. M., Valenstein, E., and Watson, R. T. (1985). The neglect syndrome. In *Clinical Neuropsychology*, ed. K. M. Heilman and E. Valenstein Amsterdam: Elsevier, pp. 153–183.

Heinemann, A. W., Roth, E. J., Cichowski, K., and Betts, H. B. (1987). Multivariate analysis of improvement and outcome following stroke rehabilitation. *Arch Neurol* **44**: 1167–1172.

Heiss, W. D., Huber, M., Fink, G. R., *et al.* (1992). Progressive derangement of periinfarct viable tissue in ischemic stroke. *J Cereb Blood Flow Metab* **12**: 193–203.

Heiss, W. D., Emunds, H. G., and Herholz, K. (1993). Cerebral glucose metabolism as a predictor of rehabilitation after ischemic stroke. *Stroke* **24**: 1784–1788.

Heiss, W. D., Grond, M., Thiel, A., von Stockhausen, H. M., and Rudolf, J. (1997). Ischaemic brain tissue salvaged from infarction with alteplase. *Lancet* **349**: 1599–1600.

Heiss, W. D., Grond, M., Thiel, A., *et al.* (1998a). Tissue at risk of infarction rescued by early reperfusion: a positron emission tomography study in systemic recombinant tissue plasminogen activator thrombolysis of acute stroke. *J Cereb Blood Flow Metab* **18**: 1298–1307.

(1998b). Permanent cortical damage detected by flumazenil positron emission tomography in acute stroke. *Stroke* **29**: 454–461.

Hennerici, M., Aulich, A., and Freund, H. - J. (1988). Carotid artery syndromes. In *Handbook of Clinical Neurology*, ed. P. J. Vinken, G. W. Bruyn, H. L. Klawans, and J. F. Toole : Amsterdam Elsevier, pp. 291–337.

Hesse, S., Bertelt, C., Jahnke, M. T., *et al.* (1995). Treadmill training with partial body weight support compared with physiotherapy in nonambulatory hemiparetic patients. *Stroke* **26**: 976–981.

Honda, M., Nagamine, T., Fukuyama, H., *et al.* (1997). Movement-related cortical potentials and regional cerebral blood flow change in patients with stroke after motor recovery. *J Neurol Sci.* **146**: 117–126.

Hopf, H. C., Schlegel, H. J., and Lowitzsch, K. (1974). Irradiation of voluntary activity to the contralateral side in movements of normal subjects and patients with central motor disturbances. *Eur Neurol* **12**: 142–147.

Hossmann, K. A. (1994). Viability thresholds and the penumbra of focal ischemia. *Ann Neurol* **36**: 557–565.

Hossmann, K. A., Fischer, M., Bockhorst, K., and Hoehn-Berlage, M. (1994). NMR imaging of the apparent diffusion coefficient (ADC) for the evaluation of metabolic suppression and recovery after prolonged cerebral ischemia. *J Cereb Blood Flow Metab* **14**: 723–731.

Hummelsheim, H., Hauptmann, B., and Neumann, S. (1995). Influence of physiotherapeutic facilitation techniques on motor evoked potentials in centrally paretic hand extensor muscles. *Electroencephalogr Clin Neurophysiol* **97**: 18–28.

Jahanshahi, M. and Rothwell, J. (2000). Transcranial magnetic stimulation studies of cognition: an emerging field. *Exp Brain Res* **131**: 1–9.

Jahanshahi, M., Jenkins, I. H., Brown, R. G., *et al.* (1995). Self-initiated versus externally triggered movements. I. An investigation using measurement of regional cerebral blood flow with PET and movement-related potentials in normal and Parkinson's disease subjects. *Brain* **118**: 913–933.

Jenkins, I. H., Brooks, D. J., Nixon, P. D., Frackowiak, R. S., and Passingham, R. E. (1994). Motor sequence learning: a study with positron emission tomography. *J Neurosci* **14**: 3775–3790.

Johansen-Berg, H., Rushworth, M. F., Bogdanovic, M. D., *et al.* (2002). The role of ipsilateral premotor cortex in hand movement after stroke. *Proc Natl Acad Sci USA* **99**: 14518–14523

Jones, R. D., Donaldson, I. M., and Parkin, P. J. (1989). Impairment and recovery of ipsilateral sensory-motor function following unilateral cerebral infarction. *Brain* **112**: 113–132.

Jorgensen, H. S., Kammersgaard, L. P., Houth, J., *et al.* (2000). Who benefits from treatment and rehabilitation in a stroke unit? A community-based study. *Stroke* **31**: 434–439.

Kalra, L., Perez, I., Gupta, S., and Wittink, M. (1997). The influence of visual neglect on stroke rehabilitation. *Stroke* **28**: 1386–1391.

Karbe, H., Kessler, J., Herholz, K., Fink, G. R., and Heiss, W. D. (1995). Long-term prognosis of post-stroke aphasia studied with positron emission tomography. *Arch Neurol* **52**: 186–190.

Karni, A., Meyer, G., Jezzard, P., *et al.* (1995). Functional MRI evidence for adult motor cortex plasticity during motor skill learning. *Nature* **377**: 155–158.

Kase, C. S., Wolf, P. A., Chodosh, E. H., *et al.* (1989). Prevalence of silent stroke in patients presenting with initial stroke: the Framingham Study. *Stroke* **20**: 850–852.

Katrak, P., Bowring, G., Conroy, P., *et al.* (1998). Predicting upper limb recovery after stroke: the place of early shoulder and hand movement. *Arch Phys Med Rehabil* **79**: 758–761.

Kidwell, C. S., Saver, J. L., Mattiello, J., *et al.* (2000). Thrombolytic reversal of acute human cerebral ischemic injury shown by diffusion/perfusion magnetic resonance imaging. *Ann Neurol* **47**: 462–469.

Knopman, D. S., Rubens, A. B., Selnes, O. A., Klassen, A. C., and Meyer, M. W. (1984). Mechanisms of recovery from aphasia: evidence from serial xenon 133 cerebral blood flow studies. *Ann Neurol* **15**: 530–535.

Kossut, M., Hand, P. J., Greenberg, J., and Hand, C. L. (1988). Single vibrissal cortical column in SI cortex of rat and its alterations in neonatal and adult vibrissa-deafferented animals: a quantitative 2DG study. *J Neurophysiol* **60**: 829–852.

Kozlowski, D. A., James, D. C., and Schallert, T. (1996). Use-dependent exaggeration of neuronal injury after unilateral sensorimotor cortex lesions. *J Neurosci* **16**: 4776–4786.

Kraemer, M., Schormann, T., Hagemann, G., Bi, Q., Witte, O. W., and Seitz, R. J. (2004). Delayed shrinkage of the brain after ischemic stroke: preliminary observations with voxel-guided morphometry. *J Neuroimaging* **14**: 265–272.

Kujirai, T., Caramia, M. D., Rothwell, J. C., *et al.* (1993). Corticocortical inhibition in human motor cortex. *J Physiol* **471**: 501–519.

Kwakkel, G., Wagenaar, R. C., Twisk, J. W., Lankhorst, G. J., and Koetsier, J. C. (1999). Intensity of leg and arm training after primary middle-cerebral-artery stroke: a randomised trial. *Lancet* **354**: 191–196.

Lafleur, M. F., Jackson, P. L., Malouin, F., *et al.* (2002). Motor learning produces parallel dynamic functional changes during the execution and imagination of sequential foot movements. *Neuroimage* **16**: 142–157.

Lee, L. J., Kidwell, C. S., Alger, J., Starkman, S., and Saver, J. L. (2000). Impact on stroke subtype diagnosis of early diffusion-weighted magnetic resonance imaging and magnetic resonance angiography. *Stroke* **31**: 1081–1089.

Lemon, R. N., Johansson, R. S., and Westling, G. (1996). Modulation of corticospinal influence over hand muscles during gripping tasks in man and monkey. *Can J Physiol Pharmacol* **74**: 547–558.

Levy, C. E., Nichols, D. S., Schmalbrock, P. M., Keller, P., and Chakeres, D. W. (2001). Functional MRI evidence of cortical reorganization in upper-limb stroke hemiplegia treated with constraint-induced movement therapy. *Am J Phys Med Rehabil* **80**: 4–12.

Lewine, J. D., Astur, R. S., Davis, L. E., *et al.* (1994). Cortical organization in adulthood is modified by neonatal infarct: a case study. *Radiology* **190**: 93–96.

Li, F., Liu, K. F., Silva, M. D., *et al.* (2000). Transient and permanent resolution of ischemic lesions on diffusion-weighted imaging after brief periods of focal ischemia in rats: correlation with histopathology. *Stroke* **31**: 946–954.

Liepert, J., Miltner, W. H., Bauder, H., *et al.* (1998). Motor cortex plasticity during constraint-induced movement therapy in stroke patients. *Neurosci Lett* **250**: 5–8.

Liepert, J., Storch, P., Fritsch, A., and Weiller, C. (2000). Motor cortex disinhibition in acute stroke. *Clin Neurophysiol* **111**: 671–676.

Lovblad, K. O., Baird, A. E., Schlaug, G., *et al.* (1997). Ischemic lesion volumes in acute stroke by diffusion-weighted magnetic resonance imaging correlate with clinical outcome. *Ann Neurol* **42**: 164–170.

Macdonell, R. A., Donnan, G. A., and Bladin, P. F. (1989). A comparison of somatosensory evoked and motor evoked potentials in stroke. *Ann Neurol* **25**: 68–73.

MacKinnon, C. D., Kapur, S., Hussey, D., *et al.* (1996). Contributions of the mesial frontal cortex to the premovement potentials associated with intermittent hand movements in humans. *Hum Brain Mapp.* **4**: 1–22.

Manganotti, P., Patuzzo, S., Cortese, F., *et al.* (2002). Motor disinhibition in affected and unaffected hemisphere in the early period of recovery after stroke. *Clin Neurophysiol* **113**: 936–943.

Manto, M., Jacquy, J., Hildebrand, J., and Godaux, E. (1995). Recovery of hypermetria after a cerebellar stroke occurs as a multistage process. *Ann Neurol* **38**: 437–445.

Marsden, C. D. (1982). Functions of the basal ganglia. *Rinsho Shinkeigaku* **22**: 1093–1094.

Marshall, R. S., Perera, G. M., Lazar, R. M., *et al.* (2000). Evolution of cortical activation during recovery from corticospinal tract infarction. *Stroke* **31**: 656–661.

McCormick, D. A. (1992). Neurotransmitter actions in the thalamus and cerebral cortex and their role in neuromodulation of thalamocortical activity. *Prog Neurobiol* **39**: 337–388.

Merzenich, M. M. and Sameshima, K. (2000). Cortical plasticity and memory. *Curr Opinion Neurobiol* **3**: 187–196.

Mesulam, M. M., Mufson, E. J., Levey, A. I., and Wainer, B. H. (1983). Cholinergic innervation of cortex by the basal forebrain: cytochemistry and cortical connections of the septal area, diagonal band nuclei, nucleus basalis (substantia innominata), and hypothalamus in the rhesus monkey. *J Comp Neurol* **214**: 170–197.

Miyai, I., Suzuki, T., Kang, J., Kubota, K., and Volpe, B. T. (1999). Middle cerebral artery stroke that includes the premotor cortex reduces mobility outcome. *Stroke* **30**: 1380–1383.

Mohr, J. P., Foulkes, M. A., Polis, A. T., *et al.* (1993). Infarct topography and hemiparesis profiles with cerebral convexity infarction: the Stroke Data Bank. *J Neurol Neurosurg Psychiatry* **56**: 344–351.

Montgomery, E. B., Jr., Nuessen, J., and Gorman, D. S. (1991). Reaction time and movement velocity abnormalities in Parkinson's disease under different task conditions. *Neurology* **41**: 1476–1481.

Moore, R. Y. (1982). Catecholamine neuron systems in brain. *Ann Neurol* **12**: 321–327.

Mori, S., Sadoshima, S., Ibayashi, S., Lino, K., and Fujishima, M. (1994). Relation of cerebral blood flow to motor and cognitive functions in chronic stroke patients. *Stroke* **25**: 309–317.

Mudie, M. H. and Matyas, T. A. (2000). Can simultaneous bilateral movement involve the undamaged hemisphere in reconstruction of neural networks damaged by stroke? *Disabil Rehabil* **22**: 23–37.

Muellbacher, W., Richards, C., Ziemann, U., *et al.* (2002). Improving hand function in chronic stroke. *Arch Neurol* **59**: 1278–1282.

Muller, F., Kunesch, E., Binkofski, F., and Freund, H. J. (1991). Residual sensorimotor functions in a patient after right-sided hemispherectomy. *Neuropsychologia* **29**: 125–145.

Naito, E., Ehrsson, H. H., Geyer, S., Zilles, K., and Roland, P. E. (1999). Illusory arm movements activate cortical motor areas: a positron emission tomography study. *J Neurosci* **19**: 6134–6144.

Nakamura, H., Kitagawa, H., Kawaguchi, Y., and Tsuji, H. (1997). Intracortical facilitation and inhibition after transcranial magnetic stimulation in conscious humans. *J Physiol* **498**: 817–823.

Nardone, R. and Tezzon, F. (2002). Inhibitory and excitatory circuits of cerebral cortex after ischaemic stroke: prognostic value of the transcranial magnetic stimulation. *Electromyogr Clin Neurophysiol* **42**: 131–136.

Nelles, G., Spiekramann, G., Jueptner, M., *et al.* (1999). Evolution of functional reorganization in hemiplegic stroke: a serial positron emission tomographic activation study. *Ann Neurol* **46**: 901–909.

Nelles, G., Jentzen, W., Jueptner, M., Muller, S., and Diener, H. C. (2001). Arm training induced brain plasticity in stroke studied with serial positron emission tomography. *Neuroimage* **13**: 1146–1154.

Netz, J., Lammers, T., and Homberg, V. (1997). Reorganization of motor output in the non-affected hemisphere after stroke. *Brain* **120**: 1579–1586.

Neumann-Haefelin, T., Wittsack, H. J., Wenserski, F., *et al.* (1999). Diffusion- and perfusion-weighted MRI. The DWI/PWI mismatch region in acute stroke. *Stroke* **30**: 1591–1597.

Neville, H. J. and Bavelier, D. (1998). Neural organization and plasticity of language. *Curr Opin Neurobiol* **8**: 254–258.

Newton, J., Sunderland, A., Butterworth, S. E., *et al.* (2002). A pilot study of event-related functional magnetic resonance imaging of monitored wrist movements in patients with partial recovery. *Stroke* **33**: 2881–2887.

Nudo, R. J., Wise, B. M., SiFuentes, F., and Milliken, G. W. (1996). Neural substrates for the effects of rehabilitative training on motor recovery after ischemic infarct. *Science* **272**: 1791–1794.

Nudo, R. J., Friel, K. M., and Delia, S. W. (2000). Role of sensory deficits in motor impairments after injury to primary motor cortex. *Neuropharmacology* **39**: 733–742.

Paolucci, S., Antonucci, G., Pratesi, L., *et al.* (1998). Functional outcome in stroke inpatient rehabilitation: predicting no, low and high response patients. *Cerebrovasc Dis* **8**: 228–234.

Pariente, J., Loubinoux, I., Carel, C., *et al.* (2001). Fluoxetine modulates motor performance and cerebral activation of patients recovering from stroke. *Ann Neurol* **50**: 718–729.

Parsons, L. M., Fox, P. T., Downs, J. H., *et al.* (1995). Use of implicit motor imagery for visual shape discrimination as revealed by PET. *Nature* **375**: 54–58.

Parsons, M. W., Barber, P. A., Desmond, P. M., *et al.* (2002). Acute hyperglycemia adversely affects stroke outcome: a magnetic resonance imaging and spectroscopy study. *Ann Neurol* **52**: 20–28.

Pascual-Leone, A., Grafman, J., and Hallett, M. (1994). Modulation of cortical motor output maps during development of implicit and explicit knowledge. *Science* **263**: 1287–1289.

Pascual-Leone, A., Wassermann, E. M., Sadato, N., and Hallett, M. (1995). The role of reading activity on the modulation of motor cortical outputs to the reading hand in Braille readers. *Ann Neurol* **38**: 910–915.

Pedersen, P. M., Jorgensen, H. S., Nakayama, H., Raaschou, H. O., and Olsen, T. S. (1998). Impaired orientation in acute stroke: frequency, determinants, and time-course of recovery. The Copenhagen Stroke Study. *Cerebrovasc Dis* **8**: 90–96.

Pineiro, R., Pendlebury, S., Johansen-Berg, H., and Matthews, P. M. (2001). Functional MRI detects posterior shifts in primary sensorimotor cortex activation after stroke: evidence of local adaptive reorganization? *Stroke* **32**: 1134–1139.

Platz, T., Denzler, P., Kaden, B., and Mauritz, K. H. (1994). Motor learning after recovery from hemiparesis. *Neuropsychologia* **32**: 1209–1223.

Pommerenke, K. and Markowitsch, H. J. (1989). Rehabilitation training of homonymous visual field defects in patients with postgeniculate damage of the visual system. *Restor Neurol Neurosci* **1**: 47–63.

Pons, T. P., Garraghty, P. E., and Mishkin, M. (1988). Lesion-induced plasticity in the second somatosensory cortex of adult macaques. *Proc Natl Acad Sci USA* **85**: 5279–5281.

Powers, W. J., Fox, P. T., and Raichle, M. E. (1988). The effect of carotid artery disease on the cerebrovascular response to physiologic stimulation. *Neurology* **38**: 1475–1478.

Price, C. J. and Friston, K. J. (1999). Scanning patients with tasks they can perform. *Hum Brain Mapp* **8**: 102–108.

Reddy, H., de Stefano, N., Mortilla, M., Federico, A., and Matthews, P. M. (2002). Functional reorganization of motor cortex increases with greater axonal injury from CADASIL. *Stroke* **33**: 502–508.

Ringelstein, E. B., Biniek, R., Weiller, C., *et al.* (1992). Type and extent of hemispheric brain infarctions and clinical outcome in early and delayed middle cerebral artery recanalization. *Neurology* **42**: 289–298.

Risedal, A., Zeng, J., and Johansson, B. B. (1999). Early training may exacerbate brain damage after focal brain ischemia in the rat. *J Cereb Blood Flow Metab* **19**: 997–1003.

Ritzl, A., Meisel, S., Wittsack, H. J., *et al.* (2004). Development of brain infarct volume as assessed by magnetic resonance imaging follow-up of DWI-lesions. *J Magn Reson Imaging* **20**: 201–207.

Rordorf, G., Koroshetz, W. J., Copen, W. A., *et al.* (1998). Regional ischemia and ischemic injury in patients with acute middle cerebral artery stroke as defined by early diffusion-weighted and perfusion-weighted MRI. *Stroke* **29**: 939–943.

Rossini, P. M., Tecchio, F., Pizzella, V., *et al.* (1998a). On the reorganization of sensory hand areas after mono-hemispheric lesion: a functional (MEG)/anatomical (MRI) integrative study. *Brain Res* **782**: 153–166.

Rossini, P. M., Caltagirone, C., Castriota-Scanderbeg, A., *et al.* (1998b). Hand motor cortical area reorganization in stroke: a study with fMRI, MEG and TCS maps. *NeuroReport* **9**: 2141–2146.

Rothwell, J. C., Traub, M. M., Day, B. L., *et al.* (1982). Manual motor performance in a deafferented man. *Brain* **105**: 515–542.

Sabatini, U., Toni, D., Pantano, P., *et al.* (1994). Motor recovery after early brain damage. A case of brain plasticity. *Stroke* **25**: 514–517.

Sadato, N., Pascual-Leone, A., Grafman, J., *et al.* (1998). Neural networks for Braille reading by the blind. *Brain* **121**: 1213–1229.

Sanes, J. N., Donoghue, J. P., Thangaraj, V., Edelman, R. R., and Warach, S. (1995). Shared neural substrates controlling hand movements in human motor cortex. *Science* **269**: 1775–1777.

Sato, K. C. and Tanji, J. (1989). Digit-muscle responses evoked from multiple intracortical foci in monkey precentral motor cortex. *J Neurophysiol* **62**: 959–970.

Schieber, M. H. and Hibbard, L. S. (1993). How somatotopic is the motor cortex hand area? *Science* **261**: 489–492.

Schiene, K., Bruehl, C., Zilles, K., *et al.* (1996). Neuronal hyperexcitability and reduction of GABAA-receptor expression in the surround of cerebral photothrombosis. *J Cereb Blood Flow Metab* **16**: 906–914.

Schlaug, G., Knorr, U., and Seitz, R. (1994). Inter-subject variability of cerebral activations in acquiring a motor skill: a study with positron emission tomography. *Exp Brain Res* **98**: 523–534.

Schmidt, R., Fazekas, F., Koch, M., *et al.* (1995). Magnetic resonance imaging cerebral abnormalities and neuropsychologic test performance in elderly hypertensive subjects. A case-control study. *Arch Neurol* **52**: 905–910.

Schneider, J. S., Diamond, S. G., and Markham, C. H. (1987). Parkinson's disease: sensory and motor problems in arms and hands. *Neurology* **37**: 951–956.

Schnitzler, A. and Benecke, R. (1994). The silent period after transcranial magnetic stimulation is of exclusive cortical origin: evidence from isolated cortical ischemic lesions in man. *Neurosci Lett* **180**: 41–45.

Schroeter, M. and Hoehn, M. (2000). Histology of MRI. *J Cereb Blood Flow Metab*

Seitz, R. J. and Azari, N. P. (1999). Cerebral reorganization in man after acquired lesions. *Adv Neurol* **81**: 37–47.

Seitz R. J. and Matyas T. (2002) Acquisition and guidance of actions: theory and neuroimaging results. In *Frontiers of Human Memory*, ed. A. Yamadori, R. Kawashima, T. Fuji, K. Suzuki. Sendai, Japan: Tohuku University Press, pp. 37–47.

Seitz, R. J. and Roland. P. E. (1992). Learning of sequential finger movements in man: a combined kinematic and positron emission tomography study. *Eur J Neurosci* **4**: 154–165.

Seitz, R. J., Schlaug, G., Kleinschmidt, A., *et al.* (1994). Remote depressions of cerebral metabolism in hemiparetic stroke: topography and relation to motor and somatosensory functions. *Hum Brain Mapp* **1**: 81–100.

Seitz, R. J., Huang, Y., Knorr, U., *et al.* (1995). Large-scale plasticity of the human motor cortex. *NeuroReport* **6**: 742–744.

Seitz, R. J., Canavan, A. G., Yaguez, L., *et al.* (1997). Representations of graphomotor trajectories in the human parietal cortex: evidence for controlled processing and automatic performance. *Eur J Neurosci* **9**: 378–389.

Seitz, R. J., Hoflich, P., Binkofski, F., *et al.* (1998). Role of the premotor cortex in recovery from middle cerebral artery infarction. *Arch Neurol* **55**: 1081–1088.

Seitz, R. J., Azari, N. P., Knorr, U., *et al.* (1999). The role of diaschisis in stroke recovery. *Stroke* **30**: 1844–1850.

Sette, G., Baron, J. C., Young, A. R., *et al.* (1993). In vivo mapping of brain benzodiazepine receptor changes by positron emission tomography after focal ischemia in the anesthetized baboon. *Stroke* **24**: 2046–2057.

Shimizu, T., Hosaki, A., Hino, T., *et al.* (2002). Motor cortical disinhibition in the unaffected hemisphere after unilateral cortical stroke. *Brain* **125**: 1896–1907.

Small, S. L., Hlustik, P., Noll, D. C., Genovese, C., and Solodkin, A. (2002). Cerebellar hemispheric activation ipsilateral to the paretic hand correlates with functional recovery after stroke. *Brain* **125**: 1544–1557.

Staines, W. R., McIlroy W. E., Graham, S. J., and Black, S. E. (2001). Bilateral movement enhances ipsilesional cortical activity in acute stroke: a pilot functional MRI study. *Neurology* **56**: 401–404.

Stephan, K. M., Netz, J., and Homberg, V. (1995a). Prognostic value of MEP and SSEP in patients with chronic UMN lesions after stroke. *Cerebrovasc Dis* **5**: 407–412.

Stephan, K. M., Fink, G. R., Passingham, R. E., *et al.* (1995b). Functional anatomy of the mental representation of upper extremity movements in healthy subjects. *J Neurophysiol* **73**: 373–386.

Stephan, K. M., Thaut, M. H., Wunderlich, G., *et al.* (2002). Conscious and subconscious sensorimotor synchronization–prefrontal cortex and the influence of awareness. *Neuroimage* **15**: 345–352.

Sultzer, D. L., Mahler, M. E., Cummings, J. L., *et al.* (1995). Cortical abnormalities associated with subcortical lesions in vascular dementia. Clinical and position emission tomographic findings. *Arch Neurol* **52**: 773–780.

Sunderland, A., Tinson, D., and Bradley, L. (1994). Differences in recovery from constructional apraxia after right and left hemisphere stroke? *J Clin Exp Neuropsychol* **16**: 916–920.

Sutherling, W. W., Levesque, M. F., and Baumgartner, C. (1992). Cortical sensory representation of the human hand: size of finger regions and nonoverlapping digit somatotopy. *Neurology* **42**: 1020–1028.

Takahashi, W., Ohnuki, Y., Ohta, T., *et al.* (1997). Mechanism of reduction of cortical blood flow in striatocapsular infarction: studies using [123I]iomazenil SPECT. *Neuroimage* **6**: 75–80.

Taub, E., Crago, J. E., Burgio, L. D., *et al.* (1994). An operant approach to rehabilitation medicine: overcoming learned nonuse by shaping. *J Exp Anal Behav* **61**: 281–293.

Taub, E., Uswatte, G., and Pidikiti, R. (1999). Constraint-induced movement therapy: a new family of techniques with broad application to physical rehabilitation – a clinical review. *J Rehabil Res Dev* **36**: 237–251.

Thaut, M. H., McIntosh, G. C., and Rice, R. R. (1997). Rhythmic facilitation of gait training in hemiparetic stroke rehabilitation. *J Neurol Sci* **151**: 207–212.

Toga, A. W., and Mazziotta, J. C. (2000). *Brain Mapping. The Systems*. San Diego, CA: Academic Press.

Tong, D. C., Yenari, M. A., Albers, G. W., *et al.* (1998). Correlation of perfusion- and diffusion-weighted MRI with NIHSS score in acute (<6.5 hour) ischemic stroke. *Neurology* **50**: 864–870.

Toni, D., Fiorelli, M., Bastianello, S., *et al.* (1997). Acute ischemic strokes improving during the first 48 hours of onset: predictability, outcome, and possible mechanisms. A comparison with early deteriorating strokes. *Stroke* **28**: 10–14.

Toni, D., Fiorelli, M., Zanette, E. M., *et al.* (1998). Early spontaneous improvement and deterioration of ischemic stroke patients. A serial study with transcranial Doppler ultrasonography. *Stroke* **29**: 1144–1148.

Traversa, R., Cicinelli, P., Bassi, A., Rossini, P. M., and Bernardi, G. (1997). Mapping of motor cortical reorganization after stroke. A brain stimulation study with focal magnetic pulses. *Stroke* **28**: 110–117.

Turton, A., Wroe, S., Trepte, N., Fraser, C., and Lemon, R. N. (1996). Contralateral and ipsilateral EMG responses to transcranial magnetic stimulation during recovery of arm and hand function after stroke. *Electroencephalogr Clin Neurophysiol* **101**: 316–328.

van Zagten, M., Boiten, J., Kessels, F., and Lodder, J. (1996). Significant progression of white matter lesions and small deep (lacunar) infarcts in patients with stroke. *Arch Neurol* **53**: 650–655.

Volpe, B. T., Krebs, H. I., Hogan, N., *et al.* (1999). Robot training enhanced motor outcome in patients with stroke maintained over 3 years. *Neurology* **53**: 1874–1876.

von Giesen, H. J., Roick, H., and Benecke, R. (1994). Inhibitory actions of motor cortex following unilateral brain lesions as studied by magnetic brain stimulation. *Exp Brain Res* **99**: 84–96.

von Monakow C. (1914). *Lokalisation im Gehirn und funktionelle Störungen induziert durch kortikale Läsionen.* Wiesbaden, Germany: Bergmann.

Warabi, T., Inoue, K., Noda, H., and Murakami, S. (1990). Recovery of voluntary movement in hemiplegic patients. Correlation with degenerative shrinkage of the cerebral peduncles in CT images. *Brain* **113**: 177–189.

Weder, B. and Seitz, R. J. (1994). Deficient cerebral activation pattern in stroke recovery 15. *NeuroReport* **5**: 457–460.

Weder, B., Knorr, U., Herzog, H., *et al.* (1994). Tactile exploration of shape after subcortical ischaemic infarction studied with PET. *Brain* **117**: 593–605.

Weiller, C., Ringelstein, E. B., Reiche, W., Thron, A., and Buell, U. (1990). The large striato-capsular infarct. A clinical and pathophysiological entity. *Arch Neurol* **47**: 1085–1091.

Weiller, C., Chollet, F., Friston, K. J., Wise, R. J., and Frackowiak, R. S. (1992). Functional reorganization of the brain in recovery from striatocapsular infarction in man. *Ann Neurol* **31**: 463–472.

Weiller, C., Ramsay, S. C., Wise, R. J., Friston, K. J., and Frackowiak, R. S. (1993). Individual patterns of functional reorganization in the human cerebral cortex after capsular infarction. *Ann Neurol* **33**: 181–189.

Weiller, C., Isensee, C., Rijntjes, M., *et al.* (1995). Recovery from Wernicke's aphasia: a positron emission tomographic study. *Ann Neurol* **37**: 723–732.

Werring, D. J., Clark, C. A., Barker, G. J., *et al.* (1998). The structural and functional mechanisms of motor recovery: complementary use of diffusion tensor and functional magnetic resonance imaging in a traumatic injury of the internal capsule. *J Neurol Neurosurg Psychiatry* **65**: 863–869.

Witte, O. W., Bidmon, H. - J., Schiene, K., Redecker, C., and Hagemann, G. (2000). Functional differentiation of multiple peri-lesional zones after focal cerebral ischemia. *J Cereb Blood Flow Metab* **20**: 1149–1165.

Wittsack, H. J., Ritzl, A., Fink, G. R., *et al.* (2002). MR imaging in acute stroke: diffusion-weighted and perfusion imaging parameters for predicting infarct size. *Radiology* **222**: 397–403.

Wolf, S. L., LeCraw, D. E., Barton, L. A., and Jann, B. B. (1989). Forced use of hemiplegic upper extremities to reverse the effect of learned nonuse among chronic stroke and head-injured patients. *Exp Neurol* **104**: 125–132.

Wunderlich, G., Knorr, U., Herzog, H., *et al.* (1998). Precentral glioma location determines the displacement of cortical hand representation. *Neurosurgery* **42**: 18–26.

Xerri, C., Merzenich, M. M., Peterson, B. E., and Jenkins, W. (1998). Plasticity of primary somatosensory cortex paralleling sensorimotor skill recovery from stroke in adult monkeys. *J Neurophysiol* **79**: 2119–2148.

Ziemann, U., Rothwell, J. C., and Ridding, M. C. (1996a). Interaction between intracortical inhibition and facilitation in human motor cortex. *J Physiol* **496**: 873–881.

Ziemann, U., Lonnecker, S., Steinhoff, B. J., and Paulus, W. (1996b). The effect of lorazepam on the motor cortical excitability in man. *Exp Brain Res* **109**: 127–135.

Zihl, J. and von Cramon, D. (1985). Visual field recovery from scotoma in patients with postgeniculate damage. A review of 55 cases. *Brain* **108**: 335–365.

Zülch, K. J. and Müller, N. (1969). *Associated Movements in Man*. Amsterdam: Elsevier.

5

Some personal lessons from imaging brain in recovery from stroke

Cornelius Weiller and Michel Rijntjes

Department of Neurology, Universitätsklinikum Hamburg-Eppendorf, Hamburg, Germany

Introduction

With imaging studies of recovery from stroke, it became clear that the brain retains a plastic potential in its motor and language domains not only in young rats or monkeys but also in adult humans and even in old and lesioned brains (Chollet *et al.*, 1991; Weiller *et al.*, 1992; 1995). This "reorganization" is individually highly variable (Weiller *et al.*, 1993a), relates to recovery of lost function (Liepert *et al.*, 1998), and can be influenced by drugs, training, and rehabilitation (Musso *et al.*, 1999; Liepert *et al.*, 2000a; Pariente *et al.*, 2001). In our opinion, there is not just one single crucial component of recovery. Rather, recovery of function seems to imply the "reconnection" or perhaps better the "recoordination" of a network of areas, each of which may be specialized in one or more aspect of the lost function but requires the coherent and timely support from others to reach a high level of proficiency (Weiller and Rijntjes, 1999). Moreover, we can learn about how the normal brain works when looking at the diseased brain.

Brain anatomy of recovery from stroke

"Plastic" changes represent a uniform reaction pattern of the brain and occur under very different conditions in the intact as well as in the lesioned brain (Merzenich *et al.*, 1982; Kaas, 1991) as a result of learning or adaptation, with or without any concomitant change in behavioral performance (Rijntjes *et al.*, 1997). After lesions, plastic changes can either be a consequence of the structural defect (e.g. diaschisis) or a result of active intervention (e.g. rehabilitational procedures) (Weiller, 1998) In animal experiments, plastic changes have been demonstrated after recovery of lost *motor* function, including peri-lesional extensions of representations, shifts from primary to secondary parallel processing systems, and recruitment of homologous areas of the unaffected hemisphere (Fries *et al.*, 1993; Nudo, 1997; Rouiller *et al.*, 1998; Darian-Smith *et al.*, 1999; Liu and

Recovery after Stroke, ed. Michael P. Barnes, Bruce H. Dobkin and Julien Bogousslavsky. Published by Cambridge University Press. © Cambridge University Press 2005.

Rouiller, 1999). Such changes have also been identified in human stroke victims (Chollet *et al.*, 1991; DiPiero *et al.*, 1992; Weiller *et al.*, 1992, 1993a; Seitz *et al.*, 1994, 1998; Weder and Seitz, 1994; Binkofski *et al.*, 1996; Dettmers *et al.*, 1997).

In most studies using functional magnetic resonance imaging (FMRI) or positron emission tomography (PET), a widespread network of neurons was activated in both hemispheres after recovery.

1. The reorganization was confined to areas activated during motor tasks under various conditions. In stroke patients, the brain seems to use the entire system to perform a relatively simple movement, as under normal conditions (Fink *et al.*, 1997), perhaps with a different weighting.

2. M1 and its major outflow pathways in the damaged hemisphere seem to remain the most important determinant of recovery of dexterity. A lateral extension of the activation (in the direction of the face area) is a robust finding in those with posterior lesions of the posterior limb of the internal capsule and this has repeatedly been found (e.g. Weiller *et al.*, 1993a; Nelles *et al.*, 1999).

3. Ipsilateral M1 (i.e. in the undamaged hemisphere) may contribute in a small percentage of subjects only, in which uncrossed (or double-crossed) corticospinal fibers may occur, as suggested by transcranial magnetic stimulation (TMS) studies (Benecke *et al.*, 1991; Palmer *et al.*, 1992; Netz *et al.*, 1997). A personal guess from the occurrence of mirror movements in the non-affected hand after stroke would be that this occurs in appoximately 10–15% (Weiller *et al.*, 1993b; Rijntjes *et al.*, 1999). Dorsal premotor cortex seems to be the most consistent ipsilateral motor area related to recovery of dexterity (Weiller *et al.*, 1992, 1993a; Seitz *et al.*, 1998; Johansen-Berg *et al.*, 2002a).

4. Secondary motor areas with direct descending corticospinal fibers (dorsal premotor cortex and supplementary motor area) (Dum and Strick, 1991; Fries *et al.*, 1993) within the damaged hemisphere seem readily able to substitute, albeit to achieve a slightly modified function (Weiller *et al.*, 1992, Binkofski *et al.*, 1995; Nudo, 1997) with lesions of the posterior limb of the internal capsule.

5. Additional motor related areas in the parietal cortex (BA 40) and the anterior part of the insula/frontal operculum are consistently found to be activated in most studies (Weiller *et al.*, 1992, 1993a; Pantano *et al.*, 1995; Dettmers *et al.*, 1997; Cao *et al.*, 1998; Seitz *et al.*, 1998; Nelles *et al.*, 1999; Marshall *et al.*, 2000), also in other conditions such as acquired dystonia (Ceballos-Baumann *et al.*, 1995).

6. Increased dorsolateral prefrontal cortex and cingulate cortex activation may be attributed to the need for increased attention and intentional load (Weiller, 1998).

7. Stroke patients usually show stronger activations than healthy controls during finger movements. This could reflect a greater effort to perform the movement

(Price *et al.*, 1994). Alternate explanations might be a lesion-induced disinhibition (Witte *et al.*, 1997; Liepert *et al.*, 2000b) through impairment of transcallosal fibers or a compensatory mechanism of the brain attempting to enhance excitability through reduction of intracortical inhibition.

Modern imaging techniques have challenged the classical view that *language* is represented only in the left hemisphere. Bilateral activations of temporal and frontal brain areas have been reported in normal subjects during various aspects of language processing (Binder, 1997; Warburton *et al.*, 1999). Early studies in aphasic patients have demonstrated reduced metabolism in those brain areas, which had been described by Broca and Wernicke to be involved in language functions (Metter *et al.*, 1981; Heiss *et al.*, 1991). However, controversial results have been published concerning which brain areas are responsible for recovery from aphasia (Lichtheim, 1885; Marie, 1926; Kinsbourne, 1971; Zaidel, 1985; Papanicolaou *et al.*, 1988; Basso *et al.*, 1989; Mesulam, 1990; Cappa and Vallar, 1992; Guerreiro *et al.*, 1995; Nagata *et al.*, 1995; Price *et al.*, 1995; Heiss *et al.*, 1999).

1. There is right hemisphere activation in recovery from aphasia. In patients who had recovered quite well from Wernicke's aphasia resulting from a large left perisylvian lesions, including Wernicke's area and its major outflow, the arcuate fascicle, a verb-generation task in a PET study showed above normal increases in homologous right hemisphere areas (superior temporal gyrus, inferior frontal gyrus, and dorsolateral prefrontal gyrus) as well as in the remaining left hemisphere language zones (frontal) (Weiller *et al.*, 1995).

2. Some studies emphasized the importance of a peri-lesional reorganization in the left hemisphere (Karbe *et al.*, 1989; Price *et al.*, 1995; Warburton *et al.*, 1999).

3. It seems rather evident that the left hemisphere is (in most subjects) best suited for many aspects of language and, therefore, is used as "first line" for recovery (Heiss *et al.*, 1999). The unanswered question is how much of the left hemisphere language network must be spared to suffice for recovery without recruiting right hemisphere substitution (Rijntjes and Weiller, 2002).

4. As yet, it is unclear if right hemispheric activations indicate a reactivation of preexisting right hemispheric language function or if they reflect a gradual development of qualitatively different language functions.

Motor and language domain are essentially different, with the motor system being more hierarchically structured with direct ascending and descending connections, while language-relevant areas are restricted to association cortex. Consequently, a different type of reorganization has to be assumed.

A number of mostly uncontrolled longitudinal studies suggest a gradual "normalization" of activation pattern over time (e.g. decrease of abnormal initially present right hemisphere activation in aphasia; Feydy *et al.*, 2002; Ward *et al.*, 2003).

Functional significance of reorganization

Apart from a few patients in whom a second stroke abolished a function recovered from a first accident (e.g. Guerreiro *et al.*, 1995), the exact relationship between reorganization and restitution of function is not known (Lemon, 1993). In stroke patients, PET data can show enhanced activation in the unlesioned hemisphere without concomitant improvement of motor function (Nelles *et al.*, 1999). Patients with peripheral facial nerve palsy (Bell's palsy) may exhibit enlarged hand representations without obvious improvement of hand motor performance (Rijntjes *et al.*, 1995), and patients with hemifacial spasm may show a decreased hand muscle representation without restriction of hand function in everyday life (Liepert and Weiller, 1999). The last two examples of reorganization may be interpreted as examples of a competitiveness inherent to the brain.

Reorganization may even be maleficient. In amputees, a positive correlation has been described between the amount of cortical reorganization and the intensity of phantom pain (Flor *et al.*, 1995; Birbaumer *et al.*, 1997).

Some longitudinal studies have correlated changes in activation pattern with (treatment-induced) improvement of function (Ohyama *et al.*, 1995; Price *et al.*, 1995; Mimura *et al.*, 1998; Nelles *et al.*, 1999; Marshall *et al.*, 2000; Feydy *et al.*, 2002). The effect of constraint-induced movement therapy (Taub *et al.*, 1994) on the brain has been examined in patients with chronic deficits after stroke (Liepert *et al.*, 2000a). After two weeks of such therapy, motor performance had improved substantially in all patients. This improvement was accompanied by an increase in motor output area size and in the amplitudes of motor evoked potentials, as well as with a shift in the center of gravity of the motor output maps. This indicated preserved neuronal excitability of the motor cortex in the damaged hemisphere, unused or little used for movement of the plegic hand for a long time, which can be brought into action by rehabilitation. Six months after the training, the functional effects persisted but motor cortex excitability returned to normal. This temporary increase of excitability may be mediated by gamma-aminobutyric acid (GABA) (Liepert *et al.*, 2001) and may suggest the utility of timely use of central-stimulating drugs.

PET and fMRI studies have been helpful in understanding the mechanisms of other physiotherapeutical interventions. Sensory stimulations and passive movements are an important feature of physiotherapy early after stroke when motor function is still strongly impaired (Johansson *et al.*, 1993). In healthy subjects, passive movements activated a widely distributed network including primary sensorimotor cortex, parts of the supplementary motor area, and cerebellum. This activation pattern is very similar to activations produced by active movements (Weiller, 1996). This similarity can be used in stroke patients to access motor areas by passive movements even if active motor performance is significantly impaired (Weiller *et al.*, 1997; Nelles *et al.*, 1999).

Brain areas activated during motor imagery in normal subjects (inferior parietal cortex, ventral opercular premotor area, insula; Stephan *et al.*, 1995) are identical to those activated by stroke patients after recovery from hemiplegia. Therefore, it seems reasonable to include motor imagery in the repertoire of physiotherapeutic techniques while the patient is still unable to perform active movements. Indeed, many hemiplegic patients retain the ability to represent accurately prehensile movements involving the impaired limb (Johnson, 2000).

Several drugs have been suggested to improve motor recovery (Small, 1994; Goldstein, 1995). Serotonergic drugs, even given in a single dose, can enhance function specific brain activation (Loubinoux *et al.*, 1999). In a single-blind, placebo-controlled, crossover trial, fluoxetine improved motor performance in stroke patients, and this was associated with an increase in brain activation (Pariente *et al.*, 2001).

Musso *et al.* (1999) investigated whether language training induced cortical reorganization in patients after aphasic stroke. Language comprehension, a function that is often abolished in aphasia but tends to recover quickly, was assessed by an exerpt from a short version of the Token Test in 12 consecutive PET scans in four patients with Wernicke's aphasia and a left perisylvian lesion. Between the scans, the patients underwent intense comprehension training sessions of eight minutes each. The training-induced improvement of language comprehension during the scanning correlated with regional cerebral blood flow changes in language-related areas in the right hemisphere only (middle, superior temporal gyrus, and supramarginal gyrus). This study strongly supports the notion of the role of the right hemisphere in recovery from aphasia and supports other evidence that reorganization is actually beneficial.

Another approach to evaluate the functional significance of activations observed in PET or fMRI is the use of repetitive TMS (Siebner *et al.*, 1998). Cohen *et al.* (1997) demonstrated that repetitive TMS over the occipital cortex impaired the ability to read Braille in blind Braille readers. Therefore repetitive TMS applied over activated areas should have some impact on performance in stroke patients if these activations are functionally relevant. Johansen-Berg *et al.* (2002b) used repetitive TMS in stroke patients to interfere with the action of brain regions that had previously been identified by fMRI as active during movement of the recovered hand. Stimulation of the ipsilateral dorsal premotor cortex impaired the function of the recovered hand in their set of patients to a higher degree than in normal subjects, illustrating the functional importance of this area in the recovery.

Few studies have assessed the predictive value of early fMRI for prognosis. A problem here, as in all longitudinal patient studies, is the dependency of the signal from the blood oxygen level-dependent contrast (BOLD) on the performance rate of the patient, which (hopefully) would improve during the recovery process. A way of dealing with this is using a "passive" paradigm that is more or less independent of the patients' performance (e.g. passive movement that activates almost identical brain areas as the corresponding active movement). Preliminary reports suggest that widespread activation is induced by passive movement of the paralytic limbs; this activation includes M1 of the damaged hemisphere and relates to a good recovery after 6 months (Weiller, 1998). An alternative approach keeps the level of individual performance constant during the process of recovery (Ward *et al.*, 2003).

Mechanisms of reorganization

The actual mechanisms underlying reorganization and therefore, recovery are not known (Lemon, 1993). Brain functions may occasionally be localized in distinct brain regions (e.g. visual perception of motion in V5 or MT; Watson *et al.*, 1993). However, more complicated abilities can only be understood if they are regarded as represented by widespread, bilateral, and parallel working networks, depending on a highly coordinated timely interaction for a proficient level of performance (Mesulam, 1981). In a current hypothesis, functional loss as in stroke can be seen as a disconnection phenomenon. Recovery may mean reconnection or better recoordination of a whole set of areas, each of which may subserve a certain aspect of the function but requires the coherent support of the others to reach a high quality (Weiller and Rijntjes, 1999). The key to investigate this idea may lie in the identification of temporal sequences of activation in the various areas.

We recently examined 13 stroke patients before, immediately after, and six months after a two-week period of constraint-induced movement therapy. All subjects improved during the treatment some deteriorated afterwards, some kept their improved in daily life, and in some further improvement occured. Besides changes in activation over time in several brain regions, changes in M1 in the lesioned hemisphere seemed remarkable. In one group, improvement of function was associated with increasing activity in this area over time. In the other group, which had substantial M1 activity, the area of activation decreased during the training but increased during the six months of follow-up (Rijntjes *et al.*, 2003). So, improvement of function could correlate either with an increase in activity or with a more U-shaped curve. We speculate that this represents two possible ways of reorganiation: the latter U-shaped one perhaps more resembling the normal learning curve (Karni *et al.*, 1995) while the former is a "pathological" way of increasing performance as measured by BOLD, which contradicts the usual notion of an economizing brain. In this group, M1 or its outflow tract was partly destroyed, which was not the case in the patients with a decrease of activity over time. Such differentiation may help in future in selecting the best rehabilitation technique and may offer better prognostic insights.

REFERENCES

Basso, A., Gardelli, M., Grass, M. P., and Mariotti, M. (1989). The role of the right hemisphere in recovery from aphasia: two case studies. *Cortex* **25**: 555–566.

Benecke, R., Meyer, B. U., and Freund, H. J. (1991). Reorganization of descending motor pathways in patients after hemispherectomy and severe hemispheric lesions demonstrated by magnetic brain stimulation. *Exp Brain Res* **83**: 419–426.

Binder, J. (1997). Functional magnetic resonance imaging. Language mapping. *Neurosurg Clin North Am* **8**: 383–92.

Binkofski, F., Seitz, R., Arnold, S., *et al.* (1995). Motor recovery after hemiparetic stroke: relation to pyramidal tract damage and thalamic hypometabolism. *Jo Cerebr Blood Flow Metab* **15**(Suppl. I): S689.

Binkofski, F., Seitz, R. J., and Arnold, S. (1996). Thalamic metabolism and corticospinal tract integrity determine motor recovery in stroke. *Ann Neurol* **39**: 460–470.

Birbaumer, N., Lutzenberger, W., Montoya, P., *et al.* (1997). Effects of regional anesthesia on phantom limb pain are mirrored in changes in cortical reorganization. *J Neurosci* **17**: 5503–8.

Cao, Y., D'Olhaberriague, L., Vikingstad, E. M., Levine, S. R., and Welch, K. M. A. (1998). Pilot study of functional MRI to assess cerebral activation of motor function after post-stroke hemiparesis. *Stroke 1998*; **29**: 112–122.

Cappa, S. F. and Vallar, G. (1992). The role of the left and the right hemisphere in recovery from aphasia. *Aphasiology* **6**: 359–372.

Ceballos-Baumann, A., Passingham, R., Marsden, C., and Brooks, D. (1995). Motor reorganization in acquired hemidystonia. *Ann Neurol* **37**: 746–757.

Chollet, F., DiPiero, V., Wise, R. J. S., *et al.* (1991). The functional anatomy of motor recovery after stroke in humans: a study with positron emission tomography. *Ann Neurol* **29**: 63–71.

Cohen, L. G., Celnik, P., Pascual-Leone, A., *et al.* (1997). Functional relevance of cross-modal plasticity in blind humans. *Nature* **389**: 180–183.

Darian-Smith, I., Burman, K., and Darian-Smith, C. (1999). Parallel pathways mediating manual dexterity in the macaque. *Exp Brain Res* **128**: 101–108.

Dettmers, C., Stephan, K. M., Lemon, R. N., and Frackowiak, R. S. J. (1997). Reorganization of the executive motor system after stroke. *Cerebrovasc Dis* **7**: 187–200.

DiPiero, V., Chollet, F., MacCarthy, P., Lenzi, G. L., and Frackowiak, R. S. J. (1992). Motor recovery after acute ischaemic stroke: a metabolic study. *J Neurol Neurosurg Psychiatry* **55**: 960–966.

Dum, R. P. and Strick, P. L. (1991). The origin of corticospinal projections from the premotor areas in the frontal lobe. *J Neurosci* **11**: 667–689.

Feydy, A., Carlier, R., Roby-Brami, A., *et al.* (2002). Longitudinal study of motor recovery after stroke: recruitment and focusing of brain activation. *Stroke* **33**: 1610–1617.

Fink, G. R., Frackowiak, R. S., Pietrzyk, U., and Passingham, R. E. (1997). Multiple nonprimary motor areas in the human cortex. *J Neurophysiol* **77**: 2164–2174.

Flor, H., Elbert, T., Knecht, S., *et al.* (1995). Phantom-limb pain as a perceptual correlate of cortical reorganization following arm amputation. *Nature* **375**: 482–484.

Fries, W., Danek, A., Scheidtmann, K., and Hamburger, C. (1993). Motor recovery following capsular stroke. *Brain* **116**: 369–382.

Goldstein, L. (1995). Common drugs may influence motor recovery after stroke. *Neurology* **45**: 865–870.

Guerreiro, M., Castro-Caldas, A., and Martins, I. (1995). Aphasia following right hemisphere lesion in a woman with left hemisphere injury in childhood. *Brain Lang* **49**: 280–288.

Heiss, W. D., Pawlik, G., and Dietz, E. (1991). Hypometabolism and functional recruitment as related to prognosis in post-stroke aphasia. *J Cerebr Blood Flow Metab* **11**, (Suppl. 2): S660.

Heiss, W. D., Kessler, J., Thiel, A., Ghaemi, M., and Karbe, H. (1999). Differential capacity of left and right hemispheric areas for compensation of post-stroke aphasia. *Ann Neurol* **45**: 430–438.

Johansen-Berg, H., Rushworth, M., Bogdanovic, M., *et al.* (2002a). The role of ipsilateral premotor cortex in hand movement after stroke. *Proc Natl Acad Sci USA* **99**: 4518–14523.

Johansen-Berg, H., Rushworth, M., and Mathews, P. A. (2002b). TMS study of the functional significance of ipsilateral motor cortical activation after stroke. *Neuroimage* **16**: S700.

Johansson, K., Lindgren, I., Widner, H., Wiklund, I., and Johansson, B. B. (1993). Can sensory stimulation improve the functional outcome in stroke patients? *Neurology* **43**: 2189–2192.

Johnson, S. H. (2000). Imagining the impossible: intact motor representations in hemiplegics. *NeuroReport* **11**: 729–732.

Kaas, J. H. (1991). Plasticity of sensory and motor maps in adult mammals. *Annu Rev Neurosci* **14**: 137–167.

Karbe, H., Holthoff, V. A., Rudolf, J., *et al.* (1989). Regional metabolic correlates of token test results in cortical and subcortical left hemispheric infarction. *Neurology* **39**: 1083–1088.

Karni, A., Meyer, G., Jezzard, P., *et al.* (1995). Functional MRI evidence for adult motor cortex plasticity during motor skill learning. *Nature* **377**: 155–158.

Kinsbourne, M. (1971). The minor hemisphere as a source of aphasic speech. *Trans Am Neurol Assoc* **96**: 141–145.

Lemon, R. N., (1993). Stroke recovery. *Curr Opin Neurobiol* **3**: 463–465.

Lichtheim, L. (1885). On aphasia. *Brain* **7**: 433–484.

Liepert, J. and Weiller, C. (1999). Mapping plastic brain changes after acute lesions. *Curr Opin Neurol* **12**: 709–713.

Liepert, J., Miltner, W. H., Bauder, H., *et al.* (1998). Motor cortex plasticity during constraint-induced movement therapy in stroke patients. *Neurosci Lett* **250**: 5–8.

Liepert, J., Bauder, H., Wolfgang, H. R., *et al.* (2000a). Treatment-induced cortical reorganization after stroke in humans. *Stroke* **31**: 1210–1216.

Liepert, J., Storch, P., Fritsch, A., and Weiller, C. (2000b). Motor cortex disinhibition in acute stroke. *Clin Neurophysiol* **111**: 671–676.

Liepert, J., Schardt, S., and Weiller, C. (2001). Orally administered atropine enhances motor cortex excitability: a transcranial magnetic stimulation study in human subjects. *Neurosci Lett* **300**: 149–152.

Liu, Y. and Rouiller, E. M. (1999). Mechanisms of recovery of dexterity following unilateral lesion of the sensorimotor cortex in adult monkeys. *Exp Brain Res* **128**: 149–159

Loubinoux, I., Boulanouar, K., Ranjeva, J. P., *et al.* (1999). Cerebral functional magnetic resonance imaging activation modulated by a single dose of the monoamine neurotransmission enhancers fluoxetine and fenozolone during hand sensormotor tasks. *J Cerebr Blood Flow Metab* **19**: 1365–1375.

Marie P. (1926). *Travaux et memoires.* Paris: Masson et Cie.

Marshall, R. S., Perera, G. M., Lazar, R. M., *et al.* (2000). Evolution of cortical activation during recovery from corticospinal tract infarction. *Stroke* **31**: 656–661.

Merzenich, M. M., Nelson, R. J., Stryker, M. P., *et al.* (1982). Somatosensory cortical map changes following digital amputation in adult monkey. *J Comp Neurol* **224**: 591–605.

Mesulam, M. M. (1981). A cortical network for directed attention and unilateral neglect. *Ann Neurol* **10**: 309–325.

(1990). Large-scale neurocognitive networks and distributed processing for attention, language, and memory. *Ann Neurol* **28**: 597–613.

Metter, E. J., Wasterlain, C. G., Kuhl, D. E., Hanson, W. R., and Phelps, M. E. (1981). [18]FDG-positron emission computed tomography in a study of aphasia. *Ann Neurol* **10**: 173–183.

Mimura, M., Kato, M., Kata, M., *et al.* (1998). Prospective and retrospective studies of recovery in aphasia. *Brain* **121**: 2083–2094.

Musso, M., Weiller, C., Kiebel, S., *et al.* (1999). Training-induced brain plasticity in aphasia. *Brain* **122**: 1781–1790.

Nagata, K., Shinohara, T., Yokoyama, E., *et al.* (1995). Possible vicarious functioning of the unaffected hemisphere for recovery from unilateral cerebral infarction. *J Cereb Blood Flow Metab* **15**(Suppl. I): S695.

Nelles, G., Spiekermann, G., Jüptner, M., *et al.* (1999). Evolution of functional reorganization in hemiplegic stroke: a serial positron emission tomographic activation study. *Ann Neurol* **46**: 901–909.

Netz, J., Lammers, T., and Hömberg, V. (1997). Reorganization of motor output in the non-affected hemisphere after stroke. *Brain* **120**: 1579–1587.

Nudo, R. J. (1997). Remodeling of cortical motor representations after stroke: implications for recovery from brain damage. *Mol Psychiatry* **2**: 188–191.

Ohyama, M., Senda, M., Terashi, A., *et al.* (1995). A follow up PET activation study in aphasia due to cerebral infarction evaluates functional reorganization. *J Cereb Blood Flow Metab* **15**(Suppl. I): S697.

Palmer, E., Ashby, P., and Hajek, V. E. (1992). Ipsilateral fast corticospinal pathways do not account for recovery in stroke. *Ann Neurol* **32**: 519–525.

Pantano, P., Formisano, R., Ricci, M., *et al.* (1995). Prolonged muscular flacidity after stroke: morphological and functional brain alterations. *J Cereb Blood Flow Metab* **15**(suppl. 1): S688.

Papanicolaou, A. C., Moore, B. D., Deutsch, G., Levin, H. S., and Eisenberg, H. M. (1988). Evidence for right-hemisphere involvement in recovery from aphasia. *Arch Neurol* **45**: 1025–1029.

Pariente, J., Loubinoux, I., Carel, C., *et al.* (2001). Fluoxetine modulates motor performance and cerebral activation of patients recovering from stroke. *Ann Neurol* **50**: 718–729.

Price, C. J., Wise, R. J., Watson, J. D., *et al.* (1994). Brain activity during reading. The effects of exposure duration and task. *Brain* **117**: 1255–1269.

Price, C. J., Warburton, E., Swinburn, K., Wise, R., and Frackowiak, R. (1995). Monitoring the recovery of aphasia using positron emission tomography. *Journal of Cerebral Blood Flow and Metab* **15**, supp. I: S696.

Rijntjes, M. and Weiller, C. (2002). Recovery of motor and language abilities after stroke: the contribution of functional imaging. *Prog Neurobiol* **66**: 109–122.

Rijntjes, M., Faiss, J., Leonhardt, G., *et al.* (1995). Motor cortex plasticity in a patient with Bell's palsy. *J Cereb Blood Flow Metab* **15**(Suppl. I): S694.

Rijntjes, M., Tegenthoff, M., Liepert, J., *et al.* (1997). Cortical reorganization in patients with facial palsy. *Ann Neurol* **41**: 621–630.

Rijntjes, M., Krams, M., Müller, S., and Weiller, C. (1999). Mitbewegungen der Gegenseite nach Schlaganfall. *Neurol Rehab* **5**: 15–18.

Rijntjes, M., Hamzei, F., Hobbeling, V., Büchel, C., and Weiller, C. (2003). Two types of reorganization in recovery from chronic stroke, depending on the involvement of primary motor cortex. *Neuroimage* **19**(Suppl. 2): S53.

Rouiller, E. M., Yu, X. H., Moret, V., *et al.* (1998). Dexterity in adult monkeys following early lesion of the motor cortical hand area: the role of cortex adjacent to the lesion. *Eur J Neurosci* **10**: 729–740.

Seitz, R., Schlaug, G., Kleinschmidt, A., *et al.* (1994). Remote depressions of cerebral metabolism in hemiparetic stroke: topography and relation to motor and somatosensory functions. *Hum Brain Mapp* **1**: 81–100.

Seitz, R. J., Höflich, P., Binkofski, F., *et al.* (1998). Role of the premotor cortex in recovery from middle cerebral artery infarction. *Arch Neurol* **55**: 1081–1088.

Siebner, H. R., Willoch, F., Peller, M., *et al.* (1998). Imaging brain activation induced by long trains of repetitive transcranial magnetic stimulation. *NeuroReport* **9**: 943–948.

Small, S. L. (1994). Pharmacotherapy of aphasia: a critical review. *Stroke* **25**: 1282–1289.

Stephan, K. M., Fink, G. R., Passingham, R. E., *et al.* (1995). Functional anatomy of the mental representation of upper extremity movements in healthy subjects. *J Neurophysiol* **73**: 373–386.

Taub, E., Crago, J. E., Burgio, L. D., *et al.* (1994). An operant approach to rehabilitation medicine: overcoming learned nonuse by shaping. *J Exp Anal Behav* **61**: 281–293.

Warburton, E., Price, C., Swinburn, K., and Wise, R. J. S. (1999). Mechanisms of recovery from aphasia: evidence from positron emission tomography studies. *J Neurol Neurosurg Psychiatry* **66**: 155–161.

Ward, N. S., Brown, M. M., Thompson, A. J., and Frackowiak, R. (2003). Neural correlates of outcome after stroke: a cross-sectional fMRI study. *Brain* **126**: 1430–1448.

Watson, J. D. G., Myers, R., Frackowiak, R. S. J., *et al.* (1993). Area V5 of the human brain: evidence from a combined study using positron emission tomography and magnetic resonance Imaging. *Cereb Cortex* **3**: 79–94.

Weder, B. and Seitz, R. J. (1994). Deficient cerebral activation pattern in stroke recovery. *Neuroreport* **5**: 457–460.

Weiller, C. (1996). Brain representation of active and passive movements. *Neuroimage* **4**: 105–110.

(1998). Imaging recovery from stroke. *Exp Brain Res* **123**: 13–17.

Weiller, C. and Rijntjes, M. (1999). Learning, plasticity and recovery in the central nervous system. *Exp Brain Res* **128**: 134–138.

Weiller, C., Chollet, F., Friston, K. J., Wise, R. J., and Frackowiak, R. S. (1992). Functional reorganization of the brain in recovery from striatocapsular infarction in man. *Ann Neurol* **31**: 463–472.

Weiller, C., Ramsay, S. C., Wise, R. J., Friston, K. J., and Frackowiak, R. S. (1993a). Individual patterns of functional reorganization in the human cerebral cortex after capsular infarction. *Ann Neurol* **33**: 181–189.

Weiller, C., Rijntjes, M., Müller, S. P., *et al.* (1993b). Associated movements during recovery after stroke relate to rCBF changes in ipsilateral sensorimotor cortex. *J Cereb Blood Flow Metab* **13**(Suppl. 1): S349.

Weiller, C., Isensee, C., Rijntjes, M., *et al.* (1995). Recovery from Wernicke's aphasia: a positron emission tomographic study. *Ann Neurol* **37**: 723–732.

Weiller C., Chollet F., and Frackowiak, R. (1997). Physiological aspects of functional recovery from stroke. In *Cerebrovascular Disease,* ed. J. Bogousslavsky, M. Ginsberg and M. Hennerici, Oxford: Blackwell Scientific, pp. 2057.

Witte, O. W., Buchkremer-Ratzmann, I., Schiene, K., *et al.* (1997). Lesion-induced network plasticity in remote brain areas. *Trends Neurosci* **20**: 348–349.

Zaidel, E. (1985). Language in the right hemisphere. In *The Dual Brain,* ed. D. F. Benson and E. Zaidel, New York: Guilford, pp. 205–231.

6

Measurement in stroke: activity and quality of life

Angus Graham

Brain Injury Rehabilitation unit, Frenchay Hospital, Bristol, UK

Introduction

Stroke is a significant cause of limitations in activity and participation in adult life. Effective rehabilitation for patients with stroke is crucial to minimize the impact of impairment and maximize the reintegration of that person into their community, with an optimal quality of life QoL. Measuring the effectiveness of intervention is essential both to demonstrate that rehabilitation has happened and, potentially, to guide practice for future management.

When considering intervention or outcome measurement, a model of illness is helpful to categorize and classify data collected. The most widely accepted model of illness is that promulgated by the World Health Organization (WHO): the International Classification of Impairments, Disabilities, and Handicaps (ICIDH) (WHO, 1980). This model differentiates the following broad categories: organ system performance, performance of activities of daily living (ADL) at the person level, and role performance as a member of society. The WHO has recently proposed a new model: the International Classification of Functioning, Disability and Health (ICF; WHO, 2001). This revision has seen the retention of these broad categories but replaced the terms *disability* and *handicap* by more positive and meaningful terms, *activity* and *participation,* respectively. It is these concepts that are used as constructs for outcome measurement in rehabilitation.

Measurement of outcome

The search for appropriate outcome measures, used to determine the intended effect of a process or treatment, continues as a focus within rehabilitation research. The goal is to develop instruments that measure and quantify the intended effect across a range of outcomes from activity to QoL and to assess and evaluate the results from instrument use and, thus, determine the effectiveness of that intervention. Such

Recovery after Stroke, ed. Michael P. Barnes, Bruce H. Dobkin and Julien Bogousslavsky. Published by Cambridge University Press. © Cambridge University Press 2005.

effectiveness is, though, subject to external variance effects of comorbidity, social, and societal factors.

A major issue in pursuing outcome measures is the adequacy of the tool, which should satisfy the following essential criteria.

Validity.   A measurement is valid if it accurately describes the underlying phenomenon or disease (Nunnally, 1978; Asplund, 1987; Spector, 1990). Three main types of validity are generally recognized: construct, criterion related, and content validity.

Reliability.   A test is reliable if the measurement error is minimal (Nunnally, 1978). There should be minimal intra- or inter-observer variability.

Sensitivity.   A chosen outcome measure is able to differentiate within a patient group and identify meaningful differences in their abilities (American Education Research Association and National Council on Research in Education, 1985).

Simplicity.   A measure should be simple and easy to use (Wade, 1992).

Communicability.   Measures should give results that are easily understood by others (Wade, 1992).

In the construction of a measure, the number of items needed to measure stroke outcome adequately in groups of patients is important. The selection of test items should be driven by the criteria mentioned above. Only highly reproducible items that are clearly related should be included. Items that lengthen the scale but add little discriminant value should be avoided as being inefficient (Prescott *et al.*, 1982). Once items are selected, comparison with several external criteria of severity, using multivariate regression, will help to clarify the accuracy of the new scale. Also, any measure should relate only to one category within the ICIDH because of the challenge of interpreting results that reflect more than a single level (Orgogozo, 1994).

Critical factors, other than the choice of a measure, must be considered in any rehabilitation study. Such factors would include the timing of the measurements, patient factors known to impact on outcome, statistical methods, and the distribution of outcomes at the chosen end points. Consensus on and consistency in the use of appropriate outcome measures, as well as careful study design, should increase information in stroke research and narrow the evidence–practice gap thereby improving stroke patient care.

Measurement in stroke: Activity as an outcome after stroke can be assessed by:

- focal activity scales
- activities of daily living scales
- instrumental activities of daily living scales,

Focal activity scales

There are a number of scales used to measure focal activity. They tend to concentrate on mobility and arm function.

The Rivermead Mobility Index

The Rivermead Mobility Index (RMI) (Collen *et al.*, 1991) measures mobility and consists of 15 subtests varying from the ability to turn over in bed to the ability to run. It has been used in a number of stroke studies (Wright *et al.*, 1998; Sommerfeld and von Arbin, 2001). The instrument is hierarchical and clinically relevant. It has been evaluated for reliability and validity and is simple to use. It has marked ceiling effects (Wright *et al.*, 1998), which have been addressed by using a modified RMI to improve sensitivity (Lennon and Johnson, 2000). It can be used in clinical practice with minimal training and has high inter-rater reliability.

The Motor Assessment Scale

The Motor Assessment Scale (MAS; Carr *et al.*, 1985) was designed to measure the functional capacities of stroke patients. It assesses the ability to perform functional motor tasks, is hierarchical, and uses criteria that address the quality of performance as well as the level of assistance required. The MAS is brief and easily administered. In stroke studies, inter-rater reliability (Carr *et al.*, 1985; Loewen and Anderson, 1988), validity (Poole and Whitney, 1988; Loewen and Anderson, 1990; Malouin *et al.*, 1994), and responsiveness (Hsueh and Hsieh, 2002) have been demonstrated for the MAS.

The Get-up and Go Test

The Get-up and Go Test (Mathias *et al.*, 1986) was designed to assess balance and basic mobility in elderly patients. It is quick and practical. The test requires a patient to stand from a chair, walk a short distance, turn around, return, and sit down again. A modified timed version has been developed as a test of basic mobility skill (Podsiadlo & Richardson, 1991). It is reliable, has obvious content validity, and correlates well with more extensive measures of balance, gait speed, and functional abilities.

Gait velocity is a widely used measure of function at the end of rehabilitation. Tests for this are simple, have obvious face validity, and are reliable (Wade *et al.*, 1987). Previous studies have shown gait velocity to be a discriminative measure (Collen *et al.*, 1990; Goldie *et al.*, 1996). To date, however, there are no simple tests of endurance with established reliability and validity.

The Action Research Arm Test

The Action Research Arm Test (ARAT; Lyle, 1981) was constructed for assessing upper extremity functional activity. The ARAT includes items in four subscales: grasp, grip, pinch, and gross movement. These items are graded on a four-point scale (0–3). The reliability and validity (Hsieh *et al.*, 1998) and responsiveness (Hsueh and Hsieh, 2002) of the ARAT are well supported.

The Nine Hole Peg Test

The Nine Hole Peg Test is used to assess upper limb function (Mathiowetz *et al.*, 1985). It has been tested for validity and reliability. It is simple and easy to use but does exhibit floor effects. It has been used in stroke studies (Sunderland *et al.*, 1989).

The Test Evaluant Les Membres Superieurs des Personnes Agees

The Test Evaluant Les Membres Superieurs des Personnes Agees (TEMPA) (Derosiers *et al.*, 1994, 1995) is a thoroughly validated timed test for upper extremity performance of tasks representing ADLs.

Summary

The value of these scales is in evaluating more specific abilities, and they may be more useful measuring activity that is relevant to the aims of therapy (Lennon, 1995). Scales, measuring focal activity may be chosen because basic ADL measurements may not provide adequate data concerning motor function for the intended study outcome.

Activities of daily living

Limitations in activity reflect the consequences a dysfunction affecting a body organ (impairment) may produce for a person's normal level of skill or ability. Activity is usually assessed through performance of routine functions and self-care measured by ADL scales.

Any index chosen to measure ADL needs to be valid and reliable, sufficiently sensitive to detect clinically relevant changes, and yet be simple to use and easily understood. There are numerous scales used to assess ADLs. The Barthel Index (BI; Mahoney and Barthel, 1965) and the Functional Independence Measure (FIM; Granger *et al.*, 1986) are the two most commonly used measures (Shah *et al.*, 1991; Heinemann *et al.*, 1993; Haigh *et al.*, 2001). The FIM is a modified BI that includes additional items designed to assess the cognition of patients (Keith *et al.*, 1987; Granger *et al.*, 1993a).

Barthel Index

The BI is a measure of severity of disability. It was designed to assess the degree of independence a patient has in performing the various self-care and mobility ADL tasks. Two versions of the original BI have been commonly used. The Wade and Collins version (Collins *et al.*, 1988) contains 10 ADL items providing a total score ranging from 0 (total dependence) to 20 (total independence). The Granger version

(Granger, 1982), includes 15 ADL items providing a total score ranging from 0 (total dependence) to 100 (total independence). The BI only takes a few minutes to administer by any healthcare professional and can be obtained by proxy and over the telephone. It has repeatedly been shown to be a reliable and valid measure of basic ADL in stroke (Gresham *et al.*, 1980; Wade and Hewer, 1987; Collin *et al.*, 1988; Loewen and Anderson, 1990; D'Olhaberriague *et al.*, 1996). The BI has demonstrated high construct validity (Wade and Hewer, 1987; Brown *et al.*, 1990), predictive and concurrent validity (Granger *et al.*, 1979a) as well as, high re-test and inter-rater reliability (Shinar *et al.*, 1987).

The scale can predict length of stay in hospital as well as the chances of independent community living (Granger *et al.*, 1979a, 1989). The rate of change of BI has also been used to predict activity outcome measure for stroke patients (McNaughton *et al.*, 2001).

The BI is intended to assess only a narrow domain of self-care and mobility, simply recording activity and estimating its extent. However, the BI has been criticized, mainly for its ceiling effects (Granger *et al.*, 1979b). The BI is less sensitive in detecting change in patients with mild stroke (Skilbeck *et al.*, 1983; Wade and Hewer, 1987). A top score of 20 (or 100) implies functional independence, not necessarily normality. The BI has also been criticized for not including domains of cognition and psychological well-being (Granger *et al.*, 1979b). However, the BI was not designed to assess cognition (Hajek *et al.*, 1997; Donkervoort *et al.*, 2002); correlations between the results of functional and cognitive tests were small, reflecting little overlap between these domains. The scale is ordinal and the weighting to each item is arbitrary; hence, parametric statistical methods should not be used. In a recent review of stroke studies (Sulter *et al.*, 1999), BI values were presented in some cases as mean or median results. These authors also noted that the criteria for classifying patients with a favorable outcome varied substantially between trials.

Overall the BI is a reliable and valid instrument to measure ADL and mobility; it is simple to administer and to score (Jacelon, 1986; Wade and Collin, 1988). However, it is less sensitive to functional change in patients with a milder stroke. If its limitations are recognized, it remains a robust tool for assessing activity.

Functional Independence Measure

The 18-item FIM (Granger *et al.*, 1986) was designed to estimate the level of physical independence and cognitive ability of stroke patients, representing a more global concept of activity. The FIM consists of 13 motor and five social–cognitive items. Each of the 18 items is assessed on a 7-point scale ranging from 1 (completely dependent) to 7 (completely independent). The total FIM score, therefore, lies between 18 and 126. The 13 items of the motor subscore can be summated as a measure of physical abilities, with a range of 13 to 91, as can the five items of the social–cognitive subscore as a measure of cognitive ability, with a range of 5 to 35. In 1989, the Functional Assessment Measure (FAM; Hall *et al.*, 1993) was developed by adding a further 12 items to the FIM because the FIM was felt to be too limited to measure the complex activities of brain injury.

The FIM was designed to provide a more detailed assessment of functional abilities than achievable with the BI. It was intended to be easy to apply and to require no specialized skills to administer. However, it requires more time than the BI and trained raters to assess the patient.

The reliability and validity of the FIM have been studied extensively (Granger *et al.*, 1993b; Hamilton *et al.*, 1995; Owen *et al.*, 1995; Cohen and Marino, 2000; Daving *et al.*, 2001); it is sensitive to change (Dodds *et al.*, 1993; Alexander, 1994) and has high inter-rater agreement (Ottenbacher *et al.*, 1994). The FIM scores are non-linear, like the BI, and require non-parametric statistical tools.

The FIM assesses the severity of stroke and has been used to divide patients into functional groups in terms of severity in a number of studies (Alexander, 1994; Ween *et al.*, 1996a, b). It quantifies a patient's level of independence (Keith, 1988; Granger *et al.*, 1986), is a predictor of long-term stroke outcome (Segal and Schall, 1994), and, to some extent, evaluates cognitive abilities, an advantage over the BI. However, the low correlation between the FIM and cognitive tests (Hajek *et al.*, 1997) would suggest that the domain of cognition is too complex to be contained in only a few items. Though the FIM cognitive subscore seems to have some validity regarding cognition, more so than the total FIM score, the cognitive components of the FIM are not representative of the patient's cognitive abilities and have little influence on the overall FIM score. A stroke patient may achieve a high physical score and a low cognitive score and still be categorized in a high functional group. Furthermore, FIM motor and not cognitive scores have been shown to be the strongest predictor of patient's ability to return home after rehabilitation (Stineman *et al.*, 1997).

The FIM, FAM, and BI have been compared for reliability, validity, and responsiveness in a number of studies (Hobart *et al.*, 2001; Hsueh *et al.*, 2002). All three instruments are rigorous measures of neurological activity, with demonstrable similar psychometric properties. The FIM and FAM are similar measures of global, physical, and cognitive activities; the motor scales in FIM, FAM, and BI are similar measures of physical activity. These findings have implications for activity measurement in neurological rehabilitation. They suggest that the newer and longer FIM and FAM tests may have few advantages, as measurement instruments, over the more practical and economical BI. The assumption that longer measures are superior, because they contain a greater number of items, may not be the case. Items in a measurement instrument should be selected on their psychometric performances in empirical field tests.

In summary, the FIM instrument is considered a reliable and valid measure of the level at which a person is functioning in task performances, vocational pursuits, social interactions, and other behaviors (Brosseau *et al.*, 1996).

The Rankin scale

The Rankin (Rankin, 1957) and modified Rankin (van Swieten *et al.*, 1988) scales are global descriptions of a patient's function based on their ability to perform ADL with reference to previous activities. They measure independence in, rather than performance of, specific tasks (van Swieten *et al.*, 1988). Both scales have had significant use in several stroke-outcome trials (Tomasello *et al.*, 1982; Bonita and Beaglehole, 1988; Roberts and Counsell, 1998; Sulter *et al.*, 1999). Investigation of the clinical meaning of the Rankin grades (de Haan *et al.*, 1995) identified that activity in ADL, and to a lesser extent instrumental ADL (IADL, see below), were the most important factors associated with the Rankin scores. The authors concluded that the Rankin scale appeared to reflect primarily a global level of activity, with a strong accent on physical activity, rather than a measure of participation.

Summary

Because several scales are highly predictive of each other, the BI has been considered by some as acceptable as any other (Gresham *et al.*, 1980; Wade and Hewer, 1987; Lindmark, 1988). It has become one of the more extensively used scales in stroke studies, research, and rehabilitation outcomes.

Instrumental activities of daily living

For patients who have had a stroke, a return to independent living in the community requires the ability to perform not only basic self-care tasks (ADL), but also the more complex daily tasks (IADL) needed to continue living, effectively, in the community. The assessment of community-based functional activities is potentially more difficult, as it may involve a complex interplay of factors such as environmental support, economic and social resources, and social, behavioral and motivational factors.

In respect of clinical evaluation, although there is a conceptual understanding of IADL, there is no agreement as to the exact items to be included in such a measure. Part of the difficulty is that the delineation between activity and participation is not clear. Nevertheless, such a measure might more accurately identify who could return safely to independent community living, and who would not. In an effort to measure these more complex functions of daily life, IADL scales have been developed.

Rivermead Activities of Daily Living Assessment

The Rivermead ADL Assessment (Whiting and Lincoln, 1980) was the first published IADL measure that was directed specifically towards the stroke population.

It is performance based, has 15 items split between two household domains, and is scored on a three-point scale.

Hamrin Activities Index

The Hamrin Activities Index (Hamrin, 1982) is a patient assessment, with or without the patient present, and is used to assess IADL before and one year after stroke. There are 22 items divided between four domains and it is scored on a four-point scale.

Frenchay Activities Index

The Frenchay Activities Index (FAI; Holbrook and Skilbeck, 1983) was developed to measure functional and social activities in people affected by stroke; it consists of 15 items using three subscales: domestic, work/leisure, and outdoors. The FAI is a self-report assessment tool that takes five minutes to complete and can be administered by interview or by mail (Holbrook and Skilbeck, 1983).

Nottingham Extended Activities of Daily Living Scale

The Nottingham Extended ADL scale (Nouri and Lincoln, 1987) is a self-reported questionnaire, based on the level of activity actually performed, one year after a stroke. There are 22 items divided between four domains and it uses a two-point scoring system that has four levels.

Assessment of motor and process skills

The assessment of motor and process skills (AMPS) was developed (Fisher, 1995) as an observational measure of functional competence in IADL. It is a performance-based test that attempts to assess why a patient might have difficulty performing a task. It is a complex and time-consuming instrument and needs to be administered by a highly trained clinician.

Summary

There is variable evidence for the reliability and validity of these IADL scales (Wade *et al.*, 1985; Towle, 1988; Lindmark and Hamrin, 1989; Lincoln and Edmans, 1990; Gompertz *et al.*, 1993; Schuling *et al.*, 1993). In a review of these scales (Chong, 1995), except for AMPS, each was identified as having its own merits and deficiencies, as well as applicability, within the purpose and population for which the measure was designed. IADL scores have been used to be significant predictors of subsequent hospitalization, home healthcare, and social services utilization (Hiroko *et al.*, 1999).

The FAI has been used in conjunction with the BI (Pederson *et al.*, 1997; Hsieh and Hsueh, 1999) to assess different activities in stroke patients. These scales could be used, in combination, to represent a comprehensive measure of activity. They are both easy to administer and so may be useful in clinics, as well as in stroke outcome and treatment-effect research.

Conclusions for activity assessments

Scales assessing varying levels of activity have been utilized in stroke-outcome measurement with much success but are, not without their limitations. Functional scales that contain only a rudimentary assessment of cognitive function should not be used to assess total disability. Many studies have different inclusion and exclusion criteria; aphasia often bars patients from being considered. Other factors include differences in sample demographics, severity of initial impairment, type of stroke, time of post-stroke evaluation, and type of scale used for measurement. The elimination of such confounding factors could be achieved by the acceptance of standard indices of activity measurement. This might improve interpretation of results, make meta-analyses easier and more powerful, and allow comparisons to be made between studies and across healthcare systems.

Measurements of quality of life

The concept of QoL comprises a broad spectrum of consequences of disease, including elements of impairments, activities and participation as well as patients' perceived health status and well-being. Several attempts have been made to define QoL, including emphasis on life satisfaction (Hornquist, 1982), psychosocial and physical well-being (Wenger et al., 1984), and health-related subjective experience (Guyatt and Jaeschke, 1990). In its original meaning, QoL was clearly related to subjectively perceived emotions of satisfaction and happiness (Campbell et al., 1976). Over time, the concept has expanded to include a complex collection of items and domains within four essential dimensions: physical, psychological, functional, and social health (de Haan et al., 1993). Although research using QoL instruments has shown a conceptual confusion, QoL has, nevertheless, become an important outcome measure in rehabilitation medicine.

Although, in general, a poorer QoL is strongly associated with the severity of neurological deficits (Jonkman et al., 1998), intuitively it is unlikely that the impairment might entirely explain a patient's QoL. Other variables commonly associated with stroke survivors' QoL, identified in numerous studies, include levels of independence and functional abilities, psychological impairment and depression, social support and healthcare, and the ability to return to work Ahlsio et al., 1984; Viitanen et al., 1988; Astrom et al., 1992; King, 1996; Duncan et al., 1997; Bays, 2001). QoL not only reflects patients' health status but also how they perceive and react to that status and other non-medical aspects of their lives (Gill and Feinstein, 1994). The need to incorporate patients' perceptions and values in QoL measures then becomes essential in constructing these scales, as several studies have shown that clinicians, and patients' judgements of QoL differ substantially (Pearlman & Uhlmann, 1988; Slevin *et al.*, 1988). Relevant patient group involvement in scale construction would make the QoL instrument more meaningful and valid.

Sanders *et al.* (1998), examined the frequency and quality of reporting on QoL in randomized controlled trials in stroke research. Few studies actually reported on QoL, and of the plethora of instruments used in different studies, the reporting of methods and results were often considered to be inadequate. There was no clear consensus as to the definition of QoL. Stroke-outcome studies ideally need a practical disease-specific QoL scale that focuses on the specific problems of stroke patients and that is valid, reliable, and sensitive to change. Unfortunately, there is no single, generally accepted method for measuring QoL after stroke. Because of the wide range of dimensions affected by stroke, different instruments are needed to assess particular aspects of this complex construct. The instruments used in QoL outcome studies are usually either generic or stroke specific.

Most researchers seem to utilize a multidimensional approach to QoL assessment (Aaronsen, 1988; de Haan *et al.* 1993). Generic scales detect relative effects of disease and treatment on different domains. They allow comparisons of QoL results across patient populations. The review by Garratt *et al.* (2002) showed that the largest number of evaluations were with generic measures. However, many generic scales are limited in assessing changes in QoL following stroke intervention, owing to a lack of sensitivity and content validity (Ebrahim, 1995). Generic measures cannot focus on the problems of a specific condition. Though stroke-specific scales should be more sensitive to QoL issues particularly relevant in this population of patients, few have used a patient-centered approach in their development, and they may not cover all the issues considered important to people with a stroke. Each approach has its advantages and disadvantages, suggesting a need for both types of instrument to be used. Not surprisingly, it has been suggested that QoL instruments should include generic items and disease-specific items responsive to QoL changes in the stroke patient population under study (Patrick and Deyo, 1989; Guyatt, 1993). Overall, the identification of an instrument that is widely accepted by stroke researchers is needed to advance the study of QoL.

There are three types of QoL instruments used in assessment of stroke patients:

- generic instruments
- stroke-specific instruments
- visual analogue scales (VAS).

Generic instruments

Short Form - 36

The Short Form-36 (SF-36) was designed to survey the health status of the general population in the Medical Outcomes Study (Stewart and Ware, 1992; Ware and Sherbourne, 1992). It is a multidimensional questionnaire that has been used for health policy evaluations, general population surveys, clinical practice, and research. The SF-36 is a subjective measure of health-related QoL (HRQL) comprising eight domains: physical functioning, role limitations-physical, bodily pain, general health, vitality, social functioning, role limitations-emotional, and mental health. Two core dimensions of health, physical and mental, can be derived from these domains. The scale consists of 36 items, one of which pertains to the patient's perception of change in health over a one-year period. The SF-36 was designed to be self-administered but can be used over the telephone (Weinberger *et al.*, 1996) and in interview (Anderson *et al.*, 1996). The SF-36 is short, comprehensive, and only requires about 10 minutes to complete.

Although internal consistency (Anderson *et al.*, 1996), validity (Dorman *et al.*, 1999), and reliability (Hays *et al.*, 1993) have generally been demonstrated for the SF-36 in stroke studies, it has been criticized for ceiling and floor effects (Kurtin *et al.*, 1992; Wade, 1992; O'Mahony *et al.*, 1998; Williams, 1998; Dorman *et al.*, 1999). Additionally, in other studies, the SF-36 has been identified as offering only limited coverage of the domains of bodily pain (McHoney *et al.*, 1993), social functioning, and general health (Hobart *et al.*, 2002). Although the SF-36 has been validated for people with stroke (Anderson *et al.*, 1996; Dorman *et al.*, 1998; Hackett *et al.*, 2000) and its use supported in stroke studies (de Haan, 2002), it may need to be supplemented by other measures for a comprehensive assessment of stroke outcome.

The SF-36 has frequently been used as a validating instrument in the psychometric evaluation of new measures and is the most commonly used generic QoL instrument (Ware and Gandek, 1998).

The Nottingham Health Profile

The Nottingham Health Profile (NHP; Hunt *et al.*, 1993) is a generic questionnaire designed to assess social and personal effects of illness. It is often regarded as a measure of general perceived health status (Walker and Rosser, 1993). There are two parts to the NHP. Part I contains 38 items measuring subjective health in six domains: energy, pain, emotional reactions, sleep, social isolation, and physical mobility. Part II of the NHP explores the impact of perceived health problems on seven areas of everyday life: work, home maintenance, social life, home life, sex life, interests and hobbies, and holidays. Items are scored dichotomously with either "yes" or "no" responses. Weightings are assigned to items to reflect varying levels of perceived distress (McKenna *et al.*, 1981). The NHP is a patient-centered instrument, the entire completion of which takes 10–15 minutes (Hunt *et al.*, 1993). It can be self- or interviewer-administered and also used as a postal questionnaire.

The NHP is reported as being valid, to have adequate test–retest reliability, and is responsive (Hunt *et al.*, 1993). The construct validity of the NHP is confirmed in the pattern of correlates among its scales with other generic instruments and criterion validity, in discriminating between major medical conditions, and in symptomatic versus non-symptomatic illness (Wiklund, 1990). However, evidence for internal consistency of some subscale items is still needed and the potential limitation in sensitivity of the NHP has been identified mainly as a large floor effect (Kind and Carr-Hill, 1987). Also, Ebrahim *et al.* (1986) identified that NHP scores for patients with a stroke did not change despite improvement in physical ability, implying the scale was measuring dimensions of illness that were independent of objective indicators of functional ability. The NHP does not consider some areas of major concern that may impact on QoL after stroke: bladder function, memory, intellectual ability, and financial difficulty. Hence, the NHP may be limited if used as a single comprehensive instrument.

The Sickness Impact Profile

The Sickness Impact Profile (SIP; Bergner *et al.*, 1976) is a generic status health questionnaire originally developed as a behaviorally based assessment of the impact of illness on everyday life. It was revised in 1981 (Bergner *et al.*, 1981) and has been used as an outcome measure, health survey, program planner, policy formulator, and monitor of patient progress (Wilkin *et al.*, 1992). The SIP is a well-evaluated 136-item measure organized into 12 domains and two main dimensions, psychosocial and physical. Domains assessing communication, cognitive alertness, emotional behavior, and social functioning may be particularly relevant for use in stroke-outcome studies. Items are weighted by severity of health impact based on equal-appearing interval scaling. Patient-centered methods have been used in the construction of the SIP. Dichotomous responses, either "yes" or "no" are used similarly as in the NHP. Interviewer, self-administered and postal versions have been developed. It has also been shown to be suitable for proxy use. The SIP takes about 30 minutes to complete, which is longer than other scales, and has been criticized as lengthy and fatiguing (Schuling *et al.*, 1993).

The SIP is reliable (Pollard *et al.*, 1976; Deyo *et al.*, 1983). The validation of general psychosocial and physical dimensions is consistent with the conceptual content of other major generic QoL measures such as SF-36 and NHP. The SIP is sensitive to change (Bergner *et al.*, 1981). Though significant ceiling and floor effects have not been reported, the sensitivity of the scale in detecting small changes has been questioned (Jette, 1980).

Although comprehensive in assessment, reliable, valid, and responsive, the length of the SIP has remained an obstacle to its routine use, both clinically and in research. Consequently, the short form SIP 68 was developed (de Bruin *et al.*, 1994a), containing 68 of the original 136 items divided over six domains rather than 12. The psychometric properties of the SIP 68 appear to be comparable to those of the longer version (de Bruin *et al.*, 1994a, b; Post *et al.*, 1996).

The SIP has been used in stroke research assessments (Bergner *et al.*, 1981; de Haan *et al.*, 1993; Carod-Artal *et al.*, 2000) and further evaluated as a measure of QoL after stroke (Buck *et al.*, 2000) unlike the SIP 68, which requires further validation in this particular population of patients.

EuroQoL

The EuroQoL (EuroQoL Group, 1990) is a generic multidimensional HRQL profile. It provides a simple descriptive profile of health in five domains: mobility, self-care, social, pain, and psychology, each with three levels. The EuroQoL also includes a VAS on which patients rate their own health between 0 and 100, giving an overall numeric estimate of their HRQL. The items were chosen from a pool of items from other HRQL indices; a patient-centered approach was not used.

The EuroQoL is short, simple to use, and can be completed in two or three minutes. It exists in self- and interviewer-administered forms. There is only moderate agreement between patient and proxy responses for the more directly observable domains of the EuroQoL; agreement is worse for the more subjective domains (Dorman *et al.*, 1997).

The EuroQoL appears to have acceptable validity for the measurement of HRQL after stroke. The EuroQoL domains of physical functioning, social functioning, pain, and overall HRQL correlate closely with those of the SF-36 in the assessment of HRQL after stroke (Dorman *et al.*, 1999). Although valid, there is less evidence for its reliability and uncertainty about its responsiveness to change. The scale is criticized for a lack of sensitivity (Williams, 1998). However, it appears to measure aspects of QoL that are highly relevant to the stroke population.

Assessment of Quality of Life Instrument

The Assessment of QoL instrument (AQoL; Hawthorne *et al.*, 1999, 2000) was designed to be generic, to meet standard psychometric requirements, and to be sensitive across the breadth of health. The AQoL includes five domains of HRQL: independent living, social relationships, physical senses, psychological well-being, and illness. Each domain is weighted to extend between death and full health. The total score yields a descriptive profile.

The AQoL occurs in self- and interviewer-administered forms and can be used by proxy. It takes about five minutes to complete.

Convergent and discriminant validity have been demonstrated (Sturm *et al.*, 2002). Despite its brevity, it is considered to capture much of the variance of participation, activity, and impairment instruments, and it returns information on broader aspects of HRQL. The AQoL clearly differentiates between patients in categories of severity of impairment and activity, and it is, therefore, considered to exhibit a degree of sensitivity. However, it does not assess upper limb and cognitive function. Initial evidence supports the validity and sensitivity of the AQoL, but further evaluation is required to examine the reliability of the scale and further validation using stroke-specific HRQL scales.

Stroke-specific instruments

Stroke Impact Scale

The Stroke Impact Scale (SIS; Duncan *et al.*, 1999) is a comprehensive stroke-specific outcome measure. The SIS incorporates meaningful dimensions of function and HRQL into one self-report questionnaire. The SIS version-3 includes 59 items and assesses eight domains: strength, hand function, ADL and IADL, mobility, communication, emotion, memory and thinking, and participation/role function. Four of the domains can be combined to produce an aggregate physical domain score. The version SIS-16, derived from the SIS physical dimension, has compared favorably with the BI, exhibiting less-pronounced ceiling effects (Duncan *et al.*, 2003). The SIS also includes a question to assess the patient's global perception of percentage of recovery, using a VAS.

The SIS was originally developed and evaluated for administration by an interviewer. The mailed SIS would also appear to be a feasible means of assessing post-stroke function (Duncan *et al.*, 2002). In this study, greater proxy agreement was observed for the assessment of the physical domains than for the more subjective domains. The measure was developed with involvement of stroke patients (Juniper *et al.*, 1996).

The SIS has undergone psychometric evaluation in stroke populations and been shown to demonstrate good reliability, validity, and responsiveness for most domains (Duncan *et al.*, 1997, 2003). The emotion domain demonstrated fewer desirable psychometric properties than the others. A more responsive measure of emotion needs to be developed, particularly as the emotion domain significantly contributes to the patient's perception of recovery (Duncan *et al.*, 1999). The instrument was developed with patients with mild-to-moderate severity of stroke, who had communication skills and cognitive function intact. Although over two-thirds of all stroke survivors have mild to moderate deficits (Jorgensen *et al.*, 1995), the usefulness of the SIS scale in more severely affected patients needs to be evaluated.

The SIS is a newly developed comprehensive measure of health after stroke and is able to capture the impact of stroke across multiple domains. It can demonstrate persisting difficulties in physical domains of stroke patients who had been considered functionally independent using ADL measures (Lai *et al.*, 2002). Using a stroke-specific outcome measure that captures a broad range of function in a population, without significant ceiling or floor effects, should improve the ability to detect change in stroke-outcome studies, allow identification of rehabilitation needs, and potentially lead to the maximization of patients' QoL.

Stroke-adapted 30-item version of the Sickness Impact Profile

The Stroke-adapted 30-item version of the SIP (SA-SIP30; van Straten *et al.*, 1997) was developed to overcome the major disadvantage of the SIP, specifically its length. The SA-SIP30 was derived from the SIP by exclusion of the least-relevant domains and items and the unreliable items. The SIP was reduced from 12 domains with 136 items, to eight domains containing 30 items. The weightings used were as for the original generic parent. The SA-SIP30 exists in self- or interviewer-administered forms. Patient-centered methods were not used in its construct.

The SA-SIP30 is both reliable and valid (van Straten *et al.*, 1997). However, its use with more severely affected stroke patients needs further study, as does its responsivity to detect clinically relevant health changes over time.

It has been concluded that the SA-SIP30 is a feasible and clinimetrically sound measure to assess QoL after stroke (van Straten *et al.*, 1997), but it clearly needs further assessment if it is to be used more frequently in future stroke studies.

Stroke-specific Quality of Life Scale

The Stroke-specific Quality of Life Scale (SS QoL; Williams *et al.*, 1999); was developed to measure stroke-specific HRQL across a range of stroke symptoms and severity. It comprises 12 domains containing 49 items. Items and domains were identified following interviews with survivors of ischemic strokes. Preliminary data concerning reliability, validity, and responsiveness are encouraging. However, many questions remain to be answered including mode of administration, proxy respondents, weighting, and performance of the scale with more severely affected stroke patients.

Quality of Life Index–Stroke Version

The Quality of Life Index–Stroke Version (QLI; Ferrans and Powers, 1985) is a stroke-specific 36-item instrument that measures QoL in terms of satisfaction and importance in four domains: health and functioning, social and economic, psychological/spiritual, and family. Modifications have been made to include communication, self-care and mobility (Ferrans and Powers, 1992). The scale is interviewer administered. It was developed without using a patient-centered approach. The average completion time is not reported. The QLI possesses strong internal consistency and validity (Ferrans and Powers, 1985) but has not been reported to be sensitive to change.

Niemi Quality of Life Scale

The Niemi Quality of Life Scale (Niemi *et al.*, 1988) employs 58 items divided between four domains: working conditions, activities at home, family/personal relationships, and leisure activities. The scale is interviewer administered, was not developed using a patient-centered approach, and average completion times have not been reported. The Niemi QoL scale demonstrates reliability and validity, but responsiveness has not been reported.

Frenchay Activities Index

The FAI (Holbrook and Skilbeck, 1983) was originally developed as an IADL measure specifically for use with stroke patients. The FAI measures lifestyle in terms of more complex physical activities and social functioning. The index is brief and can be self or interviewer administered; there is evidence for its use with proxy respondents. The psychometric properties of the FAI in QoL assessments has been reviewed (Buck *et al.*, 2000); although it demonstrates reliability, validity, and responsiveness, it was not developed as a QoL measure and maybe should not be considered as a comprehensive tool.

Visual analogue scales

Both VAS and simple single general health questions have been used to assess overall patient perception of QoL. Their value lies with brevity, minimal patient burden, and data analysis that is simpler to interpret than data from multidimensional QoL instruments. However, the information acquired is relatively crude; only a broad assessment of the QoL is obtained and outcomes in specific domains are not identified. A disease-specific VAS question cannot be used in other diagnostic groups. It has been argued that individual patients differ so much, particularly in the perception of their QoL, that a crude, yet valid measure could provide an estimate of outcome (Tukey, 1962).

Among the more commonly used questionnaires, a VAS is used in the generic EuroQoL and the stroke-specific SIS, and a single separate item assessing change in overall health over 1 year is used in the SF-36 scale. Individual VAS have been used otherwise in a number of stroke studies (Kwa *et al.*, 1996; Hop *et al.*, 1998; Indredavik *et al.*, 1998).

Summary

Zola wrote in 1983, "It is not the quantity of tasks we can perform without assistance, but the quality of life we can live without help." Since then, stroke management, from policy decision making to care of the individual patient, has undoubtedly benefited from the implementation of QoL scales. This same period has witnessed a paradigm shift in which the patient was no longer perceived as simply a recipient of services but was enabled to become actively involved, through participation, in the construction of more meaningful multidisciplinary health status instruments. Furthermore, the exclusion from many studies of patients with aphasia and significant cognitive problems led to the development of scales that effectively measured proxy respondents so that the complete breadth of stroke severity could be assessed by a QoL instrument.

The concept of QoL, is complex, and a clear definition remains elusive. The lack of clarity is demonstrated in both generic and stroke-specific scales, which utilize multiple different domains in their attempts to "capture" this concept. Until there is clarity, the interpretation and comparison of data obtained from various scales will remain challenging, as will the relation of QoL to the other dimensions of the ICF construct (WHO, 2001).

In selecting a suitable QoL instrument, some trade-off between the level of detail in the longer scales and the feasibility of the shorter scales seems inevitable. This has been addressed in some studies by simply shortening or extending existing scales, and in other studies by developing new ones. Therefore, until further evidence accrues, researchers need to be cautious in their choice of existing measures and aware of the psychometric requirements in the construction of new ones in order to be able to make a comprehensive and valid assessment of QoL after stroke.

REFERENCES

Aaronsen, N. K. (1988). Quality of life: What is it? How should it be measured? *Oncology* **2**: 69–74.

Ahlsio, B., Britton, M., Murray, V., and Theorell, T. (1984). Disablement and quality of life after stroke. *Stroke* **15**: 886–890.

Alexander, M. P. (1994). Stroke rehabilitation outcome: a potential use of predictive variables to establish levels of care. *Stroke* **25**: 128–134.

American Education Research Association and National Council on Research in Education (1985). *Standards for Education and Psychological Tests.* Washington, DC: American Psychological Association.

Anderson, C., Laubscher, S., and Burns, R. (1996). Validation of the Short Form 36 (SF-36) Health Survey Questionnaire among stroke patients. *Stroke* **27**: 1812–1816.

Asplund, K. (1987). Clinimetrics in stroke research. *Stroke* **18**: 528–530.

Astrom, M., Asplund, K., and Astrom, T. (1992). Psychosocial function and life satisfaction after stroke. *Stroke* **23**: 527–531.

Bays, C. L. (2001). Quality of life of stroke survivors: A research synthesis. *J Neurosci Nursing* **33**: 310–316.

Bergner, M., Bobbitt, R. A., Kressel, S., *et al.* (1976). The Stroke Impact Profile: conceptual foundation and methodology for the development of a health status measure. *Int J Health Serv* **6**: 393–415.

Bergner, M., Bobbitt, R. A., Cartel, W. B., and Gilson, B. S. (1981). The Sickness Impact Profile: development and final revision of a health status measure. *Med Care* **19**: 787–805.

Bonita, R. and Beaglehole, R. (1988). Recovery of motor function after stroke. *Stroke* **19**: 1497–1500.

Brosseau, L., Potvin, L., Phillipe, P., *et al.* (1996). The construct validity of the Functional Independence Measure as applied to stroke patients. *Phys Theor Pract*, **12**: 161–171.

Brown, E. B., Tietjen, G. E., Deveshwar, R. K., *et al.* (1990). Clinical stroke scales: an intra- and inter-scale evaluation. *Neurology*, **40** (Suppl. 1): 352–355.

Buck, D., Jacoby, A., Massey, A., and Ford, G. (2000). Evaluation of measures used to assess quality of life after stroke. *Stroke* **31**: 2004–2010.

Campbell, A., Converse, D. E., and Rodgers, W. L. (1976). *The Quality of American Life: Perceptions, Evaluations and Satisfactions*, New York: Sage.

Carod-Artal, J., Egido, J. A., Gonzalez, J. L., and De Seijas, V. (2000). Quality of life among stroke survivors evaluated 1 year after stroke. *Stroke* **31**: 2995–3000.

Carr, J. H., Shepherd, R. B., Nordholm, L., and Lynne, D. (1985). Investigation of a new motor assessment scale for stroke patients. *Phys Ther* **65**: 175–179.

Chong, D. K-H. (1995). Measurement of Instrumental Activities of Daily Living in stroke. *Stroke* **26**: 1119–1122.

Cohen, M. E. and Marino, R. J. (2000). The tools of disability outcomes research functional status measures. *Arch Phys Med Rehabil* **81** (Suppl. 2): S21–S29.

Collen, F. M., Wade, D. T., and Bradshaw, C. M. (1990). Mobility after stroke: reliability of measures of impairment and disability. *Int Disabil Stud* **12**: 6–9.

Collen, F. M., Wade, D. T., Robb, G. F., and Bradshaw, C. M. (1991). The Rivermead Mobility Index: a further development of the Rivermead Motor Assessment. *Int Disabil Stud* **13**: 50–54.

Collin, C., Wade, D. T., Davies, S., and Horne, V. (1988). The Barthel ADL Index: a reliability study. *Int Disabil Stud* **10**: 61–63.

Daving, Y., Andren, E., Hordholm, L., and Grimby, G. (2001). Reliability of an interview approach to the Functional Independence Measure. *Clin Rehabil* **15**: 301–310.

de Bruin, A. F., Diederiks, J. P. M., and de Witte, L. P. (1994a). The development of a short generic version of the Sickness Impact Profile. *J Clin Epidemiol* **47**: 407–418.

de Bruin, A. F., Buys, M., de Witte, L. P., and Diederiks, J. P. M. (1994b). The Sickness Impact Profile: SIP68, a short generic version. First evaluation of the reliability and reproducibility. *J Clin Epidemiol* **47**: 863–871.

de Haan, R. J. (2002). Measuring quality of life after stroke using the SF-36. *Stroke* **33**: 1176–1177.

de Haan, R. J., Aaronsen, N., Limburg, M., *et al.* (1993). Measuring quality of life in stroke. *Stroke* **24**: 320–327.

de Haan, R.,J. Limburg, M., Bossuyt, P., *et al.* (1995). The clinical meaning of Rankin 'handicap' grades after stroke. *Stroke* **26**: 2027–2030.

Derosiers, J., Herbert, R., Putil, E., *et al.* (1994). Validity of the TEMPA: a measurement instrument for upper extremity performance. *Occup Ther J Res* **14**: 267–281.

Derosiers, J., Herbert, R., Bravo, G., and Dutil, E. (1995). Upper extremity performance test for the elderly (TEMPA): normative data and correlates with sensorimotor parameters: Test d'Evaluation des Membres Superieurs de Personnes Agées. *Arch Phys Med Rehabil* **76**: 1125–1129.

Deyo, R., Invi, T., Lenninger, J., *et al.* (1983). Measuring functional outcomes in chronic disease: a comparison of traditional scales and a self-administered health status questionnaire in patients with rheumatoid arthritis. *Med Care* **21**: 180–192.

Dodds, T. A., Martin, D. P., Stolov, W. C., and Deyo, R. A. (1993). A validation of the Functional Independence Measure and its performance among rehabilitation inpatients. *Arch Phys Med Rehabil* **74**: 531–536.

D'Olhaberriague, L., Litvan, I., Mitsias, P., and Mansbrach, H. H. (1996). A reappraisal of reliability and validity studies in stroke. *Stroke* **27**: 2331–2336.

Donkervoork, M., Dekker, J., and Deelinan, B. G. (2002). Sensitivity of different ADL measures to apraxia and motor impairments. *Clin Rehabil* **16**: 299–305.

Dorman, P. J., Waddell, F., Slattery, J., *et al.* (1997). Are proxy assessments of health status after stroke with the EuroQol questionnaire, feasible, accurate and unbiased? *Stroke* **28**: 1883–1887.

Dorman, P. J., Slattery, J., Farrell, B., *et al.* (1998). Qualitative comparison of the reliability of health status measurements with the EuroQol and SF-36 questionnaires after stroke. *Stroke* **29**: 63–68.

Dorman, P. J., Dennis, M., and Sandercock, P. (1999). How do scores on the EuroQol relate to scores on the SF-36 after stroke. *Stroke* **30**: 2146–2151.

Duncan, P. W., Samsa, G. P., Weinberger, M., *et al.* (1997). Health status of individuals with mild stroke. *Stroke* **28**: 740–745.

Duncan, P. W., Wallace, D., Lai, S. M., *et al.* (1999). The Stroke Impact Scale version 2.0: evaluation of reliability, validity and sensitivity to change. *Stroke* **30**: 2131–2140.

Duncan, P. W., Reker, D. M., Horner, R. D., *et al.* (2002). Performance of mail-administered version of a stroke specific outcome measure, the Stroke Impact Scale. *Clin Rehabil* **16**: 493–505.

Duncan, P. W., Lai, S. M., Bode, R. K., *et al.* (2003). The Stroke Impact Scale-16: a brief assessment of physical function. *Neurology* **60**: 291–296.

Duncan, P. W., Bode, R. K., Lai, S. M., and Perera, S., for the GAIN Americas Investigators (2003). Rasch analysis of a new stroke specific outcome scale: the Stroke Impact Scale. **84**: 950–963.

Ebrahim, S. (1995). Clinical and public health perspectives and applications of health related quality of life measurement. *Soc Sci Med* **41**: 1383–1394.

Ebrahim, S., Barer, D., and Nouri, F. (1986). Use of the Nottingham Health Profile with patients after a stroke. *J Epidem Comm Health* **40**: 166–169.

EuroQol Group (1990). EuroQol: a new facility for the measurement of health related quality of life. *Health Policy* **16**: 199–208.

Ferrans, C. Powers, M. J. (1985). Quality of Life Index: development and psychometric properties. *Adv Nurs Sci* **8**: 15–24.

Ferrans, C. E. and Powers, M. J. (1992). Psychometric assessment of the quality of life index. *Res Nurs Health* **15**: 29–38.

Fisher, A. G. (1995). *Assessment of Motor and Process Skills*, revised edn. Fort Collins, CO: Three Star Press.

Garratt, A., Schmidt, L., Mackintosh, A., and Fitzpatrick, R. (2002). Quality of life measurement: bibliographic study of patient assessed health outcome measures. *BMJ* **324**: 1417–1419.

Gill, T. M. and Feinstein, A. R. (1994). A critical appraisal of the quality of quality of life measurements. *JAMA* **272**: 619–626.

Goldie, P. A., Matyas, T. A., and Evans, O. M. (1996). Deficit and change in gait velocity during rehabilitation after stroke. *Arch Phys Med Rehabil* **77**: 1074–1082.

Gompertz, P., Pound, P., and Ebrahim, S. (1993). Development and results of a questionnaire to measure carer satisfaction after stroke. *J Epidemiol Community Health* **47**: 500–505.

Granger, C. V. (1982). Health accounting: functional assessment of the long term patient. In *Krusen's Handbook of Physical Medicine*, ed. F. J. Koltke, G. K. Stillwell, J. F. Lehmann. Philadelphia, PA: Saunders, pp. 253–274

Granger, C. V., Albrecht, G. L., and Hamilton, B. B. (1979a). Outcomes of comprehensive medical rehabilitation: measurement of PULSES Profile and the Barthel Index. *Arch Phys Med Rehabil* **60**: 145–154.

Granger, C. V., Dewis, L. S., Peters, N. C., *et al.* (1979b). Stroke rehabilitation: analysis of repeated Barthel Index measures. *Arch Phys Med Rehabil* **60**: 14–17.

Granger, C. V., Hamilton, B. B., Keith, R. A., *et al.* (1986). Advances in functional assessment for medical rehabilitation. *Top Geriatr Rehabil* **1**: 59–74.

Granger, C. V., Hamilton, B. B., Gresham, G. E., and Kramer, A. A. (1989). The stroke rehabilitation outcome study. Part II. Relative merit of the total Barthel Index score and a four item sub-score in predicting patient outcomes. *Arch Phys Med Rehabil* **70**: 100–103.

Granger, C. V., Cotter, A. C., Hamilton, B. B., and Fielder, R. C. (1993a). Functional assessment scales: a study of persons after stroke. *Arch Phys Med Rehabil* **74**: 133–138.

Granger, C. V., Hamilton, B. B., Linacre, J. M., *et al.* (1993b). Performance profiles of the Functional Independence Measure. *Am J Phys Med Rehabil* **72**: 84–89.

Gresham, G. E., Phillips, T. E., and Labi, M. L. C. (1980). ADL status in stroke: relative merits of three standard indices. *Arch Phys Med Rehabil* **61**: 355–358

Guyatt, G. H. (1993). Measurement of health related quality of life in heart failure. *J Am Coll Cardiol* **22**: (Suppl. A): 185–191.

Guyatt, G. H. & Jaeschke, R. (1990). Measurements in clinical trials: choosing the appropriate approach. In *Quality of Life Assessments in Clinical Trials*, ed. B. Spiker. New York: Raven Press, pp. 37–46.

Hackett, M. L., Duncan, D. R., Anderson, C. S., *et al.* (2000). Health related quality of life among long-term survivors of stroke. *Stroke* **31**: 440–447.

Haigh, R., Tennant, A., Bering-Sorensen, F., *et al.* (2001). The use of outcome measures in physical medicine and rehabilitation within Europe. *J Rehabil Med* **33**: 273–278.

Hajek, V. E., Gagnon, S., and Ruderman, J. E. (1997). Cognitive and functional assessments of stroke patients: an analysis of their relation. *Arch Phys Med Rehabil* **78**: 1331–1337.

Hall, K. M., Hamilton, B. B., Gordon, W. A., and Zasler, N. D. (1993). Characteristics and comparisons of functional assessment indices: Disability Rating Scale, Functional Independence Measure and Functional Assessment Measure. *J Head Trauma Rehabil* **8**: 60–74.

Hamilton, B. B., Laughlin, J. A., Fielder, R. C., and Granger, C. V. (1995). Interrater reliability of the 7-level Functional Independence Measurement (FIM). *Scand J Rehabil Med* **27**: 253–256.

Hamrin, E. (1982). One year after stroke: a follow-up of an experimental study. *Scand J Rehabil Med* **14**: 111–116.

Hawthorne, G., Richardson, J., and Osbourne, R. (1999). The Assessment of Quality of Life (AQoL) Instrument: a psychometric measure of health related quality of life. *Qual Life Res* **8**: 209–224.

Hawthorne, G., Richardson, J., Day, N., and McNeil, H. (2000). *Technical Report 12, Using the Assessment of Quality of Life (AQoL) Instrument.* Melbourne, Australia. Centre for Health Program Evaluation.

Hays, R. D., Sherbourne, C. D., and Mazel, R. M. (1993). The RAND 36-item Health Survey 1.0. *Health Econ*, **2**: 217–227

Heinemann, A. W., Linacre, J. M., Wright, B. D., *et al.* (1993). Relationships between impairment and physical disability as measures by the Functional Independence Measure. *Arch Phys Med Rehabil* **74**: 566–573.

Hiroko, H. D., Belle, S. H., Morycz, R. K., *et al.* (1999). Functional and demographic predictors of health and human services utilization: a community based study. *J Am Ger Soc* **47**: 1271–1273.

Hobart, J. C., Lamping, D. L., Freeman, J. A., *et al.* (2001). Evidence based measurement. Which disability scale for neurological rehabilitation? *Neurology* **57**: 639–644.

Hobart, J. C., Williams, L. S., Moran, K., and Thompon, A. J. (2002). Quality of life measurement after stroke. *Stroke* **33**: 1348–1356.

Holbrook, M. and Skilbeck, C. E. (1983). An activities index for use with stroke patients. *Age and Aging* **12**: 166–170.

Hop, J. W., Rinkel, G., J. E. Algra, A., and van Gijn, J (1998). Quality of life in patients and partners after aneurysmal subarachnoid haemorrhage. *Stroke* **29**: 798–804.

Hornquist, J. O. (1982). The concept of quality of life. *Scand J Soc Med* **10**: 57–61.

Hsieh, C.-L., and Hsueh, I.-P. (1999). A cross validation of the comprehensive assessment of activities of daily living after stroke. *Scand J Rehabil Med* **31**: 83–88.

Hsueh, I. - P. and Hsich, C.-L. (2002). Responsiveness of two upper extremity function instruments for stroke inpatients receiving rehabilitation. *Clin Rehabil* **16**: 617–624.

Hsieh, C.- L., Hsueh, I.-P., Chiang, F. M., and Lin, P. S. (1998). Inter-rater reliability and validity of the Action Research Arm Test in stroke patients. *Age Aging* **27**: 107–113.

Hsueh, I.-P., Lin, J.-H, Jeng, J.- S., and Hsieh, C.- L. (2002). Comparison of the psychometric characteristics of the Functional Independence Measure, 5-Item Barthel Index and 10-Item Barthel Index in patients with stroke. *J Neurol Neurosurg Psych* **73**: 188–190.

Hunt, S. M., McEwen, J., and McKenna, S. P. (1993). *The Nottingham Health Profile User's Manual*: Manchester, UK: Galen Research.

Indredavik, B., Bakke, F., Slordahl, S. A., *et al.* (1998). Stroke unit treatment improves long-term quality of life. *Stroke* **29**: 895–899.

Jacelon, C. A. (1986). The Barthel Index and other indices of functional ability. *Rehab Nurs* **11**: 9–11.

Jette, A. M. (1980). Health status indicators: their utility in chronic disease evaluation research. *J Chron Dis* **33**: 567–579.

Jonkman, E. J., de Weerd, A. W., and Vrijens, N. L. (1998). Quality of life after a first ischaemic stroke. Long-term developments and correlations with changes in neurological deficit, mood and cognitive impairments. *Acta Neurol Scand* **98**: 169–175.

Jorgensen, H. S., Nakayama, H., Pedersen, P. M., *et al.* (1995). Outcome and time course of recovery in stroke II: time course of recovery: the Copenhagen Stroke Study. *Arch Phys Med Rehabil* **76**: 406–412.

Juniper, E., Guyatt, G., and Jaeschke, R. (1996). How to develop and validate a new health related quality of life instrument. In *Quality of Life and Pharmacoeconomics in Clinical Trials*, ed. B. Spilker. Philadelphia, PA: Lippincott-Raven. pp. 49–58.

Keith, R. A. (1988). Functional assessment measures in medical rehabilitation: current status. *Arch Phys Med Rehabil* **65**: 74–78.

Keith, R. A., Granger, C. V., Hamilton, B. B., and Sherwin, F. S. (1987). The Functional Independence Measure: a new tool for rehabilitation. In *Advances in Clinical Rehabilitation*, Vol. 1, ed. M. G. Eisenberg and R. C. Grzesiak. New York: Springer Publishing, pp. 6–18.

Kind, P. and Carr-Hill, R. (1987). The Nottingham Health Profile: a useful tool for epidemiologists. *Soc Sci Med* **25**: 905–910.

King, R. B. (1996). Quality of life after stroke. *Stroke* **27**: 1467–1472.

Kurtin, P. S., Davies, A. R., Meyer, K. B., *et al.* (1992). Patient-based health status measurements in out-patient dialysis: early experiences in developing an outcomes assessment program. *Med Care* **30** (Suppl. 5): MS136–MS149.

Kwa, V. I. H., Limburg, M., and de Haan, R. J. (1996). The role of cognitive impairment in the quality of life after ischaemic stroke. *J Neurol* **243**: 599–604.

Lai, S. M., Studenski, S., Duncan, P. W., and Perera, S. (2002). Persisting consequences of stroke measures by the Stroke Impact Scale. *Stroke* **33**: 1840–1849.

Lennon, S. (1995). Using standardized scales to document outcome in stroke rehabilitation. *Physiotherapy* **81**: 200–202.

Lennon, S. and Johnson, L. (2000). The modified Rivermead Mobility Index: validity and reliability. *Disabil Rehabil* **22**: 833–839.

Lincoln, N. B. and Edmans, J. A. (1990). A re-validation of the Rivermead ADL Scale for elderly patients with stroke. *Age Aging* **19**: 19–24.

Lindmark, B. (1988). Evaluation of functional capacity after stroke with special emphasis on motor function and ADL. *Scand J Rehabil Med* **21**: 1–40.

Lindmark, B. and Hamrin, E. (1989). Instrumental activities of daily living in two patient populations, three months and 1 year after stroke. *Scand J Caring Sci* **3**: 161–168.

Loewen, S. C., Anderson, B. A. (1988). Reliability of the Modified Motor Assessment Scale and the Barthel Index. *Phys Ther* **68**: 1077–1081.

Loewen, S. C. and Anderson, B. A. (1990). Predictors of stroke outcome using objective measurement scales. *Stroke* **21**: 78–81.

Lyle, R. C. (1981). A performance test for assessment of upper limb function in physical rehabilitation treatment and research. *Int J Rehabil Res* **4**: 483–492.

McHoney, C. A., Ware, J. E., Jr., and Raczek, A. E. (1993). The MOS 36-item short form health survey (SF-36): II. Psychometric and clinical tests of validity in measuring physical and mental health constructs. *Med Care* **31**: 247–263.

McKenna, S. P., Hunt, S. M., and McEwen, J. (1981). Weighting the seriousness of perceived health problems using Thurstone's method of paired comparisons. *Int J Epidemiol* **10**: 93–97.

McNaughton, H., Weatherall, M., Taylor, W., and McPherson, K. (2001). Factors influencing rate of Barthel Index change in hospital following stroke. *Clin Rehabil* **15**: 422–427.

Mahoney, F. I. and Barthel, D. W. (1965). Functional evaluation: the Barthel Index. *Maryland State Medical Journal* **14**: 61–65.

Malouin, F., Richard, L., Bonneau, C., *et al.* (1994). Evaluating motor recovery early after stroke: comparison of the Fugl–Meyer assessment and the Motor Assessment Scale. *Arch Phys Med Rehabil* **75**: 1206–1212.

Mathias, S., Nayak, U. S. L., and Isaacs, B. (1986). Balance in the elderly patient: the 'Get-up and Go' test. *Arch Phys Med Rehabil* **67**: 387–389.

Mathiowetz, V., Kashman, N., Volland, G., *et al.* (1985). Grip and pinch strength: normative data for adults. *Arch Phys Med Rehabil* **66**: 69–74.

Niemi, M. L., Laakonsen, M. A., Kolila, M. D., and Wallino, O. (1988). Quality of life four years after stroke. *Stroke* **19**: 1101–1107.

Nouri, F. M. and Lincoln, N. B. (1987). An extended activities of daily living scale for stroke patients. *Clin Rehab* **1**: 301–305.

Nunnally, J. C. (1978). *Psychometric Theory*. New York: McGraw-Hill.

O'Mahoney, P. G., Rodgers, H., Thomson, R. G., *et al.* (1998). Is the SF-36 suitable for assessing health status of older stroke patients? *Age Aging* **27**: 19–22.

Orgogozo, J. M. (1994). The concepts of impairment, disability and handicap. *Cerbrovasc Dis* **4** (Suppl. 2): 12–16.

Ottenbacher, K. J., Mann, W. C., Granger, C. V., *et al.*, (1994). Inter-rater agreement and stability of functional assessment in the community-based elderly. *Arch Phys Med Rehabil* **75**: 1297–1301.

Owen, D. C., Getz, P. A., and Bulla, S. (1995). A comparison of characteristics of patients with completed stroke: those who achieve continence and those who do not. *Rehabil Nurs* **20**: 197–203.

Patrick, D. L. and Deyo, R. A. (1989). Generic and disease specific measures in assessing health status and quality of life. *Med Care* **27**: 217–232.

Pearlman, R. and Uhlmann, R. (1988). Patient and physician perceptions of patient quality of life across chronic diseases. *J Gerontol* **43**: 25–30.

Pedersen, P. M., Jorgensen, H. S., Nakayama, H., *et al.* (1997). Comprehensive assessment of activities of daily living in stroke. *Arch Phys Med Rehabil* **78**: 161–165.

Podsiadlo, D. and Richardson, S. (1991). The timed 'Up and Go': a test of basic functional mobility for frail elderly persons. *J Am Geriatr Soc* **39**: 149–155.

Pollard, W. E., Bobbitt, R. A., Bergner, M., *et al.* (1976). The Stroke Impact Profile: reliability of a health status measure. *Med Care* **14**: 146–155.

Poole, J. C., and Whitney, S. C. (1988). Motor assessment scale for stroke patients: concurrent validity and interrater reliability. *Arch Phys Med Rehabil* **69**: 195–197.

Post, M. W. M., de Bruin, A. F., de Witte, L., *et al.* (1996). The Stroke Impact Profile-68: a measure of health related functional status in rehabilitation medicine. *Arch Phys Med Rehabil* **77**: 440–445.

Prescott, R. J., Garraway, M. B., and Alchtor, A. J. (1982). Predicting functional outcome following acute stroke using a standard clinical examination. *Stroke* **13**: 641–647.

Rankin, J. (1957). Cerebral vascular accidents in patients over the age of 60, II: prognosis. *Scott Med J* **2**: 200–215.

Roberts, L. and Counsell, C. (1998). Assessment of clinical outcomes in acute stroke trials. *Stroke* **29**: 986–991.

Sanders, C., Egger, M., Donovan, J., *et al.* (1998). Reporting on quality of life in randomised controlled trials: bibliographic study. *BMJ* **317**: 1191–1194.

Schuling, J., Gradanus, J., and Meijboom-De Jong, B. (1993). Measuring functional status of stroke patients with the Sickness Impact Profile. *Disab Rehabil* **15**: 19–23.

Segal, M. E. and Schall, R. R. (1994). Determining function/health status and its relation to disability in stroke survivors. *Stroke* **25**: 2391–2397.

Shah, S., Vanclay, F., and Cooper, B. (1991). Stroke rehabilitation: Australian patient profile and functional outcome. *J Clin Epidemiol* **44**: 21–28.

Shinar, D., Gross, C. R., Bronstein, K. S., *et al.* (1987). Reliability of the activities of daily living scale and its use in telephone interview. *Arch Phys Med Rehabil* **68**: 723–728.

Skilbeck, C. E., Wade, D. T., Hewer, R. L., and Wood, V. (1983). Recovery after stroke. *J Neurol Neurosurg Psych* **46**: 5–8.

Slevin, M., Plant, H., Lynch, D., *et al.* (1988). Who should measure quality of life, the doctor or the patient? *Br J Cancer* **57**: 109–112.

Sommerfeld, D. K. and von Arbin, M. H. (2001). Disability test 10 days after acute stroke to predict early discharge home in patients 65 years and older. *Clin Rehabil* **15**: 528–534.

Spector, W. D. (1990). Functional disability scales. In *Quality of Life Assessments in Clinical Trials*, ed. B. Spiker. New York: Raven Press, pp. 115–129.

Stewart, A. L. and Ware, J. E. (1992). *Measuring Functioning and Well-being: the Medical Outcomes Study Approach*. London: Duke University Press.

Stineman, M. G., Goin, J. E., Granger, C. V., *et al.* (1997). Discharge motor Functional Independence Measure-function related groups. *Arch Phys Med Rehabil* **78**: 980–985.

Sturm, J. W., Dewey, H. M., Donnan, G. A., *et al.* (2002). Handicap after stroke. How does it relate to disability, perception of recovery and stroke subtype? The North East Melbourne Incidence Stroke Study (NEMESIS). *Stroke* **33**: 762–768.

Sulter, G., Steen, C., and De Keyer, J. (1999). Use of the Barthel Index and modified Rankin Scale in acute stroke trials. *Stroke* **30**: 1538–1541.

Sunderland, A., Tinson, D., Bradley, L., *et al.* (1989). Arm function after stroke: an evaluation of grip strength as a measure of recovery and a prognostic indicator. *J Neurol Neurosurg Psych* **52**: 1267–1272.

Tomasello, F., Mariani, F., Fieschi, C., *et al.* (1982). Assessment of inter-observer differences in the Italian multi-centre study on reversible cerebral ischaemia. *Stroke* **13**: 32–34.

Towle, D. (1988). Use of the 'extended ADL scale' with depressed stroke patients. *Int Disabil Stud* **10**: 148–149.

Tukey, J. W. (1962). The future of data analysis. *Ann Math Stat* **33**: 13–14.

van Straten, A., de Haan, R. J., Limburg, M., *et al.* (1997). A stroke-adapted 30-item version of the Sickness Impact Profile to assess quality of life (SA-SIP30). *Stroke* **28**: 2155–2161.

van Swieten J. C., Koudstaal, P. J., Visser, M. C., *et al.* (1988). Inter-observer agreement for the assessment of handicap in acute stroke patients. *Stroke* **19**: 604–607.

Viitanen, M., Fugl-Meyer, K. S., Bernsprang, B., and Fugl-Meyer, A. R. (1988). Life satisfaction in long term survivors after stroke. *Scand J Rehabil Med* **20**: 17–24.

Wade, D. T. (1992). *Measurement in Neurological Rehabilitation*. New York: Oxford Medical Publications.

Wade, D. T. and Collin, C. (1998). The Barthel Index: a standard measure of physical disability? *Int Disabil Stud* **10**: 64–67.

Wade, D. T. and Hewer, R. L. (1987). Functional abilities after stroke: measurement, natural and prognosis. *J Neuro Neurosurg Psych* **50**: 177–182.

Wade, D. T., Wood, V. A., and Hewer, R. L. (1985). Recovery after stroke-the first 3 months. *J Neurol Neurosurg Psych* **48**: 7–13.

Wade, D. T., Leigh-Smith, J., and Langton-Hewer, R. (1987). Depressed mood after stroke: a community study of its frequency, prognosis and associated factors. *Br J Psychiatry* **151**: 200–205.

Walker, S. R. and Rosser, R. M. (1993). *Quality of Life Assessment: Key Issues in the 1990s*. Dordrecht, the Netherlands: Kluwer Academic.

Ware, J. E. and Gandek, B. (1998). Overview of the SF-36 health survey and the International Quality of Life Assessment (IQOLA) Project. *J Clin Epidemiol* **51**: 903–912.

Ware, J. E. and Sherbourne, C. D. (1992). The Medical Outcome Study (MOS) 36-item Short Form Health Survey (SF-36). Conceptual framework and item selection. *Med Care* **30**: 473–483.

Ween, J. E., Alexander, M., D'Esposito, M., and Roberts, M. (1996a). Incontinence after stroke in a rehabilitation setting: outcome associations and predictive factors. *Neurology* **47**: 659–663.

Ween, J. E. Alexander, M. D'Esposito, M., and Roberts, M. (1996b). Factors predictive of stroke outcome in a rehabilitation setting. *Neurology* **47**: 388–392.

Weinberger, M., Oddone, E. Z., Samsa, G. P., and Landsman, P. B. (1996). Are health related quality of life measures affected by the mode of administration? *J Clin Epidemiol* **49**: 135–140.

Wenger, N. K., Mattson, M. E., Furberg, C. D., and Elinson, J., ed. N. K. Wenger, M. E. Mattson, C. D. Furberg, and J. Elinson. (1984). In *Assessment of Quality of Life in Clinical Trials of Cardiovascular Therapies*, Washington, DC: Le Hacq, pp. xi–xv.

Whiting, S. and Lincoln, N. (1980). An ADL assessment for stroke patients. *Br J Occup Ther* **43**: 44–46.

Wiklund, I. (1990). The Nottingham Health Profile: a measure of health related quality of life. *Scand J Prim Health Care* **1**: 15–18.

Wilkin, D., Hallam, L., and Doggett, M. A. (1992). *Measures of Need and Outcome for Primary Health Care.* Oxford: Oxford University Press.

Williams, L. S. (1998). Health-related quality of life outcomes in stroke. *Neuroepidemiology* **17**: 116–120.

Williams, L. S., Weinberger, M., Harris, L. E., *et al.* (1999). Development of stroke-specific quality of life scale. *Stroke* **30**: 1362–1369.

WHO (1980). *International Classification of Impairments, Disabilities and Handicaps.* Geneva: World Health Organization.

  (2001). *The International Classification of Functioning, Disability and Health-ICF.* Geneva: World Health Organization.

Wright, J., Cross, J., and Lamb, S. (1998). Physiotherapy outcome measures for rehabilitation of elderly people: responsiveness to change of the Rivermead Mobility Index and the Barthel Index. *Physiotherapy* **84**: 216–221.

Zola, I. K. (1983). Defining Independence. In *International Perspectives about Independent Living,* ed. D. G. Tate and L. M. Chadderton. Ann Arbor, MI: Michigan State University Centre for International Rehabilitation.

7

The impact of rehabilitation on stroke outcomes: what is the evidence?

Sharon Wood-Dauphinee

McGill University, Montreal, Canada

Gert Kwakkel

VU Medical Centre and Institute for Rehabilitation "de Hoogstroat", UMC, Utrecht, the Netherlands

Introduction

The value of evidence, as one component of the clinical decision-making process, is increasingly being accepted by rehabilitation professionals (Holm, 2000; Parker-Taillon, 2002). Clearly, it is only one component. Other important elements are the knowledge, skills, and experience of the practitioner; the values, attitudes, preferences, and expectations of the patient; as well as possible treatment constraints related to safety, time, or costs (Davidoff, 1999; Sackett *et al.*, 2000). The focus of this chapter, however, is on the available research evidence that supports, or fails to support, ways of providing rehabilitation services or the use of specific interventions following stroke.

Stroke ranks as the sixth highest cause of burden of disease (Murray and Lopez, 1997) and is the leading condition for which people seek inpatient rehabilitation (Rijken and Dekker, 1998). It occurs frequently and often has lasting consequences. Common sequelae include motor and sensory impairments, visual problems such as hemianopia and unilateral neglect, and cognitive, emotional, and speech-related difficulties. Long-term deficits tend to limit usual activities, diminish participation in customary roles and life situations, and ultimately impact negatively on quality of life (Ahlsio *et al.*, 1984; Mayo *et al.*, 1999). The occurrence of stroke is, therefore, costly to persons with stroke, their families, and society. In terms of costs, it has been estimated that more than 285 billion dollars per year would be required to cover the health expenditures and loss of productivity as a result of strokes in the USA (Centers for Disease Control and Prevention, 1999). In these days of accountability and healthcare spending restraint, rehabilitation professionals must be aware of pertinent research evidence as a basis for practice. The objective of this chapter is to provide such evidence, both for and against, about the impact of different ways of organizing and delivering rehabilitation services as well as

Recovery after Stroke, ed. Michael P. Barnes, Bruce H. Dobkin and Julien Bogousslavsky. Published by Cambridge University Press. © Cambridge University Press 2005.

about the value of specific physical interventions employed in treating those with stroke.

The chapter is presented in two main sections. The first focuses on the importance of how, when, where, and with what intensity rehabilitation is delivered. The second section provides information as to the value of selected treatments at various stages of recovery. Both sections are operationalized through a series of questions much like those suggested for evidence-based practice (Rosenberg and Donald, 1995). The directive "formulate a clear clinical question from a patient's problem" was generalized to common problems of people with stroke. Taking into consideration different states of recovery and possible outcomes as well as time since stroke, questions believed to be important, timely, and feasible to answer through research evidence were written. To facilitate understanding, we have defined the acute stage as the first week after stroke, the subacute stage as the next three weeks, the post-acute stage as weeks 5 to 26, and the chronic phase as after six months. Questions are presented as subheadings in each section of the chapter.

To obtain "evidence," we first searched for carefully conducted, systematic reviews (Langhorne and Dennis, 1998) that related to the questions posed. A systematic literature review aims to provide a clear and unbiased overview of available evidence regarding a focused clinical question through systematically locating, appraising, analyzing, and synthesizing information from scientific studies. It often uses meta-analysis, a statistical technique, to combine the results of multiple studies into a single pooled estimate and to test if the estimate is statistically significant. When a review was dated prior to 2002, we searched for newly published randomized controlled trials (RCTs) and controlled clinical studies (CCSs) and critically appraised them using a quality-rating tool, the PEDro Scale (Physiotherapy Evidence Database). PEDro scores were not used as inclusion/exclusion criteria but rather as a basis for comments related to strengths and weaknesses of studies. For questions with few additional studies, results were simply used to determine if they agreed with or were contrary to conclusions of the systematic review. For other questions, one of the authors (G. K.) recombined all appropriate RCTs in which research questions, interventions, and outcomes were conceptually similar. The data were then reanalyzed by pooling the individual effect sizes using fixed (Hedges, 1994) or random (DerSimonian and Laird, 1986) effects models. Fixed effect size g^u values (Hedges's g) were calculated for each study by finding the difference between the mean changes in the experimental group and the control group and dividing this by the average population standard deviation (SD_i). To estimate SD_i for g^u values, baseline estimates and SDs of control and experimental groups were pooled. The impact of sample size was addressed by estimating a weighting factor (w_i) for each study and assigning larger weights to effects in studies with bigger samples. Subsequently, g^u values of individual studies were averaged, resulting in a weighted summary effect size (SES); the weights of each study were combined to estimate the variance in SES (Shadish and Haddock, 1994). If significant between-study variation existed, a random effects model was applied.

If no appropriate systematic review was located, we sought and appraised individual articles, again using PEDro criteria. We conducted hand searches based on references in traditional reviews and research articles and conducted electronic searches of MEDLINE, CINHAL, the Cochrane Database of Systematic Reviews, the Cochrane Controlled Trial Register and the Database of Abstracts of Reviews of Effectiveness, as well as the Practice and Service Development Initiatives, Netting the Evidence, Evidence Based Medicine Reviews, PEDro and Best Evidence.

To judge the evidence, we were guided by criteria set forth by the US Department of Health and Human Services Agency for Health Care Policy and Research (1993). These criteria, in order of decreasing strength, are evidence from a meta-analysis of RCTs, one well-designed RCT, a CCS, an experimental study, a non-experimental study, and, finally, expert committee reports and opinions of authorities.

Organization and delivery of rehabilitation services

Care in a "stroke unit"

Do people with acute stroke cared for in a "stroke unit" demonstrate better survival, independence, and return to the community than those receiving "conventional" care?

A stroke unit may be either a team of specialists who are knowledgeable about the care of stroke patients and consult throughout the hospital wherever the patient may be or a special area of the hospital that provides beds for stroke patients, who are cared for by such a team (Bonner, 1973). Different organizational structures exist for geographic units and include discrete stroke wards, acute or rehabilitation stroke units, combined acute and rehabilitation units, or mixed rehabilitation wards delivering services to patients with different diagnoses (Stroke Unit Trialists' Collaboration, 2002). The units provide comprehensive evaluation, care, and rehabilitation for those who have sustained a stroke. Typical service components include specialized medical and nursing expertise; physical, occupational, and speech therapy; social service support; an interdisciplinary approach to planning and executing care; education for patients and families; and on-going family involvement. Compared with more traditional approaches such as care on medical wards, organized stroke unit care and rehabilitation enhance survival, independence, and community reentry without increasing the length of inpatient stay after stroke (Stroke Unit Trialists' Collaboration, 2002). These results are applicable across sexes, ages, and a range of stroke severities as well as for different forms of organized care, although the dedicated stroke unit appears to achieve the best results. Moreover, there is evidence that these positive results are maintained 5 and 10 years after the stroke and that self-perceived health-related quality of life among stroke survivors at five years is better when individuals are cared for in stroke units. Finally, observational data suggest that these positive results may be obtained in routine clinical practice, although not as substantially (Stegmayr et al., 1999).

Related studies have focused on which specific components of care are effective and for whom. Suggestions as to why stroke unit care is effective have included early and standardized assessments and treatments; careful monitoring during the acute stage; a specialized workforce of professionals; early, intense, and coordinated multidisciplinary rehabilitation; and the involvement of family members. These components were viewed as facilitating appropriate investigations, accurate diagnoses, individualized patient-focused care, fewer complications, good functional outcomes, and less institutionalization. An early, secondary analysis of data (Stroke Unit Trialists' Collaboration, 1997) from the previously reported systematic review tried to identify the mechanisms through which benefits were achieved. Results suggested that common complications were lower among unit patients, perhaps contributing to better survival. Reduction in the need for institutional care was primarily a result of enhanced independence among unit patients, perhaps influenced by the integrated rehabilitation as well as by contributions of family caregivers.

More recently, Evans and colleagues (2001), using data from a RCT, demonstrated that unit patients were assessed sooner and more comprehensively, monitored more closely, and treated more aggressively. These differences were associated with fewer complications. An observational study (Edmans, 2001) also identified a number of differences between care in a stroke unit and in a rehabilitation ward. The unit had established philosophies of team care, policies, and procedures, agreed upon by all disciplines and applied consistently. Another such study (Lincoln et al. 1996) compared activities of patients cared for in a stroke unit with those admitted to hospital wards and found that unit patients spent less time by their beds and more time in rehabilitation and social areas than did ward patients. However, the proportion of time in which patients were employed in therapeutic activities was low in both locations. Lastly, Indredavik and colleagues (1999) identified treatment differences between care provided in a stroke unit and that in general wards. They found that shorter time to the start of an intensive rehabilitation program was the most important factor associated with discharge home within six weeks, but they were concerned that other characteristics of a stroke unit, such as teamwork, a specialized staff, and contributions of family members, could not be measured and might have contributed to the earlier discharge.

Role of guidelines in affecting outcomes

If service providers adhere to established clinical guidelines, do people with stroke achieve better survival or functional outcomes than when guidelines are not followed?

Two observational studies have evaluated the impact of compliance to clinical guidelines on patient outcomes. American investigators developed a method to measure compliance with guidelines (LaClair *et al.*, 2001) and conducted a prospective analysis in an inception cohort of 288 stroke patients in 11 Department of Veteran Affairs Medical Centers across the USA (Duncan *et al.*, 2002). They found that greater levels of adherence to Post Stroke Rehabilitation Guidelines (Gresham *et al.*, 1995) in post-acute inpatient settings were associated with better outcomes in terms of physical functioning six months after stroke. Compliance was particularly high for guidelines relating to baseline assessments, complication prevention, progress monitoring, rehabilitation interventions, and team coordination activities. Adherence with acute rehabilitation guidelines was unrelated to any assessed outcomes. Italian investigators (Micieli *et al.*, 2002) conducted a similar study focused on guidelines for medical care (Adams *et al.*, 1994) but included rehabilitation guidelines to prevent complications and promote function. Patients were assessed at discharge, and three and six months after stroke in terms of survival and disability. An association between guideline adherence and survival was found at each evaluation, while that with disability reduction was significant only at discharge. These studies provide early data on the impact of guidelines and may pave the way for future trials.

Intensity of therapy

Do people with stroke who receive "more-intensive" as opposed to "less-intensive" rehabilitation in all phases achieve better and faster motor and functional recovery?

Two systematic reviews (Langhorne *et al.*, 1996; Kwakkel *et al.*, 1997) suggested that an early start of intensive stroke rehabilitation may be associated with enhanced and faster improvement of activities after stroke. Both groups found small but statistically significant SES values in favor of the group that spent more treatment time focused on the activities of daily living (ADL). In a sensitivity analysis, larger overall effect sizes were found in studies that weighted individual effect sizes for the differences in amount of rehabilitation between experimental and control groups (Kwakkel *et al.*, 1997). However, methodological limitations of the primary studies, differences in organizational settings, as well as marked heterogeneity of patient characteristics proved to be major confounding factors (Kwakkel *et al.*, 1997).

To date, 16 RCTs involving 2150 patients have been conducted in the acute and subacute (Peacock *et al.*, 1972; Sivenius *et al.*, 1985; Sunderland *et al.*, 1992; Richards *et al.*, 1993; Feys *et al.*, 1998; Kwakkel *et al.*, 1999a; Lincoln *et al.*, 1999); post-acute (Stern *et al.*, 1970; Smith *et al.*, 1981; Logan *et al.*, 1997; Walker *et al.*, 1999; Partridge *et al.*, 2000; Parker *et al.*, 2001), and chronic (Wade *et al.*, 1992; Werner *et al.*, 1996; Green *et al.*, 2002.) stages after stroke. Some trials were restricted to a specific type of patient such as those with first-ever ischemic stroke, whereas others applied less-restrictive inclusion criteria with respect to type, localization, and number of previous strokes (Partridge *et al.*, 2000). Outcomes of these trials were all evaluated by standardized ADL measures. If reported differences in ADL were pooled by applying a fixed effects model, a small, but statistically significant homogeneous SES was found in favor of more intensive therapy (SES [fixed], 0.15 SD units [SDU]; 95% confidence interval [CI], 0.06–0.23; $z = 3.252$; $P < 0.001$). The SES denotes an overall change of about 5% in favor of more intensive therapy. This finding corresponds to a 1-point change out of 20 points on a Barthel Index score. While one may question the clinical significance of such a finding, even this small change in ADL score is likely to have a disproportionate impact on patients. Pound and colleagues (1999) showed that increasing the visits by therapists was an independent factor positively influencing patient satisfaction up to a year after stroke.

On average, the intensive rehabilitation groups received about 1400 minutes more training by therapists than the control groups. There were, however, considerable differences between trials with respect to the total amount of additional therapy provided, as well as in the timing and focus of interventions. Some trials concentrated on gait training, others on dexterity, and some restricted their efforts to facilitating ADL. The additional time of therapy for the experimental groups ranged from 132 (Green *et al.*, 2002) to 6186 minutes (Smith *et al.*, 1981). The association between effect size and additional time given to the experimental groups was 0.58 in favor of studies with a larger treatment contrast ($P < 0.01$), thus reinforcing the existence of a dose–response relationship between more treatment and better ADL outcomes. Differences were found, however, between studies comparing the effects of intensity in the chronic stage of stroke (SES [fixed], 0.04 SDU; 95% CI, −0.14 to 0.29; $z = 0.45$; $P = 0.29$) (Wade *et al.*, 1992; Werner *et al.*, 1996; Green *et al.*, 2002) and those comparing effects within 6 months of stroke onset (SES [random], 0.17 SDU; 95% CI, 0.02–0.26; $z = 3.49$; $P < 0.001$). The effects, consequently, appear to have a transient and limited impact (Langhorne *et al.*, 1996; Kwakkel *et al.*, 1999b, 2002). Current findings suggest that higher intensities of training are more likely to speed up functional recovery after stroke, rather than produce additional activities.

A number of factors may have contributed to these findings, including differences in experimental interventions, the way patients were treated in the control groups, how patients were selected, and which outcome measures were used. For example, most studies were pragmatic in nature and investigated the additional effects of a particular approach to treatment such as approaches specific to neurodevelopmental (Lincoln *et al.*, 1999; Partridge *et al.*, 2000; Parker *et al.*, 2001c) or task (Richards *et al.*, 1993; Kwakkel *et al.*, 1999b) activities. In all but one study, the control group received some form of therapeutic intervention. This study (Kwakkel *et al.*, 1999a) partially prevented control patients from inducing an active learning process by immobilizing the affected limbs via an inflatable pressure splint. The increased treatment contrast between the intervention and control groups may have contributed to a larger effect size for leg training in terms of the specific effect on functional recovery.

Finally, when considering the impact of intensity of rehabilitation on stroke outcome, we must think back to a prior discussion of why stroke units work. It was noted that the intensity of rehabilitation programs, even in those settings, was less intensive than expected. Another study (Tinson, 1989) showed that only 11% of patient time was spent in physical and occupational therapy, while de Weerdt and associates (2001) found that physical therapy activities accounted for 12% of the working day of people with stroke. Moreover, considerable differences exist between different settings in different countries. Given all the differences, it is not surprising that it is difficult to disentangle the contributions of the different components.

Specific modalities and treatment approaches

Electromyographic biofeedback

In *subacute*, post-acute or chronic stroke, does the addition of *electromyographic* biofeedback (EMGB) to conventional rehabilitation reduce impairments and disabilities of the affected upper and lower extremities *compared with the reduction achieved with conventional rehabilitation alone?*

EMGB is a technique that provides feedback to patients about their muscular effort. It involves applying external electrodes to the motor points of appropriate muscles to capture motor unit electrical potentials. These potentials are transformed by the biofeedback machine into auditory or visual signals that are used by the patients to increase or decrease their muscular effort. This allows the patients to have better conscious control over their voluntary contractions. Desired muscle activation can be facilitated or unwanted activation can be controlled.

Four systematic reviews with meta-analyses have been reported in the literature. Schleenbaker and Mainous (1993) included eight studies (four upper and four lower extremity) with randomized or matched controls and assessed a broad array of outcomes. While their overall results were in favor of EMGB, little attention was given to the quality of the individual studies. Glanz and his team (1995) included RCTs of both extremities as well, but performed separate meta-analyses. They selected studies by defined criteria, used only improved joint range of motion as the outcome, and failed to find a significant effect of EMGB. Moreland and colleagues conducted two reviews of RCTs on this topic: one for upper and one for lower extremities. The upper extremity review (Moreland and Thompson, 1994) compared patients receiving EBMB alone or in combination with conventional physical therapy with those receiving conventional therapy in terms of the impact on impairments and functional outcomes. Results of the meta-analysis demonstrated no significant differences in outcomes between the two groups. The review studying the lower extremity (Moreland *et al.*, 1998) was similar. Patient outcomes included a number of gait parameters, ankle muscle strength and range of motion, and gait speed. Of all outcomes assessed, only the meta-analysis estimating the impact of the intervention on dorsiflexion strength found a positive result in favor of EMGB.

Since these meta-analyses, two RCTs focusing on the use of EMGB to enhance gait recovery in the subacute phase of stroke found that control and experimental groups responded similarly (Bradley *et al.*, 1998; Geiger *et al.*, 2001). Collectively, these studies suggest that EMGB is not an effective adjunct to conventional therapy following stroke in reducing impairments or enhancing functional performance. As pointed out by Pomeroy and Tallis (2000), this conclusion seems particularly warranted as the individual studies in the reviews made different comparisons and controlled for different intensities and treatments in their analyses.

Functional electrical stimulation

Does functional electrical stimulation (FES) when used as an adjunct to exercise during any phase of the stroke rehabilitation result in better range of motion, strength, or functional performance of the affected upper or lower extremities than when it is not provided?

The FES technique delivers short, programmed bursts of electrical stimuli to a muscle group or peripheral nerve, using either surface or intramuscular electrodes, to produce or facilitate a voluntary muscle contraction (Glanz *et al.*, 1996). Application of FES to the neuromuscular body region affected by the stroke is believed to reduce spasticity, prevent or correct contractures, strengthen muscles, increase range of motion, as well as improve dexterity and gait performance. It can also be used as a supportive device for the paretic limb. There is a difference between stimulation below the motor threshold, such as with transcutaneous nerve stimulation, and higher levels of stimulation intended to induce a muscular contraction and affect motor performance (FES). In the present section, studies that applied only sensory stimulation without muscular contraction are omitted. Another form of stimulation is EMG-triggered FES, in which the stimulation is linked to generated EMG levels. Electrical stimulation is initiated only after the EMG signal exceeds a preset threshold (Kraft *et al.*, 1992). The three indications for administering FES in stroke (Glanz *et al.*, 1996) are described below.

Functional electrical stimulation for wrist and finger extension

Four RCTs involving 154 patients were identified as being relevant to assess FES therapy when provided as an adjunct treatment to promote wrist and finger extension (Bowman *et al.*, 1979; Packman-Braun *et al.*, 1988; Powell *et al.*, 1999; Chae and Yu, 2000). At baseline, most patients were able to produce some active extension of the wrist in the absence of contractures. All treatments started in the post-acute phase. Experimental patients were provided with FES from once a week for 60 minutes to three times a week for 30 minutes over a period of three to eight weeks.

Statistically significant outcomes were reported for strength (Chae *et al.*, 1998; Powell *et al.*, 1999) and range of motion (Bowman *et al.*, 1979; Chae *et al.*, 1998) in selected patients with active extension of the wrist. In one study, subgroup analysis showed better dexterity on the Action Research Arm Test in patients with more- rather than less-severe involvement (Powell *et al.*, 1999). A review of these studies, however, failed to find evidence that this improvement in motor control generalized to dexterity or was sustained after FES had ceased (de Kroon *et al.*, 2002). Additionally, the two larger studies (Chae *et al.*, 1998; Powell *et al.*, 1999) showed an extensive drop-out rate that may have biased the results. Because of the low quality of these studies, no conclusions can be drawn as to the benefits or disadvantages of FES in relation to dexterity of the paretic arm.

Functional electrical stimulation for hemiplegic shoulder subluxation and pain

Four RCTs with a total of 161 subjects have been published on the effects of FES on hemiplegic shoulder pain (Baker and Parker, 1986; Faghri *et al.*, 1994; Linn *et al.*, 1999; Wang *et al.*, 2002). The meta-analysis of Price and Pandyan (2001) included two of these RCTs but also added two others in which the effects of transcutaneous nerve stimulation as well as FES were evaluated. Patients were eligible for FES if they had a marked paresis of the shoulder musculature and a glenohumeral subluxation ranging from 5 to 9.5 mm. FES involved stimulation of the posterior deltoid and supraspinatus muscles during either the acute (Linn *et al.*, 1999) or the chronic (Wang *et al.*, 2002) phases after stroke.

Pooling data from these four RCTs showed a statistically significant overall fixed effect size for range of motion (SES [fixed], 0.55 SDU; 95% CI, 0.05–1.04) and a random effect size for amount of subluxation (SES [random], 1.41 SDU; 95% CI, 0.76–2.06). This latter finding represents a mean reduction of about 5.6 mm in subluxation. The present findings related to the value of FES confirm the results of the CCS conducted by Kobayashi and associates (1999) and that of Chantraine et al., (1999). Moreover, a significant increment in range of motion in passive humeral lateral rotation of about 13.3 degrees was found as a result of FES, but no significant effects were found for spasticity, motor function, or shoulder pain (Price et al., 2001). Mainly because of the small number of studies, the implications of shoulder FES for overall functional outcomes of the paretic arm remain inconclusive.

Functional electrical stimulation for hemiplegic gait

One systematic review (Glanz et al., 1996) and five RCTs (Merletti et al., 1978; Cozean et al., 1988; Macdonell et al., 1994; Bogataj et al., 1995; Burridge et al., 1997) investigating the effects of FES on gait have been published. All, except the trial by Merletti and colleagues (1978), studied the specific effects of FES on hemiplegic gait. Most investigated FES in conjunction with traditional physical therapy modalities and one contained FES, biofeedback, FES and biofeedback, and exercises alone (Cozean et al., 1988). In a crossover design (Bogataj et al., 1995), multichannel FES was compared with exercise therapy. FES was applied in a highly selected group of patients who were unable to elevate the affected foot during the swing phase of gait, and studies were conducted in the acute and post-acute phases after stroke.

When data from the studies were pooled for muscle strength (SES [fixed], 0.01 SDU; 95% CI, −0.51 to 0.53) (Macdonell et al., 1994; Bogataj et al., 1995) and gait speed (SES [fixed], 0.72 SDU; 95% CI, −1.08 to 2.52) (Bogataj et al., 1995; Burridge et al., 1997), no significant overall effect sizes were found, However, it may be that the few RCTs, in combination with the low numbers of patients in each study (20 to 49), were insufficient to produce adequate statistical power.

The evidence does not support the use of FES as a routine treatment modality after stroke. However, only 70 patients were included in the RCTs, indicating that all were underpowered. Finally, the value of FES as an orthosis in gait remains inconclusive.

The role of strengthening and/or aerobic exercises

Do individuals with stroke receiving strengthening and/or aerobic exercises during the sub-, post-acute, or chronic phases after stroke improve their functional abilities more than those not receiving such exercises?

Several studies have shown that most people with stroke suffer not only from hemiplegia but also from physical deconditioning when compared with age-matched controls. The health of many with stroke is also compromised by cardiac comorbidity, which by itself may limit the endurance and physical capacity to perform ADL (Roth and Noll, 1994). It is increasingly being recognized that strength and endurance training are important components of a comprehensive rehabilitation program.

Evidence for muscle strength training

Muscle strengthening has, unfortunately, been strongly discouraged in the past. Several neurological approaches assumed that strength training would increase abnormal tone and, thus, be detrimental to functional recovery. In addition, muscle weakness was often assumed to be secondary to increased muscle tone in the antagonist. Current opinions have changed in the face of growing evidence that paresis after stroke is strongly related to reduced output and that strengthening does not cause anticipated detrimental effects. There is also increasing evidence that the effects produced by strengthening programs may generalize to higher gait speeds, increased gait endurance, and improved ADL (Inaba et al., 1973; Glasser et al., 1986; Richards et al., 1993; Teixeira-Salmela et al., 1999; Dean et al., 2000; Rimmer et al., 2000). In addition, it may be hypothesized that training programs in which patients are subjected to high repetitions of functional activities (Richards et al., 1993; Engardt et al., 1995; Dean et al., 2000) are more likely to improve function than conventional lower extremity strengthening in fixed positions. Recently, a small RCT (Bourbonnais et al., 2002) detected some improvement in gait performance in those with chronic stroke who were provided with force-feedback treatment. No positive effects were found in the upper extremity. The optimal mode for training paretic muscles remains unclear.

Evidence for physical endurance training

An increasing number of studies have shown that aerobics by pedal ergometry (Potempa et al., 1995; Brown and Kautz, 1998; Duncan et al., 1998) and physical fitness programs (Teixeira-Salmela et al., 1999; Dean et al., 2000; Rimmer et al., 2000) may lead to improved strength, endurance, and locomotion in patients with subacute, post-acute and chronic stroke. For example, Potempa and colleagues (1995) demonstrated significant improvements in maximal oxygen consumption, workload, and exercise time among those with chronic stroke provided with a submaximal cycle ergometer program for 30 minutes a day, three times a week over 10 weeks. An average increment of 13% in maximal oxygen consumption was found in favor of the exercise group.

All these studies on muscle strengthening and endurance training contain small numbers of patients; several did not use random allocation of patients into groups (Butefisch *et al.*, 1995; Engardt *et al.*, 1995; Brown and Kautz, 1998; Smith *et al.*, 1999); and the outcomes were not always evaluated in terms of functional activities. More studies with strong designs are clearly needed.

Role of acupuncture

In *subacute*, post-acute, or chronic stroke, does the use of acupuncture as an adjunct to conventional therapy achieve better motor or functional recovery or health status than when only the conventional techniques are used?

For centuries, acupuncture has been used in traditional Chinese medicine to improve motor and functional outcomes following stroke. More recently, as interest in alternative or complementary therapies has grown, its use in Western countries has risen (Chen 1993a, b). There are several approaches to acupuncture but all involve needling techniques at defined acupuncture points to excite sensation. Manual stimulation is most common but electrical and other forms of acupuncture are also used. The mechanisms underlying acupuncture remain unclear.

A recent systematic review by Park and colleagues (2001) included nine RCTs in which any form of needle acupuncture was compared with any non-acupuncture control intervention for those with stroke. Different outcomes, including range of motion, motor function, balance, gait, ADL, and perceived health status, were assessed. Six studies found positive and three negative results in terms of the effectiveness of acupuncture. Because of the heterogeneity of the outcomes and the lack of methodological details, the authors were unable to conduct the planned meta-analysis. Despite the number count in favor of acupuncture, the authors concluded that current evidence does not support the use of acupuncture in stroke rehabilitation. This conclusion was based on the quality and results of the individual trials. Those that used the most rigorous methods showed no significant effects. A recent trial (Sze *et al.*, 2002) with similar inclusion criteria reported findings in agreement with this conclusion. Moreover, another adequately powered trial (Johansson *et al.*, 2001) with three arms (acupuncture, with electroacupuncture or transcutaneous nerve stimulation, as the two active intervention arm, and subliminal electrostimulation as the control arm) failed to find beneficial effects in function or perceived health status in either of the active treatment arms.

Considerable attention by a number of authors (e.g. Tang *et al.*, 1999; Linde *et al.*, 2001) has been given to the major shortcomings of studies assessing the value of acupuncture and all suggested that larger trials of better methodological quality are needed. Park and colleagues (2001) stated that the results of past studies have been sufficiently positive to warrant further investigation.

Choice of therapeutic approach

In the subacute to chronic phases of recovery following stroke, what is the evidence for selecting one therapeutic approach to exercise over another in terms motor and functional outcomes?

In 1989, Dickstein outlined and compared traditional and neurophysiological approaches to therapeutic exercises for those with stroke. Specifically, she described the methods of Brunnstrom (1970), Bobath (1990), and Rood (Stockmeyer, 1967), the approach called proprioceptive neuromuscular facilitation (Knott and Voss, 1962), and traditional therapy as a focus on the less-affected side of the body to enhance functional activities. Over the years, these approaches have evolved, incorporating new theories as well as the results from empirical research in related disciplines. Others, such as the motor relearning program (Carr and Shepherd, 1982) can be added to the list. Today in many therapy departments, specific approaches have given way to more pragmatic methods in which the restoration of meaningful movements of the more affected side as well as functional performance are therapeutic targets. Nonetheless, advocates of specific regimers exist and studies comparing one approach with another continue to appear in the literature.

In 1990, Ernst, after a critical review of studies evaluating the effectiveness of different approaches to exercise therapy, concluded that the actual choice of therapeutic approach was not important as any available method would impact positively on functional status. Since that time, the authors of several critical reviews (Wagenaar and Meijer 1991a,b; Gowland and Basmajian 1996; Duncan 1997) have agreed with this conclusion. Currently, the literature contains five RCTs (Stern *et al.*, 1970; Logigian *et al.*, 1983; Basmajian *et al.*, 1987; Jongbloed *et al.*, 1989; Langhammer and Stanghelle, 2000) and three CCSs (Dickstein *et al.*, 1986; Lord & Hall, 1986; Gelber *et al.*, 1995) that compared one of these approaches another with another therapy or with the traditional method. Not included in this list are studies testing the value of relatively new interventions, those with a primary goal of evaluating the effects of treatment intensity, or those in which the comparison group received no treatment or a placebo to control for attention.

Collectively, these studies enrolled 474 patients from the subacute to the chronic phases of stroke, most often in rehabilitation settings. They provided proprioceptive neuromuscular facilitation, Bobath (commonly termed neurodevelopmental treatment), motor learning, or traditional methods of exercise; treated patients for periods ranging from a few weeks while hospitalized to several months as outpatients; used treatment periods of 30 to 90 minutes per weekday; and assessed impairments, function, perceived health status, length of stay, and disposition for up to 12 months following stroke. With the exception of the following findings, there were no significant differences in patient outcomes between the groups being compared. Lord and Hall (1986) found that of 13 ADL skills tested, independence in feeding was better in patients treated with neuromuscular reeducation methods than in those treated with the traditional approach. Mudie and colleagues (2002) showed that the Bobath approach was more effective for retraining symmetry in seated weight distribution when assessed after treatment than either visual feedback training applied by a balance performance monitor or no training. However, 12-week follow-up effects favored the visual feedback group and could be generalized to symmetry in standing. In the RCT by Langhammer and Stanghelle (2000), functional activities were significantly better at two weeks after treatment onset in the patients receiving motor relearning than in those following the Bobath approach. However, these differences were not present at three months. Finally, several studies found that the length of institutional stay was significantly longer in patients treated with the Bobath approach (Lord and Hall, 1986; Langhammer and Stanghelle, 2000) or they showed slower improvement in ADL (Dickstein *et al.*, 1986). This suggests that methods considering the emergence of basic limb synergies as pathological and an undesirable manifestation of spasticity that should be suppressed may diminish the speed of functional recovery.

The lack of differences across approaches may result from the heterogeneity of stroke, the variable quality of the studies, small sample sizes and/or the lack of sensitivity of the outcome measures. More likely, there are no consistent differences in outcomes between treatment approaches.

Treadmill training

Do individuals with stroke receiving treadmill training, with or without body weight support, achieve better gait performance than those receiving conventional modalities?

Mastering safe walking skills is an important objective after stroke and is crucial for achieving independence in daily living. As a result, therapy is often concentrated on gait reeducation. Recently, two forms of gait training in people with hemiplegia have been investigated: body-weight-supported treadmill training (BWSTT) and unsupported treadmill training.

Body-weight-supported treadmill training

Treadmill training combined with the use of suspension to relieve some of the patient's body weight has been used, often as an adjunct to conventional therapy, to assist patients in regaining walking ability after stroke. Partial body weight support (ranging from 0 to 50% of body weight) may generate normal stepping kinematics at usual walking speeds in patients unable to walk independently. Since the mid-1990s, a number of CCSs, as well as five RCTs involving 266 stroke patients, have investigated the impact of body weight support that ranged from no support to 40% support (Visintin *et al.*, 1998; Kosak and Reding, 2000; Nilsson *et al.*, 2001; da Cunha *et al.*, 2002; Sullivan *et al.*, 2002). Two compared BWSTT with the effects of treadmill training alone (Visintin *et al.*, 1998; Nilsson *et al.*, 2001), whereas another two compared BWSTT with conventional gait training on the floor (Kosak and Reding, 2000; da Cunha *et al.*, 2002). The latest RCT investigated the effects of BWSTT at different gait speeds (Sullivan *et al.*, 2002). Among these studies, the timing of the first intervention after stroke ranged from 15 days to 26 months, and the maximum walking speed over ground at baseline varied from 0.18 to 0.71 m/s. Total treatment times were also variable, ranging from 8 to 33 hours. Finally, a number of outcomes related to gait performance were evaluated: ability to walk independently, gait speed, balance, gait endurance, and ADL. In addition, gait parameters including symmetry and motor performance measured by EMG, muscle strength, or the presence of basic limb synergies were assessed.

In spite of the different outcomes and intensities of BWSTT, pooling the individual effect sizes was possible for gait speed, gait endurance, balance, and walking ability. With respect to these functional outcomes, a statistically significant homogeneous SES was found for gait endurance (SES [fixed], 0.70 SDU; 95% CI, 0.29–1,10; $P < 0.001$), reflecting a mean difference of about 29% in favor of BWSTT. However, no significant overall effect size was found for gait speed (SES [fixed], 0.10 SDU; 95% CI, -0.17 to 0.36). Upon inspection, effect sizes appeared to be bigger in studies that included patients with no or low walking speeds at onset (Visintin *et al.*, 1998) compared with those who started with higher walking speeds (Nilsson *et al.*, 2001). Subsequent analyses of the other outcomes found no significant differences for walking ability (SES [fixed], 0.33 SDU; 95% CI, -0.09 to 0.76) (Nilsson *et al.*, 2001; da Cunha *et al.*, 2002) or balance (SES [fixed], 0.27 SDU; 95% CI, -0.07 to 0.61) (Visintin *et al.*, 1998; Nilsson *et al.*, 2001).

All these studies can be criticized for low treatment contrast since control regimens also received intense, functionally oriented training (Nilsson *et al.*, 2001). For example, one study compared BWSTT with the effects of applying an aggressive brace-assisted walking device that permitted early weight bearing on the paretic leg and control for foot extension during the swing phase of gait (Kosak and Reding, 2000). Moreover, there were methodological problems. Two studies had inadequate statistical power for demonstrating differences (Kosak and Reding, 2000; da Cunha *et al.*, 2002), and the two larger trials (Visintin *et al.*, 1998; Nilsson *et al.*, 2001) reported mean drop-out rates at the end of the intervention of 18 and 21%, respectively. The subsequent lack of intention-to-treat analyses may have biased reported effects.

Although evidence for the overall effectiveness of BWSTT is weak, it may be concluded that the use of a harness to provide partial weight support while walking on a treadmill generates additional effects on gait endurance, whereas no evidence exists for beneficial effects on gait speed, balance, and walking ability. To explain these findings, one can hypothesize that support of body weight during treadmill walking decreases the oxygen demand (Danielsson et al., 2000; Macko et al., 2001; Nilsson et al., 2001). A recent experimental study showed that ventilatory oxygen uptake during BWSTT is about 12% lower than during unsupported treadmill walking (Danielsson et al., 2000) and 20% less than peak exercise capacity (Macko et al., 2001). This suggests that, with the reduced energy costs and the lower cardiovascular demands, patients are capable of training more intensively with less fatigue (Nilsson et al., 2001). However, the benefits of BWSTT may also result from a reduction in the fear of falling provided by the support of the harness and/ or of better communication between patients and therapists in their combined efforts to restore normal gait (Hansen et al., 2002). Currently, the evidence suggests that BWSTT should be reserved for patients whose physical condition is too weak to tolerate intense training and for whom the expectation of regaining independent ambulation is unclear.

Treadmill training without body weight support

Four RCTs, enrolling 134 patients, compared treadmill training without body weight support with conventional training (Richards et al., 1993; Liston et al., 2000; Laufer et al., 2001; Pohl et al., 2002). Treatment started between 10 days and 16 weeks after stroke, in the subacute and post-acute phases. One study applied treadmill training in the chronic phase (Liston et al., 2000). Treatment intensities ranged from three to five sessions a week for three to six weeks. No overall SES was found in these RCTs with respect to gait speed (SES [random], 0.58 SDU; 95% CI, -3.45–4.61). There is no evidence, therefore, that treadmill training without body support has additional effects on walking compared with conventional gait training programs on the floor.

Utility of rhythmical auditory stimulation or positional feedback

Do individuals with stroke receiving rhythmic auditory stimulation or positional feedback during gait achieve relative better gait performance than those receiving no rhythmic facilitation?

Rhythmical auditory stimulation and rhythmical positional feedback ask patients to synchronize their arm and leg swing with an external rhythm. The rhythm functions as a timekeeper to increase stride length on the paretic side, which, in turn, enhances overall movement coordination and gait speed. Two RCTs incorporating 57 patients have provided preliminary evidence for the effectiveness of these techniques in gait training (Mandel et al., 1990; Thaut *et al.*, 1997). After pooling both studies, positive findings were found in favor of stride length (22 cm) (Thaut *et al.*, 1997) and walking speed (0.23 m/s; SES [fixed], 1.18 SDU; 95% CI, 0.54–1.84) (Mandel *et al.*, 1990; Thaut *et al.*, 1997) when patients were trained for six or 12 weeks in the subacute and chronic phases, respectively. These findings suggest that rhythmic cueing applied by a metronome or embedded in music is an effective tool to enhance spatiotemporal control of cyclic movement patterns such as gait. However, the methodological quality of both studies was low because of lack of blinding of the evaluators, number of drop-outs, and differences at baseline regarding important prognostic indicators. Further studies evaluating the effectiveness of these interventions are needed.

Utility of forced use or constraint-induced movement therapy

Does "forced use" or constraint-induced movement therapy (CIMT) improve the functional performance of the affected upper extremity in high-level functioning patients after chronic stroke patients better than other treatment approaches that do not incorporate such elements?

In 1986, CIMT was introduced to denote a combination of treatment modalities aimed at discouraging the use of the unaffected arm combined with intensive training ("shaping") of the affected arm. In the 1980s, a non-controlled study showed that this combined approach resulted in better dexterity in patients with some voluntary wrist and finger extension (Ostendorf and Wolf, 1981; Wolf *et al.*, 1989). In 1993, the first RCT of CIMT was performed in nine patients with chronic stroke (Taub *et al.*, 1993). In addition to restraining the unaffected upper extremity for more than 90% of waking time, the investigators introduced "shaping procedures" for six hours a day over 10 consecutive weekdays. These procedures consisted of training a variety of purposeful tasks such as eating with a fork and spoon, throwing a ball, and playing card games. Five control patients received physiotherapy that involved imaginary exercises for the affected limb for 10 minutes on two days and passive-range-of-movement exercises for 15 minutes each day. Outcomes were evaluated using two performance measures and the Motor Activity Log, a structured interview tapping the patient's perceptions of use of the paretic arm. One month after treatment, the four patients in the CIMT group showed an improvement of about 97% in score and a mean reduction in performance time of 28 to 38%, whereas the control group showed almost no changes. These reported differences remained two years later.

Since then, three additional RCTs demonstrating the efficacy of CIMT have been published, one in the subacute stage (Dromerick *et al.*, 2000) and two in the chronic stage after stroke (van der Lee *et al.*, 1999; Page *et al.*, 2001). Although these studies used the same inclusion criteria as Taub *et al.* (1993) (20 degrees active wrist extension and 10 degrees active finger extension), and constrained the unaffected arm for one to six hours per weekday over two consecutive weeks, the intensity and content of therapy differed markedly. For example, the intensity of training the paretic arm ranged from less than one (Page *et al.*, 2001) or two (Dromerick *et al.*, 2000) hours to more than six hours (Taub *et al.*, 1993; van der Lee *et al.*, 1999) per weekday. Moreover, the RCT of van der Lee and colleagues (1999) was designed to investigate the effects of constraining the paretic arm while offering equally intensive physical therapy to experimental and control groups. In the other studies, the treatment focused only on the paretic arm and the control groups received a much less-intensive program for two weeks. Obviously, van der Lee and colleagues (1999) found smaller effect sizes on the outcome measures than did the trial of Taub *et al.*, (1993) suggesting that the combination of the task-oriented arm training and its intensity is important for CIMT. Finally, the study of Dromerick and associates (2000) investigated the effects of CIMT in 20 subacute stroke patients and showed effects on the arm Motor Activity Test that were comparable to those of van der Lee and colleagues (1999) in chronic stroke. Despite differences in treatment contrast between experimental and control groups, as well as in the timing of interventions, a small homogeneous SES was found for dexterity in favor of CIMT (SES [fixed], 0.46 SDU; 95% CI, 0.04–0.83), suggesting a mean improvement of about 12% in dexterity.

This finding suggests that CIMT may be effective for people with stroke who display some voluntary wrist and finger extension. However, studies may be criticized for failure to use an intent-to-treat analysis (van der Lee *et al.*, 1999), lack of treatment contrast between experimental and control groups (van der Lee *et al.*, 1999), lack of objective outcome measures (Taub *et al.*, 1993), and insufficient data representing point estimates and measures of variability for key outcomes (Taub *et al.*, 1993; Dromerick *et al.*, 2000). Besides the generally poor quality, the actual number of patients in the RCTs was less than 100. This low number may reflect the strict inclusion criteria. Original estimates that 25% of stroke patients with chronic motor deficits are capable of voluntarily extension of the wrist and fingers (Wolf and Binder-MacLeod, 1983) have not materialized. Further, a recent investigation showed that 68% of 208 patients asked to participate in a CIMT program refused, and 86 participating therapists expressed concerns about patient adherence and safety. In addition, they speculated that facilities would not have the resources to provide CIMT (Page *et al.*, 2002). Finally, the optimal time window for CIMT still needs to be determined. Although the regimen has been shown to improve long-term outcomes, there are concerns about the timing of implementation. Studies in rats have shown that the exclusive use of the affected forelimb within the first week of stroke injury caused an unexpected detrimental effect on sensorimotor function, but sole use of the paretic limb after that first week did not (Humm *et al.*, 1998; Bland *et al.*,

2000). The transient period of post-ischemic, use-dependent vulnerability in rats cautions against the application of CIMT immediately after stroke in humans.

Summary

Evidence is accumulating that the organization of care and rehabilitation as well as the choice of intervention impact patient outcomes. Clearly, people with stroke cared for within the framework of a stroke unit survive more often, are more independent, and return home more frequently than those who do not receive such care, and these effects are maintained over time. People with stroke cared for by providers who adhere to established guidelines also experience better survival and demonstrate superior physical functioning after stroke. Intensity of intervention is also important in terms of speeding up functional recovery especially when activities are task orientated.

Based on evidence from available studies, EMGB is not an effective addition to conventional therapy in terms of reducing impairment or enhancing function. The impact of FES on the upper extremity remains inconclusive, whereas its use as an orthosis in hemiplegic gait requires further investigation. The value of acupuncture also remains questionable because of methodological problems, although published studies have been sufficiently positive to justify additional trials. The use of BWSTT appears to be most effective for compromised patients who do not have sufficient energy for intensive gait training. There is also preliminary evidence that rhythmic auditory or positional facilitation enhances stride length and overall gait speed. In stroke survivors who have some voluntary wrist and finger extension, CIMT may be an effective approach to treating the paretic upper extremity. Finally, there is growing evidence that muscle strengthening and physical fitness training may improve gait and endurance after stroke; however most studies are underpowered and demonstrate low methodological quality. While these questions are certainly not exhaustive many answers are positive and support the efforts of providers.

This chapter has several limitations that could affect our findings and their interpretation. First, it was written by two investigators with clinical backgrounds in physical therapy who did not have the benefit of a multidisciplinary team for discussion and consensus. Further, the data were not collected in a truly systematic manner. We did not perform the exhaustive searching for unpublished studies or the reliability checks currently expected in formal systematic reviews. Rather, we used information in the literature, updated it via restricted searching, and conducted new analyses. The focus of searching was also on the English language. Finally, from a vast array of possible questions, we selected those believed to be important, timely, and feasible to answer. Many other questions could have been asked.

Caution should be exercised, of course, when applying the results to individual patients (Evidence-based Medicine Working Group 2002). As noted in the introduction, the knowledge and skills of the clinician, the values and wishes of patients and their families, as well situations specific to the service delivery site must be considered (Davidoff, 1999). In addition, clinicians must determine if their patients are similar to those who have been studied and if published study outcomes are in line with their specific treatment goals. They may also have to decide if the size of the anticipated benefit warrants extra effort or costs for the patient or the service, or if there is a risk of an adverse event caused by treatment. Further, new studies with new evidence are appearing continuously in the literature. Their results could change the findings reported here.

ACKNOWLEDGEMENTS

We acknowledge R. van Peppen for his extensive research and synthesis of relevant publications as well B. Kollen for his suggestions. Their contributions are part of a research project supported by a grant from the Royal Dutch Society of Physical Therapy in the Netherlands. We also acknowledge D. Donnini for his assistance searching related literature and P. Hornstein for help with preparation of the manuscript.

REFERENCES

Adams, H. P., Brott, T. G., Crowelll, R. M., *et al.* (1994). Guidelines for the management of patients with acute ischemic stroke. *Stroke* **25**: 1321–1335.

Ahlsio, B., Britton, M., Murray, V., and Theorell, T. (1984). Disablement and quality of life after stroke. *Stroke* **15**: 886–890.

Baker, L. L. and Parker, K. (1986). Neuromuscular electrical stimulation of the muscles surrounding the shoulder. *Phys Ther* **66**: 1930–1937.

Basmajian, J. V., Gowland, C. A., Finlayson, M. A., *et al.* (1987). Stroke treatment: comparison of integrated behavorial physical therapy vs traditional physical therapy programs. *Arch Phys Med Rehabil* **68**: 267–272.

Bland, S. T., Schallert, T., Strong, R., *et al.* (2000). Early exclusive use of the affected forelimb after moderate transient focal ischemia in rats. *Stroke* **31**: 1144–1152.

Bobath, B. (1990). *Adult Hemiplegia: Evaluation and Treatment* 3rd edn. London: Heinemann Medical.

Bogataj, U., Gros, N., Kljajic, M., Aćimović, R., and Malezic, M. (1995). The rehabilitation of gait in patients with hemiplegia: a comparison between conventional therapy and multichannel functional electrical stimulation therapy. *Phys Ther* **75**: 490–502.

Bonner, C. D. (1973). Stroke units in community hospitals: a "how-to" guide. *Geriatrics* **28**: 166–170.

Bowman, B. R., Baker, L. L., and Waters, R. L. (1979). Positional feedback and electrical stimulation: an automated treatment for the hemiplegic wrist. *Arch Phys Med Rehabil* **60**: 497–502.

Bourbonnais, D., Bilodeau, S., Lepage, Y., et al. (2002). Effect of force-feedback treatment in patients with chronic motor deficits after a stroke. *Am J Phys Med Rehabil* **81**: 890–897.

Bradley, L., Hart, B. B., Mandana, S., et al. (1998). Electromyographic biofeedback for gait training after stroke. *Clin Rehabil* **12**: 11–22.

Brown, D. A. and Kautz, S. A. (1998). Increased workload enhances force output during pedalling exercise in persons with post-stroke hemiplegia. *Stroke* **29**: 598–606.

Brunnstrom, S. (1970). *Movement Therapy in Hemiplegia*. New York: Harper and Row.

Burridge, J. H., Taylor, P. N., Hagan, S. A., Wood, D. E., and Swain, I. D. (1997). The effects of common peroneal stimulation on the effort and speed of walking: a randomized controlled trial with chronic hemiplegic patients. *Clin Rehabil* **11**: 201–210.

Bütefisch, C., Hummelsheim, H., Denzier, P., and Mauritz, K. H. (1995). Repetitive training of isolated movements improves the outcome of motor rehabilitation of the centrally paretic hand. *J Neurol Sci* **130**: 59–68.

Carr, J. H. and Shepherd, R. B. (1982). *A Motor Relearning Program for Stroke*. Rockville, MD: Aspen.

Centers for Disease Control and Prevention(1999). Morbidity and Mortality Weekly Report. *US Depart Health Hum Serv* **40**: 649–680.

Chae, J. and Yu, D. (2000). A critical review of neuromuscular electrical stimulation for treatment of motor dysfunction in hemiplegia. *Assist Technol* **12**: 33–49.

Chae, J., Bethoux, F., Bohine, T., et al. (1998). Neuromuscular stimulation of upper extremity motor and functional recovery in acute hemiplegia. *Stroke* **29**: 975–979.

Chantraine, A., Baribeault, A., Uebelhart, D., and Gremion, G. (1999). Shoulder pain and dysfunction in hemiplegia: effects of functional electrical stimulation. *Arch Phys Med Rehabil* **80**: 328–331.

(1993a). Effective acupuncture therapy for stroke and cerbrovascular diseases. Part I. *Am J Acupunct* **21**: 105–122.

Chen, A. (1993b). Effective acupuncture therapy for stroke and cerbrovascular diseases. Part II. *Am J Acupunct* **21**: 205–218.

Cozean, C. D., Pease, W. S., and Hubbell, S. L. (1988). Biofeedback and functional electric stimulation in stroke rehabilitation. *Arch Phys Med Rehabil* **69**: 401–405.

da Cunha, I. T., Lim, P. A., Qureshy, H., et al. (2002). Gait outcomes after acute stroke rehabilitation with supported treadmill ambulation training: a randomised controlled pilot study. *Arch Phys Med Rehabil* **83**: 1258–1265.

Danielsson, A. and Sunnerhagen, K. S. (2000). Oxygen consumption during treadmill walking with and without body weight support in patients with hemiparesis after stroke and healthy subjects. *Arch Phys Med Rehabil* **81**: 953–957.

Davidoff, F. (1999). In the teeth of the evidence: the curious case of evidence based medicine. *Mt Sinai J Med* **66**: 75–83.

Dean, C., Richards, C. L., and Malouin, F. (2000). Task-related circuit training improves performance of locomotor tasks in chronic stroke: a randomized, controlled pilot trial. *Arch Phys Med Rehabil* **81**: 409–417.

de Kroon, J. R., van der Lee, J. H., Ijzerman, M. J., and Lankhorst, G. J. (2002). Therapeutic electrical stimulation to improve motor control and functional abilities of the upper extremity after stroke: a systematic review. *Clin Rehabil* **16**: 350–360.

DerSimonian, R. and Laird, N. M. (1986). Meta-analysis in clinical trials. *Control Clin Trials* **7**: 177–188.

de Weerdt, W., Nuyens, G., Feys, H., *et al.* (2001). Group physiotherapy improves time use by patients with stroke in rehabilitation. *Aust J Physiother* **47**: 53–61.

Dickstein, R. (1989). Contemporary exercise therapy approaches in stroke rehabilitation. *Clin Rev Phys Rehabil Med* **1**: 161–180.

Dickstein, R., Hocherman, S., Pillar, T., and Shaham, R. (1986). Stroke rehabilitation. Three exercise therapy approaches. *Phys Ther* **66**: 1223–1238.

Dromerick, A. W., Edwards, D. F., and Hahn, M. (2000). Does the application of constraint-induced movement therapy during acute rehabilitation reduce arm impairment after ischemic stroke? *Stroke* **31**: 2984–2988.

Duncan, P. W. (1997). Synthesis of intervention trials to improve motor recovery following stroke. *Top Stroke Rehabil* **3**: 1–20.

Duncan, P., Richards, L., Wallace, D., *et al.* (1998). A randomized controlled pilot study of a home based exercise program for individuals with mild and moderate stroke. *Stroke* **29**: 2055–2060.

Duncan, P. W., Horner, R. D., Reker, D. M., *et al.* (2002). Adherence to post-acute rehabilitation guidelines is associated with functional recovery in stroke. *Stroke* **33**: 167–178.

Edmans, J. (2001). What makes stroke units effective? *Br J Ther Rehabil* **8**: 74–77.

Engardt, M., Knutsson, E., Jonsson, E., and Sternhag, M. (1995). Dynamic muscle strength training in stroke patients: effects on knee extension torque, electromyographic activity and motor function. *Arch Phys Med Rehabil* **76**: 419–425.

Ernst, E. (1990). A review of stroke rehabiltiation and physiotherapy. *Stroke* **21**: 1081–1085.

Evans, A., Perez, I., Harraf, F., *et al.* (2001). Can differences in management process explain different outcomes between stroke unit and stroke-team care? *Lancet* **358**: 1586–1592.

Evidence-based Medicine Working Group (2002). *Users' Guides to the Medical Literature. A Manual for Evidenced-Based Clinical Practice.* Chicago: AMA Press.

Faghri, P. D., Rodgers, M. M., Glaser, R. M., *et al.* (1994). The effects of functional electrical stimulation on shoulder subluxation, arm function recovery, and shoulder pain in hemiplegic stroke patients. *Arch Phys Med Rehabil* **75**: 73–79.

Feys, H. M., de Weerdt, W. J., Selz, B. E., *et al.* (1998). Effect of a therapeutic intervention for the hemiplegic upper limb in the acute phase after stroke: a single-blind, randomized, controlled multicenter trial. *Stroke* **29**: 785–792.

Geiger, R. A., Allen, J. B., OKeefe, J., and Hicks, R. R. (2001). Balance and mobility following stroke: effects of physical therapy interventions with and without biofeedback/forceplate training. *Phys Ther* **81**: 995–1005.

Gelber, D. A., Josefczyk, P. B., Herrman, D., Good, D. C., and Verhulst, S. J. (1995). Comparison of two therapy approaches in the rehabilitation of the pure motor hemiparetic stroke patient. *J Neurol Rehabil* **9**: 191–196.

Glanz, M., Klawansky, S., Stason, W., *et al.* (1995). Biofeedback therapy in post-stroke rehabilitation: a meta-analysis of the randomized controlled trials. *Arch Phys Med Rehabil* **76**: 508–515.

Glanz, M., Klawansky, S., Stason, W., Berkey, C., and Chalmers, T. C. (1996). Functional electrostimulation in post-stroke rehabilitation: a meta-analysis of the randomized controlled trials. *Arch Phys Med Rehabil* **77**: 549–553.

Glasser, L. (1986). Effects of isokinetic training on the rate of movement during ambulation in hemiplegic patients. *Phys Ther* **66**: 673–676.

Gowland, C. and Basmajian, J. V. (1996). Stroke. In *Clinical Decision Making in Rehabilitation: Efficacy and Outcomes*, ed. J. V. Basmajian and S. R. Banerjee New York: Churchill Livingston, pp. 5–17.

Green, J., Forster, A., Bogle, S., and Young, J. (2002). Physiotherapy for patients with mobility problems more than 1 year after stroke: a randomized controlled trial. *Lancet* **359**: 199–203.

Gresham, G. E., Duncan, P. W., and Stason, W. B. (1995). *Post-stroke rehabilitation: Assessment, Referral, and Patient Management. Clinical Practice Guideline 16 (AHCPR Publication 95-0622)*. Rockville, MD: Department of Health and Human Services, Public Health Service, Agency for Health Care Policy and Research.

Hansen, P. (2002). Body-weight-support gait training. *Clin Rehabil* **16**: 343–345.

Hedges, L. V. (1994). Fixed effects models. In *The Handbook of Research Synthesis*, ed. H. Cooper and L. V. Hedges. New York: Russell Sage Foundation, pp. 285–300.

Holm, M. (2000). Our mandate for the new millennium: evidence based practice. *Am J Occup Ther* **54**: 575–585.

Humm, J. L., Kolowski, D. A., James, D. C., Gotts, J. E., and Schallert, T. (1998). Use dependent exacerbation of brain damage occurs during an early post lesion vulnerable period. *Brain Res* **783**: 286–292.

Inaba, M., Edberg, E., and Montgomery, J. (1973). Effectiveness of functional training, active exercise, and resistive exercise for patients with hemiplegia. *Phys Ther* **53**: 28–35.

Indredavik, B., Bakke, F., Slordahl, S. A., Rokseth, R., and Haheim, L. L. (1999). Treatment in a combined acute and rehabilitation stroke unit: which aspects are most important? *Stroke* **30**: 917–923.

Johansson, B. B., Hacker, E., von Arbin, M., *et al.* (2001). Acupuncture and transcutaneous nerve stimulation in stroke rehabilitation. *Stroke* **32**: 707–713.

Jongbloed, L., Stacey, S., and Brighton, C. (1989). Stroke rehabilitation: sensorimotor integrative treatment versus functional treatment. *Am J Occup Ther* **43**: 391–397.

Knott, M. and Voss, E. D. (1962). *Proprioceptive Neuromuscular Facilitation: Patterns and Techniques*. New York: Paul B. Hoeber.

Kobayashi, H., Onishi, H., Ihashi, K., Yagi, R., and Handa, Y. (1999). Reduction in subluxation and improved muscle function of the hemiplegic shoulder joint after therapeutic electrical stimulation. *J Electromyogr Kinesiol* **9**: 327–336.

Kosak, M. and Reding, M. S. (2000). Comparison of partial body weight-supported treadmill gait training versus aggressive bracing assisted walking post stroke. *Neurorehabil Neural Repair* **14**: 13–19.

Kraft, G. H., Fitts, S. S., and Hammond, M. C. (1992). Techniques to improve function of the arm and hand in chronic hemiplegia. *Arch Phys Med Rehabil* **73**: 220–227.

Kwakkel, G., Wagenaar, R. C., Koelman, T. W., Lankhorst, G. J., and Koetsier, J. C. (1997). Effects of intensity of stroke rehabilitation: a research synthesis. *Stroke* **28**: 1550–1556.

Kwakkel, G., Wagenaar, R. C., Twisk, J. W. R., Lankhorst, G. J., and Koetsier, J. C. (1999a). Intensity of leg and arm training after primary middle-cerebral-artery stroke: a randomised trial. *Lancet* **354**: 191–196.

Kwakkel, G., Kollen, B. J., and Wagenaar, R. C. (1999b). Therapy impact on functional recovery in stroke rehabilitation: a critical review of the literature. *Physiotherapy* **85**: 377–391.

Kwakkel, G., Kollen, B. J., and Wagenaar, R. C. (2002). Long term effects of intensity of upper and lower limb training after stroke: a randomised trial. *J Neurol Neurosurg Psychiatry* **72**: 473–479.

LaClair, B. J., Reker, D. M., Duncan, P. W., Horner, R. D., and Hoenig, H. (2001). Stroke care: a method for measuring compliance with AHCPR guidelines. *Am J Phys Med Rehabil* **80**: 235–242.

Langhammer, B. and Stanghelle, J. K. (2000). Bobath or motor relearning program? A comparison of two different approaches of physiotherapy in stroke rehabilitation: a randomized controlled study. *Clin Rehabil*, **14**, 361–369.

Langhorne, P. and Dennis, M. (1998). *Stroke Units: An Evidence Based Approach*. London: BMJ Books.

Langhorne, P., Wagenaar, R., and Partridge, C. (1996). Physiotherapy after stroke: more is better? *Physiother Res Int* **1**: 75–88.

Laufer, Y., Dickstein, R., Chefez, Y., and Marcovitz, E. (2001). The effect of treadmill training on the ambulation of stroke survivors in the early stages of rehabilitation: a randomized study. *J Rehabil Res Dev* **38**: 69–78.

Lincoln, N. B., Willis, D., Philips, S. A., Juby, L. C., and Berman, P. (1996). Comparison of rehabilitation practice on hospital wards for stroke patients. *Stroke* **27**: 18–23.

Lincoln, N. B., Parry, R. H., and Vass, C. D. (1999). Randomized, controlled trial to evaluate increased intensity of physiotherapy treatment of arm function after stroke. *Stroke* **30**: 573–579.

Linde, K., Jonas, W. B., Melchart, D., and Willich, S. (2001). The methodological quality of randomized controlled trials of homeopathy, herbal medicines and acupuncture. *Int J Epidemiol* **30**: 526–531.

Linn, S. L., Granat, M. H., and Lees, K. R. (1999). Prevention of shoulder subluxation after stroke with electrical stimulation. *Stroke* **30**: 963–968.

Liston, R., Mickelborough, J., Harris, B., Hann, A. W., and Tallis, R. C. (2000). Conventional physiotherapy and treadmill re-training for higher-level gait disorders in cerebrovascular disease. *Age Aging* **29**: 311–318.

Logan, P. A., Ahern, J., Gladman, J. R., and Lincoln, N. B. (1997). A randomized controlled trial of enhanced Social Service occupational therapy for stroke patients. *Clin Rehabil* **11**: 107–113.

Logigian, M. K., Samuels, M. A., Falconer, J., and Zagar, R. (1983). Clinical exercise trial for stroke patients. *Arch Phys Med Rehabil* **64**: 364–367.

Lord, J. P. and Hall, K. (1986). Neuromuscular reeducation versus traditional programs for stroke rehabilitation. *Arch Phys Med Rehabil* **67**: 88–91.

Macdonell, R. A. L., Triggs, W. J., Leikauskas, J., *et al.* (1994). Functional electrical stimulation to the affected lower limb and recovery after cerebral infarction. *J Stroke Cerebrovasc Dis* **4**: 155–160.

Macko, R. F., Smith, G. V., Dobrovolny, L., *et al.*, (2001). Treadmill training improves fitness reserve in chronic stroke patients. *Arch Phys Med Rehabil* **82**: 879–884.

Mandel, A. R., Nymark, J. R., and Balmer, S. J., (1990). Electromyographic versus rhythmic positional biofeedback in computerized gait retraining with stroke patients. *Arch Phys Med Rehabil* **71**: 649–654.

Mayo, N., Wood Dauphinee, S., Ahmed. S., *et al.* (1999). Disablement following stroke. *Disabil Rehabil* **21**: 258–268.

Merletti, R., Zelaschi, F., Latella, D., *et al.* (1978). A control study of muscle force recovery in hemiparetic patients during treatment with functional electrical stimulation. *Scand J Rehabil Med* **10**: 147–154.

Micieli, G., Cavallini, A., and Quaglini, S. for the Guideline Application for Decision Making in Ischemic Stroke (GLADIS) Study Group (2002). Guideline compliance improves stroke outcome. A preliminary study in four districts in the Italian region of Lombardia. *Stroke* **33**: 1341–1347.

Moreland, J. and Thomson, M. A. (1994). Efficacy of electromyographic biofeedback compared with conventional physical therapy for upper-extremity function in patients following stroke: a research overview and meta-analysis. *Phys Ther* **74**: 534–547.

Moreland, J. D., Thomson, M. A., and Fuoco, A. R. (1998). Electromyographic biofeedback to improve lower extremity function after stroke: a meta-analysis. *Arch Phys Med Rehabil* **79**: 134–140.

Mudie, M. H., Winzeler-Mercay, U., Radwan, S., and Lee, L. (2002). Training symmetry of weight distribution after stroke: a randomized controlled pilot study comparing task-related reach, Bobath and feedback training approaches. *Clin Rehabil* **16**: 582–592.

Murray, C. J. L. and Lopez, A. D. (1997). Global mortality, disability and contribution of risk factors: Global Burden of Disease Study. *Lancet* **349**: 1436–1442.

Nilsson, L., Carlsson, J., Danielsson, A., *et al.* (2001). Walking training of patients with hemiparesis at an early stage after stroke: a comparison of walking training on a treadmill with body weight support and walking training on the ground. *Clin Rehabil* **15**: 515–527.

Ostendorf, C. G. and Wolf, S. L. (1981). Effect of forced use of the upper extremity of a hemiplegic patient on changes in function. *Phys Ther* **61**: 1022–1028.

Packman-Braun, R. (1988). Relationship between functional electrical stimulation duty cycle and fatigue in wrist extensor muscles of patients with hemiparesis. *Phys Ther* **68**: 51–56.

Page, S. J., Sisto, S. A., Levine, P., Johnston, M. V., and Hughes, M. (2001). Modified constraint induced therapy: a randomized feasibility and efficacy study. *J Rehabil Res Dev* **38**: 583–590.

Page, S. J., Levin, P., Sisto, S. and Johnston, M. V. (2002). Stroke patients' and therapists' opinions of constraint-induced movement therapy. *Clin Rehabil* **16**: 55–60.

Park, J., Hopwood, V., White, A. R., and Ernst, E. (2001). Effectiveness of acupuncture for stroke: a systematic review. *J Neurol* **248**: 558–563.

Parker, C. J., Gladman, J. R. F., Drummond, A. E. R., *et al.* (2001). A multicentre randomized controlled trial of leisure therapy and conventional occupational therapy after stroke. TOTAL Study Group. Trial of Occupational Therapy and Leisure. *Clin Rehabil* **15**: 42–52.

Parker-Taillon, D. (2002). CPA initiatives put the spotlight on evidence-based practice in physiotherapy. *Physiother Can* **24**: 12–15.

Partridge, C., Mackenzie, M., Edwards, S., *et al.* (2000). Is dosage of physiotherapy a critical factor in deciding patterns of recovery from stroke: a pragmatic randomized controlled trial. *Physiother Res Int* **5**: 230–240.

Peacock, P. B., Riley, C. H. P., Lampton, T. D., Raffel, S. S., and Walker, J. S. (1972). The Birmingham stroke, epidemiology and rehabilitation study. In *Trends in Epidemiology*, ed. G. T. Stewart Springfield, IL: Thomas, pp. 231–345..

Pohl, M., Mehrholz, J., Ritschel, C., and Ruckriem, S. (2002). Speed-dependent treadmill training in ambulatory hemiparetic stroke patients: a randomized controlled trial. *Stroke* **33**: 553–558.

Potempa, K., Lopez, M., Braun, L. T., *et al.* (1995). Physiological outcomes of aerobic exercise training in hemiparetic stroke patients. *Stroke* **26**: 101–105.

Pound, P., Tilling, K., Rudd, A. G., and Wolfe, C. D. (1999). Does patient satisfaction reflect differences in care received after stroke? *Stroke* **30**: 49–55.

Pomeroy, V. M. and Tallis, R. C. (2000). Physical therapy to improve movement performance and functional ability post stroke. Part I: existing evidence. *Rev Clin Geronto* **10**: 261–290.

Powell, J., Pandyan, A. D., Granat, M., Cameron, M., and Stott, D. J. (1999). Electrical stimulation of wrist extensors in post-stroke hemiplegia. *Stroke* **30**: 1384–1389.

Price, C. I. M. and Pandyan, A. D. (2001). Electrical stimulation for preventing and treating post-stroke shoulder pain: a systematic Cochrane review. *Clin Rehabil* **15**: 5–19.

Richards, C. L., Malouin, F., Wood-Dauphinee, S., *et al.* (1993). Physical therapy for optimization of gait recovery in acute stroke patients. *Arch Phys Med Rehabil* **74**: 612–620.

Rimmer, J. H., Riley, B., Creviston, T., and Nicola, T. (2000). Exercise training in a predominantly African-American group of stroke survivors. *Med Sci Sport Exerc* **32**: 1990–1996.

Rijken, P. M. and Dekker, J. (1998). Clinical experience of rehabilitation therapists with chronic disease: a quantitative approach. *Clin Rehabil* **12** 143–150.

Rosenberg, W. and Donald, A. (1995). Evidence based medicine: an approach to clinical problem solving. *BMJ* **310**: 1122–1126.

Roth, E. J. and Noll, S. F. (1994). Stroke rehabilitation. 2. Comorbidities and complications. *Arch Phys Med Rehabil* **75**: S42–S46.

Sackett, D. L., Straus, S. E., Richardson, W. S., Rosenburg, W., and Haynes, R. B. (2000). *Evidence-based Medicine: How to Practice and Teach EBM*, 2nd edn. New York: Churchill Livingstone.

Schleenbaker, R. E. and Mainous, A. G. (1993). Electromyographic biofeedback for neuromuscular reeducation in the hemiplegic stroke patient – a meta-analysis. *Arch Phys Med Rehabil* **74**: 1301–1304.

Shadish, W. R. and Haddock, C. K. (1994). Combined estimates of effect size. In: *The Handbook of Research Synthesis*, ed. H. Cooper and L. V. Hedges. New York: Russell Sage Foundation pp. 261–282.

Sivenius, J., Pyorala, K., Heinonen, O. P., Salonen, J. T., and Riekkinen, P. (1985). The significance of intensity of rehabilitation of stroke. A controlled trial. *Stroke* **16**: 928–931.

Smith, D. S., Goldenberg, E., Ashburn, A., *et al.* (1981). Remedial therapy after stroke: a randomised controlled trial. *BMJ* **282**: 517–520.

Smith, G. Y., Silver, K. H. C., Goldberg, A. P., and Macko, R. F. (1999). "Task-oriented" exercise improves hamstring strength and spastic reflexes in chronic stroke patients. *Stroke* **30**: 2112–2118.

Stegmayr, B., Aspland, K., Hulter-Asberg, K., *et al.* (1999). Stroke units in their natural habitat: can the results of randomised trials be reproduced in routine clinical practice? *Stroke* **30**: 709–714.

Stern, P. H., McDowell, F., Miller, J. M., and Robinson, M. (1970). Effects of facilitation exercise techniques in stroke rehabilitation. *Arch Phys Med Rehabil* **51**: 526–531.

Stockmeyer, S. A. (1967). An interpretation of the approach of Rood to the treatment of hemiplegia. *Am J Phys Med* **46**: 900–956.

Stroke Unit Trialists' Collaboration (1997). How do stroke units improve patient outcomes? A collaborative systematic review of the randomized trials. *Stroke* **28**: 2139–2144.

(2002). Organized inpatient (stroke unit) care for stroke. In *Cochrane Database of Systematic Reviews*, Issue 2. Oxford: Update Software.

Sullivan, K. J., Knowlton, B. J., and Dobkin, B. H. (2002). Step training with body weight support: effect of treadmill speed and practice paradigms on post stroke locomotor recovery. *Arch Phys Med Rehabil* **83**: 683–691.

Sunderland, A., Tinson, D. J., Bradley, E. L., *et al.* (1992). Enhanced physical therapy improves recovery of arm function after stroke. A randomised controlled trial. *J Neurol Neurosurg Psychiatry* **55**: 530–535.

Sze, F.K-H., Wong, E., Yi, X., and Woo, J. (2002). Does acupuncture have additional value to standard post-stroke motor rehabilitation? *Stroke* **33**, 186–194.

Tang, J-L., Zhan, S-Y., and Ernst, E. (1999). Review of randomized controlled trials of traditional Chinese medicine. *BMJ* **319**: 160–161.

Taub, E., Miller, N. E., Novack, T. A., *et al.* (1993). Technique to improve chronic motor deficit after stroke. *Arch Phys Med Rehabil* **74**: 347–354.

Teixeira-Salmela, L. F., Olney, S. J., Nadeaus, S., and Brouwer, B. (1999). Muscle strengthening and physical conditioning to reduce impairment and disability in chronic stroke survivors. *Arch Phys Med Rehabil* **80**: 1211–1218.

Thaut, M. H., McIntosh, G. C., and Rice, R. R. (1997). Rhythmic facilitation of gait training in hemiparetic stroke rehabilitation. *J Neurol Sci* **151**: 207–212.

Tinson, D. J. (1989). How stroke patients spend their days. *Int Disabil Stud* **11**: 45–49.

US Department of Health and Human Services, Agency for Health Care Policy and Research (1993). *Acute Pain Management: Operative or Medical Procedures and Trauma.* 92-0023. Rockville, MD: US Department of Health and Human Services, Agency for Health Care Policy and Research.

van der Lee, J. H., Wagenaar, R. C., Lankhorst, G. J., *et al.* (1999). Forced use of the upper extremity in chronic stroke patients: results from a single-blind randomized clinical trial. *Stroke* **30**: 2369–2375.

Visintin, M., Barbeau, H., Korner-Bitensky, N., and Mayo, N. E. (1998). A new approach to retrain gait in stroke patients through body weight support and treadmill stimulation. *Stroke* **29**: 1122–1128.

Wade, D. T., Collen, F. M., Robb, G. F. and Warlow, C. P. (1992). Physiotherapy intervention late after stroke and mobility. *BMJ* **304**: 609–613.

Wagenaar, R. C. and Meijer, O. G. (1991a). Effects of stroke rehabilitation (1). *J Rehabil Sci* **4**: 61–73.

(1991b). Effects of stroke rehabilitation (2). *J Rehabil Sci* **4**: 97–109.

Walker, M. F., Gladman, J. R., Lincoln, N. B., Siemonsma, P., and Whiteley, T. (1999). Occupational therapy for stroke patients not admitted to hospital: a controlled trial. *Lancet* **354**: 278–280.

Wang, R. Y., Yang, Y. R., Tsai, M. W., Wang, W. T., and Chan, R. C. (2002). Effects of functional electric stimulation on upper limb motor function and shoulder range of motion in hemiplegic patients. *Am J Phys Med Rehabil* **81**: 283–290.

Werner, R. A. and Kessler, S. (1996). Effectiveness of an intensive outpatient rehabilitation program for post-acute stroke patients. *Am J Phys Med Rehabil* **75**: 114–120.

Wolf, S. L. and Binder-MacLeod, S. A. (1983). Electromyographic biofeedback applications to the hemiplegic patient: changes in upper extremity neuromuscular and functional status. *Phys Ther* **63**: 1393–1403.

Wolf, S. L., Lecraw, D. E., Barton, L. A., and Jann, B. B. (1989). Forced use of hemiplegic upper extremities to reverse the effect of learned non-use among chronic stroke and head-injured patients. *Exp Neurol* **104**: 125–132.

8

Is early neurorehabilitation useful?

Karin Diserens

University of Lausanne and Centre Hospitalier Universitaire Vaudois, Lausanne, Switzerland

Gerhard Rothacher

Neurological Rehabilitation Hospital, Gailingen, Germany

Introduction

A belief in the superior efficacy of early treatment has a long history in the literature of rehabilitation. This belief probably has its roots in clinical experience and logic. Wylie (1968) argued that earlier treatment is generally held to be superior in the lore of medical care. Subsequently, many investigators have studied the relationship between timing of rehabilitative efforts and patient outcome. These studies have varied greatly: the early group ranging from less than two days to up to three months post-onset. Yet, a correlation between earlier onset of rehabilitative efforts and better recovery for stroke patients has been recurrently documented, and authors have concluded that early rehabilitation is important to maximize patient recovery and to improve cost-effectiveness (Wylie, 1968; Wojner, 1996).

In order to discuss if early rehabilitation is useful, we have to distinguish rehabilitation practiced during the "acute phase" of stroke from "early rehabilitation" practiced in rehabilitation centers during the first three months. Furthermore, the organization of the rehabilitation team and the intensity of therapy has to be defined, varying from conventional wards or stroke units with only physiotherapy to stroke units with interdisciplinary teams and intensive rehabilitation programs.

In this chapter, we shall try to give an overview of the literature available describing the different definitions of early rehabilitation in order to offer some actual practical criteria for selecting patients for early rehabilitation (i.e. rehabilitation in acute phase) and give guidelines for the constitution of the interdisciplinary staff, the intensity of treatment, and the essential approaches of neurorehabilitation of the stroke patient.

Recovery after Stroke, ed. Michael P. Barnes, Bruce H. Dobkin and Julien Bogousslavsky. Published by Cambridge University Press. © Cambridge University Press 2005.

Pathophysiological aspects of activation of recovery in the acute phase

Several studies have tried to determine whether structural or functional enrichment of animals' living environment or post-ischemic training could alter the pattern of delayed neuronal cell death and influence functional impairment. Farrell *et al.* (2001) observed 84 gerbils with cerebral ischemia (some with prior ischemic conditioning) and animals with a sham procedure for 60 days in which animals were housed either in enriched animal housing with functional training or in standard (non-enriched) housing. The hippocampal neurons (CA1) were investigated in all groups by electrophysiological and histological techniques. They concluded that early, intensive intervention after ischemia can improve functional outcome but this is accompanied by increased brain damage.

These data were similar to those of Humm *et al.* (1999). In this study, the unaffected limb was placed in a plaster cast immediately after the brain lesion, thereby forcing use of the impaired limb. This intervention increased the extent of cortical injury and worsened behavioral outcome. A related experiment using a focal ischemia model demonstrated an increase in infarction volume when rats were put into an enriched environment plus training on several motor tasks beginning 24 hours after ischemia. Delaying enrichment and motor task training until seven days after ischemia had no effect on infarct volume. Interestingly, both early and late enrichment improved functional outcome even though early enrichment increased use-dependent cortical damage (Risedal *et al.*, 1999).

A question arises as to the mechanisms of use-dependent injury exacerbation. Several factors may contribute to this phenomenon. First, it is known that during and after ischemia there is a massive release of glutamate from the hippocampal and other neurons into the extracellular space and this transmitter reaches excitotoxic levels. Second, behavioral testing and spatial learning further increases glutamate release as part of the learning process. Therefore, the combination of intensive enrichment and ischemic condition enhances the damage on cerebral cells secondary to an increase of glutamate to neurotoxic levels. In contrast, less-intense stimulation (as also tested in the gerbil experiment) may not provoke such a sustained elevation of glutamate. This idea was originally proposed based on human studies which found that glutamate antagonists blocked use-dependent cortical injury following limb casting procedures (Farrell *et al.*, 2001).

Outcome research in early rehabilitation

Early rehabilitation can be regarded as a multivariant model. The results of early rehabilitation are influenced by the intensity of treatment, the organization of the rehabilitation team, the choice of the outcome measurements, the context factors of the actual rehabilitation place (e.g. general or specialized wards, stroke units), and the possibilities of post-onset inpatient ambulatory rehabilitation. The results of rehabilitation can, for instance, be measured by its efficiency or its effectiveness. *Efficiency* as defined by Paolucci *et al.* (2000) means the amount of improvements in the rating score of each scale divided by the length of rehabilitation. It represents the average increase per day obtained during rehabilitation. *Effectiveness* reflects the proportion of potential improvement achieved during rehabilitation calculated as ([discharge score − initial score]/[maximum score − initial score])×100.

The principal review studies in the literature are presented here with the main objective to evaluate usefulness of early rehabilitation.

In a case–control study with 135 patients, Paolucci *et al.* (2000) assess the specific influence of the onset–admission interval (OAI) on rehabilitation results.

The short OAI subgroup (<20 days) had significantly higher effectiveness of treatment than the medium (day 21–40) ($p < 0.50$) and longest groups (day 41–60) ($p < 0.005$). Beginning treatment within the first 20 days was associated, on the one hand, with a significantly high probability of excellent therapeutic response (odds ratio [OR], 5.18; 95% confidence interval [CI], 1.07–25.00). On the other hand, early intervention was also associated with a five times greater risk of drop-out than that seen in patients with delayed start of treatment (OR, 4.99; 95% CI, 1.38–18.034). The three subgroups were significantly ($p < 0.5$) different regarding the percentage of low and high responders.

As a rating score, Paolucci *et al.* (2000) used the Barthel Index and the Canadian Neurological Scale. The main outcome measurement concerned efficiency and effectiveness. The results showed a strong association between OAI and functional outcome in favor of the short OAI subgroup. In 2002, the Cochrane Library published two systematic reviews comparing stroke units with other concepts of care (Early Supported Discharge Trialists, 2002; Stroke Unit Trialists' Collaboration, 2002). In order to assess organized inpatient care for stroke, a total of 23 randomized and quasi-randomized trials comparing organized inpatient stroke unit care with an alternative service were evaluated (Stroke Unit Trialists' Collaboration, 2002). Organized stroke care took place in a stroke ward (with a multidisciplinary team including specialist nursing staff based in a discrete ward caring exclusively for stroke patients), a mixed rehabilitation ward (with a multidisciplinary team including specialist nursing staff in a ward providing a generic rehabilitation service but not exclusively caring for stroke patients), or in hospital wards with a mobile stroke team providing specialist care to the patient (i.e. a multidisciplinary team providing care but excluding specialist nursing staff).

Stroke wards could be acute stroke units that accepted patients acutely but discharged early, usually within 7 days (this could include an "intensive" model of care with continuous monitoring and high nurse staffing levels); a rehabilitation stroke unit that accepted patients after a delay of usually seven days or more and focused on rehabilitation; and comprehensive stroke units (i.e. combined acute and rehabilitation) that accepted patients acutely but which also provided rehabilitation for at least several weeks if necessary. Non-organized stroke care took place on general medical wards (i.e. care in acute medical ward without routine multidisciplinary input).

Compared with alternative services, stroke unit care reduced the odds of death recorded at final (median one year) follow-up (OR, 0.86; 95% CI, 0.71–0.94; $P = 0.005$), the odds of death or institutionalized care (OR, 0.80; 95% CI, 0.71–0.90; $P = 0.0002$) and death or dependency (OR, 0.78; 95% CI, 0.68–0.89; $P = 0.0003$). Stroke patients who receive organized inpatient care in a stroke unit were more likely to be alive, independent, and living at home one year after the stroke. The benefits were most apparent in units based in a discrete ward. Outcomes were independent of patient age, sex, and stroke type. There was no indication that organized stroke unit care resulted in increased hospital stay.

The second Cochrane review (Early Supported Discharge Trialists, 2002) an organized multidisciplinary or interdisciplinary rehabilitation team approach plus early discharge and further support in a community setting with conventional stroke care. Outcome data of the four trials was a comparision of available at the time showed again a net benefit for the patients treated with organized multi-disciplinary in- and outpatient care in respect of death (OR, 0.87; 95% CI, 0.39–1.93), death or institutionalization (OR, 0.69; 95% CI, 0.36–1.31) death or dependency (OR, 0.88; 95% CI, 0.49–1.57).

Anderson *et al.* (2002) systematically reviewed seven published trials (1277 patients: 54% men, mean age 73 years) with an economic analysis comparing early hospital discharge (including rehabilitation in the acute phase) and dom-iciliary rehabilitation with usual care. As the Cochrane overview (Stroke Unit Trialists' Collaboration, 2002) had suggested that organized stroke units reduced the length of hospitalization, this review evaluated (Table 8.1). The cost-effectiveness of schemes permitting earlier home-based rehabilitation in stroke. This meta-analysis concluded that a policy of early hospital discharge by an organized interdisciplinary stroke unit and rehabilitation since the acute phase permitted earlier home-based rehabilitation for patients with stroke and may reduce the use of hospital beds (13 days reduction) and the global costs (15% lower for the early-discharge inter-vention) without compromising clinical outcomes.

Organization of an early rehabilitation unit: recommendations for quality and structure

Contrary to the definition of early rehabilitation by Wylie (1968, 1970) as in the first eight weeks from stroke, modern concepts would define early rehabilitation as

Table 8.1 Randomized controlled trials of early supported discharge and domiciliary stroke rehabilitation

Reference	Study location	No. participants (early discharge/ standard care)	Time to randomization	Service	Duration of service	Duration of follow-up (months)	Unique aspects of study
Rudd *et al.* (1997)	London (UK)	331 (167/164)	Median 13 days	New multidisciplinary community therapy team (PT, OT, ST, medical)	Maximum 3 months	12	Economic analysis; caregiver assessments; patient satisfaction assessment
Rodgers *et al.* (1997)	Newcastle (UK)	92 (46/46)	Within 72 hours of stroke	New community-based hospital; inreach multidisciplinary rehab team (PT, OT, ST, SW, nurses, medical); medical support by GP and stroke physician	Median 9 weeks (range, 1–44)	3	Economic analysis; caregiver assessments; QoL assessment
Anderson *et al.* (2000)	Adelaide (Australia)	86 (42/44)	Median 13 days	Multidisciplinary community rehab team (medical, PT, OT, ST, SW, nurses); combination of hospital inreach and community outreach services.	Mean 5.4 weeks (SD, 3.7)	6	Economic analysis; caregiver assessments; QoL assessment

Table 8.1 (*cont.*)

Reference	Study location	No. participants (early discharge/ standard care)	Time to randomization	Service	Duration of service	Duration of follow-up (months)	Unique aspects of study
Widen Holmqvist et al. (1996)	Stockholm (Sweden)	83 (42/41)	Within 1 week of admission	Multidisciplinary hospital outreach early supported discharge team; therapist service (PT, OT, ST, SW: no nursing input)	14–19 weeks	12	All patients received stroke unit care; economic analysis only involved 15 intervention patients; QoL assessments
Ronning and Guldvog (1998)	Akershus (Norway)	251 (124/127)	Within 24 hours of admission	Community rehab (PT, ST, nurse) provided by variety of municipality-based services (nursing homes or ambulatory therapy); no specialist in stroke; medical input by GP; some nursing input		7	Admission to nursing home for rehab in 41%; ambulatory physiotherapy in 25%; no treatment in 30%; QoL assessment

| Mayo et al. (2000) | Montreal (Canada) | 114 | Mean 10 days | Multidisciplinary community team (nursing, PT, OT, ST, dietician), | 4 weeks | 3 | All patients had caregivers; QoL assessment; all patients received stroke unit care; 30–50% discharged to an institution |
| Indredavik et al. (2000) | Trondheim (Norway) | 320(160/160) | Within 72 hours of admission | Multidisciplinary hospital outreach mobile stroke team (nurse, PT, OT, medical) coordinating early discharge and rehab in the community | 1 month | 6 | All patients received stroke unit care; 30–50% discharged to an institution |

GP, general practicioner; medical, geriatrician, stroke physician or rehabilitation specialist with expertise in stroke medicine; OT, occupational therapist; PT, physiotherapist; SD, standard deviation; ST, speech and language therapist; SW, social worker; rehab, rehabilitation; QoL, quality of life.
From: Anderson et al. (2002).

the beginning rehabilitation efforts within 24–48 hours of the stroke (Hayes and Carroll, 1986). Unfortunately, any precision about treatment intensity has not been given. Paolucci *et al.* (2000) chose the threshold value of 20 days after stroke as the cut-off point of early intervention. Contrary to many other studies, they specified the early rehabilitation staff and the intensity of treatment: the staff included physicians (psychiatrists, neurologists, urologists, otorhinolaryngologists), neuropsychologists, nurses, physiotherapists, occupational and speech therapists, a social services care manager, dieticians, and support staff.

Individual physiotherapy was performed for 60 minutes twice a day (only once on Saturdays) six days a week. If necessary, patients had access to individual training for neglect or speech therapy, and for swallowing, bowel, and bladder dysfunctions. Physiotherapy and language treatment continued throughout the hospital stay and the training for neglect lasted for eight consecutive weeks.

Hayes and Carroll (1986) initiated "early rehabilitation" within the first 24 hours. Any precision about treatment intensity was not given.

The best documented evidence on structural and organizational issues in early rehabilitation originates from stroke unit care evaluations (Dietz-Tejedor and Fuentes, 2001). As already mentioned in the Cochrane reviews (Early Supported Discharge Trialists, 2002; Stroke Unit Trialists' Collaboration, 2002), these are characterized by a systematization in patient care, with trained staff, preestablished admission criteria, and special attention to the acute treatment and early functional and social rehabilitation of the patient. This requires precise diagnostic and therapeutic guidelines. Stroke units are geographically confined structures, with specialized staff and diagnostic neurologists expert in stroke. There is also a multidisciplinary collaboration, with the cooperation of specialists in neuroradiology, cardiology, rehabilitation, vascular surgery, and neurosurgery. Nursing staff trained in the management of these patients, with adequate knowledge in neurology and in the early detection of complications, are available, as well as physical therapists. The stroke unit is functionally integrated in the hospital and the health system. (Fig. 8.1)

The German Neurological Society recommends the following standards for structure and quality: (Ringelstein, 1998) a four to eight bed intensive care stroke unit (24 hour shift service) should have five or six physicians with special training in stroke care, one cardiologist on an "on call" basis, two nurses per bed, one physiotherapist, and a speech therapist, occupational therapist, social worker, and secretary available for 50% of time (i.e. "0.5 staffing").

The French Neurovascular Society (2001) recommends for a mixed 30-bed neurovascular unit (six intensive care beds, 24 regular beds) the presence of three neurologists trained in neurovascular medicine, 10.2 nurses during the day and 5.15 nurses during the night, two physiotherapists, one speech therapist, two psychologists (one with neuropsychology training), 0.5 social worker, and one secretary.

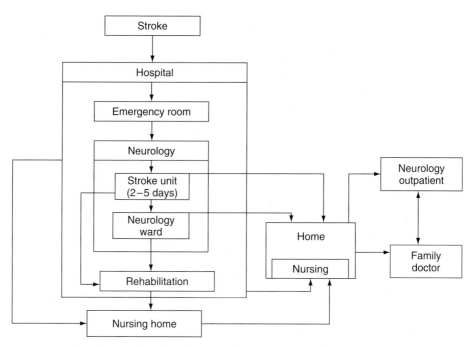

Fig. 8.1   Functional integration of stroke unit within a hospital and healthcare system. (Modified from Diez-Tejedor *et al.*, 2001.)

Proposition of selected criteria and guidelines of rehabilitation in acute phase and early rehabilitation

Based on the outcome research summarized above, we will now look at actual recommendations for organization, assessment, medical approach, and rehabilitation techniques for stroke (quality of process) in the early phase according to the Agency for Health Care Policy and Research (AHCPR) guidelines of 1997 (Stason, 1997) and accepted and published by the German Neurological Society in a synthesized form in 2002 (Steube, 2002).

Early stroke rehabilitation begins during acute hospitalization as soon as the diagnosis of stroke is established and life-threatening problems are under control. For the majority of stroke patients, rehabilitation starts two to three days after the acute stroke has occurred and before all diagnostic procedures are completed. Acute care measures and the beginning of rehabilitation will go hand in hand. In order to prevent an increase of ischemic damage, the intensity of mobilization and rehabilitation efforts during the first week should be minimal and increased thereafter. At first, the highest priorities are to prevent recurrent stroke and complications and ensure proper management of general health functions. Priorties then are to mobilize the patient, encourage resumption of self-care activities as soon as medically possible, and provide emotional support and information to the patient and family.

Clinical evaluation of patients begins with a basic examination followed by more thorough assessments and at least weekly follow-ups necessary to guide treatment decisions (Table 8.2). Information should be fully documented about medical and neurological problems, functional health patterns, complications, and social and environmental information. This will enable treatment goals and discharge decisions to be formulated. The International Classification of Functioning, Disability and Health (ICF) (Halbertsma *et al.*, 2000; Organization mondial de la Santé, 2001) can provide a framework to describe impairments, disabilities (newly called activity and participation potential), and contextual and environmental factors in respect of the resources of the patient. When possible and feasible, standardized instruments to measure function and abilities should be used.

The following aspects have to be considered: prevention of recurrence, skin protection, dysphagia, bladder control, sensorimotor rehabilitation, perceptual deficits, communication, neurophysiological alterations, and discharge planning.

Prevention of recurrence

Recurrence of stroke is considerable: 7–10% risk during the first year. The choice of therapy depends on the etiology of the stroke. For patients with subarachnoid hemorrhage, surgical treatment is effective in selected cases to prevent rebleeding. Anticoagulation therapy may be considered for a potentially cardiogenic source of embolism such as in patients with non-valvular atrial fibrillation. Antiplatelet drugs such as aspirin or clopidogrel may reduce the risk of ischemic stroke in patients with transient ischemic attacks and minor strokes. Heparin is often given during the acute phase for patients with progressive ischemic stroke or for patients with a >70% ipsilateral carotid stenosis prior to carotid endarterectomy despite lack of evidence of its benefits (Jonas, 1988; Adams *et al.*, 1994). Continuous control and start of long-term treatment of cardiovascular risk factors (e.g. hypertension, diabetes, or smoking) is mandatory.

Pulmonary embolism accounts for about 10% of deaths from stroke (Bounds *et al.*, 1981; Silver *et al.*, 1984). Therefore, all stroke patients should be screened for deep venous thrombosis (DVT). Since immobilization increases the risk of DVT (Cladgett *et al.*, 1992; Landi *et al.*, 1992), prophylaxis with heparin should be implemented soon after admission and continued until the patient is sufficiently mobile. Pooled data have shown a 45% risk reduction using low-dose heparin and a 79% risk reduction using low-molecular-weight heparin (Brandstater *et al.*, 1992; Cladgett *et al.*, 1992; Sandercock and Willems, 1992).The use of elastic stockings is also effective in preventing DVT (Cladgett *et al.*, 1992).

Table 8.2 Check-list of early rehabilitation assessment

Basic examination	Medical and neurological examination;
	evaluation of pain (e.g. shoulder–arm syndrome);
	response to commands;
	evaluation of bladder and bowel continence;
	evaluation of swallowing
Motor function	Motor control, range of movement, muscle strength;
	mobility (e.g. rolling, supine to sit, sitting, standing, transferring, walking);
	postural stability;
	balance;
	evaluation of the risk of falls;
	coordination
Communication	Spontaneous speech (e.g. fluency, word finding, naming, grammar, syntax, paraphrasia, articulation);
	repetition (see above);
	comprehension;
	reading and writing
Cognitive	Neglect (awareness of visual information or body parts);
	attention;
	orientation;
	memory;
	reasoning and judgement;
	visual fields
Emotional	Mood and motivation;
	future perspectives;
	insight and understanding of personal situation
Activities of daily living	Grooming (e.g. washing, dressing);
	eating;
	complex tasks (e.g. making a phone call, planning a day schedule, preparing a meal)
Family and caregiver	Presence of spouse or significant other;
	premorbid living situation (e.g. alone, in family, with others);
	family members who can supply support;
	family members within reasonable distance;
	physical environment of potential residence

Skin protection

Measures to maintain skin integrity should be initiated during acute care and continued throughout rehabilitation. At highest risk for skin problems are patients who are comatose, incontinent, or with high spastic muscle tone. Systematic daily inspection of the skin, paying particular attention to areas over bony prominences, gentle routine skin cleansing, protection from exposure to moisture (e.g. urine), proper positioning, regular turning, and gentle transfer techniques help to prevent skin damage. A full discussion of this problem and recommendations for prevention and treatment is found in the AHCPR-sponsored guidelines (Panel for the Prediction and Prevention of Pressure Ulcers in Adults, 1992).

Dysphagia

Dysphagia (impaired swallowing) frequently occurs in stroke patients and may lead to aspiration and pneumonia (Palmer and DeChase, 1991). Aspiration is silent in approximately 40% of patients. The goals of dysphagia management are to prevent aspiration, dehydration, and malnutrition and to restore safe swallowing. In supratentorial lesions, spontaneous improvement is frequent and often fast, while brainstem lesions have a longer time frame and worse prognosis.

The patient's ability to swallow should be assessed soon after admission and before any oral intake of fluids or food. The screening procedure itself is done in an upright position using small amounts of fluid and food, paying attention to dysfunction of the lips, mouth, tongue, palate, pharynx, larynx, or proximal esophagus (DiIorio and Price, 1990; Murray, 1999). Video fluoroscopy and/or video endoscopy allow a more differentiated analysis of the swallowing problem and may help to guide treatment decisions. Compensatory treatments involve changes in posture and the position used for swallowing, learning swallowing maneuvers, (e.g. the Mendelson maneuver or supraglottic swallowing), changes in texture of food (e.g. thickening liquids, use of pureed food), bolus size, and temperature or route of administration (e.g. by syringe). Parenteral or tube feeding may be necessary, while long-term tube feeding is preferably done by gastrostomy (Emik-Herring and Wood, 1990). Evidence of the effectiveness of treatment is mainly supported by observational studies as controlled trials are lacking (Horner et al., 1988).

Bladder control

Problems with bladder control and incontinence are common after stroke but resolve spontaneously in the majority of patients. Long-lasting incontinence infers a poor long-term prognosis for functional recovery (Jongbloed, 1986; Reding et al., 1987). Its predictive significance (78%) is higher than other factors such as consciousness or daily living skills (68%) (Wade and Hewer, 1985).

Urinary incontinence can result from bladder hypo- and hyperreflexia as well as from inattention, mental status changes, and immobility. Persistent incontinence should be evaluated in order to identify treatable medical conditions such as urinary tract infections. Indwelling catheter use should be limited to as short a time as possible because of the increasing risk of bacteriuria and urinary tract infections (Bjork et al., 1984; Sabanthan et al., 1985).

Urinary retention can be safely managed with clean intermittent catheterisation (Bennett and Diokno, 1984; Webb *et al.*, 1990). Persistent urinary incontinence after stroke should be evaluated to determine its etiology. For further discussion of the management of urinary incontinence, see the AHCPR-sponsored guidelines (Urinary Incontinence Guideline Panel, 1992). Bowel problems may include incontinence, diarrhea or constipation and impaction, the last being far more common. Assessment of constipation includes careful documentation of past and present bowel habits, dietary and fluid intake, and activity.

Sensorimotor rehabilitation

Early mobilization of the patient helps to prevent DVT, skin breakdown, contracture formation, constipation, and pneumonia. It may vary from passive range of motion to out-of-bed activities. It has positive psychological effects on both the patient and family and contributes to reduce mortality and to improved functional outcomes (Hamrin, 1982a, b; Hayes and Carroll, 1986; Asberg, 1989). Mobilization is recommended as soon as the patient's medical and neurological condition permits and, if possible, 24 to 48 hours after admission. Mobilization needs to be delayed or done with caution in patients with coma, severe obtudation, progressing neurological signs or symptoms, subarachnoid or intracranial hemorrhage, severe orthostatic hypotension, or acute myocardial infarction.

The rate of mobilization depends on the general health of the patient, the underlying cause of stroke, physical endurance, postural stability, and the extent of orthostatic hypotension.

Panajiotou *et al.* (1999) showed the main risk of orthostatic reactions is two to three weeks after stroke onset. Since a reactive increase of the systolic and diastolic blood pressure is observed during the first week post-stroke, mobilization during this first week is recommended except in those with severe vascular stenosis, very severe stroke, or severe cardiovascular disease. Observation of symptoms during exercise, fatigability, blood pressure responses, heart rate and rhythm, and respiration provides important clues to evaluate endurance and thus to decide on the rate and extent of mobilization.

The beginning of mobilization requires a careful and thorough assessment of the patient's impairments and resources. Beginning with the neurological and medical examination and basic functional observations, the assessment will gradually extend to a systematic evaluation of motor function, cognitive function, emotional state, communication abilities, activities of daily living, the patient's premorbid condition, and the potential family and caregiver support. Discharge planning should begin early. The National Institutes of Health (NIH) Stroke Scale, which measures the severity of stroke, may be used to guide selection of an appropriate discharge setting during the acute care phase of management (Table 8.3).

Table 8.3 The National Institutes of Health (NIH) Stroke Scale: a relationship with discharge disposition

Admission NIH Stroke Scale Score	Discharge disposition
0–8	Home with outpatient therapy $(P = 0.001)$
9–17	Inpatient rehabilitation $(P = 0.004)$
18+	Skilled nursing facility, subacute care, nursing home, or home custodial care $(P = 0.001)$

From: Wojner (1996).

The following sequence of mobilization may start at any point depending on the patient's condition: frequent position changes in bed and daily passive and active range-of-motion exercises of the limbs; sitting up in bed and then progress to the edge of the bed; sitting out of bed in a chair or a wheelchair; learning passive and active transfers from bed to chair, wheelchair to chair, and toilet to wheelchair; getting to a standing position; starting to walk, first with help, then on a treadmill, with an aid, and, finally, alone. Activities of daily living may start with grooming, eating, toileting, and dressing and then extend to more complex tasks.

During mobilization, falls are the most frequent cause of injury in patients hospitalized with strokes, and hip fracture is a common complication (Poplingher and Pillar, 1985).

Special attention has to be given to patients with balance problems, sensori-motor paresis, confusion, visual impairments, and communication problems. Patients with visual neglect or those who are slow in performing tasks have the highest risk of falling (Diller and Weinberg, 1970). Acute illness or drug effects may increase the risk of falls.

Perceptual deficits: unilateral neglect

Unilateral neglect or hemi-inattention is characterized by a disturbance in spatial perception affecting the contralateral side of the body. This deficit may occur in up to 50% of strokes affecting the right cerebral hemispheres and up to 25% of left hemispheric strokes (Stone et al., 1991). Neglect challenges independence in activities of daily life. Clinical improvements can be achieved either by specific activation of the right hemisphere, for instance by transcutaneous electrical stimulation (Vallar et al., 1995), or by compensatory strategies (Soderback, 1988).

Communication

Approximately 40% of stroke survivors will have a speech or language disorder (Gresham et al., 1995). The impact of alteration in speech and language function may be devastating to the patient, reducing employability and quality of life and predisposing the patient to social isolation. Fluency of speech can be altered by dysarthria; "word-finding" errors; or the presence of an expressive, receptive, or global aphasia. In this case, a speech and language pathologist should be consulted early to assist with diagnosis and treatment.

Neuropsychological alterations: affective disorders and cognitive dysfunction

The incidence of post-stroke depression has been reported to be as great as 68%, with major depressions reported in as many as 27% of stroke survivors. The origins of this depression may be organic, situational secondary to neurological dysfunction, or related to comorbid medical conditions or drug therapy. The relation to the localization of the brain infarct is discussed with controversy in the literature. Frequently, major depression occur in strokes involving left anterior cerebral cortex and the basal ganglia, whereas minor depressions and apathy occur most commonly in right posterior cerebral infarcts. Assessment for post-stroke depression should include use of standardized depression scales, behavioral observations, and interviews with both the patient and family or other significant persons. Antidepressant medications coupled with psychotherapy may be used in the treatment of major depression.

Cognitive dysfunctions affecting the patient's orientation, attention, memory, insight, judgement, and abstract reasoning skills may also increase the length of stay during both acute care and inpatient rehabilitation, contributing to limited improvement in functional outcomes (Galski et al., 1993). A cognitive evaluation performed by a neuropsychologist should guide an appropriate selection of discharge options after completion of acute care management. Compensatory techniques and cognitive retraining that includes repetitive exercises may be employed in the acute care phase of stroke management and carried through to the rehabilitation setting of choice (Gresham et al., 1995). The long-term effects of these therapies have not yet been established in the literature.

Discharge planning

Stroke is a catastrophe for patient and family. The survivors are confronted with disability and often experience a dramatic change of living situation and living plans. Families have to learn to adjust to the altered relationship and to give support to the disabled family member. It is important to provide support to the patient and family during this critical time, giving them (repeatedly) information about the nature of the disease and its consequences. A goal of education is to maintain motivation by setting up goals and the steps to reach these, explaining the nature and the expected time frame of treatments, and by providing empathy and emotional support. Effective discharge planning will contribute to better outcomes, improve efficiency,

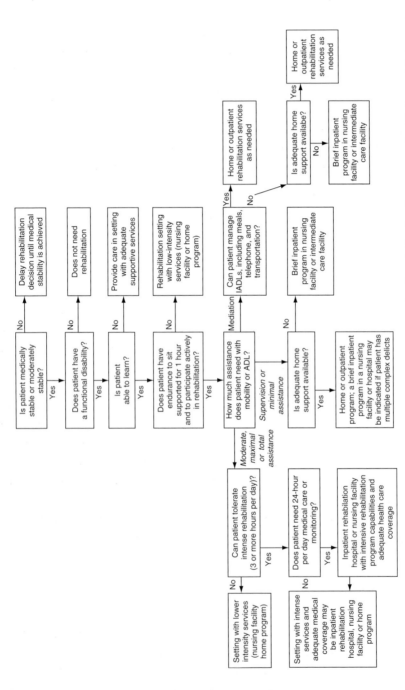

Fig. 8.2   Propositions for selection of the setting for a rehabilitation program after hospitalization for acute stroke. Under spcial circumstances, some patients with multiple, complex, functional deficits may be appropriate for inpatient programs. ADL, activites of daily living; IADL, instrumental activites of daily living. (From Gresham, 1992.)

and save costs. The patient and family should be intimately involved in the evaluation of needs and potential living options after discharge. An important goal of discharge planning is to determine the need and the best setting for rehabilitation to ensure continuity of services after discharge (Fig. 8.2).

General guidelines (Gresham *et al.*, 1995) affecting acute care discharge to an inpatient rehabilitation center after stroke include medical stability, the ability to tolerate three or more hours of continuous rehabilitation services, and the existence of more than one type of functional disability requiring interdisciplinary care. Patients with complex medical problems who require around-the-clock medical attention may be better suited for rehabilitation services provided in a skilled nursing facility or subacute care setting; reassessment of appropriateness for transfer to a comprehensive rehabilitation center should then be conducted once the patient has had the opportunity to continue convalescence. When the degree of disability is minimal, rehabilitation may best be provided on an outpatient basis (Fig. 8.2)

Summary

Early neurorehabilitation is of profound value for stroke patients and their social environment. Despite the fact that studies to prove long-term outcome benefits are scarce, there is considerable evidence that early rehabilitation improves functional outcome, reduces the social and emotional burden for the patient and family, and is cost-effective. The benefits of early rehabilitation outweigh the risk of harm the patient.

Treatment guidelines for stroke care should include medical, diagnostic, structural, and rehabilitative aspects in order to optimize the chances of stroke survival in the best conditions possible. In respect of rehabilitation, guidelines must be adapted for the individual capacity of the patient and the possibilities indentified by the interdisciplinary team, including an expert with knowledge in stroke. These are the key features for effectiveness.

Since stroke treatment is a matter of months and years rather than days or weeks, early rehabilitation is the beginning (and not the goal) of comprehensive stroke care.

REFERENCES

Adams, H. P., Brott, T. G., Cowell, R. M., *et al.* (1994). *Management of Patients with Acute Ischemic Stroke*. Dallas, TX: American Heart Association.

Anderson, C., NiMhurchu, C., Rubenach, S. *et al.* (2000). Home or hospital for stroke rehabilitation? Results of a randomised controlled trial. II: cost minimisation analysis at 6 months. *Stroke* **31**: 1032–1037.

Anderson, C., Ni Mhurchu, C., Brown, P. M., and Carter, K. (2002). Stroke rehabilitation services to accelerate hospital discharge and provide home-based care – An overview and cost analysis. *Pharmaco economics* **20**: 537–552.

Asberg, K. I. H. (1989). Orthostatic tolerance training of stroke patients in general medical wards: an experimental study. *Scand J Rehabil Med* **21**: 179–185.

Bennett, C. J. and Diokno, A. C. (1984). Clean intermittent self catheterization in the elderly. *Urology* **24**: 43–45.

Bjork, D. T., Pelletier, L. L., and Tight, R. R. (1984). Urinary tract infections with antibiotic resistant organizms in catheterized nursing home patients. *Infection Control* **5**: 173–176.

Bounds, J. V., Wiebers, D., Whisnant, J. P., and Okazaki, H. (1981). Mechanisms and timing of deaths from cerebral infarction. *Stroke* **12**: 474–477.

Brandstater, M. E., Roth, E. J., and Siebens, H. C. (1992). Venous thromboembolism in stroke: literature review and implications for clinical practice. *Arch Phys Med Rehabil* **73** (Suppl.): 379–389.

Cladgett, G. P., Anderson, F. A., Levine, M. N., Salzman, E. W., and Wheeler, H. B. (1992). Prevention of venous thromboembolism. *Chest* **102** (Suppl.): 391S–407S.

Dietz-Tejedor, E. and Fuentes, B. (2001). Acute care in stroke: do stroke units make the difference? *Cerebrovasc Dis* **11**: 31–39.

DiIorio, C. and Price, M. (1990). Swallowing: an assessment guide. *Am J Nurs* **90**: 38–46.

Diller, L. and Weinberg, J. (1970). Evidence for accident-prone behavior in hemiplegic patients. *Arch Phys Medi Rehabil* **51**: 358–363.

Early Supported Discharge Trialists (2002). Services for reducing duration of hospital care for acute stroke patients, *Cochrane Database of Systematic Reviews*, Issue 1. Oxford: Update Software, CD000443.

Emik-Herring, B. and Wood, P. (1990). A team approach to neurologically based swallowing disorders. *Rehab Nurs* **15**: 126–132.

Farrell, R., Evans, S., and Corbett, D. (2001). Environmental enrichment enhances recovery of function but exacerbates ischemic cell death. *Neuroscience* **107**: 585–592.

French Neurovascular Society (2001). Recommendations pour la création d'Unités Neurovasculaires. *Rev Neurol (Paris)* **157**: 1447–1456.

Gresham, G. E. (1992). Rehabilitation of the stroke survivor. In *Stroke: Pathophysiology, Diagnosis and Management*, ed. H. J. M. Barnett, B. M. Stein, J. P. Mohr, and F. M. Yatsu. New York: Churchill Livingstone, pp. 1189–1201.

Gresham, G. E., Duncan, P. W., and Stason, W. B. (1995). *Poststroke Rehabilitation. Clinical Practice Guideline 16* (*AHCPR Publication 95–0662*). Rockville, MD: US Department of Health and Human Services, Public Health Service, Agency for Health Care Policy and Research.

Galski, T., Bruno, R. I., Zorowitz, R., and Walker, J. (1993). Predicting length of stay, functional outcomes and after-care in rehabilitation of stroke patients. The dominant role of higher-order cognition. *Stroke* **24**: 1794–1800.

Halbertsma, J., Heerkens, Y. F., Hirs, W. M., *et al.* (2000). Towards a new ICIDH. *Disabil Rehabil* **22**: 144–156.

Hamrin, E. (1982a). Early activation in stroke: does it make a difference? *Scand J Rehabil Med* **14**: 101–109.

Hamrin, E. (1982b). One year after stroke: a follow-up of an experimental study. *Scand J Rehabil Med* **14**: 111–116.

Hayes, S. H. and Carroll, S. R. (1986). Early intervention care in the acute stroke patient. *Arch Phys Med Rehabil* **67**: 319–321.

Horner, J., Massey, E. W., Riski, J. E, Lathrop, D. L. and Chase, K. N. (1988). Aspiration following stroke: clinical correlates and outcome. *Neurology* **38**: 1359–1362.

Humm, J. L., Kozlowski, D. A., Bland, S. T., James, D. C. and Schallert, T. (1999). Use-dependent exaggeration of brain injury: is glutamate involved? *Exp Neurol* **157**: 349–358.

Indredravik, B., Fjaertoft, H., and Ekeberg, G. (2000). Benefit of an extended stroke unit service with early supported discharge; a randomised, controlled trial. *Stroke* **31**: 2989–2994.

Jonas, S. (1988). Anticoagulant therapy in cerebrovascular disease: review and meta analysis. *Stroke* **19**: 1043–1048.

Jongbloed, L. (1986). Prediction of function after stroke: a critical review. *Stroke* **17**: 765–776.

Landi, G., D'Angelo, A., Boccardi, E., *et al.* (1992). Venous thromboembolism in acute stroke: prognostic importance of hypercoagulability. *Arch Phys Med Rehabil* **73**: V414–V418.

Mayo, N. E., Wood-Dauphinée, S., Côté, R., *et al.* (2000). There's no place like home: an evaluation of early supported discharge for stroke. *Stroke* **31**: 1016–1023.

Murray J. (1999). *Manual of Dysphagia Assessment in Adults*. San Diego, CA: Singular Publishing.

Organization mondial de la Santé (2001). *Classification internationale du fonctionnement, du handicap et de la santé*. Paris: Organization mondial de la Santé; Bibliothèque de l'OMS.

Palmer, J. B. and DeChase, A. S. (1991). Rehabilitation of swallowing due to strokes. *Phys Med Rehabil Clin N Am* **2**: 529–546.

Panayiotou, B., Reid, J., Fotherby, M., and Crome, P. (1999). Orthostatic haemodynamic responses in acute stroke. *Postgrad Med J* **75**: 213–218.

Panel for the Prediction and Prevention of Pressure Ulcers in Adults (1992). *Pressure Ulcers in Adults: Prediction and Prevention. Clinical Practice Guideline 3* (AHCPR Publication 92–0047). Rockville, MD: Department of Health and Human Services, Public Health Service Agency, Agency for Health Care Policy and Research.

Paolucci, S., Antonucci, G., Grasso, M. G., *et al.* (2000). Early versus delayed inpatient stroke rehabilitation: a matched comparison conducted in Italy. *Arch Phys Med Rehabil* **81**: 695–700.

Poplingher, A. R. and Pillar, T. (1985). Hip fracture in stroke patients: epidemiology and rehabilitation. *Acta Orthop Scand* **56**: 226–227.

Reding, M. J., Winter, S. W., Hochrein, S. A., Simon, H. B., and Thompson, M. M. (1987). Urinary incontinence after unilateral hemispheric stroke: a neurologic-epidemiologic perspective. *J Neurol Rehabil* **1**: 25–30.

Ringelstein, E. B. (1998). Empfehlung für die Einrichtung von Schlaganfallspezialstationen ("Stroke Units"). *Nervenarzt* **69**: 180–185.

Risedal, A., Zeng, J., and Johansson, B. B. (1999). Early training may exacerbate brain damage after focal brain ischemia in the rat. *J Cereb Blood Flow Metab* **19**: 997–1003.

Rodgers, J., Soutter, J., Kaiser, W., *et al.* (1997). Early supported hospital discharge following acute stroke: pilot study results. *Clin Rehabil* **11**: 280–287.

Ronning, O. M. and Guldvog, B. (1998). Outcome of subacute stroke rehabilitation: a randomised controlled trial. *Stroke* **29**: 779–784.

Rudd, A. G., Wolfe, C. D., Tilling, K., *et al.* (1997). Randomised controlled trial to evaluate early discharge scheme for patients with stroke. *BMJ* **315**: 1039–1044.

Sabanthan, K., Castleden, C. M., and Mitchell, C. J. (1985). The problem of bacteriuria with indwelling urethral catheterization. *Age Aging* **14**: 85–90.

Sandercock, P. and Willems, H. (1992). Medical treatment of acute ischemic stroke. *Lancet* **339**: 537–539.

Silver, F. L., Norris, J. W., Lewis, A. J., and Hachinski, V. C. (1984). Early mortality following stroke: a prospective study. *Stroke* **25**: 666.

Soderback, I. (1988). The effectiveness of training intellectual functions with acquired brain damage: an evaluation of occupational therapy methods. *Scand J Rehabil Med* **20**: 47–56.

Stason, W. B. (1997). Can clinical practice guidelines increase the effectiveness and cost-effectiveness of post-stroke rehabilitation? *Top Stroke Rehabil* **4**: 1–16.

Steube, D. (2002). Neuropädagogkik in der Rehabilitation von Patienten mit erworbenen Hirnschäden. *Neurol Rehabil* **8**: 148–152.

Stone, S. P., Wilson, B., Wroot, A., *et al.* (1991). The assessment of viso-spatial neglect after acute stroke. *J Neurol Neurosurg Psychiatry* **54**: 345–350.

Stroke Unit Trialists' Collaboration (2002). Organized inpatient (stroke unit) care for Stroke. In *Cochrane Database of Systematic Reviews*, Issue 2. Oxford: Update Software.

Urinary Incontinence Guideline Panel (1992). *Urinary Incontinence for Adults. Clinical Practice Guideline 2 (AHCPR Publication 92–0038)*. Rockville, MD: Department of Health and Human Services, Public Health Service Agency, Agency for Health Care Policy and Research.

Vallar, G., Rusconi, M. L., Barozzi, S., *et al.* (1995). Improvement of left visio-spatial hemineglect by left-sided transcutaneous electrical stimulation. *Neuropsychologia* **33**: 73–82.

Wade, D. T. and Hewer, R. L. (1985). Outlook after an acute stroke: urinary incontinence and loss of consciousness compared in 532 patients. *Q J Med* **56**: 601–608.

Webb, R. J., Lawson, A. L., and Neal, D. E. (1990). Clean intermittent self-catheterization in 172 adults. *Br J Urol* **65**: 20–23.

Widen Holmqvist, L., de Pedro Cuesta, J., Moller, G., *et al.* (1996). A pilot study of rehabilitation at home after stroke: a health-economic appraisal. *Scand J Rehabil Med* **28**: 9–18.

Wojner, A. W. (1996). Optimizing ischemic stroke outcomes: an interdisciplinary approach to post-stroke rehabilitation in acute care. *Crit Care Nurs Q* **19**: 47–61.

Wylie, C. M. (1968). Early rehabilitation promises greater improvements to stroke parents. *Hospitals J A H A* (**42**): 100–104.

(1970). The value of early rehabilitation in stroke. *Geriatrics* **42**: 107–113.

9

Community rehabilitation after stroke: is there no place like home?

Michael P. Barnes

Hunter Moor Regional Rehabilitation centre, Newcastle upon Tyne, UK

Introduction

Many hospitals in the western world now have a dedicated stroke unit. There is no doubt that such units provide an important role in the overall management of stroke and there is now hard evidence of their efficacy (see Ch. 8). However, while people who survive stroke may have a slightly shorter life expectancy than the general population, they will often still have many years of life back at home, back at work, and back in the community. The stroke unit may have maximized their recovery in the few months after the stroke but it is likely that there is still further recovery potential in the months and years after discharge from hospital. It would also be important to avoid unnecessary complications, such as muscle contractures secondary to spasticity or problems with incontinence. In worldwide terms, those admitted to a stroke unit are in the lucky minority and most people will not be admitted to hospital or, if they are admitted to acute medical ward, will probably be discharged quite quickly. These people will be in need of active rehabilitation in a community setting. Consequently, virtually all disabled survivors of stroke will need some form of community-based rehabilitation. Such support is sadly lacking across the world.

There are some indications that health systems around the world are beginning to recognize the longer-term health and rehabilitation needs of disabled people who are living at home. In many countries, particularly in Europe, government resources are beginning to be directed away from acute, and expensive, hospitals towards a health system that is delivered within the local community. There is increasing emphasis on the family physician and the primary care team. There are now a number of initiatives that help to support disabled people within their own homes and indeed prevent unnecessary admission or readmission to hospital. There are also a number of other schemes that facilitate early discharge from hospital. There are slowly increasing numbers of health professionals who have a remit to work in the community. The nursing profession has long had this

Recovery after Stroke, ed. Michael P. Barnes, Bruce H. Dobkin and Julien Bogousslavsky. Published by Cambridge University Press. © Cambridge University Press 2005.

tradition, but there are a number of schemes that are placing expert rehabilitation nurses in the community. More slowly, there are signs that the medical profession and the therapy professions are also beginning to develop community roles. There are now, for example, a few community-based geriatricians in the UK who have a full-time remit to work with elderly disabled people in their homes. This is a trend that should be encouraged and is certainly a trend that is compatible with the disabled people's movement, which has long encouraged a community- and home-based focus for health services. This chapter reviews the need for community rehabilitation and describes some of the schemes that are now in existence to support stroke survivors at home. The chapter will also review the, albeit sparse, evidence for the efficacy of some of these schemes.

The case for community rehabilitation

Other chapters in this book have highlighted the large numbers of people who have a stroke each year. The prevalence of individuals who have had a stroke in the community is around 600 per 100 000 population and approximately half of these people will have a significant residual disability (Wade and Langton-Hewer, 1987). Langton-Hewer and Tennant (2003) estimated that approximately 25% of all severely disabled people living in the community have had a stroke. There are no global figures for the number of people who have a stroke who are admitted to a hospital stroke unit. In the UK, there is now a government target that every hospital that admits people with a stroke must have a stroke unit by 2004. In the UK, the great majority of people with a stroke (in excess of 80%) are admitted to hospital. This is probably the same situation in most of Western Europe, USA, Canada, and Australia. Regrettably, in Eastern Europe and most of the rest of the world, the situation is reversed and the great majority of people with a stroke are not admitted to hospital or if they are then there is little concept of multidisciplinary stroke unit rehabilitation. Therefore, in global terms, the overwhelming majority of people who have a stroke will either remain at home or return home quite quickly after the acute event – and obviously all those who have not made a quick and complete recovery will be in need of active ongoing rehabilitation. There can be no doubt about the numbers of people with stroke who are in need of a community-based rehabilitation service. If it is accepted that there are sufficient numbers of disabled stroke survivors in need of a community service, what are the key drivers that should move rehabilitation towards the community?

The later problems of disability

Many of the longer-term problems associated with disability come after discharge from hospital. This is particularly true for acute-onset disabilities, including stroke and traumatic brain injury. The disabled person and the family often make a surprisingly good adjustment to the physical disability but the neuropsychological, emotional, and behavioral problems that commonly follow stroke are more difficult to manage. The potential range of problems are wide and include difficulties with immobility, incontinence, eyesight, perception, mood, and behavior, as well as social isolation, alienation from previous friends and relatives, and difficulties with employment. These problems may not have been obvious in the early stages while the individual was in hospital. In the post-acute stage, there is a natural tendency to focus on physical disability with a lack of emphasis on potential later-stage cognitive, intellectual, emotional, and behavioral problems. When these problems emerge in the home setting, the necessary community support has often been withdrawn. Pressure on hospital beds may precipitate early discharge at a time when the individual is still in an active recovery phase. The lack of continuity after discharge and often the lack or complete absence of ongoing rehabilitation can lead to unnecessary complications. Classic examples would be the development of muscle contractures following poorly treated spasticity, the lack of further training with regard to mobility and unnecessary confinement to a wheelchair, sparse attention to issues of sexuality, and lack of recognition and treatment of anxiety and depression. After discharge home, the carers themselves, usually the other spouse and/or their children, will also need continuing advice, guidance, information, and support.

Increasing autonomy of non-medical health practitioners

In many countries, there are now increasing numbers of health professionals working in the community. In most countries, nurses have long worked alongside the general practitioner/family physician. However, many countries, particularly in northern Europe, are now seeing the growth of the specialist nurse. These people are usually trained in specific subjects, such as multiple sclerosis, Parkinson's disease, epilepsy, or stroke. The growth of these nurse practitioners has been somewhat haphazard and the training and quality standards have not generally been subject to much scrutiny. However, the situation is improving and a number of appropriately monitored training programs are now in existence. In addition to developments in nursing, there are now more physical therapists working in the community setting. Physiotherapists, occupational therapists, and chiropodists have had a long history of community working but these individuals have usually had generic, broad-based skills as opposed to being specially trained in the management of people with more complex neurological problems. The medical profession has generally been slower at developing such initiatives. A general practitioner is obviously community based but will usually lack specific knowledge in neurological rehabilitation. In some countries, there are now a few consultant specialists who have a part-time or even full-time remit to work in the community. Pediatric colleagues have been at the forefront of these developments, but now there are a small but increasing number of community-based geriatricians and rehabilitation physicians. In this way, many health systems, mainly in the developed world, have seen a steady growth of community rehabilitation, particularly with regard to non-medical health professionals. The slowly increasing number, as well as the independence and autonomy of these individuals, is a further key driver for the development of community rehabilitation. It is a trend that should be encouraged.

Developments in health services

In recent years, many countries have witnessed a radical change in health politics with a clear shift away from acute hospitals and towards the community. In the UK, for example, the majority of health commissioning is now conducted through Primary Care Trusts, which are semi-autonomous bodies within the umbrella of the National Health Service. These Trusts have a responsibility for commissioning health services in their locality both in the community and in the hospital. The directors of these Trusts are mainly community practitioners, particularly general practitioners/family physicians. This change has naturally resulted in greater resources being placed within the community, with less emphasis towards acute hospital care. This, in turn, has resulted in many hospitals, particularly in larger conurbations, seeing a significant reduction in bed numbers and, therefore, a major drive to keep people out of hospital if at all possible and if they are admitted then to discharge them back home much more quickly.

Views of disabled people

Recent years have also seen the development of an effective and coherent disabled person's movement – particularly in the USA and parts of Europe. In a study by Sabari and colleagues (2000), members of a community-based stroke club found that "specific issues of major concern to the stroke survivors and their care givers included a lack of individualised treatment, a tendency for professionals to disregard issues related to stroke survivors' general quality of life, inadequate home care services and insensitive healthcare workers." Frustration particularly surrounded the rehabilitation services, which were concentrated during the first weeks after the stroke at a time when many were not ready to take full advantage of the therapists' expertise. As Newborn (1998) stated "how can any survivor adapt and learn everything in that brief period of time, while going through confusing changes in body and mind?" The participants in the study of Sabari et al. (2000) felt ill-equipped for their transition back to community living. In a further study by McKevitt and Wolfe (2000), interviewees were asked to identify the main problems they faced after a stroke and to give their views on what a stroke-specific community service should offer. The overwhelming view was that participants wanted more information, particularly about the implications of having had a stroke, as well as ongoing access to therapy in the community. In addition this and other studies (e.g. Sabari *et al.*, 2000) also confirmed that, in general, rehabilitation professionals pay inadequate attention to the social and psychological consequences of stroke after discharge to the community. The clear consensus of the disabled people's movement is that support should be available from the acute event into the long term and certainly when the individual is being discharged from hospital. The emphasis at this point needs to be more on the psychosocial consequences of the stroke rather than the purely physical consequences. Such information and support should be provided in a way that empowers disabled people and their families.

Consequently, there are four main drivers that are moving services towards the community. First, an evidence-based realization that most problems associated with stroke occur when the individual is back at home. Second, the trend towards increasing autonomy of therapists and nurses, who are becoming more prevalent in the community. Third, government-backed changes to the health service, which are placing more emphasis on commissioning and provision of services in the local setting. Fourth, the clear view of disabled people and their lobby organizations that more resources should be placed in the community.

Theoretical models

This section illustrates some of the theoretical models that may underpin a community-rehabilitation program. Further specific examples and their evidence base are reviewed later in this chapter. This section will simply describe some theoretical possibilities and outline some of the advantages and disadvantages associated with these options.

Hospital outpatients

Most rehabilitation resources are concentrated in hospital rehabilitation departments. One model would be to establish a proper outpatient follow-up system based within the same department or rehabilitation center. Indeed this is the most prevalent model as most hospital units have some form of outpatient follow-up system. The outpatient department can certainly act as a source of advice and information, act as a social center for the gathering of people with similar problems, and act as a focal base for self-help groups. It also makes some sense for the same staff to provide continuity from the hospital stroke unit into the community. There are also logistic advantages in that many more people can be seen in a single outpatient clinic compared with the number of people who could be seen in their own homes in the same period of time. However, while there are some obvious advantages to such a system, there are many significant disadvantages. Obviously, the main disadvantage is the fact that the disabled person has to travel to the clinic, which may be impractical and will certainly be tiring. It is most unlikely that a properly coordinated active rehabilitation program within the home can be monitored from an outpatient setting. Time constraints will allow only a relatively brief period of consultation, probably with several months' gap between appointments.

Disease-specific clinics

An adaptation of the outpatient system would be the use of disease- or symptom-based clinics. In the context of this textbook, a stroke follow-up clinic would have the advantage of acting as a convenient base for self-help and support groups. People with similar problems could gather together for discussion and mutual support. However, other than this advantage there is really no particular benefit to the disease-specific clinic over the straightforward hospital outpatient system. Obviously, this system still does not fulfill the requirement for providing proper coordinated multidisciplinary rehabilitation in the community.

Hospital outreach teams

The hospital-based multidisciplinary rehabilitation team could, in theory, provide outreach work into the community. Individual team members could continue to work with the same disabled person whether they are in hospital or in the community, and this obviously has some advantages with regard to continuity. There are a number of examples of such teams, particularly the early-discharge stroke teams, which are described later in this chapter. However, there are clear logistic disadvantages. The management of a proper team in the community will require a significant increase in resources, and the team may well have a very large geographical area to cover with consequent problems of travelling time and the logistical difficulties of organizing appropriate team members to be in the right place at the right time. It is a concept that is used in some developing countries when the hospital-based team effectively performs an outpatient function in the surrounding villages and smaller towns, visiting each locality on a regular basis.

Extension of the primary care team

In many countries, the general practitioner/family physician has a range of primary care staff based in the so-called primary care team. This will usually include nurses and often therapists, particularly physiotherapists. A typical primary care team, at least in the UK, covers a population of around 10 000 people and, therefore, the number of stroke survivors is reduced to a more practical level. However, there are clear disadvantages. The general practitioner and the primary care team are unlikely to be expert in the management of complex physical and neuropsychological disabilities after stroke. It is a specialist field and to fulfill this function the team would need extensive specialist training. The other main disadvantage is that many experts, particularly in the therapy professions, are few and far between and it is very unlikely that the necessary expertise will be found to support adequately each primary care team, both in terms of hands-on therapy as well as education and training. It may be theoretically possible for the primary healthcare team to be supported by occasional visits and training by members of the specialist unit. It would, for example, be quite practical for specialist stroke nurses to advise the local district nurse on particular problems that may arise in a given individual.

Community-based teams

The ideal model would probably be an expert multidisciplinary team actually based in the community, covering a geographical area that was sensible and practicable both in terms of the number of stroke survivors and the geographical spread. Such teams would need to maintain links with the local stroke unit, and possibly with a regional center, for adequate audit, education, and training. An example, in a different context, is the Newcastle-upon-Tyne Community Multiple Sclerosis Team (Makepeace *et al.*, 2001). This is a self-contained expert team led by a physiotherapist and based in a local disabled-living center. The team has managerial and professional links with the regional rehabilitation center based in the same city and indeed the team is able to access beds within that center for emergency or respite purposes or for periods of rehabilitation. In a larger geographical area, a number of such teams could interlink and thus share educational opportunities, training, and research. This concept of a managed clinical network is gaining some favor in a number of localities. One disadvantage of a health-based team is that necessary social support may be lacking, and indeed the team may not have sufficient expertise in other important areas, such as employment rehabilitation. Therefore, if possible, healthcare expertise should be combined with social service-based expertise to provide comprehensive rehabilitation.

Individual practitioners in the community

There are a number of new initiatives in the UK with regard to the development of nurse practitioners, nurse consultants, and therapy consultants; in addition, as referred to above, increasing autonomy and independence is being given to such individuals. This is a trend to be encouraged as it provides locally based expertise. However, no matter how good the individual practitioner, there is the loss of the added advantage of the multidisciplinary team. The evidence base is that it is the multidisciplinary ethos that produces benefits over and above the skill of the individual practitioner.

Independent living movement

If the ultimate aim of community rehabilitation is to empower the disabled person then it is logical that the disabled person should be able to organize their own rehabilitation services. The independent-living movement supports the concepts behind the devolvement of resources to disabled people, allowing them to buy in the necessary services and rehabilitation staff as required. This may be a sensible option for many, although it can have significant resource implications and it may not be possible to enact in cash-starved health services. Care will needed to ensure that the disabled person was fully informed and aware of the necessary services. The person would need to be cognitively intact and able to make appropriate decisions. Obviously, the appointment of a trained advocate or an appropriate family member may get round such problems. This model is certainly firmly supported by many groups of disabled people (e.g. Brisenden, 1986).

Evidence base for community rehabilitation

The literature regarding community rehabilitation mainly focuses on three main areas. The first could be described as "hospital at home" schemes, which aim to provide rehabilitation in the home as a direct alternative to hospital admission. The second area concerns people who are already receiving hospital treatment and focuses on reducing their time in hospital. These schemes tend to be referred to as "early discharge." The third area in which community teams provide an input is when people are already established in their homes and do not need any acute medical intervention but may benefit from further rehabilitation. The evidence behind such schemes both in neurological rehabilitation in general and in stroke in particular will now be discussed.

Hospital at home

Hospital at home schemes are largely designed to act as an alternative to hospital admission. Shepperd and Iliffe (2000) have proposed a definition as "a service that provides active treatment by healthcare professionals in the patient's home of a condition that otherwise would require acute hospital inpatient care, always for a limited period." The literature is limited but a few schemes are worthy of further discussion. In 1985, Wade and colleagues (1985) described a study in which 49 out of 96 general practitioners in a district in the southwest of England were asked to refer their acute stroke patients either to a nurse-led multidisciplinary home care team or, if they preferred, to the hospital in the normal fashion. The acute stroke patients of the other 47 general practitioners formed the control group who had access to standard hospital and community services. Rehabilitation at home was provided by an interdisciplinary team consisting of a district nurse, a physiotherapist, an occupational therapist, a speech therapist, and a social worker. This was a large study (400 people recruited in each group). At the end of six months, the authors found no difference in functional recovery, emotional adjustment, or differences in the stress levels of carers between the two groups. Indeed, the trial group, even though they had more participants at home, had a slightly higher hospital admission rate. Overall, the study raised doubt about the benefit of domiciliary services to reduce hospital usage. However, these were early days of community care, and apprehensiveness on behalf of the general practitioners, who continued to have a choice of whether to refer to the home team or the hospital, may have biased the results. The services provide in the home care group were also rather similar to the community-based services provided to the control group. Nevertheless, this was the first attempt to evaluate any form of hospital at home scheme for people with stroke.

In the context of other diseases, further studies have shown that there is increased client satisfaction with hospital at home schemes and most studies have shown few significant differences in health outcome between a hospital at home group and a hospital admission group. Such a conclusion was reached by Pozzilli and colleagues (1999) in a study of patients with multiple sclerosis and by Wilson and colleagues (1999) in a study of patients with cardiovascular and respiratory disorders. However, in the context of stroke, the emergence of strong evidence for the efficacy of admission to hospital and appropriate management in a stroke unit has probably now made evaluation of hospital at home schemes for stroke undesirable and unethical. There can be little doubt from the literature that an individual with a stroke should be admitted as soon as possible to hospital, undergo appropriate scanning for confirmation of the diagnosis, and then be immediately put on appropriate treatment and managed in a multidisciplinary setting. Therefore, at least in the context of stroke, there are unlikely to be many further studies of such schemes. However, this should not reduce the importance of community management in societies where admission to hospital remains impractical because of cost, geography, or simple lack of resources. This situation prevails in many developing counties, and the best way to organize community stroke care in such circumstances should still be properly investigated and the results published.

Early discharge

Early-discharge teams are probably of more relevance for stroke. If people with stroke are quickly admitted for diagnosis, acute management, and early intensive rehabilitation, then the question that needs to be answered is "when is an optimal time for discharge?" Finance and political pressures are beginning to dictate discharge times rather than clinical evidence. These pressures have led to the formulation of various models of early-discharge teams and some of these studies have been properly evaluated. In general terms, studies have shown that early-discharge teams are able to reduce admission times and provide a cost-effective alternative to longer-term hospital care. More importantly, the studies have generally confirmed that there is little difference in functional outcome in those who stay in hospital longer compared with those who are discharged earlier to an appropriate community team. Therefore, the individual is no worse off and indeed in psychological terms is usually more satisfied with early discharge back home; at the same time, acute hospital beds and associated costs are saved. In one of the early studies in London (Rudd *et al.*, 1997; Beech *et al.*, 1999), 136 people with stroke were discharged after an average stay of 12 days and received rehabilitation at home for three months. In the control group, 126 people remained in hospital for about 18 days and thereafter only continued outpatient hospital treatment. The total therapy time received by each group was equal. At 12 months, there were no differences between the two groups with regard to activities of daily living. The authors concluded that early discharge was as clinically effective as conventional hospital care but reduced costs in terms of the use of hospital beds and was acceptable to patients.

In an important study by Rodgers and colleagues (1997), 92 individuals who were medically stable at 72 hours after a stroke were randomized into two groups. One group received early supported discharge and the other conventional care in hospital. The median length of stay in hospital was 13 days for the discharge group but 22 days for the control group. The community team was involved with individuals for a median of nine weeks. The control group received hospital and then standard outpatient rehabilitation. At three months, there were no differences between the two groups in terms of functional ability, handicap, health status, carer stress, readmission rate, or mortality. The early-discharge group participated more in activities of daily living. The cost analysis showed that the cost of the discharge team was balanced by reduced hospital bed costs (McNamee *et al.*, 1998). A similar study in Stockholm reached similar conclusions (Widen Holmqvist *et al.*, 1998). This study was similarly designed and the early-discharge group received three or four months of continued rehabilitation at home. At six months, there were no statistically significant differences in outcome; however, a more detailed analysis suggested a positive effect of home rehabilitation on social activity, activities of daily living, motor capacity, manual dexterity, and walking (von Koch *et al.*, 2000; Widen Holmqvist *et al.*, 2000). For example, death or dependency in activities of daily living was 24% in the intervention group and 44% in the control group. There was a reduction in hospital days from 29 in the control group to just 14 in the home rehabilitation group. These were positive results but it is fair to point out that both the study of Rodgers *et al.* (1997) and that of Widen Holmqvist *et al.* (1998) involved relatively small sample sizes and so there must be some doubts about the generalizability of the results.

Richards and colleagues (1998) performed a larger-scale study in 241 elderly hospitalized people but this was not exclusively in stroke disease. Once the individuals were medically stable, they were randomized to receive either ongoing hospital care or home care. The home care service was provided by a nurse coordinated team, which provided interim support before transfer to local community services. The length of health contact was actually less in the hospital-based group compared with the total time of contact in the home-based group. The hospital care and the home care were equally effective and acceptable to the two groups three months later. In addition, although the hospital scheme provided longer contact, it was less costly than the hospital-based care.

The whole subject of early discharge has recently been reviewed from an economic viewpoint by Anderson and colleagues (2002). They reviewed the evidence for the cost-effectiveness of services designed to accelerate hospital discharge and provide home-based rehabilitation for people after acute stroke. They analyzed seven published trials involving a total of 1277 patients. The pooled data showed that overall a policy of early hospital discharge and domiciliary rehabilitation reduced total length of stay by 13 days. There was no significant effect on mortality or other clinical outcomes. The overall mean costs were approximately 15% lower for the early-discharge intervention (US$9941 compared with US$11 390 for standard care). The authors concluded that the policy of early hospital discharge and home-based rehabilitation reduced the use of hospital beds without compromising clinical outcomes and at the same time was a cost-saving alternative to longer-term conventional hospital care. The same broad conclusions were reached by a Cochrane review from the Early Supported Discharge Trialists (2002). The group concluded that early discharge of patients after stroke reduced length of hospital stay by approximately nine days. However, they felt that the relative risks and benefits and overall costs of such early-discharge services remained unclear on the basis of the current literature. A slightly more positive conclusion was reached in a study by Mayo and colleagues (2000). Once again, individuals medically ready for discharge were randomly allocated to either a home intervention group or to a usual care group. The home group received a four-week tailored program of rehabilitation and nursing services whereas the other group continued to receive normal hospital services. The total length of stay for the home group was around 10 days, which was six days shorter than the usual care group. Interestingly, there was significantly beneficial effect in the home group in terms of activities of daily living and reintegration into normal living at one and three months. At three months, the home intervention group also showed a significantly higher score on the Short Form 36 (SF-36) physical health component. Obviously, further studies are required to delineate the place of early supported discharge schemes in the overall context of stroke care.

A final factor that needs to be determined is whether there are any longer-term differences following early supported discharge. Can, for example, a coordinated community rehabilitation program in the shorter term lead to gains in the longer term when compared with standard hospital care? This question is largely unanswered but a single study by von Koch and colleagues (2001) has addressed the question. A total of 83 patients were included in the original randomized controlled trial, 42 being allocated to the interventional group and 41 to routine hospital rehabilitation. These individuals were followed for one year. Analysis showed that the intervention had a significant and positive effect on independence and activities of daily living. The control group registered more outpatient visits to hospital, occupational therapy departments, private physical therapists, and day hospital attendance. Overall, they concluded that early supported discharge with continued rehabilitation at home proved no less beneficial as a rehabilitation service and was able to provide rehabilitation for five moderately disabled stroke patients over 12 months for the cost of four patients in routine rehabilitation.

In conclusion, the majority of studies support the use of early-discharge schemes in terms of reduced the number of hospital bed days and thus making cost savings without any functional detriment to the patient and with the added benefit of returning an individual to the home and family as soon as possible.

Longer-term community support

Longer-term community support can be defined as rehabilitation after stroke for those who may or may not have been admitted to hospital and do not require any further acute medical treatment but still need active rehabilitation, information, and social support. Regrettably, the literature on such longer-term support is generally poor. Geddes and Chamberlain (2001) compared six community services providing coordinated, multidisciplinary rehabilitation across England and Northern Ireland. Regrettably, no hard conclusions could be drawn because the teams all differed in their target populations and in their timing, duration, and style of intervention. They found that these rather diverse community services had some impact on the Barthel Index score (median of 15 at the beginning of intervention to a median of 18 at the end of intervention, with a median duration of such intervention of 12 weeks). However, no real conclusions could be drawn from such a heterogeneous array of services. Plant and colleagues (2000) showed that short-term intervention (12 weeks) by a community stroke rehabilitation team resulted in significant improvements in adults under the age of 65 years with regard to patient-reported performance and satisfaction in activities of daily living. This team was managed by a coordinator (a physiotherapist) and consisted of a physiotherapist, an occupational therapist, a speech and language therapist, and a rehabilitation assistant. It is interesting to note that the patients had the right to choose the location of therapy (either outpatient department or home) and many preferred to have their physiotherapy within an outpatient setting. If the hospital-based studies can be extrapolated into the community, then it would be expected that a multidisciplinary community-based team would produce added benefit over individual therapists working in the community. However, at present, there is little supporting evidence for this statement. Nevertheless, there are a number of studies that indicate the efficacy of individual therapists working in the community. Young and Forster (1991, 1992, 1993) have done much work on this subject. In one study, they compared day-hospital attendance and physiotherapy at home for people with stroke after discharge from hospital (Young and Forster, 1993). The participants attended the day hospital for two days a week or received home treatment from a community physiotherapist. Of the 124 people recruited, 108 were able to be fully assessed at six months. Both arms of the study showed significant improvement in functional abilities between discharge and six months, but the improvements were significantly greater for those treated at home. This was despite the fact that those treated at home received less actual treatment. The authors suggested that home-based post-stroke therapy should be the preferred long-term method of physical rehabilitation.

In a similar study, 327 people discharged from medical or geriatric wards were randomized into two groups (Gladman *et al.*, 1993; Gladman and Lincoln, 1994). One group received domicilary rehabilitation at home from physiotherapy, occupational therapy, and other relevant professionals. The other group received hospital-based rehabilitation in both an outpatient and a day unit setting. At six months, the outcome was similar for both groups in terms of functional disability, perceived health, social engagement, and life satisfaction, which slightly contradicts the work by Young and Forster (1993). It is worth noting that approximately 15–20 therapy contacts were required per month within a six-month timescale to obtain any significant functional benefit. Although some studies have not been able to show any difference between outpatient-based therapy and home-based therapy, a few studies have shown an increased level of satisfaction in a home-based group. For example, Gilbertson and colleagues (2000) described a six-week domiciliary intervention program run by an occupational therapist; activities of daily living were increased at eight weeks compared with those having routine follow-up, but this difference was not maintained at six months. However, an increased level of satisfaction was reported in the intervention group at six months.

A recent Cochrane review of the subject by Outpatient (2003) assessed the effects of therapy-based rehabilitation services targeted towards stroke patients resident in the community within one year of stroke onset or discharge from hospital. The author identified a heterogeneous group of 14 trials that were properly randomized controlled trials of a community therapy service compared with conventional or no care. The results indicated that the therapy-based rehabilitation services reduced the odds of poor outcome and increased scores for personal activities of daily living. Overall, for every 100 stroke patients resident in the community receiving therapy rehabilitation services, seven patients would be spared a poor outcome by such intervention. However, the author was once again critical of the nature of the evidence available.

It is obvious that most rehabilitation needs to be delivered in the first few months after the stroke. It is sometimes thought that later-stage rehabilitation many months or even years after the stroke may not be worthwhile. Once again, there are few studies to confirm or refute this statement, but there is some evidence that this is not necessarily the case. Werner and Kessler (1996), for example, delivered rehabilitation to 28 people after stroke with 16 controls. These people were approximately three years post-stroke and participated in an outpatient program consisting of an hour of physiotherapy and an hour of occupational therapy five times weekly for a total of 12 weeks. This group had clinically relevant functional gains as well as improvements in self-esteem and reduced depression. It is probably true, although unproven, that intermittent review by a multidisciplinary team may be worthwhile after stroke in order to ensure that otherwise unrecognized post-stroke complications have not arisen, either physical (e.g. muscle contracture, ongoing incontinence, etc.) or psychological (e.g. unrecognized and untreated depression). The same team could monitor the ongoing effect on the family and, in particular, on the main carer. Respite breaks or other longer-term support services could be organized and delivered in this fashion. Some studies have evaluated the value of a care manager as a longer-term support agent. The care manager is often factored into legal settlements, usually in the context of traumatic brain injury, as a useful individual for coordinating a complex array of home care services. While common sense would dictate that coordination of a complex care package is necessary, there is only limited literature to show a benefit. However, Goldberg and colleagues (1997) offered elderly individuals post-stroke a system of home-based care management. The team comprised a project physician, psychologist, recreational therapist, and the care manager, who was also a social worker. The care manager's role was to address psychosocial needs, ensure access to information, and identify any problems in the early stage. This was done via weekly telephone contact and monthly visits. The individuals in the intervention group showed improvements in social activities and in activities of daily living at six months, although the differences were no longer significant at 12 months. The telephone contact was perceived to be as efficacious as the home visits, which perhaps indicates that it is the coordination role that may produce benefit rather than a physical presence. A number of the other studies referred to above incorporated care management in the rehabilitation program, but regrettably the published details of the studies do not allow for a description of the exact role of the care manager or coordinator. The care managers seem to work at a number of different levels, sometimes being part of the professional team while at other times just acting in an administrative and coordinating capacity. It would be useful if further studies on community rehabilitation identified more clearly the role of any case manager or coordinator.

Summary

There is increasing literature on various aspects of community rehabilitation after stroke. However, it is still fair to say that good-quality studies are sparse and often involve only small sample sizes. Consequently, any conclusions must be tentative. However, there does seem to be an emerging evidence base for the efficacy of early-discharge stroke teams in terms of being able to discharge individuals safely from hospital earlier and to provide rehabilitation that is at least as good as ongoing hospital care. There is a trend to support active ongoing rehabilitation into the longer term, at least by individual therapists if not by a full multidisciplinary coordinated rehabilitation team. This is probably the case whether the individual has been admitted to hospital or not, although the very clear evidence regarding the efficacy of hospital-based stroke units indicates that most people after stroke should be admitted to hospital for initial diagnosis, management, and post-acute rehabilitation. However, the lesson from the literature is that a comprehensive stroke care service should involve not just an efficient admission and acute rehabilitation service but also longer-term community support. Such support will need to involve an active array of therapists in a properly coordinated multi-disciplinary team in the shorter term. As the individual improves from the physical point of view, then the individual and the family need to be fully supported in order to ensure that good-quality information is always available and good-quality health and social care support is also available when required. In this way, it can be hoped that natural recovery can be maximized and unnecessary disability and handicap minimized, thus improving the quality of life for not only the person with the stroke but also their family.

REFERENCES

Anderson, C., Ni Mhurchu, C., Brown, P. M., and Carter, K. (2002). Stroke rehabilitation services to accelerate hospital discharge and provide home based care: an overview and cost analysis. *Pharmacoeconomics* **20**: 537–552.

Beech, R., Rudd, A. G., Tilling, K., and Wolfe, C. D. A. (1999). Economic consequences of early inpatient discharge to community based rehabilitation for stroke in an inner London teaching hospital. *Stroke* **30**: 729–735.

Brisenden, S. (1986). Independent living in a medical model of disability. *Disabil Handicap Soc* **1**: 173–181.

Early Supported Discharge Trialists (2002). Services for reducing duration of hospital care for acute stroke patients. *Cochrane Database of Systematic Reviews*, Issue 1. Oxford: Update Software, CD000443.

Geddes, J. M. and Chamberlain, M. A. (2001). Home-based rehabilitation for people with stroke: a comparative study of six community services providing co-ordinated, multidisciplinary treatment. *Clin Rehabil* **15**: 589–599.

Gilbertson, L., Langhorne, P., Walker, A., *et al.* (2000). Domiciliary occupational therapy for patients with stroke discharged from hospital: randomised controlled trial. *BMJ* **320**: 603–606.

Gladman, J. R. F. and Lincoln, N. B. (1994). Follow-up of a controlled trial of domiciliary stroke rehabilitation (DOMINO Study). *Age Aging* **23**: 9–13.

Gladman, J. R. F., Lincoln, N. B., and Barer, D. H. (1993). A randomised controlled trial of domiciliary and hospital-based rehabilitation for stroke patients after discharge from hospital. *J Neurol Neurosurg Psychiatry* **56**: 960–966.

Goldberg, G., Segal, M. E., Berk, S. N., *et al.* (1997). Stroke transition after inpatient rehabilitation. *Top Stroke Rehabil* **4**: 64–79.

Langton Hewer, R. and Tennant, A. (2003). The epidemiology of disabling neurological disorders. In *Neurological Rehabilitation*, eds. R. Greenwood, M. Barnes, T. McMillan, C. Ward. Hove, UK: Psychology Press.

Makepeace, R. W., Barnes, M. P., Semlyen, J. K., and Stevenson, J. (2001). The establishment of a community multiple sclerosis team. *Int J Rehabil Res* **24**: 137–141.

Mayo, N. E., Wood-Dauphinee, S., Cote, R., *et al.* (2000). There's no place like home: the evaluation of early supported discharge for stroke. *Stroke* **31**: 1016–1023.

McKevitt, C. and Wolfe, C. (2000). Community support after stroke: patient and carer views. *Br J Ther Rehabil* **7**: 6–10.

McNamee, P., Christensen, J., Soutter, J., *et al.* (1998). Cost analysis of early supported hospital discharge for stroke. *Age Aging* **27**: 345–351.

Newborn, B. (1998). Quality of life for long term recovery in stroke. *Top Stroke Rehabil* **5**: 61–63.

Outpatient, S. E. (2003). Therapy based rehabilitation services for stroke patients at home. *Cochrane Database of Systematic Reviews*, Issue 1. Oxford: Update Software, CD002925.

Plant, R., Tait, B., Dawson, P., and Buri, H. (2000). *Community Stroke Rehabilitation Team Evaluation Project: Executive Summary*. Newcastle upon Tyne: Institute of Rehabilitation.

Pozzilli, C., Pisani, A., Palmisano, L., *et al.* (1999). Service location in multiple sclerosis: home or hospital? In *Advances in Multiple Sclerosis: Clinical Research and Therapy,* ed. S. Fredrickson and H. Link. London: Martin Dunitz, pp. 173–180.

Richards, S. H., Coast, J., Gunnell, D. J., *et al.* (1998). Randomised controlled trial comparing effectiveness and acceptability of an early discharge, hospital at home scheme with acute hospital care. *BMJ* **316**: 1796–1801.

Rodgers, H., Soutter, J., Kaiser, W., *et al.* (1997). Early supported hospital discharge following acute study: pilot study results. *Clin Rehabil* **11**: 280–287.

Rudd, A. G., Wolfe, C. D. A., Tilling, K., and Beech, R. (1997). Randomised controlled trial to evaluate early discharge scheme for patients with stroke. *BMJ* **315**: 1039–1044.

Sabari, J. S., Meisler, J., and Silver, E. (2000). Reflections upon rehabilitation by members of a community based stroke club. *Disabil Rehabil* **22**: 330–336.

Shepperd, S. and Iliffe, S. (2000). Hospital at home versus inpatient hospital care. *Cochrane Database of Systematic Reviews,* Issue 2. Oxford: Update Software, CD000356.

von Koch, L., Widen Holmqvist, L., Kostulas, V., *et al.* (2000). A randomised controlled trial of rehabilitation at home after stroke in Southwest Stockholm: outcome at six months. *Scand J Rehabil Med* **32**: 80–86.

von Koch, L., de Pedro-Cuesta, J., Kostulas, V., Almazan, J., and Widen Holmqvist, L. (2001). Randomised controlled trial of rehabilitation at home after stroke: one year follow-up of patient outcome, resource use and cost. *Cerebrovasc Dis* **12**: 131–138.

Wade D. T. and Langton-Hewer, R. (1987). Epidemiology of some neurological diseases with specific reference to work load on the NHS. *Int Rehabil Med* **8**: 129–137.

Wade D. T., Langton-Hewer, R., Skilbeck C. E., *et al.* (1985). Controlled trial of a home care service for acute stroke patients. *Lancet* **1**: 323–326.

Werner, R. A. and Kessler, S. (1996). Effectiveness of an intensive outpatient rehabilitation program for post-acute stroke patients. *Am J Phys Med Rehabil* **75**: 114–120.

Widen Holmqvist, L., von Koch, L., Kostulas, V., *et al.* (1998). A randomised controlled trial of rehabilitation at home after stroke in Southwest Stockholm. *Stroke* **29**: 591–597.

Widen Holmqvist, L., von Koch, L., and de Pedro-Cuesta, J. (2000). Use of healthcare, impact on family caregivers and patient satisfaction of rehabilitation at home after stroke in Southwest Stockholm. *Scand J Rehabil Med* **32**: 173–179.

Wilson, A., Parker, H., Wynn, A., *et al.* (1999). Randomised controlled trial of effectiveness of Leicester hospital at home scheme compared with hospital care. *BJM* **319**: 1542–1546.

Young, J. and Forster, A. (1991). The Bradford community stroke trial: eight week results. *Clin Rehabil* **5**: 283–292.

(1992). The Bradford community stroke trial: results at six months. *BMJ* **304**: 1085–1089.

(1993). Day hospital and home physiotherapy for stroke patients: a comparative cost effectiveness study. *J R Coll Physicians Lond* **27**: 252–258.

10

Physical therapy

Gillian D. Baer and Frederike M. J. van Wijck

Queen Margaret University College, Edinburgh, UK

Introduction

The aim of this chapter is to present an overview of different physical therapy strategies for the rehabilitation of people who have had a stroke. We will start with a brief historical outline of the classic physiotherapy approaches and the evidence currently available regarding their efficacy. Next, we will discuss a number of current and emerging physiotherapy interventions. Since physiotherapy encompasses a wide variety of treatment modalities – a comprehensive description of which is beyond the scope of this chapter – we have selected strategies that are particularly relevant to the management of movement problems in stroke rehabilitation. Specific issues related to orofacial, bowel, bladder, and sexual function are discussed in chapters 14–16, while pain management is discussed in chapter 12. For a more comprehensive account of neurological physiotherapy in general, the reader is referred to other textbooks (e.g. Ada and Canning, 1990; Edwards, 2002; Stokes, 2004). Finally, the chapter presents a case study that illustrates a range of physiotherapy strategies which could be provided from the acute to the chronic stage after stroke.

Physical therapy in stroke rehabilitation: a historical overview

The development of neurological physiotherapy was given impetus in the late nineteenth century by a growing interest in cerebral palsy. Alongside rehabilitation for children with cerebral palsy, rehabilitation for stroke patients developed in the twentieth century on the basis of emerging orthopedic, educational, and neurophysiological research. Although some of the original schools of thought have undergone considerable change, they still serve as the foundations for neurological physiotherapy today. Below, a brief description is given of the orthopedic, neuro-facilitation, and motor learning approaches. For a further discussion of their historical development and theoretical underpinnings, the reader is referred to Gordon (2000).

Recovery after Stroke, ed. Michael P. Barnes, Bruce H. Dobkin and Julien Bogousslavsky. Published by Cambridge University Press. © Cambridge University Press 2005.

Orthopedic approach

Physiotherapy before the 1950s was mainly concerned with the treatment of poliomyelitis (Gordon, 2000). According to the "muscle re-education approach," the focus was on strengthening isolated paretic muscles. Exercises for patients with hemiplegia was supplemented with orthotics (e.g. calipers) to prevent or correct ʾhnormalities of the musculoskeletal system. This approach – also termed a ʾnal" approach – was perceived by some as a negative influence in that ʾncorporating braces, walking aids, and splints might promote xpense of perceived quality of movement. Furthermore, ch yielded limited results for patients with lesions leading ɔ syndrome, as its focus was restricted to the biomechanical primarily affected in its organization of the control of is approach fell from favour in the ensuing decades with ofacilitation approach.

opment in children in the 1940s to 1960s and pioneering ysiology of the nervous system in the early to mid 1900s led levelop entirely new ways of working with patients with a m (CNS) lesion. The so-called "neurofacilitation" approach sumptions that the CNS operates in a hierarchical, top-down terns of movement may be altered by applying sensory stimula-)00). This led to the development of a number of different schools 'uding Bobath or neurodevelopmental treatment (Bobath, 1990), awner and LaVigne, 1992), Rood (Rood, 1956) and proprioceptive r facilitation (Knott and Voss, 1968). With "Bobath" probably being ely practiced approach in many countries (Nilsson and Nordholm, al., 1994; Sackley and Lincoln, 1996; Davidson and Waters, 2000; ıl., 2001; Pomeroy and Tallis, 2002a), this approach will be described in more ɑ ıl below.

According to Bobath, the CNS controls the "normal postural reflex mechanism," which is responsible for normal postural tone, reciprocal innervation, and automatic movement patterns (Bobath and Bobath 1954, 1964; Bobath, 1971). Consequently, a lesion leading to upper motor neuron syndrome was thought to cause a disruption of this mechanism, resulting in a release of "lower patterns" of activity from "higher inhibitory control." This manifested itself in abnormalities in postural tone (e.g. hypertonia), reciprocal innervation (e.g. excessive co-contraction), and abnormal movement patterns (Bobath, 1971).

The aim of the original Bobath approach was to prepare the patient for functional activity by inhibiting "abnormal" movement patterns and facilitating more "normal" movement, thereby enhancing the quality of movement (Bobath, 1969, 1990). Originally, this was primarily achieved by providing the patient with the sensation of more normal movement through skilful handling by the therapist and by placing the patient in so-called "reflex-inhibiting postures" to reduce spasticity (Bobath and Bobath, 1957). However, carry-over into functional abilities was limited (Mayston, 1992). As the approach evolved, handling became focused on the use of so-called "key points of control": i.e. areas of the body that were thought to influence movement (Bobath and Bobaih, 1964; Bryce, 1972). In addition, appropriate tactile and proprioceptive stimulation was advocated (Bobath, 1971).

Nowadays, the focus on spasticity, righting, and equilibrium reactions is considered to be outdated (Mayston, 2002). The initial emphasis on quality of movement has shifted and it is now recognized that, with the optimization of "function" being the primary goal in rehabilitation, it may be necessary to accept a reduction in movement quality and invoke compensatory strategies (Edwards, 2002). Despite claims, however, that the Bobath approach has now become more functional and problem orientated (Mayston, 1992), Lennon *et al.* (2002) suggested that more emphasis could be placed on the practice of actual functional tasks rather than on the preparation of function.

Bobath practitioners emphasize how the approach has continued to change (Mayston, 1992, 2002; see http://www.bobath.org.uk/concept.html). However, despite an ongoing training program for therapists, there is a lack of up-to-date literature (Davidson and Waters, 2000; Mayston, 2002), evidence-based publications (Paci, 2003), and documentation of the underpinning theories and current intervention strategies. As a result, it appears that there are diverging interpretations of "the Bobath approach," a problem that is beginning to be addressed but which requires further work (Lennon and Ashburn, 2000).

While the Bobaths have made a significant contribution to the understanding and management of stroke patients, the approach has been criticized on a number of grounds, including the lack of clear operational definitions (e.g. "quality of movement") and the validity of the "normality" concept as the gold standard for treatment (Van Sant 1991), while the assumption that physical exertion would exacerbate spasticity has been challenged by more recent evidence (Badics *et al.*, 2002). Furthermore, the evidence from a review of 15 studies evaluating the efficacy of the Bobath approach for stroke patients was inconclusive (Paci, 2003), highlighting the necessity for further research.

Educational approach

Conductive Education was developed after the Second World War by the physician and neuropsychologist András Petö, with the aim of teaching adults and children with motor disorders to function independently in society (Read, 1992). Conductive education is now practiced in a number of different countries and is delivered by "conductors," who integrate teaching, speech and language therapy, and physical and occupational therapy into a comprehensive, group-based approach (Brown and Mikula-Toth, 1997). Since conductive education requires skills across different healthcare professions, it will not be further discussed here and readers are referred to the National Library for Conductive Education for further information (http://www.conductive-education.org.uk/html/national_library.html).

Motor learning approach

Carr and Shepherd (1987, 1989, 2003) developed a motor relearning program for stroke that provided guidelines for a training program for stroke patients based on principles of neuroscience, motor control and learning, biomechanics, exercise physiology, cognitive psychology, and human ecology. This program differed from the Bobath approach at that time, in which patients were often predominantly passive recipients of treatment, by promoting an active role for the patient. The main assumptions underpinning this approach are that regaining activities of daily living after stroke requires a relearning process that is similar to the learning process for non-impaired people. In addition, practice needs to be task and context specific. Normal movement is thought to consist of essential components (i.e. the invariant kinematics of an activity) that are used to perform many different activities (Carr and Shepherd, 1987).

The aims of the motor relearning program are for the patient to relearn every day tasks, such as reaching and manipulation, balanced sitting and standing, walking, standing up and sitting down, bed mobility, and orofacial function. This requires the patient to regain controlled muscle activity and normalization of movement components into functional synergies (Carr and Shepherd, 1998). In order to achieve this, the program also aims to restore or maintain soft tissue extensibility, muscle strength as well as fitness.

Training involves task- and context-specific activities: in other words, functional tasks in functional settings. The main role of the therapist is to facilitate the motor relearning process by identifying the patient's problems and by analyzing movement through observation and comparison with normal movement. The therapist also identifies those components that are thought to be "missing" or poorly controlled. Using goal setting, instruction, feedback and manual guidance, the therapist teaches the patient to perform these so-called "missing components." These are then practiced, followed by training of the task in a more functional context to promote transfer (or carry-over). The patient is encouraged to practice relevant tasks extensively, not only under supervision of the therapist but also independently, using both physical and mental practice in a variety of environments.

Regarding the evidence supporting the motor learning approach, Dean *et al.* (2000) found that exercising leg strength and lower limb functional activities in the format of circuit training, three times a week for four weeks, improved walking speed and endurance as well as other outcomes related to lower limb function compared with patients who trained only upper limb function. These effects were retained at follow-up two months later. In a task-related program of 10 sessions over two weeks in which stroke patients trained seated reaching tasks, Dean and Shepherd (1997) found that the speed and distance over which patients reached, loading of the affected lower limb and sit-to-stand improved, compared with a control group that carried out cognitive–manipulative tasks with the unaffected hand within arm's length.

There is little evidence supporting a more general skill acquisition paradigm for stroke rehabilitation (i.e. not necessarily part of the motor learning approach), as most research on skill acquisition has been based on studies with non-impaired adults (e.g. Schmidt and Lee, 1999; Magill, 2001). Although many authors have emphasized the potential of a motor learning paradigm for neurological rehabilitation (e.g. Marteniuk, 1979; Lee *et al.*, 1991; Winstein, 1991a, b; Majsak, 1996; Hochstenbach and Mulder, 1999), to date very few studies have actually been conducted with patients with neurological deficits (Pollock, 1998). Winstein *et al.* (1999) showed that, compared with non-impaired controls, patients with anterior circulation infarct were impaired in the control of rapid movement but not in the acquisition of it. These preliminary findings support the potential of implementing motor learning principles in neurological rehabilitation. However, the optimum structure of skill acquisition programs for patients with a CNS deficit requires further research (Fuhrer and Keith, 1998).

Evidence of the efficacy of traditional physiotherapy approaches

Several reviews have highlighted the lack of evidence in favor of any of the traditional physiotherapeutic approaches for stroke patients (e.g. Wagenaar *et al.*, 1990; Ashburn *et al.*, 1993; Duncan, 1997; Kwakkel *et al.*, 1999; Pollock *et al.*, 2003). In addition to other methodological weaknesses, this stems primarily from poorly described interventions. Although therapeutic processes are not easy to describe, as they revolve around procedural skills and are tailored to the individual (a point made by Bobath in 1990), this may have led to considerable differences in what is often referred to in the literature as "standard" or "traditional" physiotherapy (Pollock *et al.*, 2003).

In order to strengthen the necessary evidence base, we would, therefore, like to further the argument that physiotherapists need to move away from rigid "approaches" to neurological physiotherapy and towards the evaluation of specific and clearly described interventions. In addition, appropriate and valid outcome measures that are sufficiently sensitive to clinically relevant change are required to document efficacy of treatment (Kwakkel *et al.*, 1999).

The next section addresses a range of current and emerging intervention strategies that feature a specific type of therapeutic input.

Current and emerging physiotherapy strategies for stroke rehabilitation

Strength training and physical conditioning

In the past, many proponents of the neurofacilitation approach used to argue that the apparent loss of strength following stroke was not a problem of muscle force *per se*, but rather a symptom of a dysfunctional postural reflex mechanism (Bobath, 1990). Furthermore, it was thought that the effort involved in strengthening exercises would be detrimental and would result in marked abnormal reflex activity and increased muscle tone. These views were articulated despite any objective evidence to support them and were predominant until recently, when evidence about the effects of physical activity, strength training, and circuit training in stroke patients began to challenge these assumptions. The uncertainty regarding unwanted effects of increasing muscle tone following vigorous exercise are beginning to be addressed.

Dawes *et al.* (2000) used a single case study to investigate whether the effort induced by high-intensity cycling would result in increased muscle tone or involuntary muscle activity. A single subject, in the chronic stage after stroke, took part in a cycling program for two weeks and demonstrated improved active elbow extension and a reduction in pain and fatigue, while no change in muscle tone was found.

Badics *et al.* (2002) carried out a non-randomized study into the effects of a strength training program for 56 stroke patients (three weeks to 10 years after a cerebro vascular accident [CVA]) on muscle tone. Leg and arm presses were practised for four weeks. Although this study was not placebo controlled and there was no long-term follow-up, two important findings emerged. First, strength gains (mean 31% increase in leg strength and mean 37% increase in arm strength) could be achieved in patients several years after a CVA. Second, strength training did not appear to have a detrimental effect on the Ashworth scores, which suggested that strength training did not increase resistance to passive movement.

Morris *et al.* (2004) carried out a systematic review of studies that investigated the effects of progressive resistance training after stroke. One of the inclusion criteria was that the training should have been administered in isolation, as opposed to being one component of intervention. Only eight trials out of a total of 350 met the inclusion criteria for the review. The authors noted that there was considerable variability between studies in terms of the frequency, duration, intensity, and content of the training programs. Despite this variation, strength training appeared to have a positive effect on muscle strength, while adverse reactions were few and only minor. The belief that strength training leads to increased spasticity was again not supported by the literature. All in all, while the review highlighted the lack of research into the effects of strength training following stroke, studies that have been carried out suggest that the effect size of progressive resistance training on muscle strength is considerable. Further research on this topic is required, especially in relation to the effects of such training on activity limitations and participation restrictions.

Saunders *et al.* (2004) argued that impaired physical fitness, strength, and mobility in stroke patients may be a consequence of normal aging. It was also noted that bilateral limb weakness may be manifest after stroke, although the paretic limbs are more severely affected. These findings may support the view that immobility after stroke may compound deterioration of muscle tissue and diminish a patient's general functional ability (Andrews, 2000).

It has been suggested that aerobic exercise after stroke is related to improved functional ability (Potempa *et al.*, 1996). In a small study, Teixeira-Salmela *et al.* (2001) investigated the effects of a physical conditioning and strengthening regimen in chronic stroke. Thirteen subjects participated and following a 10 week program (three days a week); improvements in muscle strength and gait parameters were found.

Saunders *et al.* (2004) carried out a systematic review of randomized controlled trials (RCTs) investigating the effectiveness of physical fitness training following a CVA. Twelve trials were included, featuring cardiorespiratory training (involving lower limb musculature) and/or strength training (targeting upper and/or lower limb musculature). The effects of physical fitness training on activity limitations, cardiorespiratory fitness, and strength were equivocal. Walking training resulted in a significant improvement in the functional ambulation categories scores, while cardiorespiratory training had a beneficial effect on maximum walking speed and some aspects of lower limb function, but not on cardiorespiratory fitness. No effects on upper limb function were found. There was insufficient information to determine whether strength training resulted in improved force production. All in all, the authors concluded there is not enough evidence at present to support the implementation of physical fitness training in stroke rehabilitation.

In summary, although the evidence is only starting to emerge, there are some positive indications that a controlled strengthening and fitness program has beneficial effects for patients suffering chronic stroke problems. Because of the muscle and soft tissue shortening that is thought to occur within the first 24 hours following inactivity (Goldspink and Williams, 1990), it is probably prudent that any strengthening and fitness regimen be combined with an appropriate stretching program.

Stretching, orthotics, and positioning

Disorders of tone are common following a lesion of the (normalization) CNS and an important component of neurological physiotherapy is the normalization of muscle tone, in conjunction with reeducation of movement. Following an acute CNS lesion, hypotonia or flaccidity tends to be observed, which often changes into hypertonia (Edwards, 2002). "Tone" is a concept that is difficult to define; according to Bernstein (1967), it reflects a state of readiness, whilst Brooks (1986) defined it as *"the resistance offered by muscles to continuous passive stretch."* A different but related phenomenon is spasticity, which is most commonly defined as *"a motor disorder, characterised by a velocity – dependent increase in tonic stretch reflexes (muscle tone) with exaggerated tendon jerks, resulting from hyper-excitability of the stretch reflex as one component of the upper motor neurone (UMN) syndrome"* (Lance, 1980). Although there is a lack of agreement in both the literature and within clinical practice on what hypertonia and spasticity actually are, the definitions above suggest that hypertonia may be interpreted as a result of tonic muscle contractions in static conditions (Edwards, 2002), while spasticity is specifically velocity dependent. The situation is further complicated by the fact that both phenomena involve neural (e.g. hyperreflexia) as well as non-neural components (e.g. soft-tissue changes). For an excellent discussion on the neurophysiology of spasticity, the reader is referred to Sheean (2001).

Given the general lack of agreement on the definitions of tone and spasticity, it follows that the operationalization of these definitions (i.e. the methods to assess spasticity and tone) is also a matter of great debate. Reviewing these methods and suggesting ways to standardize the assessment of spasticity is the aim of an interdisciplinary EU Thematic Network (http://www.ncl.ac.uk/spasm). In summary, there is a lack of understanding with regards to the processes that are responsible for spasticity and disorders of tone, which led Sheean (2001) to suggest that spasticity may be a heterogeneous condition. In clinical practice, the concepts "hypertonia" and "spasticity" are commonly used interchangeably, with "spasticity" often being employed to refer to the entire upper motor neurone syndrome instead of just one component of it (Edwards, 2002). In order to be able to make a rational decision on the most appropriate form of treatment however, it is important to establish the nature of the clinical phenomenon and determine the contribution of neural and non-neural components.

Numerous forms of intervention are available that are thought to influence tone and reduce spasticity. These include stretching, mobilization, casting, splinting, orthotics, posture management, pharmacological interventions, and surgery. These – predominantly passive – forms of treatment need to be complemented with active treatment whenever possible, in order to improve motor control and enhance more long-term and functional carry-over. Below, only a brief outline is given for these passive forms of treatment, while the reader is referred to excellent textbooks (Barnes and Johnson, 2001; Edwards, 2002; Carr and Shepherd, 2003) for further details.

An important aspect of therapeutic management of patients with a neurological deficit and tone abnormalities is to ensure optimal positioning throughout the day, particularly when therapeutic intervention is not taking place. To achieve this, a multidisciplinary team approach is required (Kirkwood and Bardsley, 2001). This may include the input from a physiotherapist, an occupational therapist, and a wheelchair engineer to ensure appropriate seating in a chair and positioning in bed. Seating and positioning is a specialist subject, a full discussion of which is beyond the remit of this chapter. For further details on seating, the reader is referred to Kirkwood and Bardsley (2001), while further information on posture and seating can be found in Pope (2002).

It is of utmost importance to monitor muscle tone and range of movement immediately after the acute event (Carr and Shepherd, 2003). In animal studies, a reduction of sarcomere numbers has been found within 24 hours (Gossman *et al.*, 1982). Further animal work has also shown that prolonged immobilization of a muscle in a shortened position (e.g. foot held in plantarflexion) resulted in a loss of sarcomere numbers and, therefore, muscle extensibility (Taylor *et al.*, 1990). It is important that a multidisciplinary team approach be used to ensure consistency in positioning and handling of the patient. Therefore, physiotherapists are often involved in training nurses, occupational therapists, family, and other carers in procedures that aim to normalize muscle tone, posture and maintain joint and muscle range of movement.

Stretching may influence both biomechanical and neurophysiological properties of soft tissues. Experimental animal models have shown that repeated, short-duration (30 second) stretches result in a reduction of peak tension within four stretches in normally innervated muscles, after which no significant changes occur (Taylor *et al.*, 1990). Although these data are difficult to extrapolate to humans, particularly those with CNS lesions, there are some studies that have found similar changes in humans with brain injury (Moseley, 1993). In a study with adults with a range of CNS lesions, Hale *et al.* (1995) compared the efficacy of stretching the quadriceps femoris muscles for 2, 10, and 30 minutes. More statistically significant improvements were found for the 10-minute stretch condition, although it was unclear whether these differences were large enough to be clinically significant. Al-Zamil *et al.* (1995) placed a 2.3 kg (5lb) sand bag on the anterior aspect of the forearm for 30 minutes; this significantly reduced the amplitude of the EMG response to passive stretch of the elbow flexors. However, it is questionable whether such a procedure would be clinically acceptable. Altogether, it is clear that more research is needed to establish clinical guidelines for optimum soft tissue stretching in adults with a lesion of the CNS.

Orthoses, defined as external devices used to "modify the structural or functional characteristics of the neuromuscular system," include splints, casts, and braces (Charlton and Ferguson, 2001). In practice, however, "orthoses" are usually made by an orthotist, whereas splints (usually made from low-temperature plastics) and casts (made from plaster or casting tape) may be made by therapists. The main aims for using these devices are primarily to promote more normal posture and movement and to prevent secondary complications (e.g. contractures and pain). However, not all therapists agree on whether splints are beneficial, especially in patients with hypertonia (Edwards and Charlton, 2002). If an orthosis is prescribed, it is important that it be reassessed on a regular basis to ensure that optimal fit and, therefore, optimal benefit are maintained. Further guidelines for splinting adults with neurological deficits have been drawn up by a physiotherapy specialist interest group in the UK (ACPIN, 1998).

Probably the most commonly prescribed orthosis to improve gait after a stroke is the ankle–foot orthosis (AFO) (Carr and Shepherd, 2003). AFOs come in many different designs, ranging from rigid to hinged (Charlton and Ferguson, 2001; Edwards and Charlton, 2002). In their systematic review of the effects of AFOs on gait and leg muscle activity in stroke patients, Leung and Mosely (2003) found that these devices may be effective in improving a number of gait parameters in patients who were able to walk without an AFO and who demonstrated a dynamic foot drop. However, the evidence regarding the effects of AFOs on lower limb paresis was inconclusive. The authors highlighted the methodological problems within some of the studies and the lack of standardization (e.g. regarding the type of AFO and selection of gait parameters) between studies, which hampers the formulation of clinical guidelines regarding the prescription of AFOs in hemiplegic patients.

Hand splints may be prescribed where patients have spasticity or hypertonia of their finger and/or hand muscles. In addition to maintaining soft tissue length, hand splints may make it easier for patients or carers to clean the hand and cut finger nails in those with little functional use of their hands. Although physiotherapists may be involved in hand splinting in some cases, this is often the specialist remit of the occupational therapist and will not be further discussed in this chapter.

Casting or serial casting may be applied where a definitive device is not appropriate or not available. A description of different casting techniques is provided by Stoeckman (2001), while an excellent overview of a range of applications may be found in Edwards and Charlton (2002). Serial casting, which involves the progressive immobilization of a limb at increasing muscle and joint ranges, may be effective in managing contractures. The biomechanical and neurophysiological processes thought to be promoted by these procedures have been addressed by Watkins (1999).

As mentioned above, pain and instability of the glenohumeral joint are common problems following a stroke, and a number of different supports have been developed (see Edwards and Charlton [2002] for an overview). However, their use is still controversial, and there is also a lack of agreement on the optimum type of support. A study by Zorowitz *et al.* (1995) compared the effects of four different shoulder supports on vertical, horizontal, and total asymmetry of glenohumeral subluxation within six weeks of stroke onset. The results showed that each support had a different effect on specific measures of asymmetry. The authors suggested that patients should try a range of supports to identify the most appropriate one. They also cautioned that some forms of support may actually increase measures of asymmetry. It was further suggested that both biomechanical factors and the patient's cognitive and psychosocial circumstances should be considered for the device to be used properly and safely. In conclusion, Jackson (1998) suggested that the application of supports for shoulder subluxation cannot be justified on the basis of the current evidence.

Electrical stimulation

Electrical stimulation involves the application of an electrical current to the skin, to elicit muscle contraction, to maintain range of movement, to reduce pain or to reduce spasticity. There are different types of electrical stimulation, which are described in more detail by Jackson (1998). Electrical stimulation may be used to strengthen weakened muscles or to stimulate contraction if muscles are too weak to generate any observable contraction.

A specific application of electrical stimulation in stroke rehabilitation is the prevention or reduction of subluxation of the glenohumeral joint, which may occur in up to 81% of patients. Ada and Foongchomcheay (2002) carried out a meta-analysis on the effects of electrical stimulation, applied to produce a motor response in the deltoid and supraspinatus muscles. The evidence suggested that, in the early stage following stroke (i.e. 2–49 days), electrical stimulation combined with conventional physiotherapy was more effective in preventing subluxation and improving upper limb function than conventional physiotherapy alone. In the late stage following stroke (i.e. 60–434 days), electrical stimulation was effective in reducing shoulder pain, while the reduction of subluxation was minimal. The authors, however, commented on the poor quality as well as quantity of the evidence base: only seven trials could be included in the analysis.

de Kroon *et al.* (2002) systematically reviewed the efficacy of therapeutic Electrical stimulation on motor control and functional abilities of the upper limb following stroke. "Motor control" was described as the ability to perform voluntary movements, as assessed in terms of strength, active range of movement, Fugl–Meyer (upper extremity part), and other outcome measures. "Functional ability" was referred to as the "ability to perform purposeful activities," which was reflected in outcome measures such as the Action Research Arm Test and other dexterity tests. The evidence emerging from the six RCTs that met the inclusion criteria suggested that Electrical stimulation had a positive effect on motor control, although it was not possible to determine the clinical significance of these effects. Regarding the effects of Electrical stimulation on functional ability, the evidence was inconclusive since it had only been assessed in two studies. Overall, the authors emphasized that no firm conclusions could be drawn, because of the limitations of the evidence currently available.

Another example of electrical stimulation to enhance motor control and function is the Odstock Dropped Foot Stimulator (ODFS), which is a device that stimulates the common peroneal nerve during the swing phase of gait. In an RCT, Burridge *et al.* (1997) investigated the effects of ODFS in patients who were at least six months post-stroke and whose gait was impaired by a drop foot. The ODFS improved both speed and the effort of walking considerably when the device was worn, whereas conventional physiotherapy was ineffective. However, in general, no carry-over was observed when the device was not worn. Despite its efficacy, the authors explained why the ODFS may not be suitable for some patients: effective use of the device requires the patient to understand the way it is to be applied as well as to be able to apply it either by themselves or with a carer. Taylor *et al.* (1999), in a survey gauging patients' opinion on the ODFS, added that a dedicated and comprehensive clinical service is needed to ensure that patients can continue to reap the benefits of the ODFS.

Regarding the use of electrical stimulation in the management of pain, Price and Pandyan (2001) reviewed the literature on the efficacy of surface electrical stimulation for preventing and treating post-stroke shoulder pain. Studies involving any type of electrical stimulation were screened, but only four were eligible for inclusion in the review. The results showed that, compared with control treatment, there was no significant effect of electrical stimulation on pain incidence or pain intensity. However, there was a significant effect of electrical stimulation on improvement of pain-free passive range of lateral rotation of the humerus, as well as degree of glenohumeral subluxation. Given the paucity of data, the authors concluded that there was insufficient evidence to support or refute the application of electrical stimulation for post-stroke shoulder pain, but that risks involved appear to be sufficiently low as to allow application of electrical stimulation at any time post-stroke. However, there was insufficient evidence to recommend the optimum type or dosage of electrical stimulation.

Recent developments in neuromuscular electrical stimulation technology include semi-implanted or fully implantable systems, which may be part of neuroprosthetics. A description of the development of these systems and their current applications in clinical practice may be found in Chae and Yu (2000, 2002).

Biofeedback

Biofeedback may be defined as "the technique of using equipment (usually electronic) to reveal to human beings some of their internal physiological events, normal and abnormal, in the form of visual and auditory signals in order to teach them to manipulate these otherwise involuntary or unfelt events by manipulating the displayed signals" (Basmajian, 1989). Biofeedback may be implemented in several different ways in neurological rehabilitation; probably one of the most frequently applied techniques is electromyographic biofeedback. This can demonstrate to the patient levels of muscular activation that are too subtle to be observed in an unaided manner. Several RCTs and meta-analyses have been carried out, which have been summarized in the National Clinical Guidelines for Stroke (www.rcplondon.ac.uk/pubs/books/stroke/ceeu_stroke_tab9_5.htm). On the basis of the available evidence, these guidelines suggest that there is insufficient justification for electromyographic biofeedback and, therefore, it will not be further discussed here.

Constraint-induced therapy

The idea for constraint-induced therapy (CIT) is based on observations of monkeys after experimentally induced deafferentation (Taub, 1980; Taub and Uswatte, 2003 [citing Ogden and Franz 1917]), which resulted in the animals making less use of their affected upper limb. Attempting to promote recovery, the researchers then constrained the non-affected upper limb of the monkeys and noted that this reduced the non-use of the affected upper limb. CIT, or forced use, appears to have first been investigated in stroke in a single patient in 1981 (Ostendorf and Wolf, 1981). The aim is to force the patient to use the more affected limb by constraining the lesser or unaffected upper extremity. This requires the latter to be restrained for a prolonged period of time, up to 90% of "waking hours" (Taub et al., 1999). In conjunction with the constraint, patients need to participate in intensive repetitive training of the "free limb" for at least six hours a day. Taub and Uswatte (2003), in their synthesis of research on CIT, explained how three important processes could lead to learned non-use: punishment for using the affected limb (e.g. discomfort, loss of food objects), positive reinforcement for using the non- or less-affected side, and cortical reorganization following the natural or iatrogenic lesion, which involved shrinkage of the cortical representation area for the affected limb.

The rationale for CIT is based on both neurophysiological and motor learning literature. CIT involves massed practice of tasks: the time spent practicing the tasks exceeds the time spent resting. Not only does this reinforce the use of the affected arm, but it is also postulated to promote functional reorganization of brain areas in chronic stroke (Taub et al., 1993, 1999). Liepert et al. (2001) used focal transcranial magnetic stimulation to investigate changes in motor output areas

12 training sessions of TTBWS and varying treadmill speed in 24 chronic stroke subjects resulted in improved overground walking velocity that persisted at three months' follow-up.

While most of the work on TT has been undertaken with chronic stroke patients and concentrated on the question of whether or not to use TTBWS, there is more recent work looking at the effects of TT in the earlier rehabilitation phase. Laufer *et al.* (2001) claimed that stroke patients may tolerate TT early on in rehabilitation and that this modality may be more effective than conventional gait training for improving parameters such as stride length and percentage of paretic single-stance periods. Positive findings of early intervention using stepwise speed progression on the treadmill have also been demonstrated by Pohl *et al.* (2002)

In general, claims in favor of the use of TT for stroke include an improvement in weight-bearing ability, and, therefore, stance phase of gait (Mudge *et al.*, 2001) and improved neural adaptation as a result of repetitive training of cyclical activity; TTBWS enables the patient to retrain control of the gait cycle without having to concentrate on limb loading and balance. This means that patients can relearn walking within days of stroke onset. Recent work also suggests that TT may be useful in improving fitness capacity of chronic stroke subjects (Macko *et al.*, 2001).

One issue regarding TT is its ecological validity; locomotion in real-life conditions usually involves a stable surface and a dynamic optic flowfield and the need to deal with perturbations and obstacles. Therefore, it is unlikely that TT is sufficient for training safe locomotion in real-life conditions. The alternative argument is that TT is more similar to walking than part-practice of task components (e.g. heel strike), which is common in the context of conventional physiotherapy. In general, while the evidence appears to lend some support to TT, there are very few large-scale studies in this area. Two recent systematic reviews of current evidence identified that, in general, studies on TT have been conducted with varied interventions, undertaken at different times within the rehabilitation period, and used a diversity of outcome measures (Manning and Pomeroy, 2003; Moseley *et al.*, 2003). Moseley *et al.*, concluded that among ambulant stroke patients TTBWS may improve walking speed. Manning, 2003 concluded that there is little evidence to suggest that current practice should be abandoned in favor of TT and that further larger-scale studies are required before a rational decision can be made. In practical terms, although the equipment for TT is rather costly, the physical demands on the treating therapist(s) may be lower than with conventional gait training.

Botulinum toxin

Botulinum toxin (BT) is a relatively new pharmacological agent for the reduction of focal spasticity (Barnes and Johnson, 2001). For a comprehensive overview of the use, effects and side-effects of BT in stroke, the reader is referred to Davis and Barnes (2001); however, since its application in the UK is increasingly involving physiotherapists (Stark, 2001), a brief overview of its use is included here.

BT, injected intramuscularly, prevents the release of presynaptic acetylcholine, thus causing selective paresis. Following the chemical denervation, axonal sprouting and gradual reinnervation take place, resulting in full recovery of the neuro-muscular junctions usually after a period of two to six months (Davis and Barnes, 2001). In practice, this short-term benefit means that many chronic patients require to be reinjected on a regular basis. Obviously, this has important cost implications, which have, to the authors' knowledge, not been investigated so far.

The effectiveness of BT in reducing focal spasticity has been documented in several studies (e.g. Simpson *et al.*, 1996; Simpson, 1997; Richardson and Thompson, 1999; Brashear, *et al.*, 2002). BT may also be instrumental in reducing pain associated with spasticity (Wissel *et al.*, 2000), as well as the burden of care (Bhakta *et al.*, 2000), although the evidence is mixed. To date, the effects of BT on function have not been investigated extensively. Bhakta *et al.* (1996, 2000) reported that BT was effective in reducing disability, while Pandyan *et al.* (2002) showed that, following BT injected into the elbow flexors, electromyographic activity of the elbow flexors was reduced and upper limb function improved, despite most patients having elbow contractures.

Since BT primarily targets muscle tone, it is generally recommended that it be part of a comprehensive rehabilitation program to enhance functional carry-over (e.g. Sheean, 1997; Richardson and Thompson, 1999; Bhakta; 2000, Hesse, 2000; Hesse *et al.*, 2001), which is reflected in the relevant guidelines (Barnes *et al.*, 2001). However, there is a dearth of evidence regarding the additional benefits of other treatment modalities when given with BT. The addition of short-term electrical stimulation treatment to BT injected into the ankle plantar flexors resulted in a significant improvement in a number of gait parameters (Hesse *et al.*, 1995b) when compared with BT alone. Similarly, short-term electrical stimulation to the upper limb flexor muscles following BT injection made a significant improvement in terms of maintaining hand hygiene and upper limb resting position (Hesse *et al.*, 1998). Reiter *et al.* (1998) combined a single BT injection of the musculus tibialis posterior with ankle strapping and found that this combination was as effective for this purpose as conventional BT intervention, which typically involves multiple injections. To date, however, there do not appear to be any published studies on the additional effects of exercise or motor learning when administered together with BT in stroke patients (van Wijck *et al.*, 2004).

In conclusion, there is encouraging evidence regarding the effectiveness of BT in reducing focal spasticity. However, studies demonstrating the effects of BT on spasticity must be interpreted with caution, since many have used the Ashworth or modified Ashworth scales, which have both been criticized for their poor validity (Pandyan *et al.*, 1999). In general, research on the effects of BT tends to be hampered by limited sample size, variation in dosage and injection site between studies, predominantly qualitative outcome measures, and, often, inappropriate statistical analysis (Richardson and Thompson, 1999). Further research is required to guide clinicians regarding optimum combinations of treatment to enhance functional carry-over of BT.

Mental practice

Mental practice, also referred to as "movement imagery," "covert practice," involves the cognitive rehearsal of movement in the absence of overt activity (reviewed by Martin *et al.*, 1999). It is used extensively in sports and dance to enhance performance (Magill, 2001). Although the integration of mental practice in rehabilitation has been advocated by various authors (e.g. Decety, 1993; van Leeuwen and Inglis, 1998; Jackson *et al.*, 2001), there are very few empirical studies on the effectiveness of mental practice in people with CNS lesions. In an RCT, Page *et al.* (2001b) examined the efficacy of mental practice in patients 2–11 months after stroke. Therapy was provided for one hour, three times per week for six weeks, after which patients listened to a 10-minute audiotape. For the experimental group, this tape gave instructions for mental practice, guiding patients in the use of their affected arm; the tape for the control group provided general information about their stroke. Patients using mental practice showed considerably better scores on arm function tests than did the control group: in the latter, outcomes remained virtually the same. One limitation of this study was the variability in time after stroke, given that most recovery of upper limb function takes place in the first three months after a stroke (Wade *et al.*, 1983). Hence, in this small cohort, time after stroke could have influenced the results.

An understanding of the effects of mental practice has been greatly facilitated by neuroimaging and techniques such as transcranial magnetic stimulation (Jeannerod and Frak, 1999). Although many aspects of mental practice still require further research, the most commonly accepted explanation at present, is that it involves brain areas, neural pathways, and cognitive processes similar to those involved in the actual production of movement (Magill, 2001). Several studies have shown that mental practice increases the excitability of areas within the motor cortex, involved in the activation of muscles required for the execution of a particular movement (Tremblay *et al.*, 2001; Facchini *et al.*, 2002). The specific modification of activity in primary sensorimotor areas is the basis for imagery-directed brain–computer interfaces to steer a hand orthosis (Pfurtscheller and Neuper, 2001) or virtual keyboard (Obermaier *et al.*, 2001) in tetraplegic patients.

The advantages of mental practice are that it is well tolerated, easy to perform, and (provided that adequate instructional material is available and the patient is able to use this independently) it can be undertaken outwith therapy time. Given the fact that practice time is restricted in most rehabilitation settings, this is an important consideration. A limitation of this technique, however, is that it is virtually impossible to monitor the way it is carried out. Therefore, the information input needs to be carefully formulated in order to guide the process. An important question is whether a stroke affects the ability to engage in mental practice. Johnson (2000) suggested that lesions affecting the right posterior parietal or left frontal lobes may affect the ability to use mental practice. At present, however, there is insufficient evidence to suggest for which patients the technique may or may not be suitable. It is reasonable to suggest that, because of the verbal–cognitive content of the instructions, mental practice may not be suitable for patients with severe attentional, cognitive, and/or certain speech and language disorders, but this requires further investigation.

Emerging technologies

Interventions that are currently in a more experimental stage include virtual reality (e.g. Holden *et al.*, 2002; Merians *et al.*, 2002; Sisto *et al.*, 2002) and robotics (e.g. Krebs *et al.*, 1999, 2000, 2002; Volpe *et al.*, 2000). Coote and Stokes (2003) explored patients' and therapists' attitudes with regards to the first prototype of the GENTLE/s robot-mediated therapy system (http://www.gentle.rdg.ac.uk/) and found generally positive results. While the efficacy of treatment is being evaluated, further user input is sought to continue to develop this technology.

Provided of course that health and safety requirements are met, these technologies may provide valuable opportunities for patients to relearn perceptuo-motor skills in an enriched, interactive, yet controllable environment with extended scope for practice. The optimum patient conditions in which these technologies should be applied and the barriers and opportunities for their implementation in routine clinical practice, however, is an issue of debate (Volpe *et al.*, 2001).

Physiotherapy in stroke rehabilitation: looking ahead

Research into the efficacy of physiotherapy in stroke rehabilitation has been hampered by a number of problems, including poor methodologies, low sample sizes, a myriad of diverse outcome measures, and a lack of information regarding the content of therapeutic interventions (Kwakkel *et al.*, 1999; Pollock *et al.*, 2003). Regarding the last, many authors have emphasized that therapeutic input – alluded to by some as the "black box of therapy" (Ballinger *et al.*, 1999; Pommeroy and Tallis, 2002a) – needs to be described more clearly and in more detail (Pommeroy *et al.*, 2000; Partridge, 2002; Pommeroy and Tallis, 2002b). The outcome measures selected have often been unable to detect subtle, yet perhaps clinically relevant, change; a particular problem with questionnaires concerning activities of daily living (van der Lee *et al.*, 2001). Not surprisingly, it has been very difficult to establish the relationship between input and output in neurological physiotherapy – a problem compounded by the heterogeneity of patient populations included in research. Furthermore, RCTs in neurological physiotherapy are few and far between, with the result that many studies may not have been included in meta-analyses. This, in turn, has made it difficult to establish evidence-based physiotherapy strategies.

While functional recovery may largely result from spontaneous recovery in the early stages post-stroke (Kwakkel *et al.*, 1999), further improvement in the chronic stage can be obtained through targeted rehabilitation (e.g. Tangeman *et al.*, 1990; Wade *et al.*, 1992). Several reviews have shown that patients may benefit from physiotherapy that starts early after stroke, encourages active patient participation, involves resistance training, incorporates task-orientated practice, and provides ample opportunity for practice (Duncan, 1997; Kwakkel *et al.*, 1999; van der Lee *et al.*, 2001; Pomeroy and Tallis, 2002a). Further research is required into the efficacy of specific forms of treatment targeted at clearly defined patient populations.

A whole new impetus has been given to neurological physiotherapy by studies using techniques such as transcranial magnetic stimulation, functional magnetic resonance imaging and position emission tomography to monitor recovery and response to treatment after a CNS lesion. Work with non-human primates and patients has provided evidence for the neuroplastic changes associated with recovery from brain damage (reviewed by Johansson, 2000). In general, an enriched environment, social interaction, and physical activity may all be instrumental in modifying the anatomical structure and physiological processes of neural networks. With regards to task-orientated upper limb training, Nelles *et al.* (2001) reported an increase in regional cerebral blood flow bilaterally in the inferior parietal cortex, premotor cortex, and in the contralateral sensorimotor cortex, changes in brain activation associated with CIT have been described above. Despite the limitations of many of these studies (e.g. small sample size and limited follow-up time), the results are encouraging and suggests that – provided there is sufficient stimulation in terms of appropriate activity and amount of practice at the right time – positive changes can be enhanced by physiotherapy.

The following case study illustrates an approach to management based on current literature that could be adopted during the course of stroke rehabilitation. The assessment sections are written in a short-hand form similar to that which might be used in a practical setting.

A case study

History

Mr. M is a 56-year-old taxi driver who presented to the A and E department of the local hospital four months previous with acute onset of right-sided weakness affecting limbs, trunk, and face, in addition to slurred speech. He was diagnosed as having had a left hemisphere CVA, which was confirmed by a computed tomography scan showing a partial anterior circulation infarction.

Mr. M lives with his wife and 2-year-old baby. Mr. M's wife works part-time in a nursing home and he has two days off to look after his son while his wife is at work. They live in a first floor apartment with steps leading to the front door. All rooms are on one level. No close family live nearby. His hobbies include playing darts and playing the guitar in a local pub.

Examination by a physiotherapist in the neurological assessment ward

Large man with ruddy complexion, obese (weight: 150 kg). BP (blood pressure): 180/100. Slumped in bed, lying on back. Good comprehension and orientation to place, time, and person. Speech: hesitant and slightly dysarthric – requiring referral to speech and language therapist.

Physical assessment on admission

No movement to command of right limbs. Slow to respond but able to move left arm and leg. Requiring the assistance of one person to perform all bed mobility activities, tending to pull excessively with left arm when trying to assist. Slumped, kyphotic posture in sitting, with more weight bearing on left side. Unable to reach forward or to the right without losing balance. Able to stand up from a chair with assistance of one person on either side, but no weight taken through right foot. No independent standing balance. Unable to walk. Requiring help from one person to assist upper limb and trunk dressing. Unable to reach forward to put on socks, shoes, or trousers. Low tone in right leg but some flickers of quadriceps and hamstring activity. Little muscle activity around right shoulder. Only hand to mouth movement when yawning.

Initial management

The aims of treatment and initial management strategies at this stage were to:
- maintain a clear chest and respiratory status: monitoring and chest physiotherapy as required
- maintain muscle and soft tissue length and joint integrity by passive and assisted active movements, plus careful positioning in bed (involving education with nurses and carers regarding handling techniques to avoid inducing pain)

- avoid pressure areas: regular turning and changing position
- reeducate functional movements: rehabilitation encompassing bed mobility and sitting transfers from bed to chair; only to be sitting out of bed for short periods on the ward, with careful monitoring of his blood pressure
- prevent glenohumeral subluxation through education of the multidiscipinary team regarding handling and support of upper limb on pillows and wheelchair laptray.

The multidisciplinary team met at the end of his first week to determine short-term and long-term rehabilitation goals before his transfer to the stroke rehabilitation unit.

Assessment of progress at two weeks

Progress was reassessed after one week in a general ward and one week in the stroke recovery unit.

Some recovery of right limbs noted. Able to perform all bed mobility activities independently but with minimal right-sided involvement and persisting tendency to overuse left side. Still requiring assistance of one person to move from lying into sitting. Asymmetry and unequal weight bearing gradually resolving in sitting and standing. Able to take 10 steps with the assistance of one person. Minimal hip and knee flexion on right side and tending to weight bear on right hyperextended knee. Able to step onto a small (2 cm) block but unable to clear right foot above this height. Referral to orthotist for custom-made ankle–foot orthosis to assist foot clearance. Able to dress top half independently with vest and T-shirt but cannot perform any dextrous tasks. Still requiring help to complete some aspects of lower body dressing. Lower limb function improving, with more normal muscle tone on the right and some ability to move against gravity in supine and standing. Low tone persisting proximally in the right shoulder with some complaints of a painful shoulder during exercise, but no subluxation noted. Orofacial function: right-sided facial weakness improving, with only occasional problems when drinking.

Management at two weeks after the stroke

Mr. M attended the gym for 45 minutes per day. The agreed focus of treatment was to provide task-orientated training of bed mobility tasks, sitting to standing and sitting down again, balance in standing and walking, and reaching. The integrity of his right shoulder continued to be monitored and electrical stimulation was applied to strengthen further the paretic musculature around the glenohumeral joint.

Simple verbal feedback was given to Mr. M in order to aid learning of the components required to complete tasks appropriately. In addition, Mr. M was given a booklet of exercises to promote self-practice of achievable functional tasks: weight transfer and reaching in sitting, and facial muscle practice using word sounds and expressions (smiling, frowning, etc.). He was encouraged to use mental practice for these tasks outwith therapy time.

Assessment of progress at three months

Now independent in bed mobility, able to sit unsupported for a minute and reach in all directions, stand up independently (although more weight bearing on left side) and maintain standing balance. Able to walk 10 m in 28 seconds and climb four stairs with a handrail. Active shoulder shrugging and flexion to 90 degrees, improved strength of deltoid and supraspinatus muscles, full elbow flexion but reduced extension, able to grasp objects although having difficulties in letting go. Increased tone in wrist and finger flexors. Difficulty with active and passive straightening of 3rd, 4th, and 5th fingers. Facial weakness and comprehension problems resolved.

Management at three months

After three months, Mr. M was attending the gym twice daily for 45 minutes. In the morning a physiotherapist helped him to stretch upper limb muscles affected by increased tone and worked on specific movement problems. In addition, 30 minutes in the afternoon were used for self-directed circuit training, including upper- and lower-limb strengthening exercises and walking endurance. With the physiotherapist, Mr. M undertook TT three times a week with 20% BWS to facilitate correct limb loading. Self-practice activities included sitting to standing with equal weight bearing; stepping on and off a small step; upper limb stretches; reaching, and pointing to encourage weight transfer in the trunk and extensor activity in the arm. Practice involved both physical and mental practice. A night splint was worn to maintain length of wrist and finger flexors.

Discharge at four months

On discharge, Mr. M was instructed to continue with his exercises at home with bimonthly monitoring. It was agreed that if the upper-limb recovery plateaued, he would undergo a two week program of CIT six to eight months after his stroke. The option of BT was considered if hypertonia of the finger flexors were to interfere with function. Mr. M had to give up active taxi driving but was able to undertake the role of radio-controller for the taxi fleet. Although unable to continue all the child-care roles previously undertaken, Mr. M continued these responsibilities with the assistance of a child minder.

Summary

In general, stroke rehabilitation requires a problem-solving approach (Edwards, 2002). New therapeutic developments are likely to arise from interdisciplinary collaborations (e.g. between various healthcare professions, engineering and neuroscience), embracing the opportunities offered by emerging technologies. As far as evidence-based practice is concerned, physiotherapy is a new discipline and many aspects of physiotherapy are currently not supported by research (Partridge, 2002). However, rather than "evidence of absence" of therapeutic efficacy, this tends to constitute "absence of evidence", owing to a paucity of information. Further resources are required to generate and support clinical research that will enable therapists to provide patients with optimal treatment based on current clinical and research evidence.

ACKNOWLEDGEMENTS

The authors would like to sincerely thank Christopher Price for his thoughtful comments on an earlier version of the manuscript.

REFERENCES

ACPIN (Association of Chartered Physiotherapists Interested in Neurology) (1998). *Clinical Practice Guidelines on Splinting Adults with Neurological Dysfunction*. London: Chartered Society of Physiotherapy.

Ada, L. and Cannin, C. (ed.) (1990). *Key Issues in Neurological Physiotherapy*. Oxford: Butterworth-Heinemann.

Ada, L. and Foongchomcheay, A. (2002). Efficacy of electrical stimulation in preventing or reducing subluxation of the shoulder after stroke: a meta-analysis. *Aus J Physiother* **48**: 257–267.

Al-Zamil, Z. M., Hassan, N., and Hassan, W. (1995). Reduction of elbow flexor and extensor spasticity following muscle stretch. *J Neurol Rehabil* **9**: 161–165.

Andrews, A. W. (2000). Effect of physical therapy intervention on muscle strength and functional limitations in a patient with chronic stroke. *Phys Ther Case Rep* **3**: 17–21.

Ashburn, A., Partridge, C., and de Souza, L. (1993). Physiotherapy in the rehabilitation of stroke: a review. *Clin Rehab* **7**: 337–345.

Badics, E., Wittmann, A., Rupp, M., Staubauer, B., and Zifko, U. A. (2002). Systematic muscle building exercises in the rehabilitation of stroke patients. *Neurorehabil* **17**: 211–214.

Ballinger, C., Ashburn, A., Low, J., and Roderick, P. (1999). Unpacking the black box of therapy: a pilot study to describe occupational therapy and physiotherapy interventions for people with stroke. *Clin Rehabil* **13**: 301–309.

Barnes, M. P. and Johnson, G. R. (eds.) (2001). *Upper Motor Neurone Syndrome and Spasticity. Clinical Management and Neurophysiology*. Cambridge, UK: Cambridge University Press.

Basmajian, J. V. (1989). *Biofeedback Principles and Practice for Clinicians*, 3rd edn. Baltimore, MD: Williams and Wilkins.

Bernstein, N. (1967). *The Co-ordination and Regulation of Movements*. Oxford: Pergamon.

Bhakta, B. B., Cozens, J. A., Bamford, J. M., and Chamberlain, M. A. (1996). Use of botulinum toxin in stroke patients with severe upper limb spasticity. *J Neurol Neurosurg Psychiatry* **61**: 30–35.

Bhakta, B. B., Cozens, J. A., Chamberlain, M. A., and Bamford, J. M. (2000). Impact of botulinum toxin type A on disability and carer burden due to arm spasticity after stroke: a randomised double blind placebo controlled trial. *J Neurol Neurosurg Psychiatry* **69**: 217–221.

Bobath, B. (1969). The treatment of neuromuscular disorders by improving patterns of coordination. *Physiotherapy* **55**: 18–22.

(1990). *Adult Hemiplegia: Evaluation and Treatment*, 3rd edn. Oxford: Butterworth-Heinemann.

(1971). The normal postural reflex mechanism and its deviation in children with cerebral palsy. *Physiotherapy* **57**: 515–525.

Bobath, K. and Bobath, B. (1954). The treatment of cerebral palsy by the inhibition of abnormal reflex action. *Br Orthop J* **11**: 88–98.

(1957). Control of motor function in the treatment of cerebral palsy. *Physiotherapy* **43**: 295–303.

(1964). The facilitation of normal postural reactions and movements in the treatment of cerebral palsy. *Physiotherapy* **50**: 246.

Brashear, A., Gordon, M., Elovic, E., Kassicieh, V., and Marciniak, C. (2002). Intramuscular injection of botulinum toxin for the treatment of wrist and finger spasticity after stroke. *N Engl J Med* **347**: 395–400.

Brooks, V. (1986). *The Neural Basis of Motor Control*. Oxford: Oxford University Press.

Brown, M. and Mikula-Toth, A. (1997). *Adult Conductive Education*. Cheltenham, UK: Stanley Thomes.

Bryce, J. (1972). Facilitation of movement: the Bobath approach. *Physiotherapy* **58**: 403–408.

Burridge, J. H., Taylor, P. N., Hagan, S. A., Wood, D. E., and Swain, I. D. (1997). The effects of common peroneal stimulation on the effort and speed of walking: a randomized controlled trial with chronic hemiplegic patients. *Clin Rehabil* **11**: 201–210.

Carr, J. H. and Shepherd, R. B. (1987). *A Motor Learning Model for Stroke*, 2nd edn. Oxford: Butterworth Heinemann.

(1989). A motor learning model for stroke rehabilitation *Physiotherapy* **75**: 372–380.

(1998). *Neurological Rehabilitation. Optimizing Motor Performance*. Oxford: Butterworth Heinemann.

(2003). *Stroke Rehabilitation. Guidelines for Exercise and Training to Optimize Motor Skill*. London: Butterworth Heinemann.

Carr, J. H., Mungovan, S. F., Shepherd, R. B., Dean, C. M., and Nordholm, L. A, (1994). Physiotherapy in stroke rehabilitation: bases for Australian physiotherapists' choice of treatment. *Physiother Theory Pract* **10**: 201–209.

Chae, J. and Yu, D. (2000). A critical review of neuromuscular electrical stimulation for treatment of motor dysfunction in hemiplegia. *Assis Technol* **12**: 33–49.

(2002). Neuromuscular electrical stimulation for motor restoration in hemiparesis. *Top Stroke Rehabil* **8**: 24–39.

Charlton, P. T. and Ferguson, D. W. N. (2001). Orthoses, splinting and casting in spasticity. In, *Upper Motor Neurone Syndrome and Spasticity. Clinical Management and Neurophysiology*, ed. M. P. Barnes and G. R. Johnson, Cambridge, UK: Cambridge University Press, pp. 142–164.

Coote, S. and Stokes, E. K. (2003). Robot mediated therapy: attitudes of patients and therapists towards the first prototype of the GENTLE/s system. *Technol Disabil* **15**: 27–34.

Davidson, I. and Waters, K. K. (2000). Physiotherapists working with stroke patients: a national survey. *Physiotherapy* **86**: 69–80.

Davis, E. C. and Barnes, M. P. (2001). The use of botulinum toxin in spasticity. In *Upper Motor Neurone Syndrome and Spasticity: Clinical Management and Neurophysiology*, ed. M. P. Barnes and G. R. Johnson. Cambridge, UK: Cambridge University Press, pp. 206–222.

Dawes, H., Bateman, A., Wade, D., and Scott, O. M. (2000). High intensity cycling exercise after a stroke: a single case study. *Clin Rehabil* **14**: 570–573.

Dean, C. M. and Shepherd, R. B. (1997). Task-related training improves performance of seated reaching tasks after stroke. A randomized controlled trial. *Stroke* **28**: 722–728.

Dean, C. M., Richards, C. L., and Malouin, F. (2000). Task-related circuit training improves performance of locomotor tasks in chronic stroke: a randomized controlled pilot trial. *Arch Phys Med Rehabil* **81**: 409–417.

de Kroon, J. R., van der Lee, J. H., IJzerman, M. J., and Lankhorst, G. J. (2002). Therapeutic electrical stimulation to improve motor control and functional abilities of the upper extremity after stroke: a systematic review. *Clin Rehabil* **16**: 350–360.

Decety, J. (1993). Should motor imagery be used in physiotherapy? Recent advances in cognitive neurosciences *Physiother Theory Pract* **9**: 193–203.

Dromerick, A. W. (2003). Guest editorial. Evidence-based rehabilitation: the case for and against constraint-induced movement therapy. *J Rehabil Res Dev* **40**: vii–ix.

Dromerick, A. W., Edwards, D. F., and Hahn, M. (2000). Does the application of constraint induced movement therapy during acute rehabilitation reduce arm impairment after ischemic stroke? *Stroke* **31**: 2984–2988.

Duncan, P. W. (1997). Synthesis of intervention trials to improve motor recovery following stroke. *Top Stroke Rehabil* **3**: 1–20.

Edwards, S. (ed.) (2002). *Neurological Physiotherapy*, 2nd edn. Edinburgh: Churchill Livingstone.

Edwards, S. and Charlton, P. T. (2002). Splinting and the use of orthoses in the management of patients with neurological disorders. In *Neurological Physiotherapy*, 2nd ed. Edwards. Edinburgh: Churchill Livingstone, pp. 219–254.

Facchini, S., Muellbacher, W., Battaglia, F., Boroojerdi, B., and Hallett, M. (2002). Focal enhancement of motor cortex excitability during motor imagery: a transcranial magnetic stimulation study. *Acta Neurol Scand* **105**: 146–151.

Fuhrer, M. J. and Keith, R. A. (1998). Facilitating patient learning during medical rehabilitation. A research agenda. *Am J Phys Med Rehabil* **77**: 557–561.

Goldspink, G. and Williams, P. (1990). Muscle fiber and connective tissue changes associated with use and disuse. In *Key Issues in Neurological Physiotherapy*, ed. L. Ada and C. Canning. Oxford: Butterworth-Heinemann.

Gordon, J. (2000). Assumptions underlying physical therapy intervention: theoretical and historical perspectives. In *Movement Science. Foundations for Physical Therapy in Rehabilitation*, 2nd edn. ed. J. Carr and R. Shepherd. Gaithersburg, MD: Aspen pp. 1–32.

Gossman, M. R., Sahrmann, S. A., and Rose, S. J., (1982). Review of length associated changes in muscle. *Phys Ther* **62**: 1799–1808.

Hale, L. A., Fritz, V. U., and Goodman, M. (1995). Prolonged static muscle stretch reduces spasticity. *S Afr J Physiother* **51**: 3–6.

Hesse, S. (2000). Botulinum toxin A in the treatment of spasticity after stroke. *Akt Neurol* **27**: 412–417.

Hesse, S., Bertelt, C., Schaffrin, A., Malezic, M., and Mauritz, K. H. (1994). Restoration of gait in nonambulatory hemiparetic patients by treadmill training with partial body-weight support. *Arch Phys Med Rehabil* **75**: 1087–1093.

Hesse, S., Bertelt, C., Jahnke, M. T., *et al.* (1995a). Treadmill training with partial body weight support compared with physiotherapy in nonambulatory hemiparetic patients. *Stroke* **26**: 976–981.

Hesse, S., Jahnke, M. T., Luecke, D., and Mauritz, K. H. (1995b). Short-term electrical stimulation enhances the effectiveness of Botulinum toxin in the treatment of lower limb spasticity in hemiparetic patients. *Neurosci Lett* **201**: 37–40.

Hesse, S., Reiter, F., Konrad, M., and Jahnke, M. T. (1998). Botulinum toxin type A and short-term electrical stimulation in the treatment of upper limb flexor spasticity after stroke: a randomized, double-blind, placebo-controlled trial. *Clin Rehabil* **12**: 381–388.

Hesse, S., Konrad, M., and Uhlenbrock, D. (1999). Treadmill walking with partial body weight support versus floor walking in hemiparetic subjects. *Arch Phys Med Rehabil* **80**: 421–427.

Hesse, S., Brandl-Hesse, B., Bardeleben, A., Werner, C., and Funk, M. (2001). Botulinum toxin A treatment of adult upper and lower limb spasticity. *Drugs Aging* **18**: 255–262.

Hochstenbach, J. and Mulder, T. (1999). Neuropsychology and the relearning of motor skills following stroke. *Int J Rehabil Res* **22**: 11–19.

Holden, M. K. and Dyar, T. (2002). Virtual environment training: a new tool for neurorehabilitation. *Neurol Report* **26**: 62–71.

Jackson, J. (1998) Specific treatment techniques. In *Neurological Physiotherapy*, ed. M. Stokes. London: Mosby, pp. 299–311.

Jackson, P. L., Lafleur, M. F., Malouin, F., Richards, C., and Doyon, J. (2001). Potential role of mental practice using motor imagery in neurological rehabilitation. *Arch Phys Med Rehabil* **82**: 1133–1141.

Jeannerod, M. and Frak, V. (1999). Mental imaging of motor activity in humans. *Curr Opin Neurobiol* **9**, 735–739.

Johansson, B. B. (2000). Brain plasticity and stroke rehabilitation. The Willis lecture. *Stroke* **31**: 223–230.

Johnson, S. H. (2000). Imagining the impossible: intact motor representations in hemiplegics. *Neuroreport* **11**: 729–732.

Kirkwood, C. A. and Bardsley, G. I. (2001). Seating and positioning in spasticity. In *Upper Motor Neurone Syndrome and Spasticity. Clinical Management and Neurophysiology*, eds. M. P. Barnes and G. R. Johnson. Cambridge: Cambridge University Press, pp. 122–141.

Knott, M. and Voss, D. (1968). *Proprioceptive Neuromuscular Facilitation: Patterns and Techniques*. New York: Harper and Row.

Krebs, H. I., Hogan, N., Volpe, B. T., *et al.* (1999). Overview of clinical trials with MIT-MANUS: a robot-aided neuro-rehabilitation facility. *Technol Health Care* **7**: 419–423.

Krebs, H. I., Volpe, B. T., Aisen, M. L., and Hogan, N. (2000). Robotic applications in neuro-motor rehabilitation. *Top Spinal Cord Inj Rehabil* **5**: 50–63.

Krebs, H. I., Volpe, B. T., Ferraro, M., *et al.* (2002). Robot-aided neurorehabilitation: from evidence-based to science-based rehabilitation *Top Stroke Rehabil* **8**: 54–70.

Kwakkel, G., Wagenaar, R. C., Twisk, J. W., Lankhorst, G. J., and Koetsier, J. C. (1999). Intensity of leg and arm training after primary middle-cerebral-artery stroke: a randomised trial. *Lancet* **354**: 191–196.

Lance, J. (1980). Pathophysiology of spasticity and clinical experience with baclofen. In *Spasticity: Disordered Motor Control*, ed. J. W. Lance, R. G. Feldman, R. R. Young, and W. P. Koella. Chicago: Yearbook, pp. 185–204.

Laufer, Y., Dickstein, R., Chefez, Y., and Marcovitz, E. (2001). The effect of treadmill training on the ambulation of stroke survivors in the elderly stages of rehabilitation: a randomized study. *J Rehabil Res Dev* **38**: 69–78.

Lee, T. D., Swanson, L. R., and Hall, A. L. (1991). What is repeated in a repetition? Effects of practice conditions on motor skill acquisition. *Phys Ther* **71**: 150–156.

Lennon, S. and Ashburn, A. (2000). The Bobath concept in stroke rehabilitation: a focus group study of the experienced physiotherapists' perspective. *Disabil Rehabil* **22**: 665–674.

Lennon, S., Baxter, D., and Ashburn, A. (2001). Physiotherapy based on the Bobath concept in stroke rehabilitation: a survey within the UK. *Disabil Rehabil* **23**: 254–262.

Lennon, S., Ashburn, A., and Baxter, D. (2002). Gait outcome in acute patients following physiotherapy based on the Bobath concept. In *Proceedings of the 3rd World Congress on Neurology and Rehabilitation*, Venice, Italy, p. 251.

Leung, J. and Moseley, A. (2003). Impact of ankle–foot orthoses on gait and leg muscle activity in adults with hemiplegia: systematic literature review. *Physiotherapy* **89**: 39–55.

Levy, C. E., Nichols, D. S., Schmalbrock, P. M., Keller, P., and Chakeres, D. W. (2001). Functional MRI evidence of cortical reorganization in upper-limb stroke hemiplegia treated with constraint-induced movement therapy. *Am J Phys Med Rehabil* **80**: 4–12.

Liepert, J., Bauder, H., Wolfgang, H. R., *et al.* (2000). Treatment-induced cortical reorganization after stroke in humans. *Stroke* **31**: 1210–1216.

Liepert, J., Uhde, I., Gräf, S., Leidner, O., and Weiller, C. (2001). Motor cortex plasticity during forced-use therapy in stroke patients: a preliminary study. *J Neurol* **248**: 315–321.

Macko, R. F., Smith, G. V., Dobrovolny, L., *et al.* (2001). Treadmill training improves fitness reserve in chronic stroke patients. *Arch Phys Med and Rehabil* **82**: 879–884.

Magill, R. A. (2001). *Motor Learning: Concepts and Applications*, 6th edn. Madison, WI: WCB Brown and Benchmark.

Majsak, M. J. (1996). Application of motor learning principles to the stroke population. *Top Stroke Rehabil* **3**: 27–59.

Manning, C. D. and Pomeroy, V. M. (2003). Effectiveness of treadmill training on gait of hemiparetic stroke patients: systematic review of current evidence. *Physiotherapy* **89**: 337–349.

Marteniuk, R. G. (1979). Motor skill performance and learning: considerations for rehabilitation. *Physiother Can* **31**: 187–201.

Martin, K. A., Moritz, S. E., and Hall, C. R. (1999). Imagery use in sport: a literature review and applied model. *Sport Psychol* **13**: 245–268.

Mayston, M. J. (1992). The Bobath concept: evolution and application. In *Movement Disorders in children*, ed. H. Forssberg and H. Hirschfeld. Basel, Karger.

(2002). Problem solving in neurological physiotherapy: setting the scene. In *Neurological Physiotherapy*, 2nd edn, ed. S. Edwards. Edinburgh: Churchill Livingstone, pp. 3–19.

Miltner, W. H. R., Bauder, H., Sommer, M., Dettmers, C., and Taub, E. (1999). Effects of constraint-induced movement therapy on patients with chronic motor deficits after stroke: a replication. *Stroke* **30**: 586–592.

Merians, A. S., Jack, D., Boian, R., *et al.*, (2002). Virtual reality-augmented rehabilitation for patients following stroke. *Phys Ther* **82**: 898–915.

Morris, S. L., Dodd, K. J., and Morris, M. E. (2004). Outcomes of progressive resistance strength training following stroke: a systematic review. *Clin Rehabil* **18**: 27–39.

Moseley, A. (1993). The effect of a regimen of casting and prolonged stretching on passive ankle dorsiflexion in traumatic head-injured adults. *Physiother Theory Pract* **9**: 215–221.

Moseley, A. M., Stark, A, Cameron., I. D., and Pollock., A. (2003). Treadmill training and body weight support for walking after stroke. In *Cochrane Database of Systematic Reviews*, Issue 2: CD 002840. Chichester, UK: Wiley.

Mudge, S. and Rochester, L. (2001). Neurophysiological rationale of treadmill training: evaluating evidence for practice. *NZ J Physiother* **29**: 7–17.

Nelles, G., Jentzen, W., Jueptner, M., Müller, S., and Diener, H. C. (2001). Arm training induced brain plasticity in stroke studied with serial positron emission tomography. *Neuroimage* **13**: 1146–1154.

Nilsson, L. M. and Nordholm, L. A. (1992). Physical therapy in stroke rehabilitation: bases for Swedish physiotherapists' choice of treatment *Physiother Theory Pract* **8**: 49–55.

Obermaier, B., Muller, G., and Pfurtscheller, G. (2001). "Virtual keyboard" controlled by spontaneous EEG activity. *Lect Notes Comp Sci* **2130**: 636–641.

Ostendorf, C. G. and Wolf, S. L. (1981). Effect of forced use of the upper extremity of a hemiplegic patient on changes in function *Phys Ther* **61**: 1022–1028.

Paci, M. (2003). Physiotherapy based on the Bobath concept for adults with post-stroke hemiplegia: a review of effectiveness studies. *J Rehabil Med* **35**: 2–7

Page, S. J., Sisto, S. A., Levine, P., Johnston, M. V., and Hughes, M. (2001a). Modified constraint induced therapy: a randomized feasibility and efficacy study. *J Rehabil Res Dev* **38**: 583–590.

Page, S. J., Levine, P., Sisto, S. A., and Johnston, M. V. (2001b). A randomized efficacy and feasibility study of imagery in acute stroke. *Clin Rehabil* **15**: 233–240.

Page, S. J., Levine, P., Sisto, S., Bond, Q., and Johnston, M. V. (2002a). Stroke patients' and therapists' opinions of constraint-induced movement therapy. *Clin Rehabil* **16**: 55–60.

Page, S. J., Sisto, S. A., and Levine, P. (2002b). Modified constraint-induced therapy in chronic stroke. *Am J Phys Med Rehabil* **81**: 870–875.

Pandyan, A., Johnson, G., Price, C., *et al.* (1999). A review of the properties and limitations of the Ashworth and modified Ashworth Scales as measures of spasticity. *Clin Rehabil* **13**: 373–383.

Pandyan, D., Vuadens, P., van Wijck, F., *et al.* (2002). Are we underestimating the clinical efficacy of botulinum toxin (type A)? Quantifying changes in spasticity, strength and upper limb function after injections of Botox to the elbow flexors in a unilateral stroke population. *Clin Rehabil* **16**: 654–660.

Partridge, C. (2002). The way forward. In *Neurological Physiotherapy*, 2nd edn., ed. S. Edwards., Edinburgh: Churchill Livingstone, pp. 275–284.

Pfurtscheller, G. and Neuper, C. (2001). Motor imagery and direct brain-computer communication. *Proc IEEE* **89**: 1123–1134.

Pohl, M., Mehrholz, J., Ritschel, C., and Rickriem, S. (2002). Speed-dependent treadmill training in ambulatory hemiparetic stroke patients: a randomized controlled trial. *Stroke* **33**: 553–558.

Pollock, A. (1998). An investigation into independent practice as an addition to physiotherapy intervention for patients with recently acquired stroke. Ph. D. Thesis, Queen Margaret University College, Edinburgh, UK.

Pollock, A., Baer, G., Pomeroy, V., and Langhorne, P. (2003). Physiotherapy treatment approaches for the recovery of postural control and lower limb function following stroke *Cochrane Database of Systematic Reviews*, CD 001920.

Pomeroy, V. M. and Tallis, R. C. (2002a). Restoring movement and functional ability after stroke: now and the future. *Physiotherapy* **88**: 3–17.

Pomeroy, V. and Tallis, R. (2002b). Neurological rehabilitation: a science struggling to come of age. *Physiother Res Int* **7**: 76–89.

Pomeroy, V. D., D. Sykes, L. Faragher, *et al.* (2000). The unreliability of clinical measures of muscle tone: implications for stroke therapy. *Age Ageing* **29**: 229–233.

Pope, P. M. (2002). Posture management and seating. In *Neurological Physiotherapy*, 2nd edn. ed. S. Edwards. Edinburgh: Churchill Livingstone, pp. 189–218.

Potempa, K., Braun, L. T., Tinknell, T., and Popovitch, J. (1996). Benefits of aerobic exercise after stroke. *Sports Med* **21**: 337–346.

Price, C. I. M. and Pandyan, A. D. (2001). Electrical stimulation for preventing and treating post-stroke shoulder pain: a systematic Cochrane review. *Clin Rehabil* **15**: 5-19.

Read, J. (1992). *Conductive Education 1987–1992: The Transitional Years*. Birmingham, UK: The Foundation for conductive Education.

Reiter, F., Danni, M., Lagalla, G., and Ceravolo, G. (1998). Low-dose botulinum toxin with ankle taping for the treatment of spastic equinovarus foot after stroke. *Arch Phys Med Rehabil* **79**: 532–535.

Richardson, D. and Thompson, A. J. (1999). Botulinum toxin, its use in the treatment of acquired spasticity in adults. *Physiotherapy*, **85**: 541–551.

Rood, M. S. (1956). Neurophysiological mechanisms utilized in the treatment of neuromuscular dysfunction. *Am J Occup Ther* **10**: 220–224.

Sackley, C. M. and Lincoln, N. B. (1996). Physiotherapy for stroke patients: a survey of current practice. *Physiother Theory Pract*: **12**: 87–96.

Saunders, D. H., Greig, C. A., Young A., and Mead, G. E. (2004). Physical fitness training for stroke patients. *Cochrane Database of Systematic Reviews*, Issue 1. CD003316. pub2.

Saunders, D. H., Greig, C. A., Young, A., and Mead, G. E. (2004). Physical fitness training for stroke patients. In *Cochrane Database of Systematic Reviews*, Issue 2. Chichester, UK: Wiley.

Sawner, K. A. and LaVigne, J. M. (1992). *Brunnstrom's Movement Therapy in Hemiplegia: A Neurophysiological Approach*, 2nd edn. New York: Lippincott.

Schmidt, R. A. and Lee, T. D. (1999). *Motor Control and Learning, a Behavioral Emphasis*. Champaign, IL: Human Kinetics.

Sheean, G. L. (1997). The management of spasticity with botulinum toxin. *Eur J Neurol* **4** (Suppl. 2): S41–S44.

(2001). Neurophysiology of spasticity. In *Upper Motor Neurone Syndrome and Spasticity. Clinical Management and Neurophysiology*, ed. M. P. Barnes and G. R. Johnson. Cambridge, UK: Cambridge University Press, pp. 12–78.

Simpson, D. A., O'Brien, D. N., Tagliati, C. F., *et al.* (1996). Botulinum toxin type A in the treatment of upper extremity spasticity: a randomized, double-blind, placebo-controlled trial. *Neurology*; **46**: 1306–1310.

Simpson, D. M. (1997). Clinical trials of botulinum toxin in the treatment of spasticity. *Muscle Nerve Suppl* **6**: S169–S175.

Sisto, S. A., Forrest, G. F., and Glendinning, D. (2002). Virtual reality applications for motor rehabilitation after stroke. *Top Stroke Rehabil* **8**: 11–23.

Stark, S. C. (2001). Product focus. Physiotherapy and botulinum toxin in spasticity management. *B. J. Ther Rehabil* **8**: 386–392.

Stoeckmann, T. (2001). Casting for the person with spasticity. *Top Stroke Rehabil* **8**: 27–35.

Stokes, M. (2004). *Neurological Physiotherapy*, 2nd edn. London: Mosby, in press.

Sullivan, K. J., Knowlton, B. J., and Dobkin, B. H. (2002). Step training with body weight support: effect of treadmill speed and practice paradigms on post-stroke locomotor recovery. *Arch Phys Med Rehabil* **83**: 683–691.

Tangeman, P. T., Banaitis, D. A., and Williams, A. K. (1990). Rehabilitation of chronic stroke patients: changes in functional performance. *Arch Phys Med Rehabil* **71**: 876–880.

Taub, E. (1980). Somatosensory deafferentation research with monkeys: implications for rehabilitation medicine. In *Behavioral Psychology in Rehabilitation Medicine: Clinical Applications*. New York: Williams and Wilkins, pp. 371–401.

Taub, E. and Uswatte, G. (2003). Constraint-induced movement therapy: bridging from the primate laboratory to the stroke rehabilitation laboratory. *J Rehabil Med* **41**(Suppl.): 34–40.

Taub, E., Miller, N. E., Novack, T. A., *et al.* (1993). Technique to improve chronic motor deficit after stroke. *Arch Phys Med Rehabil* **74**: 347–354.

Taub, E., Uswatte, G., and Pidikiti, R. (1999). Constraint induced movement therapy: a new family of techniques with broad application to physical rehabilitation : a clinical review. *J Rehabil Res Dev* **36**: 237–251.

Taylor, D. C., Dalton, J. D., Seaber, A. V., and Garrett, W. E. (1990). Viscoelastic properties of muscle–tendon units. *Am J Sports Med* **18**: 300–309.

Taylor, P. N., Burridge, J. H., Dunkerley, A. L., *et al.* (1999). Patients' perceptions of the Odstock Dropped Foot Stimulator (ODFS). *Clin Rehabil* **13**: 439–446.

Teixeira-Salmela, L. F., Nadeau, S., McBride, I., and Olney, S. J. (2001). Effects of muscle strengthening and physical conditioning training on temporal, kinematic and kinetic variables during gait in chronic stroke survivors. *J Rehabil Med* **33**: 53–60.

Tremblay, F, Tremblay, L. E, and Colcer, D. E. (2001). Modulation of corticospinal excitability during imagined knee movements. *J Rehabil Med* **33**: 230–234.

van der Lee, J. H, Snels, I. A, Beckerman, H., *et al.* (2001). Exercise therapy for arm function in stroke patients: a systematic review of randomized controlled trials. *Clin Rehabil* **15**: 20–31.

van der Lee, J. H., Wagenaar, R. C., Lankhorst, G. J., *et al.* (1999). Forced use of the upper extremity in chronic stroke patients; results from a single blind randomised clinical trial. *Stroke* **30**: 2369–2375.

van Leeuwen, R. and Inglis, J. T. (1998). Mental practice and imagery: a potential role in stroke rehabilitation. *Phys Ther Rev* **3**: 47–52.

Van Sant, A. F. (1991). Neurodevelopmental treatment and pediatric physical therapy: a commentary. *Pediatr Phys Ther* **3**: 137–141.

van Wijck, F., Mackenzie, J., Hooper, J., Barnes, M. P., and Johnson, G. R. (2004). Improving arm function in patients with chronic spasticity: combining botulinum toxin with a task-orientated motor learning program. *Int J Rehabil Res* **27**(Suppl.1): 109.

Visintin, M., Barbeau, H., Korner-Bitensky, N., and Mayo, N. E. (1998). A new approach to retrain gait in stroke patients through body weight support and treadmill stimulation. *Stroke* **29**: 1122–1128.

Volpe, B. T., Krebs, H. I., Hogan, N., *et al.* (2000). A novel approach to stroke rehabilitation: robot-aided sensorimotor stimulation. *Neurol* **54**: 1938–1944.

Volpe, B. T., Krebs, H. I., and Hogan, N. (2001). Is robot-aided sensorimotor training in stroke rehabilitation a realistic option? *Curr Opin Neurol* **14**: 745–752.

Wade, D. T. (1999). Goal planning in stroke rehabilitation: evidence. *Top Stroke Rehabil* **6**: 37–42.

Wade, D. T., Langton-Hewer, R., Wood, V. A., Skilbeck, C., and Ismail, H. M. (1983). The hemiplegic arm after stroke: measurement and recovery. *J Neurol Neurosurg Psychiatry* **46**: 521–524.

Wade, D. T., Collen, FM, Robb, G. F., and Warlow, C. P., (1992). Physiotherapy intervention late after stroke: and mobility. *BMJ* **304**: 609–613.

Wagenaar, R. C., Meijer, O. G., van Wieringen, P. C. W., *et al.* (1990). The functional recovery of stroke: a comparison between neuro-developmental treatment and the Brunnstrom method. *Scand J Rehabil Med* **22**: 1–8.

Watkins, C. A. (1999). Mechanical and neurophysiological changes in spastic muscles: serial casting in spastic equinovarus following traumatic brain injury *Physiotherapy* **85**: 603–609.

Winstein, C. J. (1991a). Knowledge of results and motor learning : implications for physical therapy. *Phys Ther* **71**: 140–149.

(1991b). Designing practice for motor learning: clinical implications. In *Proceedings of the II STEP Conference Contemporary Management of Motor Control Problems* ed. M. J. Lister. Alexandra, VA: Foundation for Physical Theropy, pp. 65–76.

Winstein, C. J., Merians, A. S., and Sullivan, K. J. (1999). Motor learning after unilateral brain damage. *Neuropsychologia* **37**: 975–987.

Wissel, J., Muller, J., Dressnandt, J., *et al.* (2000). Management of spasticity associated pain with botulinum toxin A. *J Pain Symptom Manage* **20**: 44–49.

Wolf, S. L., Lecraw, D. E., Barton, L. A., and Jann, B. B. (1989). Forced use of hemiplegic upper extremities to reverse the effect of learned nonuse among chronic stroke and head-injured patients. *Exp Neurol* **104**: 125–132.

Zorowitz, R. D., Idank, D., Ikai, T., Hughes, M. B., and Johnston, M. V. (1995). Shoulder subluxation after stroke: a comparison of four supports. *Arch Phys Med Rehabil* **76**: 763–771.

11

Abnormal movements after stroke

Joseph Ghika

Centre Hospitalier Universitaire Vaudois, Lausanne, Switzerland

Introduction

Acute, paroxysmal, recurrent, transient, permanent, progressive, or delayed movement disorders have been occasionally reported in the acute phase of stroke as well as after a delay of up to months or years (Kitanaka *et al.*, 1995; Scott and Jankovic, 1996). Almost any type of hyperkinetic or hypokinetic movement disorder has been reported, most commonly as hemi- or focal dyskinesia. Only isolated case reports or very small series can be found in the literature, and few epidemiological studies (D'Olhaberriague *et al.*, 1995; Ghika-Schmid *et al.*, 1997) have been performed to estimate the prevalence of movement disorders in cerebrovascular disease. However, what is clear in all studies is that any kind of dyskinesia can be found with lesions at any level of the motor frontosubcortical circuits of Alexander *et al.*, (1986), including the sensorimotor cortex, caudate, putamen, pallidum, subthalamic nuclei, thalamus, brainstem and interconnecting pathways (reviewed by Bhatia and Marsden, 1994).

Hypokinetic syndromes

Vascular parkinsonism

Critchley (1929) introduced the concept of arteriosclerotic parkinsonism, characterized by clinical and pathological criteria, but his definition of this "disorder of the pallidal system" with "general rigidity of non-pyramidal type, weakness and slowness of movement" is somewhat different from what is accepted in the definition of the parkinsonian syndrome (requiring at least two items of bradykinesia, tremor, rigidity, and loss of balance or postural responses).

Parkinsonism of vascular origin is a controversial entity. Only 2% of patients with cerebral infarcts may have a parkinsonian syndrome (Takeuchi *et al.*, 1992). Acute hemiparkinsonism has been recently reported with infarcts in the area of

Recovery after Stroke, ed. Michael P. Barnes, Bruce H. Dobkin and Julien Bogousslavsky. Published by Cambridge University Press. © Cambridge University Press 2005.

the anterior cerebral artery (Kim, 2001a), large infarcts in the territory of the lenticulostriate arteries, sometimes in association with stereotyped movements (Kulisevsky *et al.*, 1996), and exceptionally, in bilateral vascular lesions of the substantia nigra (Inoue *et al.*, 1997). Subacute or delayed parkinsonism can occur after anoxia (postanoxic parkinsonism is also a well-known entity (Li *et al.*, 2000) but it is rare to happen after a unilateral striatal infarct (Lazzarino *et al.*, 1990).

In the 1960s and 1970s, the concept of vascular parkinsonism was discarded (reviewed by Parkes *et al.*, 1974). However, it is well recognized (since the advent of computed tomography [CT] and magnetic resonance imaging [MRI]) that diffuse lesions of the hemispheric white and/or gray matter, lacunar states, senile or hypertensive leukoencephalopathy, or multiple infarcts can present with bradykinesia, akinesia, mixed features of rigidity and spasticity, loss of balance or gait disorder; these can easily be confused with a parkinsonian syndrome. As pointed out by Critchley (1929), incomplete forms are more common but generalized rigidity, pure akinesia, or bradykinesia can be found. The "*syndrome strié du vieillard*" of Lhermitte (1922), or "arteriosclerotic pseudoparkinsonism" (Critchley, 1981) has also been widely reported by others (Yamanouchi and Nagura, 1997, van Zagten *et al.*, 1998), but the border between this entity and the ill-defined "senile gait disorders" or "lower body parkinsonism" still remains to be delimited (Nutt *et al.*, 1993). However, strategic infarcts or hemorrhage in the mesencephalon can lead to true vascular parkinsonism (Inoue *et al.*, 1997).

Wide variation in case definitions do not allow a precise delineation of prevalence of vascular parkinsonism (Foltynie *et al.*, 2002). The association of "arteriosclerosis" and parkinsonism has been studied but does not seem to be significant (Horner *et al.*, 1997; Homann and Ott, 1997). The parkinsonism reported in association with cerebrovascular lesions corresponds to a clinical entity that differs from the parkinsonian syndrome of degenerative origin. Generally, the symptoms tend to be generalized and not lateralized initially, with ictal, slowly progressive (Nakamura *et al.*, 1999a, b), stepwise or insidious onset or progression. Pseudobulbar signs, brisk reflexes, Babinski signs, sphincter incontinence, and dementia are commonly associated, but ataxia is less frequent. Tremor is characteristically absent unless the patient has essential tremor (Critchley, 1981), but it has been reported (Holmes, 1904). The rigidity is generally of "sticky" or "lead pipe type" with no cogwheel, and characteristically variable in degree (with paratonia or *gegenhalten*), and the topographic distribution of the hypertonia is more suggestive of spastic antigravity muscles than in parkinsonism. Bradykinesia, akinesia, and hypokinesia are typically found. Micrography has also been reported, but frequent synkineses or mirror movements are common when patients are performing rapid alternating movements. Hypophonic, dysarthric, monotonous, pallilalic, monosyllabic or elliptic speech may be present, and sometimes frank mutism. Features of bulbar speech can be found. A "mask facies with an expression of bewilderment, elevated eyebrows, retracted lids and gaping mouth, accounting for a mixture of spastic and extrapyramidal face" (Critchley, 1929) has been reported, but sebaceous secretion is generally absent. The "*marche à petits pas*" or Petren gait (Petren 1901, 1902) can sometimes be confused with parkinsonian gait; however, stooped posture and excessive flexion of hip and knee are usually absent; both arms are frequently held rigidly away from the sides, with variable loss of armswing. Associated movements occur at the shoulder joint, and en-bloc turn is present, the steps being exceptionally short and the feet are not lifted from the ground. However, festination and propulsion generally do not occur, and the base is not massively increased. Apraxia and magnetism of the feet to the ground can be found. Tandem gait is generally impossible. Retropulsion can be massive. The overall extrapyramidal syndrome predominates in the lower body and in the proximal segments of the limbs, usually symmetrically. Dubinsky and Jankovic (1987), Winitakes and Jankovic (1994), and others (Josephs *et al.*, 2002) have described a syndrome resembling progressive supranuclear palsy in a patient with a multiinfarct state, sometimes called "vascular supranuclear palsy" or multiinfarct Progressive Supranucleat Palsy (Dubinsky and Jankovic, 1987).

A history of hypertension and/or diabetes mellitus is present in most patients and CT or MRI images clearly show multiple small deep infarcts and white matter changes. Convincing cases of sudden parkinsonian syndrome of vascular etiology with bilateral basal ganglia ischemic lesions have been described in patients with bilateral thalamic infarcts, and bilateral putaminal infarcts, and bilateral caudate infarcts (Tolosa and Santamaria, 1984).

In any event, while the clinical picture of atypical parkinsonian syndromes in a patient with multiple vascular lesions on CT and MRI does exist, the diagnosis of vascular parkinsonism is essentially made by exclusion, and the final diagnosis can only be made on pathological examination. Few pathological studies show ischemic involvement of the substantia nigra in status cribrosus, multilacunar state, and hypertensive or senile leukoencephalopathy, but the striatum is generally involved (Jellinger, 1996). Denny-Brown (1962) reported vascular lesions in the putamen in one-third of patients with "diffuse microangiopathic disease." In other studies, however, there were Lewy bodies in the substantia nigra of patients with cerebrovascular disease and parkinsonism, illustrating the difficulty in separating the entities without pathological studies (Escourolle *et al.*, 1970). The absence of response to antiparkinsonian medication relates to postsynaptic damage with involvement of striatopallidal structures, making it difficult to differentiate this condition from multiple system atrophy.

Senile gait disorders

Higher level gait disorders (Nutt *et al.*, 1993; Thajeb, 1993) can be found in patients with generalized small vessel disease.

"Subcortical disequilibrium" is characterized by disequilibrium with absent or inefficient postural responses and hyperextension of axial muscles with retropulsion, but stepping is possible. Astasia-abasia, thalamic astasia (Masdeu and Gorelick, 1988), or tottering are synonymous for this type of gait disorder, which can be acute or insidious with lesions in basal ganglia, thalamus, and midbrain.

"Frontal disequilibrium," also known as trunk or gait apraxia, frontal apraxia of Bruns, or astasia-abasia, is defined by disequilibrium; inappropriate or counterproductive postural and locomotor synergies; and inability to stand, sit, or to rise from a chair, with severe retropulsion and crossing of the legs. These patients cannot walk and step or turn. Bilateral corticospinal signs, corticobulbar and frontal syndromes as well as incontinence are frequently associated.

In "isolated gait ignition failure" (also known as gait apraxia, magnetic gait, slipping clutch gait, lower body parkinsonism, trepidant abasia, Petren's gait, or isolated progressive freezing, the steps are short; shuffling occurs, with hesitation in starting and turning, variable freezing, and variable base. Once this difficulty in starting to walk has been overcome, the gait is almost normal, with normal posture, stride base, stride length, and armswing, until the need to turn. Isolated freezing, start hesitation, or turn hesitation can be found.

Frontal gait disorder or *marche à petits pas* is characterized by variable base, hesitation in starting or turning, and short steps with shuffling and disequilibrium. Apraxia of sitting can be isolated. Cautious gait (elderly gait or senile gait) is defined by shortened stride with slowing, mild disequilibrium, difficulty in balancing on one foot, normal or wide base, and en bloc turn, but there is no hesitation, shuffling, or freezing. The stance phase is longer, with short swing phase, increased number of steps anteroposterior swinging, and preserved rhythm, but loss of postural responses. Mixed peripheral and central nervous system disorders are frequently found. Posture, standing from a sitting position, equilibrium, postural reflexes, and protective reactions are normal.

Catalepsy, motor neglect and hypokinesia, and other akinetic syndromes

Asymmetric cataleptic posturing, more prominent in the left side, was found in a patient with a large frontoparietal infarct (Saver *et al.*, 1993) and has been frequently observed in parietal strokes (Ghika *et al.*, 1998). The patient maintains for minutes postures passively produced by the examiner or actively performed, even though they are uncomfortable. Hemihypokinesia is also found in right hemispheric strokes (von Giesen *et al.*, 1994) as part of motor hemineglect, in basal ganglia strokes (von Giesen *et al.*, 1994), including the thalamus (Verret and Lapresle, 1986), and with catatonia in biparietal infarcts (Howard and Low-Beer, 1989). Isolated micrographia has been described in a lenticular hematoma (Martinez-Vila *et al.*, 1988; Derkindeeren *et al.*, 2002). Motor impersistance can also be seen in right hemisphere strokes (de Renzi *et al.*, 1986).

Athymormia, loss of self-autoactivation, apathy, abulia, and other akinetic syndromes such as akinetic mutism can be found in association with bilateral basal ganglia infarcts, hemorrhage, or deep venous thrombosis (Mega and Cohenour, 1997; Laplane and Dubois 1998), with thalamic infarcts (Tanaka *et al.*, 1986; Bogousslavsky *et al.*, 1991), with uni- or bilateral capsular genu infarcts (Yamanaka *et al.*, 1996), with midbrain infarcts or bilateral cingulate hemorrhage (Miyashi *et al.*, 1995; von Domburg *et al.*, 1996), with vertebrobasilar transient ischemic attacks (Price *et al.*, 1983), or with basal forebrain or frontal strokes (Okawa *et al.*, 1980; Calvanio *et al.*, 1993).

Hyperkinetic mutism is also reported (Hesselink *et al.*, 1987).

Hyperkinetic movement disorders

Dystonia

Dystonia is defined as a persistent inappropriate posture (dystonic posture) at rest or on action, in overflexion, overextension, or rotation by prolonged co-contraction of antagonist muscles or simply by tonic contraction of focal muscles, sometimes associated with tremor-like motion (dystonic tremor), myoclonic or athetotic snake-like movements (dystonic movements).

Acute dystonia

Acute hemidystonia has been reported in association with acute strokes. On CT, MRI, or pathology, large parietal or frontal infarcts have been reported (Marsden *et al.*, 1985). Small infarcts or hematomas have also been found in the motor frontosubcortical circuit including the caudate and lenticular nuclei (pallidum and putamen) (Kostic *et al.*, 1996; Kelley *et al.*, 2000), but particularly in the putamen (Bhatia and Marsden, 1994; Casas-Parera *et al.*, 1994; Girlanda *et al.*, 1997). Lesions have also been reported in posterior and lateral thalamic nuclei (Ghika *et al.*, 1998; Kim, 2001b), in the parietal and frontal cortex (Ghika-Schmid *et al.*, 1997), in brainstem (Kulisevky *et al.*, 1993), and in cerebellar infarction (Rumbach *et al.*, 1995).

Focal hand or foot dystonia has been found in patients with lacunar infarctions in the lenticular or caudate nuclei (Karsidag *et al.*, 1998; Deleu *et al.*, 2000) in the thalamus (the "thalamic hand or "*signe de la main creuse*") (Karsidag *et al.*, 1998), in superficial parietal lobe infarcts (Ghika *et al.*, 1998; Burguera *et al.*, 2001), and less frequently, in the territory of the anterior cerebral artery. Shoulder girdle dystonia has been associated with thalamic infarcts (Wali, 1999). Posthemiplegic focal hand dystonia is frequent but not well studied (Apaydin *et al.*, 1998; Factor *et al.*, 1988).

Focal foot dystonia after an infarct in the territory of the anterior cerebral artery has been reported in one patient (Boisson *et al.*, 1981). One patient with focal facial and lingual dystonia was reported by Zeman and Whitlock (1968); cephalic dystonia (Meige syndrome or jaw-opening dystonia) has been reported in association with a brainstem (Dietrichs *et al.*, 2000), thalamic (Domzal and Zaleska, 2001), or caudate (Arunabh *et al.*, 1992) infarcts, and jaw dystonia has been found together with basilar artery thrombosis (Nishi *et al.*, 1985) or, less frequently, parietal infarcts (Jacob and Chand, 1997). So-called "apraxia of lid opening" is probably also a focal blepharospasm and is associated with vascular lesions of the basal ganglia (Lepore and Duvoisin 1985). Keane and Young (1985) and others (Larumbe *et al.*, 1993) have reported a blepharospasm in bilateral basal ganglia infarcts and Kulisevsky *et al.*, (1993) described it in a thalamomesencephalic stroke.

Patients with cervical dystonia of acute onset have also been reported (LeDoux and Brady 2003).

Generalized dystonia after a stroke has been reported, with or without concomitant choreoathetosis (Zeman and Whitlock, 1968).

Painful repetitive tonic spasms, described as "sudden, vigorous muscle spasm, preceded or accompanied by pain in the same limb" affecting the arm more often than the leg and facial grimacing, lasting a few seconds to minutes, have been reported in patients with putaminal infarcts from various etiologies (lupus erythematosus and other vasculitis; Merchut and Brumlik, 1986). The spasms can be spontaneous or triggered by various stimuli (anxiety, hyperventilation, physical activity, or sensory stimuli). Various generalized "tetanic postures" of the limb can be found during the spasm.

Paroxysmal kinesigenic dystonia has been described in a medullary infarct (Riley, 1996) and a thalamocapsular infarct (Uterga *et al.*, 1999), and action-induced rhythmic dystonia in a thalamic stroke (Sunohara *et al.*, 1984).

Delayed hemidystonia

Posthemiplegic hemidystonia may develop months or years after hemiplegia of vascular origin (Chuang *et al.*, 2002) in association with putaminocaudate infarcts on CT (Choi *et al.*, 1993) and on MRI (Burton *et al.*, 1984) and, less frequently, with capsulothalamic lesions (Ghika *et al.*, 1995a; Ghika-Schmid *et al.*, 1997).

Chorea and ballism

Hemichorea–hemiballism

Hemichorea–hemiballism is certainly the most frequently reported movement disorder in acute stroke. It can be acute or delayed after stroke (Kim, 2001b).

Hemiballism is defined as a severe, involuntary, very fast, arrhythmic, explosive, large-amplitude excursion of the limb at proximal joints, with an element of rotation in the movement; it is possibly present at rest but is increased by any attempt to move. Patients may attempt to fixate the affected limb with the uninvolved side and can be exhausted by these explosive motions, especially if they have chronic cardiac failure. The movements generally predominate in one limb and may be strictly unilateral. They disappear during sleep.

Hemichorea is characterized by unilateral rapid involuntary motion with flexion and extension, rotation or crossing; it may involve all body parts but predominantly distal areas, with fluent distal-to-proximal or proximal-to-distal march. There may be some grimacing of the face, tongue protrusion, and vocalization. Patients frequently use the involuntary movement in a semipurposeful manner, as if they were hiding them, or will hold the moving limb with the good one.

Kase *et al.* (1981) proposed the name hemichorea–hemiballism.

Some degree of dystonia (persistent postures in overflexion, overextension, or torsion), and athetosis (inability to maintain fixed postures with slow snake-like motions) can be added. Patients have been described with associated corticospinal, sensory, ataxic, neuropsychological, or even psychiatric features (like mania) (Kulisevsky *et al.*, 1993).

The syndrome of hemichorea–hemiballism is generally transient, lasting a few days or, less commonly, weeks (Reimer and Knuppel, 1963); it can, rarely, be persistent (Lang, 1985) or recurring (Goldblatt *et al.*, 1974). It responds well generally to neuroleptic drugs (Klawans *et al.*, 1976).

Classically, acute hemichorea and its variants are found after an acute small deep infarct or hemorrhage in the contralateral subthalamic nucleus (Bhatia and Marsden 1994; Lee and Marsden, 1994), sometimes ipsilaterally (Crozier *et al.*, 1996); however, it can occur any location in the motor frontosubcortical circuit of Alexander *et al.* (1986) (i.e. from the caudate to putamen), pallidum (Kelley *et al.*, 2000; Ballassoued *et al.*, 2001), bilateral pallidum (Ichikawa *et al.*, 1980), thalamus (Kim *et al.*, 1999; Lera *et al.*, 2000), and pathways interconnecting these nuclei, including corona radiata (Fukui *et al.*, 1993). It is also seen with frontal lobe (Papez *et al.*, 1942), parietal lobe (Rossetti *et al.*, 2003), or watershed infarcts (Lee *et al.*, 2000a). It is seen less often in those with primary hemorrhage or hemorrhagic infarcts in the same loci than in those with ischemic strokes

(Ghika-Schmid *et al.*, 1997). Exceptionally, an angioma can be discovered (Tamaoka *et al.*, 1987). Hemichorea associated with ipsilateral chronic subdural hematoma has also been reported (Yoshikawa *et al.*, 1992).

Transient or paroxysmal hemiballism can be found in association with a stroke (Blakeley and Jankovic, 2002). It has been considered as a vertebrobasilar transient ischemic attack by a few authors (Margolin and Marsden, 1982) and a patient with transient hemiballismus associated with subclavian steal syndrome has been reported (Calzetti *et al.*, 1980).

Paraballism, diballism, generalized choreo-ballism

Paraballism (biballism, diballism, or generalized choreo-ballism) has been reported in patients with bilateral deep hemorrhage (Lodder and Baard, 1981) or infarcts (Vila and Chamorro 1997): sometimes in substantia nigra bilaterally (Caparros-Lefebvre *et al.*, 1994), bilateral thalamus (Rondot *et al.*, 1986), unilateral caudate (Goldblatt *et al.*, 1989), or subcortical white matter near the subthalmic nucleus (Nicolai and Lazzarino, 1994). One patient presented a clinical picture suggestive of Huntington's disease (Folstein *et al.*, 1981). On postmortem examination, he had multiple small infarcts in the caudate, putamen, and internal capsule.

Monochorea and monoballism

Monochorea or monoballism confined to one limb have been reported (Ikeda and Tsukagoshi, 1991) in association with striatal, subthalamic, or thalamic infarcts (Ito *et al.*, 2000).

Delayed hemichorea

Delayed posthemiplegic hemichorea is a rare entity. It has been reported years after a stroke involving the basal ganglia (Dooling and Adams, 1975). It should be considered in patients with transient hemichorea.

Athetosis

Athetosis is rarely found in association with acute stroke. Delayed syndromes after perinatal anaoxia are well recognized (Dooling and Adams, 1975). Athetosis is now considered as the distal presentation of slow dystonic movements and postures. It can be associated with chorea. It can be paroxysmal (Blakeley and Jankovic, 2002), uni- or bilateral or focal (Ito *et al.*, 2000) or, rarely, acute (Clark *et al.*, 1995). Striatal (Ghika *et al.*, 1998; Kim, 2001a), thalamic (Tan *et al.*, 2001a, b), parietal (Ghika *et al.*, 1998), and watershed (Lee *et al.*, 2000a, b) infarcts are mostly reponsible for this symptomatology. Thalamic hand is probably one of the presentations.

Pseudoathetosis

Pseudoathetosis (dystonic distal movements as a result of severe loss of proprioception) can be found in association with lesions in the parietal lobe, thalamus, brainstem, or spinal cord and causes severe proprioceptive deficits (Ghika *et al.*, 1995b, 1998; Kim *et al.*, 1999).

Tremor

Acute tremor

Tremor is exceptionally reported as an acute event in strokes. Rarely, it can be very violent (Frates *et al.*, 2001) or delayed (Kim, 2001b). Most of the time, the tremor is contralateral to the lesion, but ipsilateral tremor has been reported (Imai *et al.*, 1997). Benedikt's syndrome (1989), associating a resting and action tremor of 3–4 Hz with a contralateral corticospinal deficit, is rarely seen in small mesencephalic infarcts or hemorrhage (Kalita *et al.*, 1999). Pontine strokes with tremor are exceptional (Shepherd *et al.*, 1997). An acute resting tremor has been reported in a patient with a lacunar infarction at the border between the thalamus and the internal capsule (Lee *et al.*, 1993) in patients with an infarct in the lateral or posterior thalamus (Frates *et al.*, 2001; Tan *et al.*, 2001a, b) and, more exceptionally, in the anterior thalamus (Cho and Samkoff, 2000). Postural tremor has also been reported after thalamic infarction (Soler *et al.*, 1999). Subthalamic infarcts can be accompanied by an acute resting and action tremor (Febert and Gerwig, 1991) or by myoclonus (Kao *et al.*, 1999). Rarely, caudate or striatum (Brannan *et al.*, 1999), frontal, parietal (Ghika *et al.*, 1998), corona radiata (Dethy *et al.*, 1993), thalamus border with the internal capsule (Lee *et al.*, 1993), or cerebellar strokes are reported (Yanagisawa *et al.*, 1999). Most are children, or adults with stroke, in whom tremor develops during the acute phase or within weeks (Quaglieri *et al.*, 1977) or years (Burke *et al.*, 1980) after the ischemic lesion.

Palatal tremor generally occurs after laterobulbar or cerebella–brainstem posterior inferior cerebellarn arterial strokes or hemorrhages (Yanagisawa *et al.*, 1999). Head tremors described as "yes–yes" or tremor-like movement of the neck have been reported in bilateral cerebellar (Finsterer *et al.*, 1996), thalamic, or midbrain (Otto *et al.*, 1995) infarcts. Writing tremor after a cortical frontal infarct can rarely occur (Kim and Lee, 1994).

Delayed tremor

Progressive tremor, chorea, and dystonia seven years after stroke has been reported by Burke *et al.* (1980) in a boy. Intention, action, and postural tremor was found in a boy with venous sinus thrombosis with bilateral thalamic involvement (Solomon *et al.*, 1982). Delayed tremor has also been reported after a stroke in posterior thalamic nuclei (Ferbert and Gerwig, (1991), and in the cerebellar outflow tracts in the brainstem (Scott and Jankovic, 1996). Delayed tremor, with choreo-athetotic and ballistic features, has been described months after a stroke in patients with posterior thalamic infarcts in the territory of the posterior choroidal artery (Ghika et al., 1994; Ghika-Schmid et al., 1997), the thalamogeniculate artery (Ghika-Schmid et al., 1997), and, exceptionally, in the territory of the anterior choroidal artery (Bogousslavsky and Regli 1986). Delayed tremor has also been described in giant cell arteritis (Caselli et al., 1988), rarely in cortical frontal or parietal strokes (Ghika et al., 1998), in cerebellar infarcts (Louis et al., 1996), and, less frequently, after parieto-occipital strokes (Dove et al., 1994).

Transient, paroxysmal, and episodic dyskinesia

Paroxysmal, episodic or transient dyskinesia can be symptoms of transient cerebral ischemia in the territory of the internal carotid artery or the vertebrobasilar system. Repetitive stereotyped, often complex, involuntary limb movements have been reported in the literature as associated with carotid transient ischemic attacks. The movements are described as rhythmic or arrhythmic, uncontrollable, transient, and lasting a few seconds to minutes; they are elicited by sitting, standing, or stress, rarely kinesigenic (Loiseau, 1969) or progressive (Solomon et al., 1982). Orthostatic "limb shaking" spells have been described, with involuntary, uncontrollable shaking, coarse irregular wavering, flapping, circling, flailing-type lateral excursions, drawing up or trembling of the upper and/or lower extremity on one hemibody or bilaterally, sometimes with pseudo-jacksonian march, sometimes difficult to be distinguished from epileptic seizures (Schulz and Rothwell 2002). Flexion and pronation of the wrist, movements of the hand behind the neck, and transient hemichoreo–athetoid, writhing, snake-like, gyratory or hemiballic movements lasting a few minutes have also been reported, without accompanying neuroimaging, by Margolin and Marsden, (1982), in association with severe uni- or bilateral carotid stenosis, basilar artery stenosis, or occlusion and vertebrobasilar thrombosis (Gordon and Lendon, 1985). Transient weakness and transient sensory, visual, or aphasic symptoms can coexist with these movements. Painful tonic spasms (Merchut and Brumlik, 1986) or transient abnormal movements in patients with thalamic infarcts (Milandre et al., 1993) can be of difficult differential diagnosis. Electroencephalography performed during the paroxysmal movements showed slow waves without paroxysms, and cerebral blood flow studies demonstrated transient hypoperfusion in contralateral frontoparietal regions (Michel et al., 1989).

Paroxysmal complex dyskinesias with elements of dystonia, ballism, chorea, jerks and stereotypies have been described in a posterolateral thalamic infarct (Camac et al., 1990).

Myoclonus

Myoclonus is exceptionally seen in patients with strokes, although generalized myoclonus has never been reported. The anoxic action myoclonus of Lance and Adams (1963) has been reported in association with multiple lacunar lesions in the basal ganglia. Intention and action myoclonus was found in a patient with a thalamic angioma (Avanzani *et al.*, 1977). Focal reflex myoclonus has been reported by Sutton and Mayer (1974) in a patient with a superficial sylvian stroke involving the frontoparietal lobes, and later by others (Bartolomei *et al.*, 1995). Nagura *et al.* (1987) reported a mixed rhythmic and arrhythmic unilateral myoclonus that occurred at rest and increased on action and reflex stimuli, disappearing during sleep. Cortical action tremor is also sometimes encountered in parietal infarcts (Schulze-Bonaheg and Ferbert, 1998). Segmental myoclonus has been reported in association with basilar lesions (Ghika-Schmid *et al.*, 1997), midbrain or pontine strokes (Palmer *et al.*, 1991), basal ganglia infarcts (Scott and Jankovic, 1996), cerebellar infarcts (Sutton and Meyer, 1974), and spinal cord ischemia (Polo *et al.*, 1994).

Facial myoclonus is infrequent in strokes (Finsterer *et al.*, 1996). Palatal myoclonus is generally found in association with pontine or bulbar strokes (Sumer, 2001). Intractable hiccup has similar topography (Al Deeb *et al.*, 1991). Laryngeal nystagmus as been reported as a symptom of a cerebellar and brainstem infarct (Kisselbach and Kaps, 1985).

Convulsive movements have been reported in brainstem strokes (Saposnik and Caplan, 2001) and myoclonic status epilepticus in multiple cerbrovascular accidents (Garcia *et al.*, 1983).

Clonic perseveration (rythmic persevering, stereotyped, repetitive, clonic movements of upper and lower limbs) after infarcts of the thalamus and basal ganglia have been reviewed in a short series of four patients (Fung *et al.*, 1997).

Myorrhythmia

Myorrhythmia has been found in thalamic (Lera *et al.*, 2000) or bulbar strokes (Wu *et al.*, 2000).

Asterixis

Bilateral asterixis (negative myoclonus) is associated with diffuse encephalopathy (metabolic, toxic, or infectious). Clinically, asterixis is a failure to sustain muscle contraction in postures, and electrophysiological studies show a negative myoclonus (paroxysmal, brief [less than 200 milliseconds] loss of muscular activity in muscles of the upper or lower extremity, axial muscles, or tongue). Unilateral asterixis has been reported with contralateral lesions involving any of the possible structures involved in motion (frontoparietal cortex, basal ganglia, cerebellum, thalamus, brainstem, but not yet in the spinal cord) (Tatu *et al.*, 1996), and, exceptionally, in ipsilateral brainstem lesion (Peterson and Peterson, 1987) or the anterior or posterior cerebral artery territory (Lazzarino and Nicolai 1992). Sensory, motor, ataxic, eye movement, or neuropsychological disturbances can be associated. Ischemic or hemorrhagic lesions have been found on CT, MRI, or pathology, involving the parietal lobe (Ghika *et al.*, 1998) and in the territory of the lenticulostriate artery from the middle cerebral artery (head of caudate, lenticular nuclei, internal capsule) (Mizutani *et al.*, 1990). Thalamic ischemic or hemorrhagic lesions (posterior cerebral artery territory) can cause acute unilateral asterixis (Ghika-Schmid *et al.*, 1997). The lesions involved the paramedian nuclei (Donat, 1980), the lateral nuclei (thalamogeniculate territory; Mizutani *et al.*, 1990), posterior nuclei (Trouillas *et al.*, 1990), the mesothalamic region (Lee and Marsden, 1994), or both thalami (Rondot *et al.*, 1986). Bril *et al.* (1979) reported patients with unilateral acute asterixis in association with midbrain infarct, but no topographic correlate was described. Asterixis has been reported in patients with mesencephalic pontine or bulbar strokes in the posterior fossa (Shepherd *et al.*, 1997).

Stereotypies

Complex stereotypies have been found in associated with an infarct in the territory of the lenticulostriate arteries on the right side (Maranganore *et al.*, 1991), with bilateral thalamocapsular infarcts (Combarros *et al.*, 1990), and with parietal strokes (Ghika *et al.*, 1998). (Wallesh *et al.*, 1983) reported stereotypies of speech in a patient with aphasic stroke. Unilateral parkinsonism and stereotyped movements have also been described in association with a right lenticular infarct (Kulisevsky *et al.*, 1996).

Mirror movements

Mirror movements have been described in strokes and recently studied (Newton *et al.*, 2002). They can also occur together with anterior cerebral artery infarcts, sometimes associated with alien hand syndrome (Hanakita and Nishi 1991) or during the recovery from subcortical strokes (Wittenberg *et al.*, 2000).

Hyperekplexia

Hyperekplexia, exacerbated by the occlusion of posterior thalamic arteries, has been described (Farriello *et al.*, 1983).

Akathisia, maniform agitation, and compulsive motor behaviors

Akathisia per se has not been reported in association with stroke, except in one patient with unilateral akathisia associated with a posterior thalamic infarct

(Ghika *et al.*, 1995a). Agitation or agitated confusional state have been reported in association with lesions in various locations, especially subthalamic infarcts (Bogousslavsky *et al.*, 1988a,b) but also caudate hemorrhagic and ischemic strokes (Milhaud *et al.*, 1994), mesencephalic, substantia nigra, and thalamic strokes (Lauterbach, 1996), right hemispheric strokes (Migliorella *et al.*, 1993), or multiple lacunar strokes (Fujikawa *et al.*, 1996). Akathisia can be precipitated by neuroleptic drugs after pallidal infarct (Auzou *et al.*, 1996).

Hypergraphia (Yamadori *et al.*, 1986), graphomania (Williams *et al.*, 1988), logorrhea (Trillet *et al.*, 1995), compulsive grasping or manipulation (Sandson *et al.*, 1991), or obsessive–compulsive behaviors have been described associated with basal ganglia (Tonkonogy, 1989), thalamic (Sandson *et al.*, 1991), subthalamic (Trillet *et al.*, 1995), temporoparietal (Bogousslavsky *et al.*, 1995) and cingulate (Paunovic, 1984) strokes.

Agitated delirium can occur with posterior cerebral (Verslegers *et al.*, 1991) or right middle cerebral (Schmidley and Messing, 1984) strokes.

Tourettism

Tourettism or tics associated with attentional deficit disorders or obsessive–compulsive disorders, or both, secondary to subcortical strokes have been recently reported in children (Kwak and Jankovic, 2002).

Hemifacial spasm and blepharospasm

Hemifacial spasm is generally caused by the impingement of a posterior fossa artery on the facial nerve. Blepharospasm or hemifacial spasm can rarely occur as the presenting lesion of a caudate infarct (Arunabh *et al.*, 1992).

Hyperkinesia contralateral to hemiplegia

We have reported a series of patients with hemiplegic strokes who presented various types of hyperkinetic motor behaviors contralateral to the motor deficits (Ghika *et al.*, 1995b), including compulsive grasp reaction associated with frontal strokes (Castaigne *et al.*, 1970), but also generalized non-goal-directed hypermotility and stereotypies. More complex behavior has also been reported (Rosolacci *et al.*, 1999) and this motor behavior has also been reported after bilateral infarcts (Chang and Spokoyny, 1996).

Complex hyperkinesias

The most complex hyperkinesia associated with stroke is found in association with posterolateral thalamic strokes, mostly posterior choroidal or thalamogeniculate. A mixture of rubral tremor, chorea, pseudoathetosis, myoclonus, dystonia, and ataxia is regularly found, which has been called the "jerky dystonic unsteady hand syndrome " by our group (Ghika *et al.*, 1994, 1995b). It has also been described in bilateral paramedian thalamic or bilateral cerebellar infarcts (Tan *et al.*, 2001b). When associated with a painful syndrome, this is well known as the Dejerine–Roussy syndrome (1906). Very complex dyskinesia with dystonia, avoidance, and withdrawal behaviors, hypertonia (poikilotonia), persistence of awkward postures (hemicatalepsy, levitation), akinesia, multiple apraxias, ataxia, and sensorimotor deficits are found in the parietal lobe motor syndrome (Ghika *et al.*, 1998), but also in temporoparietal (Bogousslavsky *et al.*, 1995), and basal ganglia (Williams *et al.*, 1988) strokes.

Alien hand syndrome

Three varieties of alien hand syndrome have been reported. Lesions of the corpus callosum (anterior variant), sometimes associated with the medial frontal cortex, is responsible for the "anarchic," "wayward" hand with autonomous undesired activity that is felt as involuntary and purposeless by the patient, or with a failure to recognize ownership with reflexive grasping or compulsive manipulation of tools (Suwanwela and Leelacheavasit, 2002), instinctive reaching or grasp reaction (Chan and Ross, 1997), impulsive groping (Wu *et al.*, 1999), involuntary hand levitation (Carrilho *et al.*, 2001), choking or hitting the face, creeping and crawling (Nicholas *et al.*, 1998), or even a Nazi salute ("Dr Strangelove syndrome" of Peter Sellers; Banks *et al.*, 1989). Automatic gestures increase during stress or conversations. A recent report mentions involuntary masturbation after right anteromedial frontal and anterior cingulate infarct in the territory of the anterior cerebral artery (Ong and Odderson, 2000). Chan and Liu (1999) insist on the presence of an additive medial frontal lesion to the corpus callosum. When the corpus callosum is included, bimanual coordination, intermanual conflict, ideomotor and construction apraxia of the right hand or bilateral, left agraphia, tactile anomia, hemihypokinesia, spatial dyscaculia, speech or motor perseverations, anomia of the left hemifield, adynamic aphasia, or mirror writing can occur (McNabb *et al.*, 1998). The activity generally involves one hand only, less frequently the leg (alien foot) (Banks *et al.*, 1989). The autonomous motor activity of the hand disturbs and disrupt daily life.

The posterior variant, including a subcortical variant, is characterized by a feeling of strangeness of the limb, which may be felt as belonging to another person and can be denied or aggressively considered by the patient. Alien hand syndromes with autonomous activity of the hand can be found in association with both frontal and parietal strokes. The posterior variant of alien (capricious) hand with autonomous movements, foreign feeling of the limb, and personification of the affected extremity can be found with thalamic (Marey-Lopez *et al.*, 2002) or parietal (right more than left) (Ghika *et al.*, 1998) lesions or, less frequently, with posterior cerebellar artery strokes (Groom *et al.*, 1999). The leg is rarely involved (Chan *et al.*, 1996). The role of neglect on the clinical presentation has been stressed (Chan and Ross, 1997).

The last form is diagonistic apraxia, antagonistic behavior of both hands or intermanual conflict: one limb undoes what the other one does and performs no other activity but the contrary of the opposite limb. Diagonistic apraxia has been reported with lesions of the striatum, premotor lateral cortex, and callosal fibers after an infarct in the territory of the anterior cerebral artery (Chan and Ross, 1997).

Utilization behavior and compulsive manipulation of tools can also been found in right thalamic lesions (Hashimoto *et al.*, 1995). This is sometimes considered as a white matter disconnection syndrome in strokes (Ishihara *et al.*, 2002), especially in the territory of the anterior cerebral artery, uni- or bilaterally (Boccardi *et al.*, 2002).

Avoidance or withdrawal/rejection phenomena of the dystonic type, initial avoidance, or nociceptive-like retraction of the hand, arm, and trunk are sometimes elicited in parietal lesions (Ghika *et al.*, 1998).

Orofacial dyskinesias

Oral dyskinesias are exceptionall reported in association with vascular lesions. One case with bilateral thalamo-capsular infarcts has been reported (Combarros *et al.*, 1990).

Modification of previous movement disorders by strokes

Strokes can be a "treatment" for essential tremor contralaterally to a thalamic (Barbaud *et al.*, 2001), subthalamic (Struck *et al.*, 1990), or pontine (Nagaratnam and Kalasabil, 1997) strokes. Improvement of parkinsonian signs after vascular lesions of the basal ganglia (Krauss *et al.*, 1997) or ipsilateral cerebellum (Rivest *et al.*, 1990) have been reported. Chorea may also be altered by a stroke in Huntington's disease (Bassi *et al.*, 1984). Hyperekplexia exacerbated by the occlusion of posterior thalamic arteries has been described (Farriello *et al.*, 1983).

Summary

In conclusion, acute hypo- or hyperkinetic syndromes can occur in people with acute strokes occurring at any levels of the motor frontosubcortical circuit of Alexander. The majority of such movement disorders hemichorea and hemiballism, but acute unilateral asterixis, dystonia, or, less frequently, myoclonus, stereotypy, or complex motor behaviors including akinetic states can be found. Most of them are transient and are not specific for any vascular topography or anatomical structure, but the majority are caused by a lesion in the basal ganglia or thalamus. Exceptional complex recurring acute movement disorders like "limb shaking" can be found in transient ischemic attacks and are important to recognize early. Delayed or recurring hyperkinetic syndromes can be found months or years after a stroke. Parkinsonism-like syndromes in association with diffuse small artery disease are common, usually not asymmetrical, and resistent to treatment.

REFERENCES

Al Deeb, S. M., Sharif, H., Al Motahery, K., and Biary, N. (1991). Intractable hiccup induced by brainstem lesion. *J Neurol Sci* **103**: 144–150.

Alexander, G. E., Delong, M. R., and Strick, P. L. (1986). Parallel organization of functionally segregated circuits linking basal ganglia and cortex. *Annu Rev Neurosci* **9**: 357–381.

Apaydin, H., Ozekmeckci, S., and Yeni, N. (1998). Posthemiplegic focal limb dystonia: a report of two cases. *Clin Neurol Neurosurg* **100**: 46–50.

Arunabh Jain, S. and Maheshwari, MC. J. (1992). Blepharospasm and hemifacial spasm and tremors possibly due to isolated caudate nucleus lesions. *Assoc Physicians India* **40**: 687–689.

Auzou, P., Ozsancak, C., Hannequin, D., and Augustin, P. (1996). Akathisia induced by low doses of neuroleptics after pallidal infarction. *Presse Med* **25**: 260.

Avanzani, G., Bruggi, G., and Caraceni, T. (1977). Intention and action myoclonus from thalamic angioma. *Eur Neurol* **15**: 194–202.

Ballassoued, M., Mhiri, C., Triki, C., and Abid, M. (2001). Hemichorea caused by striatal infarct in a young type 1 diabetic patient. *Rev Neurol* **157**: 1287–1289.

Banks, G., Short, P., Martinez, L., *et al.* (1989). The alien hand syndrome. Clinical and postmortem findings. *Arch Neurol* **46**: 456–459.

Barbaud, A., Hadjout, K., Blard, J. M., and Pages, M. (2001). Improvement in essential tremor after pure sensory stroke due to thalamic infarction. *Eur Neurol* **46**: 57–79.

Bartolomei, F., Bureau, M., Paglia, C., Genton, P., and Roger, J. (1995). Myoclonus d'action focal et lésion hémisphérique localisée. Etude polygraphique et pharmacologique. *Rev Neurol* **151**: 311–315.

Bassi, S., Frattola, L., Sbacchi, M., and Trabucchi, M. (1984). Motor behavior modifications after a stroke in a patient with Huntington's disease. *J Neurol Neurosurg and Psychiatry* **47**: 1358–1359.

Benedikt, M. (1989). Tremblement avec paralysie croisée du moteur oculaire commun. *Bull Med* **3**: 547–548.

Bhatia, K. P. and Marsden, C. D. (1994). The behavioral and motor consequences of focal lesions of the basal ganglia in man. *Brain* **117**: 859–894.

Blakeley, J. and Jankovic, J. (2002). Secondary causes of paroxysmal dystonia. *Adv Neurol* **89**: 401–420.

Boccardi, E., Della Salla, S., Motto, C., and Spinnler, H. (2002). Utilisation behavior consequent to bilateral SMA softening. *Cortex* **38**: 289–308.

Bogousslavsky, J. and Regli, F. (1986). Unilateral watershed infarcts. *Neurology* **36**: 373–377.

Bogousslavsky, J., Regli, F., and Uske, A. (1988a). Thalamic infarction: clinical syndromes, etiology and prognosis. *Neurology* **38**: 837–848.

Bogousslvsky, J., Ferrazzini, M., and Regli, F. (1988b). Manic delirium and frontal lobe syndrome with paramedian infarction of the right thalamus. *J Neurol Neurosurg Psychiatry* **51**: 116–119.

Bogousslavsky, J., Regli, F., Delaloye Bischof, A., Assal, G., and Uske, A. (1991). Loss of psychic self-activation with bithalamic infarction. Neurobehavioral, CT, MRI and SPECT correlates. *Acta Neurol Scand* **83**: 309–316.

Bogousslavsky, J., Kumral, E., Regli, F., Assal, G., and Ghika, J. (1995). Acute hemiconcern: a right anterior parietotemporal syndrome. *J Neurol Neurosurg Psyychiatry* **58**: 428–432.

Boisson, D., Confavreux, C., Eyssette, M., Aimard, G., and Devic, M. (1981). Isolated tonic ambulatory flexion of the foot. *Rev Neurol* **137**: 807–815.

Brannan, T. and Yahr, M. D. (1999). Focal tremor following striatal infarct: a case report. *Mov Disorders* **14**: 368–370.

Bril, V., Sharpe, J. A., and Ashby, B. (1979). Midbrain asterixis. *Ann Neurol* **6**: 362–364.

Burguera, J. A., Bataller, L., and Valero, C. (2001). Action hand dystonia after cortical parietal infarction. *Mov Disord* **16**: 1183–1185.

Burke, R. E., Stanley, F., and Gold, A. P. (1980). Delayed onset dystonia in patients with "static" encephalopathy. *J Neurol Neurosurg Psychiatry* **43**: 789–797.

Burton, K., Farrel, K., Li, D., and Calne, D. B. (1984). Lesions of the putamen in dystonia: CT and magnetic resonance imaging. *Neurology* **34**: 962–965.

Calvanio, R., Levine, D., and Petrone, P. (1993). Elements of cognitive rehabilitation after right hemisphere stroke. *Neurol Clin* **11**: 25–57.

Calzetti, S., Morett, G., Gemignati, F. *et al.* (1980). Transient hemiballismus and subclavian steal syndrome. *Acta Neurol Belg* **80**: 829–831.

Camac, A., Greene, P., and Khandji, A. (1990). Paroxysmal kinesigenic dystonic choreoathetosis associated with a thalamic infarct. *Mov Disord* **5**: 235–238.

Caparros-Lefebvre, D., Deleume, J. F., Bradai, N., and Petit, H. (1994). Biballism caused by bilateral infarction in the substantia nigra. *Mov Disord* **9**: 108–110.

Carrilho, P. E., Caramelli, P., Cardoso, F., *et al.* (2001). Involuntary hand levitation associated with parietal damage: another alien hand syndrome. *Arq Neuropsyiquiatr* **59**: 521–525.

Casas-Parera, I., Gatto, E., Fernandez Pardal, M. M., *et al.* (1994). Neurological complications by cocaine abuse. *Medicine* **54**: 35–41.

Caselli, R. J., Hunder, C. G., and Whisnant, J. P. (1988). Neurological disease in biopsy-proven giant cell (temporal) arteritis. *Neurology* **38**: 352–359.

Castaigne, P., Cambier, J., Escourolle, R., and Dehen, H. (1970). Le comportement de préhension pathologique (à propos de 4 observations anatomo-cliniques). *Rev Neurol* **123**: 5–15.

Chan, J. L. and Liu, A. B. (1999). Anatomical correlates of alien hand syndromes. *Neuropsychiatry Neuropsychol Behav Neurol* **12**: 149–155.

Chan, J. L. and Ross, E. D. (1997). Alien hand syndrome: influence of neglect on the clinical presentation of frontal and callosal variant. *Cortex* **33**: 287–299.

Chan, J. L., Chen, R. S., and Ng, K. K. (1996). Leg manifestation in alien hand syndrome. *J Formos Med Assoc* **95**: 342–346.

Chang, G. Y. and Spokoyny, E. (1996). Hyperkinetic motor behavior in bihemispheric stroke. *Eur Neurol* **35**: 27–32.

Cho, C. and Samkoff, L. M. (2000). A lesion of the anterior thalamus producing dystonic tremor of the hand. *Arch Neurol* **57**: 1353–1355.

Choi, Y. C., Lee, M. S., and Choi, I. S. (1993). Delayed-onset focal dystonia after stroke. *Yonsei Med J* **34**: 391–396.

Chuang, C., Fahn, S., and Frucht, S. J. (2002). The natural history and treatment of acquired hemidystonia: report of 33 cases and review of the literature. *J Neurol Neurosurg Psychiatry* **72**: 59–67.

Clark, J. D., Pahwa, R., Koller, C., and Morales, D. (1995). Diabetes mellitus presenting as paroxysmal kinesigenic dystonic choreoathetosis. *Mov Disord* **10**: 353–355.

Combarros, O., Gutierrez, A., Pascual, J., and Berciano, J. (1990). Oral dyskinesia associated with bilaeral thalamo-capsular infarction. *J Neurol Neurosurg Psychiatry* **53**: 168–169.

Crozier, S., Lahercy, S., Vresichtel, P., Masson, C., and Masson, M. (1996). Transient hemiballsim/hemichorea due to ipsilateral subthalamic infarction. *Neurology* **46**: 267–268.

Critchley, M. (1929). Arteriosclerotic parkinsonism. *Brain* **52**: 82–83.

Critchley, M. (1981). Atherosclerotic pseudoparkinsonism. In *Progress in Parkinson's disease*, ed. F. Clifford Rose, R. Copildeo. London: Pitmann Med, pp. 40–42.

Déjérine, J. and Roussy, G. (1906). Le syndrome thalamique. *Revue Neurol* **14**: 521–532.

Deleu, D., Lagopoulos, M., and Lounon, A. (2000). Thalamic hand dystonia: an MRI anatomoclinical study. *Acta Neurol Belg* **100**: 237–241.

Denny Brown D. (1962). *The Basal Ganglia and their Relation to Disorders of Movement*. London: Oxford University Press, pp. 55–56.

de Renzi, E., Gentilini, M., and Bazolli, C. (1986). Eyelid movement disorders and motor impersistance in acute hemisphere disease. *Neurology* **36**: 414–418.

Derkinderen, P., Dupont, S., Vidal, J. S., Chedru, F., and Vidailhet, M. (2002). Micrographia secondary to lenticular lesions. *Mov Disord* **17**: 835–837.

Dethy, S., Luxen, A., Bidaut, L. M., and Goldman, S. (1993). Hemibody tremor related to stroke. *Stroke* **24**: 2094–2096.

Dietrichs, E., Hiere, M. S., and Nakstad, P. H. (2000). Jaw-opening dystonia presumably caused by a pontine lesion. *Mov Disord* **15**: 1026–1028.

D'Olhaberrigue, L., Arboix, A., Marti-Vilalta, J. L., Mora, A., and Massons, J. (1995). Movement disorders in ischemic stroke: clinical study of 22 patients. *Eur J Neurol* **2**: 553–557.

Domzal, T. M. and Zaleska, B. (2001). Blepharospasm and Meige's syndrome: a contribution to its pathogenesis. *Pol Merkuruisz Lek* **10**: 98–100.

Donat, J. R. (1980). Unilateral asterixis due to thalamic hemorrhage. *Neurology* **30**: 83–84.

Dooling, E. C. and Adams, R. D. (1975). The pathological anatomy of posthemiplegic athetosis. *Brain* **98**: 29–48.

Dove, C. A., Vezzetti, D., and Escobar, N. (1994). Metoprolol for action tremor following intracerebral hemorrhage. *Arch Phys Med Rehab* **75**: 1011–1014.

Dubinsky, R. M. and Jankovic, J. (1987). Progressive supranuclear palsy and a multiinfarct state. *Neurology* **37**: 570–576.

Escourolle, R., de Recondo, J., and Gray, F. (1970). Aspects neuropathologiques des syndromes parkinsoniens. *Rev Prat* **20**: 5175.

Factor, S. A., Sanchez-Ramos, J. and Weiner, W. J., (1988). Delayed-onset dystonia associated with corticospinal tract dysfunction. *Mov Disord* **3**: 201–203.

Fariello, R. G., Schwartzman, R. J., and Beall, S. S. (1983). Hyperekplexia exacerbated by occlusion of posterior thalamic arteries. *Arch Neurol* **40**: 244–246.

Ferbert, A. and Gerwig, M. (1991). Non-rubral tremor of vascular origin. *Mov Disord* **6**: 276.

Ferbert, A.(1993). Tremor due to stroke. *Movement Disord* **8**: 179–182.

Finsterer, J., Muellbacher, W. and Mamli, B. (1996). Yes/yes head tremor without appendicular tremor after bilateral cebellar infarction. *J Neurol Sci* **139**: 242–245.

Folstein, S., Abbott, M., Moser, R., *et al.* (1981). Phenocopy of Huntington's disease: lacunar infartcs of the corpus striatum. *Johns Hopkins Med J* **148**: 104–113.

Foltynie, T., Barker, R., and Brayne, C. (2002). Vascular parkinsonism: a review of the precision and frequency of the diagnosis. *Neuroepidemiology* **21**: 1–7.

Frates, E. P., Burke, D. T., Chae, H., and Ahangar, B. (2001). Post-stroke violent adventitial movement responsive to levodopa/carbidopa therapy. *Brain Inj* **15**: 911–916.

Fukui, T., Hasegawa, Y., Seriyama, S., *et al.* (1993). Hemiballism–hemichorea indiced by subcortical ischemia. *Can J Neurol Sci* **20**: 324–328.

Fujikawa, T., Yamawaki, S., and Touhouda, Y. (1996). Silent cerebral infarctions in patients with late-onset mania. *Stroke* **26**: 946–949.

Fung, V. S., Moris, J. G., Leicester, J., Soo, Y. S., and Davies, L. (1997). Clonic perseveration following thalamofrontal disconnection: distinctive movement disorders. *Mov Disord* **12**: 378–385.

Garcia, F., Romero, J., Rallo, B., and Gonzalez-Elipe, J. (1983). Myoclonic status epilepticus in an adult with multiple cerebrovascular accidents. *Rev Clin Esp* **171**: 355–356.

Ghika, J., Bogousslavsky, J., Henderson, J. and Regli, F. (1994). The "jerky dystonic unsteady hand", a delayed complex hyperkinetic syndrome in posterior thalamic infarcts. *J Neurol* **241**: 537–542.

Ghika, J., Bogousslavsky, J., and Regli, F. (1995a). Delayed unilateral akathisia with posterior thalamic infarct. *Cerbrovasc Dis* **5**: 55–58.

Ghika, J., Bogousslavsky, J., and Regli, F. (1995b). Hyperkinetic motor behaviors contralateral to acute hemiplegia. *Eur Neurol* **35**: 27–32.

Ghika, J., Ghika-Schmid, F., and Bogousslavsky, J. (1998). Parietal motor syndrome: a clinical description of 32 patients in the acute phase of pure parietal strokes studied prospectively. *Clin Neurol Neurosurg* **100**: 271–282.

Ghika-Schmid, F., Ghika, J., Regli, F., and Bogousslavsky, J. (1997). Hyperkinetic movement disorders during and after acute stroke. *J Neurol Sci* **146**: 109–116 *[Erratum in J. Neurol Sci* (1997). **152**: 234–235.]

Girlanda, P., Quartarone, A., Simicropi, S., *et al.* (1997). Botulinum toxin in upper limb spasticity: astudy of reciprocal inhibition between forearm muscles. *NeuroReport* **8**: 3039–3044.

Goldblatt, D., Markesbery, W., and Reeves, A. G. (1974). Recurrent hemichorea following striatal lesions. *Arch Neurol* **31**: 51–54.

Goldblatt, J., White, N. W., and Wright, M. G. (1989). Bilateral chorea associated with caudate lacunar infarct. A case report. *S Afr J Med* **6**: 443–444.

Gordon, N. and Lendon, M. (1985). Vertebro-basilar thrombosis and involuntary movements. *Dev Med Child Neurol* **37**: 664–674.

Groom, K. N., Ng, W. K., Keborkian, C. G., and Levy, J. K. (1999). Ago-syntonic alien hand syndrome after right posterior cerebral artery stroke. *Arch Phys Med Rehabil* **80**: 162–165.

Hanakita, J. and Nishi, S. (1991). Left alien hand sign and mirror writing after left anterior cerebral artery infarction. *Sur Neurol* **35**: 290–293.

Hashimoto, R., Yoshida, M., and Tanaka, Y. (1995). Utilization behavior after right thalamic infarction. *Eur Neurol* **5**: 58–62.

Hesselink, K., van Gijn, J., and Verwey, J. C. (1987). Hyperkinetic mutism. *Neurology* **37**: 1566.

Holmes, G. (1904). On certain tremors in organic lesions. *Brain* **27**: 327–375.

Horner, S., Niederkorn, K., Ni, X. S., Homann, N., and Ott, E. (1997). Evaluation of risk factors in patients with Parkinson's syndrome. *Nervenarzt* **68**: 967–971.

Howard, R. and Low-Beer, T. (1989). Catatonia following biparietal infarction with spontaneous recovery. *Postgrad Med J* **65**: 316–317.

Ichikawa, K., Kim, R. G., and Givelbet, H. (1980). Chorea glavidium Report of a fatal case with neuropathological observations. *Arch Neurol* **37**: 429–432.

Ikeda, M. and Tsukagoshi, H. (1991). Monochorea caused by striatal lesion. *Eur Neurol* **31**: 257–258.

Imai, N., Hara, A., Miyata, K., Terayama, Y., and Ishihara, N. (1997). A case of midbrain infarction with ipsilateral hand tremor. *No To Shinkei* **49**: 1033.

Inoue, H., Udaka, F., Takahashi, M., Nishinaka, K., and Kameyama, M. (1997). Secondary parkinsonism following midbrain hemorrhage. *Rinsho Shinkeigaku* **37**: 266–269.

Ishihara, K., Nishino, H., Maki, T., Kawamura, M., and Murayama, S. (2002). Utilization behavior as a white matter disconnection syndrome. *Cortex* **38**: 379–387.

Ito, T., Jijiwa, M., Ando, Y., *et al.* (2000). A patient with choreoathetosis of the left upper extremity due to acute cerebral infarction. *Rinsho Sinkeigaku* **40**: 184–186.

Jacob, P. C. and Chand, R. P. (1997). Blepharospasm and jaw closing dystonia after parietal infarct. *Mov Disord* **12**: 262–263.

Jellinger, K. (1996). Parkinsonism due to Binswanger's subcortical arteriosclerotic encephalopathy. *Mov. Disord* **11**: 461–462.

Josephs, K. A., Ishizawa, T., Tsuoboi, Y., Cookson, N., and Dickson, D. W. (2002). A clinicopathological study of vascular supranuclear palsy: a multi-infarct disorder presenting as progressive supranuclear palsy. *Arch Neurol* **59**: 1597–1601.

Kalita, J., Bansal, R., Ayagiri, A., and Misra, U. K. (1999). Midbrain infarction: a rare presentation of cryptococcal meningitis. *Clin Neurol Neurosurg* **101**: 23–25.

Kao, Y. F., Shih, P. Y., and Chen, W. H. (1999). An unusual concomitant tremor and myoclonus after a contralateral infarct and subthallamic nucleus. *Kaohsiung J Med Sci* **15**: 562–566.

Karsidag, S., Ozer, F., Sen, A., and Arpaci, B. (1998). Localization in developing postroke hand dystonia. *Eur Neurol* **40**: 99–104.

Kase, C. S., Maulsby, G. O., De Juan, E., and Mohr, J. P. (1981). Hemichorea–hemiballism and lacunar infarction in the basal ganglia. *Neurology* **31**: 452–455.

Keane, J. R. and Young, J. A. (1985). Blepharospasm associated with bilateral basal ganglia infarction. *Arch Neurol* **42**: 1237–1240.

Kelley, R. E. and Jain, P. K. (2000). Hyperkinetic movement disorders caused by corpus striatum infarcts: brain MRI/CT findings in three cases. *J Neuroimaging* **10**: 22–26.

Kim, J. S. (2001a). Involuntary movements after anterior cerebral artery territory infarction. *Stroke* **32**: 258–261.

Kim, J. S. (2001b). Delayed onset mixed involuntary movements after thalamic stroke: clinical, radiological and pathophysiological findings. *Brain* **124**: 299–309.

Kim, J. S. and Lee, M. C. (1994). Writing tremor after discrete cortical infarction. *Stroke* **25**: 2280–2282.

Kim, J. W., Kim, S. H., and Cha, J. K. (1999). Pseudochoreoathetosis in four patients with hypesthetic ataxiac hemiparesis in a thalamic lesion. *J Neurol.* **246**: 1075–1079.

Kisselbach, G. and Kaps, M. (1985). So-called laryngeal nystagmus. Progressive myoclonus as a symptom of a cerebellar and brainstem infarct. *Laryngol Rhinol Otol* **64**: 306–308.

Kitanaka, C. and Teraoka, A. (1995). Clinical features of preogressive lacunar infarction:retrospective analysis of patients with motor syndromes. *Neurol Med Chir* **35**: 663–666.

Klawans, H. L., Moses, H., Nausieda, P. A., Bergen, D., and Weiner, W. J. (1976). Treatment and prognosis of hemiballismus. *New Engl J Med* **295**: 1348–1350.

Kostic, V. S., Stojanovic-Svetel, M., and Kacar, A. (1996). Symptomatic dystonias associated with structural brain lesions. *Can J Neurol Sci* **23**: 53–56.

Krauss, J. K., Grossmann, R. G., and Jankovic, J. (1997). Improvement of parkinsonian signs after vascular lesions of the basal ganglia circuitry. *Mov Disord* **12**: 124–126.

Kulisevsky, J., Avila, A., Roig, C., and Escarfin, A. (1993). Unilateral blepharospasm stemming from a thalamomesencephalic lesion. *Mov Disord* **8**: 239–240.

Kulisevsky, J., Berthier, M. I., Avila, A., and Roig, C. (1996). Unilateral parkinsonism and stereotyped movements following right lenticular infarction. *Move Disord* **11**: 752–754.

Kwak, C. H. and Jankovic, J. (2002). Tourettism and dystonia after subcortical stroke. *Mov Disord* **17**: 821–825.

Lance, J. W. and Adams, R. D. (1963). The syndrome of intention or action myoclonus as a sequel to hypoxic encephalopathy, *Brain* **86**: 111–136.

Lang, A. E. (1985). Persistent hemiballismus with lesions outside the subthalamic nucleus. *Can. J Neurol Sci* **12**: 125–128.

Laplane, D. and Dubois, B. (1998). Les troubles affectifs de la perte d'auto-activation psychique. Comparaison avec l'athymormie. *Rev Neurol* **154**: 35–39.

Larumbe, R., Vaamonde, J., Artieda, J., Zubieta, J. L., and Obeso, J. A. (1993). Reflex blepharospasm associated with bilateral basal ganglia lesion. *Mov Disord* **8**: 1980–200.

Lauterbach, E. C. (1996). Bipolar disorder, dystonia and compulsion after dysfunction of the cerebellum, dentatorubrothalmic tract, and substantia nigra. *Biol Psychiatry* **15**: 726–730.

Lauterbach, E. C., Price, S. T., Wilson, A. N., Kavali, C. M., and Jackson, J. G. (1994). Post-stroke bipolar disorders : age and thalamus. *Biol Psychiatry* **35**: 681.

Lazzarino, L. G. and Nicolai, A. (1992). Late onset unilateral asterixis secondary to posterior cerebral artery infarction. *Ital J Neurol Sci* **13**: 361–364.

Lazzarino, L. G., Nicolai, A., and Toppani, D. (1990). Subacute parkinsonism forms a single lacunar infarct in the basal ganglia. *Acta Neurol* **12**: 292–295.

LeDoux, M. S. and Brady, K. A. (2003). Secondary cervical dystonia associated with structural lesions of the central nervous system. *Mov Disord* **18**: 60–69.

Lee, M. S. and Marsden, C. D. (1994). Movement disorders following lesions of the thalamus and subthalamic region. *Mov Disord* **9**: 493–507.

Lee, M. S., Lee, S. A., Heo, J. H., and Choi, I. S. (1993). A patient with resting tremor and a lacunar infarction at the border between the thalamus and the internal capsule. *Move Disord* **8**: 244–246.

Lee, M. S., Lyoo, C. H., Lee, H. H., and Kim, Y. D. (2000a). Hemicoreoathetosis following posterior parietal watershed infarction: was striatal hypoperfusion really to blame? *Mov Disord* **15**: 178–179.

Lee, M. S., Kim, Y. D., Kim, J. T., and Lyoo, C. H. (2000b). Abrupt onset of transient pseudo-choreoathetosis associated with proprioceptive sensory loss as a result of a thalamic infarction. *Disord* **13**: 184–186.

Lepore, F. E. and Duvoisin, R. C. (1985). "Apraxia" of eyelid opening: an involuntary levator inhibition. *Neurology* **35**: 423–427.

Lera, G., Scipioni, O., Cammarota, A., Fischbein, G., and Gershanik, O. (2000). A combined pattern of movement disorders resulting from posterolateral thalamic lesions of a vascular nature. A syndrome with clinico-radiologic correlation. *Mov Disord* **15**: 120–126.

Lhermitte, J. (1922). Les syndromes anatomo-cliniques du corps strié chez le vieillard. *Rev Neurol* **29**: 406–432.

Li, J. Y., Lai, P. H., Chen, C. Y., Wang, J. S., and Lo, Y. K. (2000). Postanoxic parkinsonism: clinical, radiologic and pathological correlation. *Neurology* **55**: 591–593.

Lodder, J. and Baard, W. C. (1981). Paraballism caused by hemorrhagic infarction in the basal ganglia. *Neurology* **31**: 484–496.

Loiseau, P. (1969). Crises provoquées par les mouvements. *Agrégés* **2**: 273–280.

Louis, E. D., Lynch, T., Ford, B., *et al.* (1996). Delayed-onset cerebellar syndrome. *Arch Neurol* **53**: 450–454.

Maranganore, D. M., Lees, A. J., and Marsden, C. D. (1991). Complex stereotypies after right putaminal infarcts: a case report. *Move Disord* **6**: 358–361.

Marey-Lopez, J., Rubio-Nazabal, E., Alonso-Magdalena, L., *et al.* (2002). Posterior alien hand syndrome after a right thalamic infarct. *J Neurol Neurosurgery and Psychiatry* **73**: 447–449.

Margolin, D. I. and Marsden, C. D. (1982). Episodic dyskinesia and transient cerebral ischemia. *Neurology* **32**: 1379–1380.

Marsden, C. D., Obeso, J. A., Zarranz, J. J., and Lang, A. E. (1985). The anatomical basis of symptomatic hemidystonia. *Brain* **108**: 463–483.

Martinez-Vila, E., Artieda, J., and Obeso, J. (1988). Micrographia secondary to lenticular hematoma. *J Neurol Neurosurg Psychiatry* **51**: 1353.

Masdeu, J. C. and Gorelick, P. B. (1988). Thalamic astasia: inability to stand after unilateral thalamic lesions. *Ann Neurol* **23**: 596–603.

McNabb, A. W., Carroll, W. M., and Mastaglia, F. L. (1998). "Alien hand" and loss of bimanual coordination after dominant anterior cerebral artery territory infarction. *J Neurol Psychiatry* **51**: 218–222.

Mega, M. S. and Cohenour, R. C. (1997). Akinetic mutism: disconnection of fronto-subcortical circuitry. *Neuropsychiatry Neuropsychol Behav Neurol* **10**: 254–259.

Merchut, M. P. and Brumlik, J. (1986). Painful tonic spasms caused by putaminal infarction. *Stroke* **17**: 1319–1321.

Michel, B., Lemarquis, P., Nicoli, F., and Gastaut, J. L. (1989). Mouvements involontaires positionnels: accès ischémiques carotidiens. *Rev Neurol* **12**: 853–855.

Migliorelli, R., Starkstein, S. E., Teson, A., *et al.* (1993). SPECT findings in patients with primary mania. *J Neuropsychiatry Clin Neurosci* **5**: 379–383.

Milandre, L., Brosset, C., Gabriel, B., and Khalil, R. (1993). Mouvements involontaires transitoires et infarctus thalamiques. *Rev Neurol* **149**: 6–7, 402–406.

Milhaud, D., Magnin, M. N., Roger, P. M., and Bedouda, P. (1994). Infarctus du noyau caudé ou infarctus striato-capsulaire antérieur. *Rev Neurol* **150**: 286–291.

Miyashi, S., Watanabe, M., Okamura, K., *et al.* (1995). Acute neovascularization for bihemispheric anterior cerebral artery. *Neurologia Medico-Chirurgica* **35**: 369–372.

Mizutani, T., Shiozawa, R., Nozawa, T., and Nozawa, Y. (1990). Unilateral sterixis. *J Neurol* **237**: 480–482.

Nagaratnam, K. and Kalasabil, G. (1997). Contralateral abolition of essential tremor following a pontine stroke. *J Neurol Sci* **149**: 195–196.

Nagura, H., Kuzuhara, S., and Yamanouchi, H. (1987). Unilateral myoclonus induced by hypocalcemia in a case of cerebral infarction. *Rinsho Shinkeigaku* **27**: 1200–1202.

Nakamura, K., Saku, Y., Ibayashi, S., and Fujishima, M. (1999a). Progressive motor deficits in lacunar infarction. *Neurology* **52**: 29–33.

Nakamura, Y., Miura, K., Yamada, I., and Takada, K. (1999b). Disappearance of essential tremor after thalamic infarction. *Rinsho Sinhkeigaku* **39**: 340–342.

Newton, J., Sunderland, A., Butterworth, S. E., *et al.* (2002). A pilot study of event-related functional magnetic resonance imaging of monitored movements in patients with partial recovery. *Stroke* **33**: 2881–2887.

Nicolai, A. and Lazzarino, L. G. (1994). Paraballism associated with anterior opercular syndrome: a case report. *Clin Neurol Neurosurg* **96**: 145–147.

Nicholas, J. J., Wichner, M. H., Gorelick, P. B., and Ramsey, M. M. (1998). "Naturalization" of the alien hand: case report. *Arch Phys Med Rehabil* **79**: 113–114.

Nishi, K., Nagoaku, M., Sugita, Y., *et al.* (1985). A case of jaw opening phenomenon associated with basilar artery thrombosis. *No To Shinkei* **37**: 127–132.

Nutt, J. G., Marsden, C. D., and Thompson, P. (1993). Human walking and higher level gait disorders, particularly in the elderly. *Neurology* **43**: 268–279.

Okawa, M., Maeda, S., Nujui, H., and Kawafuchi, J. (1980). Psychiatric symptoms in ruptured anterior communicating aneurysms: social prognosis. *Acta Psychiatr Scand* **61**: 308–312.

Ong Hai, B. G. and Odderson, I. R. (2000). Involuntary masturbation as a manifestation of stroke-related hand syndrome. *Am J Psychiatry* **79**: 395–398.

Otto, S., Buttner, T., Schols, L., Windmeyer, D. T., and Przuntek, H. (1995). Head tremor due to bilateral thalamic and midbrain infarct. *J Neurol.* **242**: 698–610.

Papez, J. W., Benett, A. E., and Cash, P. T. (1942). Hemichorea (hemiballism). Association with pallidal lesions involving afferent and efferent connections of subthalamic nucleus: curare therapy. Arch Neurol Psychiatr **47**: 667–676.

Palmer, J. B., Tippett, D. C., and Wolf, J. S. (1991). Synchronous positive and negative myoclonus due to pontine hemorrhage. *Muscle Nerve* **14**: 124–132.

Parkes, J. D., Marsden, C. D., Rees, J. E. *et al.* (1974). Parkinson's disease, cerebroarteriosclerosis, and senile dementia. *Q J Med* **43**: 49–61.

Paunovic, V. R. (1984). Syndrome obsessionnel au decours d'une atteinte cérébrale organique. *Ann Med Psychol* **142**: 377–382.

Peterson, D. I. and Peterson, G. W. (1987). Unilateral asterixis due to ipsilateral lesions in the pons and medulla. *Ann Neurol* **22**: 661–663.

Petren, K. (1901). Ueber den Zusammenhang zwischen anatomisch bedingter und functioneller Gangstörung (besonders in der Form von trepidanter Abasie) im Grisenalter. Part 1. *Arch Neurol Psychiatr Nervenkr* **33**: 818–871.

Petren, K. (1902). Ueber den zusammenhang zwischen anatomisch bedingter und functioneller Gangstörung (besonders in der Form von trepidanter Abasie) im griisenalter. Part 2. *Arch Neurol Psych Nervenkr* **34**: 444–489.

Polo, K. B. and Jabbari, B. (1994). Effectiveness of botulinium toxin type A against painful limb myoclonus of spinal cord origin. *Mov Disord* **9**: 233–235.

Price, J., Whitlock, F. A., and Hall, R. T. (1983). The psychiatry of vertebrobasilar insufficiency with the report of a case. *Psychiatria Clin* **16**: 26–44.

Quaglieri, C. E., Chun, R. W., and Cleeland, C. (1977). Movement disorders as a complication of acute hemiplegia in childhood. *Am J Dis Child* **131**: 1009–1010.

Reimer, F. and Knüppel, H. (1963). Uber Hemiballism. Ein Beitrag zur Prognose der vaskülären Formen. *Psychiatr Neurol* **145**: 211–222.

Riley, D. E. (1996). Paroxysmal kinesigenic dystonia associated with a medullary lesion. *Mov Disord* **11**: 738–740.

Rivest, J., Quinn, N., Gibbs, J., and Marsden, C. D. (1990). Unilateral abolition of extrapyramidal rigidity after ipsilateral cerebellar infarction. *Mov Disord* **5**: 328–330.

Rondot, P., de Recondo, J., Davous, P., Bathien, N., and Gignet, A. (1986). Infarctus thalamique bilateral avec mouvements anormaux et amnésie durable. *Rev Neurol* **142**: 398–405.

Rosolacci, T., Neuville, V., Huric, R., and Dobbelaere, P. (1999). Complex hyperkinesia ipsilateral to right frontoparietal infarction. *Mov Disord* **14**: 879–882.

Rossetti, A. O., Ghika, J. A., Vingerhoets, F. and Novy, J. Bogousslavsky, J. (2003). Neurogenic pain and abnormal movements contralateral to an antemos pariental artery stroke. *Arch Neurol* **60**: 1004–1006.

Rumbach, L., Barth, P., and Costaz, A. and Mas, J. (1995). Hemidystonia consequent upon ipislateral vertebral artery occlusion and cerebellar infarction. *Mov Disord* **10**: 522–525.

Sandson, T. A., Daffber, K. R., Carvalho, P. A. *et al.* (1991). Frontal-like dysfunction following infarction of the left-sided medial thalamus. *Arch Neurol* **48**: 1300–1303.

Saposnik, G. and Caplan, L. R. (2001). Convulsive-like movements in brainstem stroke. *Arch Neurol* **58**: 654–657.

Saver, J. L., Greenstein, P., Ronthal, M., and Mesulam, M. M. (1993). Assymmetric catalepsy after right hemispheric stroke. *Move Disord* **8**: 69–73.

Schmidley, J. W. and Messing, R. O. (1984). Agitated confusional state in patients with right hemisphere infarctions. *Stroke* **15**: 883–885.

Schulz, U. G. and Rothwell, P. M. (2002). Transient ischemic attacks mimicking focal motor seizures. *Postgrad Med J* **78**: 246–247.

Schulze-Bonaheg, A. and Ferbert, A. (1998). Cortical action tremor and focal motor seizures after parietal infarction. *Mov Disord* **12**: 356–358.

Scott, B. L. and Jankovic, J. (1996). Delayed-onset progressive movement disorders after static brain lesions. *Neurology* **46**: 68–74.

Shepherd, G. M., Tauboll, E., Bakke, S. J., and Nyberg-Hansen, R. (1997). Midbrain tremor and hypertrophic olivary degeneration after pontine hemorrhage. *Mov Disord* **12**: 432–437.

Soler, R., Vivancos, F., Munoz-Torrero, J. J., Arpa, J., and Barreiro, P. (1999). Postural tremor after thalamic infarction. *Eur Neurol* **42**: 180–181.

Solomon, G. E., Engel, M., Hecht, H. L., and Rapoport, A. R. (1982). Progressive dyskinesia due to internal cerebral vein thrombosis. *Neurology* **32**: 769–772.

Struck, L. K., Rodnizky, R. L., and Dobson, J. K. (1990). Stroke and its modification in Parkinson's disease. *Stroke* **21**: 1395–1399.

Sumer, M. (2001). Symptomatic palatal myoclonus: an unusual cause of respiratory difficulty. *Acta Neurol Belg* **101**: 113–115.

Suwanwela, N. C. and Leelacheavasit, N. (2002). Isolated corpus callosal infarction secondary to pericallosal artery disease presenting as alien hand syndrome. *J Neurol Neurosurg Psychiatry* **72**: 533–536.

Sunohara, N., Mukoyama, M., Mano, Y., and Satoyoshi, E. (1984). Action-induced rythmic dystonia: an autopsy case. *Neurology* **34**: 321–327.

Sutton, G. G. and Meyer, R. F. (1974). Focal reflex myoclonus. *J Neurol Neurosurg and Psychiatry* **37**: 207–217.

Takeuchi, K., Matsubayashi, K., Kimura, S., *et al.* (1992). Silent lacunes in the elderly: Parkinson's disease correlated with ambulatory blood pressure. *Nippon Ronen Igakkai Zhassi* **29**: 549–553.

Tamaoka, A., Sakuta, M., and Yamada, H. (1987). Hemichorea-hemiballism caused by ateriovenous malformations in the putamen. *J Neurol* **234**: 124–125.

Tan, H., Turanli, G., and Saatci, I. (2001a). Rubral tremor after thalamic infarction in childhood. *Pediatr Neurol* **25**: 409–412.

Tan, E. K., Chan, L. L., and Auchus, A. P. (2001b). Complex movement disorders following bilateral paramedian thalamic and bilateral cerebellar infarcts. *Mov Disord* **16**: 968–970.

Tanaka, K., Fujishima, H., Motomura, S., *et al.* (1986). Acase of dural arterioverous malformation with bilateral thalmic infarction. *No To Shinkei* **38**: 1005–1010.

Tatu, L., Moulin, T., Martin, V., *et al.* (1996). Unilateral asterixis and focal brain lesions. 12 cases. *Rev Neurol* **152**: 121–127.

Thajeb, P. (1993). Gait disorders of multi-infarct dementia. CT and clinical correlation. *Acta Neurol Scandinavica* **87**: 239–242.

Tolosa, E. S. and Santamaria, J. (1984). Parkinsonism and basal ganglia infarcts. *Neurology* **34**: 1516–1518.

Tonkonogy, J. and Barreira, P. (1989). Obsessive–compulsive disorder and caudate–frontal lesion. *Neuropsychiatry Neuropsychol Behav Neurology* **2**: 203–209.

Trillet, M., Vighetto, A., Croisile, B., Charles, N., and Aimard, G. (1995). Hémiballisme avec libération thymo-affective et logorrhée par lésion du noyau sous-thalamique gauche. *Rev Neurol* **151**: 416–419.

Trouillas, P, Nighoghossian, N., and Maughière, F. (1990). Syndrome cérébelleux et asterixis unilatéral par hematome thalamique. Mécanismes présumés. *Rev Neurol* **146**: 484–489.

Uterga, J. M., Portillo, M. F., Iriondo, I., *et al.* (1999). Symptomatic paroxysmal dystonia (non-kinesigenic forms) new cases. *Neurologia* **14**: 190–192.

van Zagten, M., Lodder, J., and Kessels, F. (1998). Gait disorder and parkinsonian signs in patients with stroke related to small deep infarcts and white matter lesions Mov *Disord* **13**: 89–95.

Verret, J. M. and Lapresle, J. (1986). Séméiologie motrice du thalamus. *Rev Neurol* **142**: 368–374.

Verslegers, W., De Deyn, P. P., Saerenes, J., *et al.* (1991). Slow progressive bilateral posterior artery infarction presenting as agitated delirium, complicated with Anton's syndrome. *Eur Neurol* **31**: 216–219.

Vila, N. and Chamorro, A. (1997). Ballistic movements due to ischemic infarcts after intravenous heroin overdose: report of two cases. *Clin Neurol Neurosurg* **99**: 259–262.

von Domburg, P. H., ten Donkelaar, H. J., and Notermans, J. L. (1996). Akinetic mutism with bithalamic infarction. Neurophysiological correlates. *J Neurol Sci* **139**: 58–65.

von Giesen, H. J., Schlaug, G., Steinmetz, H., *et al.* (1994). Cerebral network underlying unilateral motor neglect: evidence from positron emission tomography. *J Neurol Sci* **125**: 29–38.

Wali, G. M. (1999). Shoulder girdle dyskinesia associated with a thalamic infarct. *Mov Disord* **14**: 375–377.

Wallesch, C. W., Brunner, R. J., and Seemuller, E. (1983). Repetitive phenomena in the spontaneous speech of aphasic patients: perseverations, stereotypy, echolalia, automatism and recurring utterance. *Fortschr Neurol Psychiatr* **51**: 427–430.

Williams, A. C., Owen, C., and Heath, D. A. (1988). A complex movement disorder with cavitation of the caudate nucleus. *J Neurol Neurosurg Psychiatry* **51**: 447–448.

Winitakes, J. and Jankovic, J. (1994). Vascular progressive supranuclear palsy. *J Neural Transm* **42**: 189–201.

Wittenberg, G. F., Bastian, A. J., Dromerick, A. W., Thach, W. T., and Powers, W. (2000). Mirror movements complicate interpretation of cerebral activation changes during recovery from subcortical infarcts. *Neurorehabil Neural Repair* **14**: 213–221.

Wu, F. Y., Leong, C. P., and Su, T. L. (1999). Alien hand syndrome: report of two cases. *Changgeng Yi Xue Za Zhi* **22**: 660–665.

Wu, J. C., Lu, C. S., and Ng, S. H. (2000). Limb myorythmia in association with hypertrophy of the inferior olive. Report of two cases. *Changgeng Yi Xue Za Zhi chang-gung Med J chang-gung Memorial Hosp* **23**: 630–635.

Yamanaka, K., Fukuyama, H., and Kimura, J. (1996). Abulia from unilateral capsular genu infarct: report of two cases. *J Neurol Sci* **143**: 181–184.

Yamadori, A., Mori, E., Trabuchi, M, Kudo Y., and Mitami, Y. (1986). Hypergraphia. A right hemisphere syndrome. *J Neurol Neurosurg and Psychiatry* (1986). **49**: 1160–1164.

Yamanouchi, H. and Nagura, H. (1997). Neurological signs and frontal white matter lesions in vascular parkinsonism. A clinicopathologic study. *Stroke* **28**: 965–969.

Yanagisawa, T., Sugihara, H., Shibahara, K., Kamo, T., Fujisawa, K., and Murayama, M. (1999). Natural course of combined limb and palatal tremor caused by cerebellar brainstem infarction. *Mov Disorders* **14**: 851–854.

Yoshikawa M, Yamamoto M, Shibata K, *et al.* (1992). Hemichorea associated with ipsilateral chronic subdural hematoma: case report. *Neurol Med Chir* (Tokyo) 32: 769–772.

Zeman, W. and Whitlock, C. C. (1968). Symptomatic dystonia. In *Handbook of Neurology*, vol. 6, ed. P. T. Viken and G. W. Bruyn. Amsterdam North Holland, pp. 554–566.

12

Spasticity and pain after stroke

Philippe Vuadens

Clinique Romande de Réadaptation, Sion, Switzerland

Michael P. Barnes

Hunters Moor Regional Neurorehabilitation Centre, Newcastle upon Tyne, UK

R. Peyron and B. Laurent

Hôpital de Bellevue, Saint-Etienne, France

Introduction

Since the studies of Sherrington(1947) on decerebrate rigidity in the cat, evidence has shown that spasticity is the result of modification of the sensitivity of the central reflex pathways. Lance defined spasticity in 1980 as a velocity-dependent increase in muscle tone in response to muscle stretch. This resistance to muscle stretch may also result in soft tissue modifications and eventually muscle and soft tissue contractures (Goldspink and Williams, 1990). In this way, it may limit movement and be a significant cause of disability and handicap. Usually spasticity is simply one part of the upper motor neuron syndrome and the other elements of the syndrome are responsible for further disability (Table 12.1).

Spasticity is a dynamic feature that can vary with the position of the limb or trunk, with time, with medication, and with a variety of other factors. Consequently, it is often difficult to evaluate the real impact of spasticity as an independent factor in its own right. The treatment must take into account all the features of the upper motor neuron syndrome, only some of which are responsive to clinical management. The main goal, as always in rehabilitation practice, is to identify the function limited by spasticity and introduce appropriate measures to improve that function. Sometimes a secondary goal can be simply to avoid unnecessary future complications associated with spasticity, such as contractures.

The aim of the first part of this chapter is to discuss the overall context of spasticity in terms of treatment decisions and outcome measures. The general management of spasticity will then be discussed both in terms of physical therapy and orthotic management as well as in terms of oral antispastic medication, focal

Recovery after Stroke, ed. Michael P. Barnes, Bruce H. Dobkin and Julien Bogousslavsky. Published by Cambridge University Press. © Cambridge University Press 2005.

Table 12.1 Features of the upper motor neurone syndrome

Positive	Negative
Spasticity (hypertonia)	Paresis
Clonus	Muscle weakness
Positive Babinski sign	Loss of dexterity and slow initiation
Extensor and flexor spasms	Fatigability
Hyperreflexia and clonus	Loss of cutaneous reflexes
Mass reflex	
Dyssynergic patterns of co-contraction during movement	
Associated reactions and other dyssynergic and stereotypical spastic patterns	

treatments, and surgery. We will then discuss the management of various types of post-stroke pain, including hemiplegic shoulder pain.

Spasticity

Definition

Lance (1980) defined spasticity as *"a motor disorder characterised by a velocity dependent increase in tonic stretch reflexes (muscle tone) with exaggerated tendon jerks, resulting from hyperexcitability of the stretch reflex, as one component of the upper motor neurone syndrome."* There are three main mechanisms that induce spasticity: modification of the muscle, new nerve collaterals at the spinal level, and exaggeration of the spinal reflexes, which are not appropriately modulated by the supraspinal pathways (Brown, 1994; Young, 1994). It is likely that the perturbations of several of these mechanisms are necessary to produce clinical spasticity. Moreover, according to the level of the lesion, spasticity can be manifest in different ways and this may be one explanation for the variable response to treatment (Faist *et al.*, 1994; Aymard *et al.*, 2000). The degree of presynaptic inhibition differs between the spine and the brain, and the absence of a relationship between the degree of clinical spasticity and the level of presynaptic inhibition implies a multifactorial origin of spasticity. These different physiopathological aspects may be important for the choice of treatment. For example, a medication that has an action on presynaptic inhibition is in theory likely to be less useful for a person with stroke because in cerebral lesions the presynaptic inhibition should be normal. However, in clinical practice the theory does not necessarily match reality.

As Lance (1980) commented, spasticity is simply one part of the upper motor neuron syndrome. Therefore, it is only one factor that can contribute to the overall motor dysfunction. In the upper motor neuron syndrome, enhanced stretch reflexes are accompanied by increased muscle tone (tonic stretch reflex activity), hyperreflexia of tendon jerks (phasic stretch reflex activity), spread or radiation of phasic stretch reflexes, and clonus (Lance, 1984) (Table 12.1). These phenomena can be explained by dysfunction of the mechanism of reciprocal inhibition at the spinal level owing to lack of control by supraspinal pathways (Pierrot-Deseilligny, 1990). However, depending on how the peripheral afferent activity is handled centrally, two types of spasticity can be described: spinal and central (Herman *et al.*, 1973). In the cerebral model, the transmission of primary ending spindle discharges occurs through monosynaptic pathways whereas this transmission is polysynaptic in the spinal model. Moreover, at the segmental level, impaired reciprocal inhibition also occurs and explains the presence of antagonistic activity, which can interfere with movement. This antagonistic contraction can mask agonist-induced motion during voluntary movement. It is essential before introducing therapeutic procedures to determine if the activity of agonist muscles is restrained by spastic activity in the antagonists. This chapter does not allow for detailed discussion of the neurophysiology of spasticity and the reader is referred to an excellent recent review of the subject by Sheean (2001a).

Spasticity rating scales

At the bedside, spasticity is characterized by the sensation of resistance felt as one moves a joint through a range of motion. This resistance depends on the physical inertia of the extremity, the mechanicoelastic characteristics of muscles and connective tissues, and reflex muscle contraction (Hufschmidt and Mauritz, 1985). Spasticity can be influenced by many factors (Table 12.2), especially the position of the limb against gravity. Therefore it is vital to be precise concerning in which particular condition and position of the limb spasticity is measured. On subsequent occasions, the limb needs to be placed in a similar position and as many external factors as possible also need to be similar on each measurement occasion.

Tone intensity scales

The most well-known spasticity rating scale is the original or modified Ashworth scale (Ashworth, 1964; Bohannon and Smith, 1987) (Table 12.3). Either version is a simple ordinal scale and easy to use if the recommendations of Pandyan and colleagues are followed (1999). The main disadvantages of these scales are that they combine the effects of both mechanical and neural components of tone and that the performance parameters are not standardized. In fact, the scale does not take

Table 12.2 External factors that may exacerbate spasticity

Pain
Decubitus ulcers, skin irritations
Seizures
Fecal impaction
Limb and body position
Deep venous thrombosis
Fever
Fractures
Urinary retention or infection
Increased sensory stimuli (orthoses, splint, ingrown toe nails, etc.)

Table 12.3 The original and modified Ashworth scales

Score	Original scale	Modified scale
0	No increase in tone	No increase in tone
1	Slight increase in tone giving a catch when the limb is moved in flexion or extension	Slight increase in muscle tone, manifested by a catch and release or by minimal resistance at the end of the ROM when the affected part(s) is moved in flexion or extension
1+	–	Slight increase in muscle tone, manifested by a catch, followed by minimal resistance throughout the remainder (less than half) of the ROM
2	More marked increase in tone but limb easily flexed	More marked increase in muscle tone through most of the ROM but affected part(s) easily moved
3	Considerable increase in tone, passive movement difficult	Considerable increase in muscle tone, passive movement difficult
4	Limb rigid in flexion or extension	Affected part(s) rigid in flexion or extension

ROM, range of motion.

positioning of the limb or the speed of the movement into consideration. Although the Ashworth scales are commonly used, they are probably best avoided. Both these aspects are considered in the scale devised by Tardieu *et al.*, 1959). In fact, resistance is measured at slow and at rapid speed. It has been validated in English and has a better inter-rater reliability than the Ashworth scale.

An alternative is the Oswestry Scale of Grading, which is also an ordinal scale and considers the influence of posture and descending brainstem and spinal reflexes (Goff, 1976). However, at present, this scale has not been properly validated.

Measurement of range of movement

To evaluate the response to treatment, the measurement of range of movement of the limb by goniometry is useful. It is usually performed by a hand-held goniometer but care should be taken to make sure that the goniometer is correctly placed on the limb and the measurement should be made according to standardized positions (Norkin and White, 1995).

Electrophysiological or biomechanical evaluation

If combined with clinical examination, electrophysiological or biomechanical measurements may help to analyze spasticity and impaired control of movement. These techniques are useful but the procedures need experience and sophisticated equipment, such as dynamic electromyography (EMG), computer-based systems, force platforms, and gait analysis facilities. Consequently, both electrophysiological and biomechanical evaluations are usually reserved for a research setting and are not really practical measures in a clinical setting (Johnson, 2001).

Measurement of disability and handicap caused by spasticity

As already mentioned, spasticity is only one of the features of the upper motor neuron syndrome and it should not be analyzed in isolation. Therefore, the evaluation of disability (activity) and handicap (participation) related to spasticity should include the effect of other positive and negative features of the syndrome on the overall control of voluntary movement. The most commonly used measurement tools of functional abilities are the Barthel Index and the Functional Independence Measure, but there are a large variety of general disability and quality of life scales that can include an assessment of motor abilities. The correct scale for a particular circumstance in a particular patient needs to be chosen with care. It should be remembered that treatment of spasticity in isolation may have only a limited overall impact on general disability and, therefore, may not produce much actual movement on a more general daily living or quality of life scale. However, it remains paramount that the impact of the spasticity treatment on the individual is given due consideration in the clinical setting, and the patient's own subjective opinion should not be discounted simply because there has been little change in the chosen scale. It may be the scale that is wrong and not the patient!

Treatment decisions

The key goal of spasticity treatment is clearly the improvement of motor function leading to improved independence in activities of daily living. However, there can be other goals of treatment. Occasionally, spasticity can be painful and a goal may simply be to reduce the pain associated with muscle spasticity. An important long-term goal is the prevention of unnecessary complications of spasticity, particularly muscle and soft-tissue contracture. Other goals that may be relevant for the individual include the preservation of skin hygiene to avoid maceration and pressure sores, the prevention of dysphagia, particularly caused by trunk and neck spasticity, and the preservation of sexual functioning. Unusually the treatment of spasticity can be justified to ease elements of nursing care. An individual, for example, may not be too troubled by their own spasticity but the spasticity and muscle spasms can make transferring, hygiene, washing, and dressing, for example, particularly difficult for the carers. Therefore, the treatment goal, and consequently the outcome measure, needs to be chosen carefully. The treatment should obviously take into account the effect of the spastic muscles on joint movement, positioning at rest, and inaction. The clinical examination may help to predict whether the limb could be made more functional, whether the deformity is caused by contractures, or whether it is still alleviable by spasticity management. It may sometime be helpful to determine which muscles are causing adverse motor patterns, and the use of EMG, dynamic EMG, gait analysis, and nerve blocks can all be helpful in particular individuals. A number of authors have attempted to describe the various commoner patterns of spasticity (e.g. Winters *et al.*, 1987; Mayer *et al.*, 1997; Rodda and Graham, 2001). It is important to emphasize once again the dynamic nature of spasticity and the fact that the spastic patterns can readily change according to the position of the patient, the time of day, timing of medication, and a variety of other factors, even including the weather. Therefore, sometimes a prolonged period of observation is necessary in order to initiate the correct treatment strategy. It is undoubtedly worth spending some time in the initial assessment phase, particularly for people who are still mobile and who may exhibit a whole variety of different spastic patterns in different circumstances.

General management

In general terms, spasticity is a disabling symptom. Feldman and colleagues (1980) showed that individuals with spasticity spent three times longer in rehabilitation units than stroke patients without hypertonia. However, it must be emphasized that the presence of spasticity is not always a reason for treatment. Sometimes, spasticity can be beneficial for patients. It can be useful, for example, for weight bearing during ambulation or to stabilize the knees for transfers and walking. Spasms can sometimes be functionally utilized for dressing. The negative effects of treatment need also to be borne in mind. Oral antispastic medication, for example, can induce weakness and so have a negative impact on functional abilities. It is, as always in rehabilitation, a matter of balance between potential functional benefit and functional loss.

Assuming that spasticity needs treatment, however, then it is first important to exclude all the non-neurological factors that may increase spasticity (Table 12.2). Education of the carers is vital at this stage as, inadvertently, the carers or even the individual themselves can make matters worse by, for example, inappropriate positioning or tightly fitting appliances. Family education is a vital prerequisite of treatment.

The positioning of the individual is of primary importance. Spasticity can often be eliminated, or at least the functional impact significantly reduced, by appropriate positioning and appropriate seating (Pope, 1992, 1996; Edwards, 1996). Correct positioning, for example, reduces the risk of algodystrophy (Katz, 1988). In the lying position, it is often helpful for the knees to be in flexion to reduce the extensor tone of the trunk and lower limbs. To minimize hypertonia in the seated position, stability at the hips and pelvis must be ensured. Wheelchairs often need to be individually tailored. Standing should be initiated as soon as possible after stroke to reduce flexor tone and encourage extensor activity. The input of a physiotherapist is vital both in the acute and chronic phases of spasticity management.

Physiotherapy

Rehabilitation of people with spasticity needs a multidisciplinary approach. In this context, the role of the physiotherapist is vital. The physiotherapist will usually lead the team in terms of advice with regard to posture, seating, and correct mobilization in order to reduce spasticity in specific muscles and realign the muscles. Treatment should start as soon as possible to avoid inappropriate patterns developing and unnecessary complications arising. It is particularly important for the physiotherapist, with others, to prevent the development of contractures (O'Dwyer and Ada, 1996; O'Dwyer *et al.*, 1996). Early intervention is important even if the patient is non-responsive, such as in a coma, as spasticity and contractures can still develop in such circumstances.

There are many different methods of physiotherapy that have been proposed over the years. Each one emphasizes mobilization and serves to improve motor control into effective function even if some of the approaches are not orientated towards the inhibition of spasticity (Perry, 1980). Brunnstrom's method (1970), for example, utilizes reflex tensing and synergistic patterns of hemiplegia to improve motor control. In Rood's paradigm (1956), the correction of tone is obtained through the use of appropriate sensory stimuli. Proprioceptive neuro-muscular facilitation attempts to teach normal patterns of movement (Knott and

Voss, 1968). It assumes that motor recovery follows a pattern similar to that of the developing nervous system.

The concept of the Bobath approach (e.g. Bobath, 1990), is based on the idea that there is a relationship between spasticity and movement, and weakness of muscles results from opposition by spastic antagonists. However, this idea has been refuted by several other studies (Landau, 1974; Sahrmann and Norton, 1977; Fellows and Thilmann, 1994). The response of a spastic muscle to stretch is different during passive and active movement; moreover, resistance to movement incorporates not only neural components but also non-neural ones, especially altered soft-tissue compliance (Dietz *et al.*, 1981; Hufschmidt and Mauritz, 1985). The Bobath method is certainly the most widely used, even if it is empirical, and no study has yet been able to demonstrate its real superiority over other techniques.

The Perfetti method is a sensory motor technique developed for controlling spasticity, especially in the arm (Perfetti *et al.*, 2001). It is based on tactile recognition from passive exploration and manipulation to active manipulation. This technique needs relative preservation of cognition. One study has shown a better recovery of upper limb function with the Perfetti method compared with the Bobath method (Rousseaux *et al.*, 2002a).

A popular approach proposed by Carr and Shepherd (1982) is to analyze each particular function so that the components that cannot be performed because of spasticity can be determined. The patient is trained in those components and the task for the physiotherapist is to ensure both appropriate training and generalization of this training into tasks of daily living.

Many modern neurological physiotherapists will now tend to be eclectic in their approach and pick and choose various physiotherapy methods that are appropriate for that individual in a given circumstance. Strict adherence to a particular physiotherapy school is an approach that has now largely vanished.

Orthotic management

Orthoses can undoubtedly be useful for restoring deformity induced by spasticity and for improving motion and function (Fig. 12.1). Orthoses obviously need to be prescribed alongside other therapies. Their prescription requires selection of appropriate objectives and periodical assessment of the patient to monitor treatment goals. Although orthoses have been used for many years, there are relatively few studies that have documented their efficacy for the management of spasticity (Kaplan, 1962; Charait, 1968; Neuhaus *et al.*, 1981; Edwards and Charlton, 1996). When an orthosis seems necessary, a Technical Analysis Form, developed by the American Academy of Orthopedic Surgeons, may be helpful for decided the nature of the prescription (McCollough, 1985).

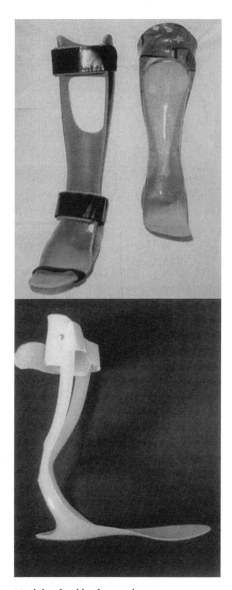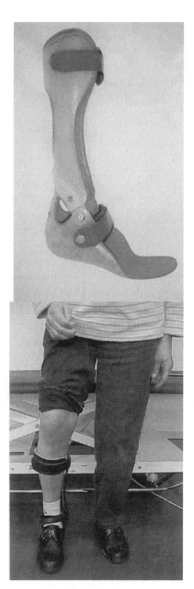

Fig. 12.1   Models of ankle–foot orthoses.

Orthoses can be useful for controlling deformity by prolonged stretch, which permits an increased range of motion and reduction of tone. They can also be useful for preventing contractures and for stabilizing a limb in a physiological position. The use of botulinum toxin can sometimes ease the fitting of an orthosis, which obviously needs to be comfortable otherwise it will not be worn (Kottke *et al.*, 1966; Tabary *et al.*, 1972; McPherson *et al.*, 1985; Hylton and Allan, 1997).

Pharmacological treatments

Progress in our understanding of the pathophysiology and neurochemistry of spasticity has offered a large variety of potential medical or even surgical possibilities for treatment (Losseff and Thompson, 1995; Spasticity Study Group, 1997; Barnes and Johnson, 2001; Pérennoud *et al.*, 2001). Before a more detailed discussion on pharmacological approaches, it is important to emphasize that it would be unusual for a medical treatment to be the only modality used in the management of spasticity. Medical approaches will nearly always need to be combined with other measures, particularly physiotherapy. The drugs described below are all efficacious in reducing spasticity, but none is clearly superior in reducing disability (Ward and Ko, 2001). In general terms, the oral antispastic drugs, such as baclofen, dantrolene, or tizanidine, are most effective in mild spasticity. As the spasticity becomes more severe, then it is usually more appropriate for focal treatments to be initiated, such as local nerve blockade or the use of botulinum toxin. Before any oral medication is initiated, the potential negative effects of such treatment, particularly muscle weakness and fatigability, need to be borne in mind and actively monitored during ongoing treatment. It is often the emergence of adverse effects that limits the dose, sometimes prior to the emergence of any functionally significant antispastic effects.

Benzodiazepines

Benzodiazepines are the oldest antispastic drugs and continue to be prescribed even though there are now preferable drugs available (Randall, 1982). In 1961, Randall and colleagues showed a decrease in rigidity and flexor reflexes in decerebrate cats given diazepam. This effect was confirmed in humans with hemiplegia (Kendall, 1964). Since this first positive report, many further studies have confirmed the benefit of diazepam for the relief of spasticity. Biochemically, benzodiazepines increase the affinity of gamma-aminobutyric acid (GABA) type A (GABA$_A$) receptors for the endogenous neurotransmitter. This leads to an increase of the chloride current and augmentation of presynaptic inhibition in the spinal cord. In turn, a reduction in the release of excitatory transmitters from afferent sensory pathways induces a reduction of the gain of the stretch reflex and of spasticity (Randall, 1982).

Among the different benzodiazepines used for the management of spasticity and associated spasms, diazepam is the most common. It is metabolized by the liver and has a long half-life of 20–80 hours. Clonazepam, usually used for the treatment of epileptic seizures, is sometimes prescribed for the treatment of nocturnal spasms. Chlorazepate has an antispastic effect that is longer than that of diazepam or clonazepam. Few studies have really evaluated the effect of benzodiazepines in the stroke population. After the first study of Kendall 1964), a double-blind cross-over study evaluated the effects of diazepam, phenobarbital, and placebo on 19 hemiplegic patients, 16 with stroke (Cocchiarella *et al.*, 1967). The outcome measures revealed no significant effects on such measures as grip strength and timed maze walk; indeed, the performance of grip and walk were worse on diazepam. In a group of 51 patients with spasticity caused by spinal and supraspinal lesions and treated with four different antispastic drugs (diazepam, baclofen, tizanidine, and idrocilamide), diazepam enhanced vibratory inhibition of tendon reflexes and baclofen, in other patients, normalized the H-reflex recovery curves (Delwaide *et al.*, 1980). Glass and Hannah (1974) compared the effects of dantrolene and diazepam. The improvement of a mixed population, including stroke patients, was the same for each drug used alone. However, the results were better for treatment with both drugs together. Clonazepam seemed to be equally effective as diazepam but was less well tolerated in one study because of increased sedation (Cendrowski and Sobczyk, 1977).

The efficacy of benzodiazepines in the treatment of spasticity resulting from cerebral lesions is, in general terms, poor, and the utilization is often limited by adverse effects, particularly sedation and drowsiness. It is for this reason that clinicians would generally prefer baclofen (Roussan *et al.*, 1987). The adverse effects are dose dependent, particularly in elderly people; somnolence, dizziness, and ataxia are particularly troublesome. Moreover, benzodiazepines may impair coordination, intellect, attention, and memory. Physiological dependence can also occur, especially when high doses are used and over longer periods of time. Therefore, there is a risk of a withdrawal syndrome. Benzodiazepines should always be used with caution and initiated at a low dose. It is now reasonable to state that benzodiazepines should probably be in the last line of drugs when other medications have failed to have the necessary effects.

Baclofen

Baclofen is one of the most powerful antispastic drugs and probably the most widely used. It is an analogue to GABA and acts on $GABA_B$ receptors. At the spinal cord level, these receptors are mainly located presynaptically on afferent neurons and GABAergic interneurons. Some postsynaptic receptors are present on the Ia sensory afferent terminals (Davidoff, 1985; Rice, 1987; Bowery, 1989; Dressnandt *et al.*, 1995). Through this GABAergic stimulation, baclofen increases presynaptic inhibition, leading to a reduction in activity of mono- and polysynaptic reflexes. There is a large intersubject variation in absorption and elimination. The mean half-life of baclofen is approximately 3.5 hours and it is secreted by the kidney. It is partially metabolized in the liver. Consequently, liver function parameters should be checked and doses must be reduced in the presence of renal and liver insufficiency.

The efficacy of baclofen on spasticity has been evaluated in patients with multiple sclerosis or spinal cord injury (Bastings and Malapira, 2002). It seems most effective in spinal cord spasticity. It can reduced slow passive stretch responses, increase muscle tone and ankle clonus, and has been shown to reduce the number and intensity of painful spasms (Duncan et al., 1976; McLellan, 1977; Milanov, 1992). There is not yet evidence that baclofen can have a real functional benefit and there are no published studies that show improvement in gait or manual dexterity (Pedersen et al., 1970; Basmajan, 1975; McLellan, 1977; Young and Delwaide, 1981). Baclofen, like other drugs, probably does have a significant impact on spasticity-associated disability but this is yet to be shown in the published literature with any degree of robustness. In some people, baclofen can worsen ambulation by increasing muscle weakness. Baclofen seems to be less effective in spasticity resulting from cerebral lesions, which includes stroke patients. These individuals tend to benefit less and experience more side-effects (Pedersen et al., 1974; van Hemert, 1980). In a review of European clinical trials of baclofen, Hattab (1980) reported 53 publications covering 2284 patients with an incidence of unwanted effects of 42%. This incidence was higher in cerebral spasticity; problems included daytime sedation, confusion, euphoria, and muscular weakness.

Dantrolene

Dantrolene is an antispastic drug that is rather different from most others available in that it acts directly on the muscle. It inhibits the release of intramuscular calcium from the sarcoplasmic reticulum of striated muscles. This induces a reduction of strength by excitation–contraction uncoupling (Ward et al., 1986).

Placebo-controlled trials with dantrolene sodium have demonstrated a reduction of muscle tone, tendon reflexes, and clonus and an increase in range of passive movement (Pinder et al., 1977; Katrak et al., 1992). It can be used for all causes of spasticity and, therefore, may be especially useful for stroke patients (Chyatte and Bergman, 1971; Katrak et al., 1992). However, the actual efficacy of dantrolene in the management of spasticity is still unproven. Some studies have reported improvement with dantrolene and others have failed to document any functional improvements (Chyatte and Bergman, 1971). Moreover, in one study, weakness and difficulty in climbing stairs was reported during dantrolene treatment (Chyatte and Bergman, 1971). There have been a few trials that have compared dantrolene and diazepam in patients with spinal or cerebral spasticity (Glass and Hannah, 1974; Nogen, 1976; Schmidt et al., 1976). It seems that dantrolene was better tolerated in these studies. It also seems that a combination of the two drugs increased the efficacy.

The adverse effects are mainly nausea, vomiting, diarrhea, dizziness, and par-esthesiae (Schmidt *et al.*, 1976). Sedation is less frequent than with benzodiaze-pines or baclofen. However, the most serious adverse effect is hepatotoxicity, leading to hepatonecrosis – particularly in females (Ward *et al.*, 1986). Therefore, it is vital for liver function to be checked regularly.

Tizanidine

Tizanidine is an agonist of the α_2-adrenoceptors (spinal and supraspinal nor-adrenergic activity) that inhibits the release of glutamate and aspartate from spinal interneurons and decreases the action of excitatory neurotransmitters at their receptors (Newman *et al.*, 1982). The efficacy of tizanidine is similar to baclofen, at least in people with multiple sclerosis and spinal cord injury (Newman *et al.*, 1982; Stein *et al.*, 1987; Bes *et al.*, 1988; Eyssette *et al.*, 1988; Wallace, 1994). However, tizanidine seems to be more effective than the other drugs in reducing clonus and is probably better tolerated and there seems to be less risk of muscle weakness (Lataste *et al.*, 1994). In one trial, tizanidine was compared with diazepam and was found to have a better effect with regard to walking distance and was better tolerated (Bes *et al.*, 1988). Another study confirmed the positive effect of tizani-dine in stroke patients. In 47 people treated for 16 weeks there was a reduction in muscle tone measured by the modified Ashworth scale and improvement in pain and a trend towards improvement in functional abilities (Gelber *et al.*, 2001). Treatment needs to be initiated at a low dose and progressed slowly up to a maximum of approximately 36 mg per day. A longer-lasting form of 6 mg tablets allows dosing once or twice daily, which may be useful for those who are disturbed by nocturnal spasms. The principal adverse effects of tizanidine are dry mouth and sedation. Sometimes individuals complain of drowsiness, tiredness, and dizziness; symptomatic hypotension may also occur, especially if tizanidine is combined with clonidine. Visual hallucinations and confusion have been reported. Liver dysfunction is also possible but rare; nevertheless, liver function need to be monitored at regular intervals.

Other alternative medications

There are a large number of other potential medications that can be used for the treatment of spasticity (Table 12.4). The efficacy is mainly demonstrated for spinal spasticity or for those with severe and generalized spasticity. However, in general terms, these other agents have not been subject to rigorous evaluation and few have been evaluated in the context of stroke. Probably most studies have been conducted on gabapentin. The role of cannabinoids and indeed cannabis itself is currently undergoing evaluation in a number of multicenter trials.

Table 12.4 Alternative antispastic drugs

Drug	Dose	Main side-effects
Clonidine	0.05–0.4	Postural hypotension, lethargy, dizziness
Valproic acid	250–1000	Nausea, vomiting, drowsiness
Gabapentin	100–3600	Drowsiness
Piracetam	50 (per kg body weight)	Nausea, vomiting
Progabide	10–45 (per kg body weight)	Drowsiness, dizziness, nausea, elevation of liver enzymes
Cyproheptadine	12–24	Sedation, dry mouth
Cyclobenzaprine	30–60	Sedation, dry mouth
Cannabinoids	5–10	Long-term tolerance, addiction

Focal pharmacological treatments

Nerve blocks

Focal antispastic treatment is often of particular help in people with more severe spasticity after stroke as such treatment can often reduce the need for oral antispastic medications with their associated side-effects. Nerve blocks have a long history of usage in the management of focal spasticity (Khalili and Betts, 1967; Braun et al., 1973; Bakheit et al., 1996). Proper evaluation is obviously essential prior to nerve blocks. It is important to determine precisely the severity and location of spasticity, the relative strength of the muscles, and the passive and active range of motion of the affected joint in order to predict the potential gain after the block. The success of the block often depends on the presence or absence of contractures. Sometimes a nerve block with a local anesthetic agent can be useful to evaluate the effect of a more prolonged block. The longer-acting neuro-lytic agents used are usually phenol or alcohol, and these should be injected as close as possible to the nerve trunk or to the motor points. The procedure can be rather prolonged but with perseverance the results can be good (Skeil and Barnes, 1994). Side-effects of the procedure can be local infection, edema, and, if mixed sensory motor nerves are injected, painful dysesthesae. The clinical duration is variable and probably depends on the proximity of the neurolytic agent to the nerve trunk. It can vary from a few hours to several months; occasionally the effect can be permanent. Obviously such clinical variability can be a disadvantage. Although the procedure can be time consuming, it has the advantage of being cheap and so it is particularly applicable in countries or health systems where more expensive alternatives, such as botulinum toxin, may not be available.

Botulinum toxin

The paralytic effect of botulinum toxin has become useful for the treatment of focal spasticity in the last few years. Injections of the toxin induce irreversible chemodenervation and paralysis through blockade of acetylcholine release at the presynaptic nerve terminal (Burgen *et al.*, 1949). The denervation can occur in both the alpha motor innervated extrafusal fibers and the gamma motor inner-vated intrafusal fibers (Rosales *et al.*, 1996). Some central effect may be possible as a result of retrograde axonal transport (Wiegand *et al.*, 1976). The technique requires injection into the muscle and a paralytic effect appears usually after 48–72 hours and the duration of response is usually around three months, with a range of 2–6 months. However, the injection technique itself is relatively simple and not too painful. The toxin is reconstituted with normal saline and injected into the affected muscles. Most authorities would now suggest that EMG guidance is not essential, although it can be used – particularly if smaller muscles, such as in the hand or feet, are being injected. The exact localization of the toxin is not too important as it diffuses along the muscle planes (Borodic *et al.*, 1992; Park, 1995). A large variety of muscles can be injected. There is no generally accepted maximum dose of botulinum toxin at one session, but most authorities would suggest a maximum of approximately 2000 Dysport units or 600 Botox units. At this point, it is important to emphasize that botulinum toxin type A is made by two different manufacturers: Ipsen (product: Dysport) and Allergan (product: Botox). The units used are different and approximately 3.5 Dysport units is equivalent to 1 Botox unit. Botulinum type B is now available (Elan Pharmaceuticals: Neurobloc/Myobloc). The injection technique is identical but once again the toxin units are different (available in 2500, 5000, 10 000 unit ready prepared ampules).

In the stroke population, a number of studies have now demonstrated a significant improvement in muscle tone. Functional benefit has been less consistently proven, but once again this probably reflects lack of studies rather than lack of efficacy. There may also be a factor regarding the use of global outcome measures when a more focal and functional outcome measure may be more appropriate (Sheean, 2001b). Some studies have shown an improvement in daily activities and others have failed to show a significant functional benefit (Hesse *et al.*, 1992; Mémin *et al.*, 1992; Dunne *et al.*, 1995; Reiter *et al.*, 1996; Simpson *et al.*, 1996; Sampaio *et al.*, 1997; Bakheit *et al.*, 2000; Richardson *et al.*, 2000; Smith *et al.*, 2000; Rousseaux *et al.*, 2002b). Other studies in the legs have once again shown improvements in impairment in the Ashworth scale and often improvement in gait velocity (Dengler *et al.*, 1992; Hesse *et al.*, 1994; Burbaud *et al.*, 1996; Reiter *et al.*, 1998).

However, the current consensus is that botulinum toxin has an important and significant role to play in the management of focal spasticity (Davis and Barnes, 2000)

A number of questions remain. The exact dose and dilution and the role of EMG needs to be clarified. However, in particular, the role of botulinum toxin in conjunction with other therapies needs further elucidation. For example, there is some indication that, short-term electrical stimulation may enhance the effectiveness of the toxin (Hesse *et al.*, 1998).

Botulinum toxin has a further advantage of being remarkably safe. There are very few side-effects. A small proportion of people (around 1%) complain of a influenza-like illness for a few days but otherwise there are virtually no reported systemic effects. Spread of the toxin can, of course, cause local and neighboring muscle weakness, which, for a patient who is still mobile or has functional use of the arm, may be problematic.

In general, botulinum toxin has proved a remarkable and useful advance in the overall management of spasticity.

Intrathecal baclofen

A number of studies have now confirmed the efficacy of intrathecal baclofen as a treatment of spinal spasticity. It can not only improve spasticity but also alleviate pain associated with muscle spasm and alleviate pain of musculoskeletal origin (Meythaler *et al.*, 1996). Successful treatment has been reported for spasticity of cerebral origin (Meythaler *et al.*, 1996; Becker *et al.*, 1997). However, in these circumstances, dosage needs to be about twice that required for spinal spasticity and there is a higher risk of epileptic seizures (Saltuari *et al.*, 1992; Rifici *et al.*, 1994). The treatment is not often used in people after stroke, but one recent study enrolled 59 patients with spastic hemiplegia. There was a significant decrease of spasticity with modification of strength. A functional benefit measured by the Functional Independence Measure and the Sickness Impact Profile was also apparent after treatment (Francisco 2002).

The technique obviously involves a surgical procedure to insert the intrathecal catheter and the automatic pump under the skin. The pump will need to be refilled at intervals. A test dose is normally required to determine the eventual pump dosage. The pump can be externally programed to adjust the infusion rate as required. Pump complications are possible, such as catheter blockage, pump failure, and infection, but such complications are relatively unusual.

Surgical management of spasticity

When spasticity is excessive, harmful, and not sufficiently controlled by physical and pharmacological treatments, surgery, especially neurosurgical procedures, can be appropriate and useful (Keenan, 1987; Sindou *et al.*, 1991; Hysey and Keenan,

1999). There are several orthopedic surgical techniques that can modify muscle function, including denervation, tendon release, tendon lengthening, and tendon transfer. Denervation or selective neurotomies can be helpful in focal spasticity: particularly obturator neurectomy and/or adductor tenotomy. Tendon or muscle release will correct a static contracture. Lengthening of a muscle tendon unit is preferred when muscle exhibits volitional control with dyssynergy. In order to redirect a muscle force, a tendon transfer can be used. Neuroablative or neurosurgical techniques can be chosen if spasticity is localized to muscle groups or affects an entire limb. The techniques are rarely used in stroke patients except for very severe bilateral spasticity. Posterior rhizotomy attempts to abolish the afferent input to the monosynaptic stretch and polysynaptic withdrawal reflexes by sectioning selectively and partially the lumbosacral roots. Percutaneous radiofrequency rhizotomy produces the same effect by heat lesions from L1 to S1. Different types of myelotomy or selective spinal cordectomy are invasive and radical surgical procedures that can be used in extreme circumstances. The use of intrathecal phenol is also a possibility for individuals with the most severe forms of spasticity. The surgical detail is beyond the scope of this chapter, but the reader is referred to a useful review of the subject (Mertens and Sindou, 2001).

Conclusions

The management of spasticity is an ideal example of the importance of the multidisciplinary rehabilitation team. The involvement of the physiotherapist, orthotist, and doctor, amongst others, is vital to the overall management. Often successful treatment can be relatively simple and just involve removal of external exacerbating factors and proper seating and positioning. If treatment is needed, then there is now a wide choice of other physical therapeutic techniques, orthoses, oral medications, and focal treatments, particularly the use of nerve blocks and botulinum toxin. Overall, the management of spasticity can often produce rewarding results and significant reductions in unnecessary disability.

Pain after stroke

Spasticity can be painful, and adequate treatment of spasticity can obviously reduce such pain. However, there are other causes of pain after a stroke and this part of the chapter will deal with the assessment and treatment of other causes of post-stroke pain. Pain can be defined as an unpleasant sensory and/or emotional experience associated with actual or potential tissue damage (Justins *et al.*, 2003): Merskey and Bogduk, 1994). There are a number of different types of pain
- allodynia: pain from a stimulus that does not normally provoke pain
- dysesthesia: an unpleasant abnormal sensation whether spontaneous or evoked

- hyperalgesia: an increased response to a stimulus that would normally be painful
- hyperesthesia: an increase in severity (sensitivity) to stimulation
- hyperpathia: a painful syndrome characterized by an increased reaction to a stimulus, especially a repetitive stimulus, as well as an increased threshold to such stimulus
- paresthesia: an abnormal sensation, whether abnormal or provoked.

Pain in the context of stroke is mainly generated directly by the damaged nervous system. However, other non-stroke causes of pain should be taken into account, particularly musculoskeletal problems secondary to joint disorders, which are often secondary to abnormal postures induced by the stroke. Other causes of continuing pain should not be forgotten, such as bladder disease, pressure ulcers, or even, in those with severe cognitive impairment, fractured limbs or abdominal emergencies. The assessment of pain can be complicated and time consuming as often there is an associated psychological element to pain or to coping with the pain. An assessment of someone with long-term neurological pain needs to be multidisciplinary and will often utilize, for example, neurologists, neurosurgeons, orthopedic surgeons, anesthetists with a special interest in chronic pain, and rehabilitation physicians, as well as physiotherapists, occupational therapists, clinical psychologists, specialist nurses, and complementary medicine practitioners, particularly those specializing in acupuncture.

It is not appropriate in this chapter to cover the management of non-neurological causes of pain. It is simply important to note that non-neurological causes of pain exist in the individual after stroke. This is particularly true of osteoarthritic pain which, given the general age of the stroke population, is likely to be already present in the individual at the time of the stroke. Obviously postural changes in the limbs or the need for prolonged periods in bed or in a wheelchair can worsen such musculoskeletal and arthritic pain. This chapter will not discuss the assessment or the management of pain from peripheral structures, such as pain secondary to peripheral neuropathy or muscle disorders, except for the management of spasticity outlined in the earlier part of the chapter. This section will concentrate on the assessment and management of central pain syndromes as well as making a brief mention of complex regional pain syndrome (CRPS) type 1 and type 2.

Central pain syndromes

Central post-stroke pain (CPSP) used to be known as a thalamic syndrome. However, the latter title is inappropriate as many cases are now known to have an origin in extrathalamic structures. Dejerine and Roussy (1906) were the first authors to describe the thalamic syndrome. In the laterobulbar brainstem syndrome (Wallenberg's syndrome), the incidence of central pain is thought to be approximately 70%. CPSP can also occur in spinal cord syndromes, such as the anterior spinal artery syndrome: more frequently found at incomplete lesions rather than complete lesions (Davidoff *et al.*, 1987). Other brain areas involved in causation of CPSP include the parietal cortex, which is clearly implicated in sensory processing (Peyron *et al.*, 1999) as confirmed by positron emission tomography (PET) and functional magnetic resonance imaging (FMRI) studies. Nevertheless, in most cases, central pain is found in the presence of lesions involving the posterior parietal cortex, thalamoparietal radiations, or the thalamus itself.

The incidence of CPSP post-stroke varies considerably in the literature but probably the incidence is approximately 2–8% (Andersen *et al.*, 1995; Kumral *et al.*, 1995). It may affect younger people rather than older people and may also occur more commonly in those with relatively mild motor deficits. The onset of CPSP can either be immediately after the stroke or delayed for several months. Description of the pain is also variable, but the commonest descriptor is of a burning sensation made worse by a number of factors, including movement, touch, and cold. Other descriptors include such terms as "shooting," "lancinating," "stabbing," and "jolting" pain. The pain is often associated with various combinations of allodynia, hyperalgesia, hyperpathia, and hyperesthesia. Occasionally, the pain can be exacerbated by emotions. Often individuals have concurrently both superficial and deep pain. Usually the pain is constant but occasionally (perhaps approximately 15%) the pain is intermittent. Sometimes, there is an abnormal radiation of pain from a specific location to another bodily location. The terms allochiria or Mitempfindung can be used to describe this sensation. An example would be light stroking of the upper thigh resulting in a similar sensation of light stroking in the ankle or foot (Gonzales and Casey, 2003).

Pathophysiology

The pathophysiology of CPSP is basically unknown. Ansreddine and Saver (1997) demonstrated that right-sided thalamic lesions were more common than left-sided lesions. Otherwise, clinical evidence shows that damage to the spinothalamic tract or its major thalamocortical projections is a critical feature in the pathophysiology. There are a number of hypothetical mechanisms that may not be mutually exclusive.

Disinhibition

One theory is that disinhibition may result from lesions of the spinothalamic tract, leading to loss of feedback control over nociceptive inputs to the spinal dorsal horn (Craig and Bushnell, 1994). However, such disinhibition caused by damage to the spinothalamic tract does not explain some of the clinical phenomenon, such as delayed onset. Other authors have suggested that denervation and supersensitivity may play a role. Spinal thalamic tract denervation, perhaps by altering membrane neurotransmitter receptor sensitivity, may alter the firing of thalamic cells, which may play some role in the perception of pain. Bowsher (1996) suggested that one critical factor in CPSP is a receptor or metabolically based reduction in the nociceptive inhibitory action of noradrenergic neurotransmitters. Deficiencies in GABA-mediated inhibition have been demonstrated in animal models. The clinical effectiveness of lamotrigine, for example, suggests that enhanced glutaminergic activation of N-methyl-D-aspartate (NMDA) receptors may be the critical abnormality in some cases of CPSP. Finally, other authors have suggested that there may be some maladaptive process with regard to neural plasticity following stroke. The long-term reorganizational processes may be important in some patients as suggested by the latency between injury and symptom onset in a number of people. Spinothalamic or spinoreticulothalamic inputs ascending from an injured spinal cord, for example, may be perceived as painful because of maladaptive reorganizations within the forebrain (van den Pol 1997). Overall, it is likely that CPSP is not caused by a single critical abnormality but by several mechanisms acting either individually or together to produce a spectrum of CPSP syndromes. The advent of PET scanning and fMRI after stroke should rapidly improve our knowledge of underlying pathophysiological mechanisms of central pain (Craig *et al.*, 1996; Peyron *et al.*, 1999).

Treatment

The adequate treatment of CPSP can be very difficult. A reasonable goal to aim for is pain reduction rather than complete pain removal. In some individuals, CPSP is a self-limiting problem occurring during the recovery phase after stroke and the pain can spontaneously resolve. However, in many people it remains a long-term problem. Treatment must also bear in mind the significant range of adverse effects that can be associated with the various treatment entities: particularly sedation, nausea, vomiting, and constipation. Finally, it should be remembered that there are a number of other physical conditions that can initiate or exacerbate chronic pain, including pressure sores, spasticity, bladder infections, etc.

Overall resolution of the pain over a period of years has been reported in approximately 20% of patients with CPSP, and another 30% report some spontaneous pain reduction (Leijon and Boivie, 1996).

Physiotherapy

Physiotherapy is important after stroke to ensure correct seating and posture. Incorrect positioning can not only exacerbate post-stroke musculoskeletal pain but also worsen CPSP. Therefore, as always in rehabilitation, proper regarding to appropriate posture is vital.

Psychological input

There is a significant risk of depression in central CPSP. A number of individuals have significant difficulty in coping with chronic pain, which begins to have an overwhelming effect on their lifestyle and quality of life. Consequently, appropriate psychiatric or psychological intervention for the treatment of depression and/or anxiety is an important parallel treatment. Obviously, antidepressant medication, which may have a role in its own right in the treatment of pain (see below), may be useful. Relaxation training can be helpful, and mental imagery to induce a relaxed state of mind has been used (Benson *et al.*, 1989). More direct approaches to pain management itself are also possible. There are various direct cognitive strategies that help to address the patient's thoughts about pain and its impact on his or her life. Individuals can be taught to focus on avoiding unhelpful and maladaptive ways of thinking about the pain and replacing such thinking strategies with more positively adapted thoughts. There is some evidence of benefit from such an approach in individuals with chronic pain, although no hard direct evidence in the context of CPSP (Rosenstiel and Keefe, 1983). There are also specific behavioral approaches to pain management that, simplistically, include non-reinforcement of pain behaviors in association with positive reinforcement of 'wellness' behaviors. There is now good evidence that a consistent behavioral approach can be helpful (Kerns *et al.*, 1986). Therefore, the involvement of a properly trained clinical psychologist or psychiatrist with an interest in pain can be an important component in the overall treatment strategy for CPSP. Indeed a report of the Working Party of the Pain Society (1997) recommended that a pain management program should include posture retraining, relaxation, education about pain and pain management, regular review of medication, psychological assessment and intervention, and a graded return to activities of daily living. While drug and surgical management of pain are important, it is equally important to remember the broader psychological and social consequences of chronic pain.

Pharmacological management of central pain

Regrettably, there is little literature on the pharmacological management of central pain (Schwartzman *et al.*, 2001). There are relatively few controlled studies and such studies that have been performed have often included only small numbers of people. However, there are now a number of drugs that have been shown to be useful in the management of CPSP and that have a reasonably robust evidence base.

Antidepressants

A variety of antidepressants have now been shown to have some success in the management of CPSP. Amitriptyline has been studied more than most other drugs. Other cyclic compounds have also been shown to produce some benefit, including nortriptyline, imipramine, disipramine, and doxepin. The newer selective serotonin-reuptake inhibitors have been studied rather less but nevertheless there is evidence of the efficacy of fluoxetine and sertraline and further evidence regarding other antidepressant compounds such as trazodone. (Leijon and Boivie, 1989a; Cobbel, 1986).

Anticonvulsant drugs

There are now some reasonable studies of the use of anticonvulsant drugs in CPSP. Probably the most studied drug is carbamazepine, but there is also evidence of the efficacy of phenytoin as well as GABAergic agents, including clonazepam and valproate (Agnew and Goldberg, 1976; Swerdlow and Cundill, 1981). A number of studies have indicated the efficacy of gabapentin at a dosage of up to 2.4 g per day. It seems to have antihyperalgesic and antiallodynic effects and is equally effective in reducing pain for peripheral nerve injuries as well as central lesions and paroxysmal pain (Attal et al., 1998). Likewise, studies have shown the efficacy of lamotrigine (Harbison et al., 1997).

Opioid analgesics

The use of opioids for CPSP is fraught with problems and it is generally recommended that they should be avoided if at all possible. However, some patients do report some analgesic effects from relatively low doses of opioids but regrettably most need relatively high doses, with associated difficulties (Hammond, 1991).

Adrenergic agents

Clonidine and propanolol are known to have some analgesic properties but regrettably there have been no definitive studies in CPSP. Tizanidine, an antispastic agent, may have some direct analgesic properties.

Other agents

Some studies have shown the efficacy of the anesthetic agents lidocaine and mexiletine in the context of deafferented pain. However, there have been no definitive studies in the context of central pain.

Naloxone has also been reported to be very useful but only in small studies with few patients (Budd and Follows, 1987; Bainton et al., 1992).

Phenothiazines, particularly chlorpromazine, have been successfully used in at least one study (Margolis and Gianascol, 1956).

Other treatments

Transcutaneous electrical nerve stimulation

Transcutaneous electrical nerve stimulation (TENS) has been reported to be useful for post-stroke pain but regrettably there are few studies. The treatment at least has the benefit of few side-effects and the further advantage of allowing the individual to control the electrical input and modulate the pain according to personal need. It is regrettable that there are no good-quality long-term studies (Leijon and Boivie, 1989b).

Central nervous system stimulation

There are a few reports of intracerebral or posterior column stimulation for pain alleviation. The intracerebral stimulation is usually in the thalamic region, but techniques involving spinal cord stimulation have also been developed. Undoubtedly, spinal cord stimulation can be a very useful procedure for pain caused by peripheral nerve lesions, but there has been little reported success in the context of central pain syndromes. The advent of deep brain stimulation may produce some better-quality studies involving reasonable numbers of people but at the moment efficacy in central pain syndromes is still lacking.

Ablative procedures on the nervous system

Over the years, there have been a number of neurosurgical operations developed for the relief of various pain syndromes. Such procedures should be avoided if at all possible because of their irreversible nature. In addition, individuals may not be particularly fit for neurosurgical procedures after stroke. There are a number of ablative procedures on the spinal cord and brain. However, many are helpful only in the context of pain of peripheral origin rather than central pain. Dorsal route entry-zone lesions can sometimes be useful but usually in the context of significant spasticity and associated pain. More central procedures such as thalamotomy, post-central gyrectomy, frontal leukotomy, and cingulotomy were in vogue a number of years ago but should be rarely, if ever, used these days. It is more likely that deep brain stimulation rather than ablative procedures will be useful in the future (Sjolund, 1991).

Conclusions

There are clearly a number of treatment methodologies for the management of chronic central pain. The evidence is rather patchy for the efficacy of a number of agents and there is certainly no clear hierarchy of strategies that should be tried. Most individuals would start with antidepressant and/or anticonvulsant medication with psychosocial support. Adrenergic agents, opioid analgesics and TENS may be used as a second line with or without neuropsychiatric intervention as appropriate. Various neurosurgical, stimulative, and ablative procedures should be reserved for the more severe and resistant cases.

Complex regional pain syndromes

The sympathetic nervous system has an important role in the generation and maintenance of chronic pain. Nerve damage can lead to a disturbance in sympathetic activity, which, in turn, can lead to a group of conditions now termed complex regional pain syndrome (CRPS) type 1 and type 2. These syndromes were previously called reflex sympathetic dystrophy or causalgia. These syndromes mainly follow relatively mild trauma but can rarely follow fracture, soft-tissue lesions and immobilization or other medical events, including stroke. Usually symptoms occur within a month or so of the initial trauma. The pain is described as burning or continuous and is often exacerbated by movement. The pain is usually disproportionate to the initiating lesion and associated with evidence of edema, changes in skin blood flow, abnormal sudomotor activity, allodynia, and hyperalgesia. Impairment of motor function can follow and there are often other signs, such as atrophy of the nails and skin and alterations in the hair growth. Treatment is usually unsatisfactory and focuses on a similar range of options as outlined for the management of CPSP. Regional infusions of sympatholytic agents, such as guanethidine or reserpine, are obviously more likely to be helpful in CRPS than in CPSP, as are other local treatments, including lidocaine, either topically or intravenously. Surgical sympathetic nerve blockades can be helpful. Stimulation analgesia, such as TENS or spinal cord stimulation, is also more likely to help chronic CRPS than CPSP. The reader is referred to an up-to-date review of the subject written by Sandroni and colleagues (2003).

Hemiplegic shoulder pain

Although this chapter has not concentrated on musculoskeletal and arthritic pain, it is appropriate to discuss the prevention, diagnosis, and management of hemiplegic shoulder pain as it is such a common problem after stroke. Shoulder pain occurs in up to 84% of hemiparetic stroke patients (Vuagnat and Chantraine, 2003). There are a number of causes of shoulder pain and the commonest are shoulder dysfunction secondary to imbalance of tone around the shoulder muscles, biceps tendonitis, rotator cuff tear, frozen shoulder, inferior subluxation, and CRPS.

The shoulder is a complex joint with a fairly wide range of motion stabilized mainly by surrounding muscles. The absence of motor activity during the flaccid stage of hemiplegia prevents proper stabilization of the shoulder, which becomes very vulnerable to strain and injury. Under the action of gravity, the humerus slips downwards, stretching the joint capsule, the glenohumeral ligaments, and the rotator cuff muscles. The resulting inferior subluxation of the glenohumeral joint is very commonly seen but is thought to be painless unless the shoulder is further traumatized by tissue damage to tendons, ligaments, and capsules (Braus *et al.*, 1994; Zorowitz *et al.*, 1996). The usual cause of such traumatization of the tissues is improper handling of the shoulder, which in turn leads to capsulitis, bursitis, and even lesions of the brachial plexus, subscapular nerve, or axilliary nerve (Moskowitz and Porter, 1963).

Such injuries to the shoulder should be preventable. It is vital that the shoulder is kept correctly positioned at all times in order to minimize the subluxation by supporting the weight of the arm. Proper transfer and handling techniques should be used to move the patient. Pulling on the paretic arm, lifting the patient by holding underneath their axilla, or letting the arm move passively around without control will disrupt the shoulder and should be avoided. It is important to emphasize that the prevention of such injuries is not limited to the ward but to the therapy areas and during transportation, imaging procedures, and relative's visits, etc. Teaching everyone involved with the individual, including the family, reduces the incidence of such complications (Braus *et al.*, 1994). The use of slings to reduce subluxation is controversial. Their efficiency is limited and the weight of the arm has to be supported by the neck. Tapes may provide a better solution but need to be constantly renewed (Ancliffe, 1992). In order to be efficient, the tapes have to fit tightly on to the arm and there may be a risk of interfering with venous and lymphatic drainage and thus increasing edema. A lapboard fixed onto a wheelchair may be another solution, with the arm placed on it slightly externally rotated with the elbow joint partly extended. Such position should give support to the humerus. However, there is no evidence to confirm the efficacy of any such technique.

Despite controversy over the mechanism to prevent such problems, prevention is far better than cure. Once the hemiplegic shoulder has developed, then it can be extremely resistant to treatment. Functional electrical stimulation to the supra-spinatus and deltoid muscle can produce a lasting reduction of subluxation (Chantraine *et al.*, 1999). Intra-articular steroid injections can reduce the pain (Dekker *et al.*, 1997). There is no evidence from systematic reviews that physiotherapy has any effect on the long-term outcome (van der Heijden *et al.*, 1997). Non-steroidal anti-inflammatory agents are probably helpful at least in the short term. Local TENS has been shown to lead to prolonged pain relief and increased range of movement (Leandri *et al.*, 1990). Other treatment modalities for CPSP may be used if all else fails but there is little evidence of efficacy for centrally acting analgesic agents such as anticonvulsants and antidepressants.

Overall it is important to emphasize that proper instructions to all involved, including the family, on handling the arm is important in preventing the problem in the first place. Indeed one controlled clinical trial in 86 patients (Braus *et al.*, 1994) demonstrated a reduction of hemiplegic shoulder pain from 27% to 8% in the educated group.

Summary

Spasticity after stroke is a common and often disabling problem. Appropriate treatment needs to be initiated early in order to prevent unnecessary complications such as muscle and soft-tissue contracture.

Pain after stroke is quite common and can be secondary to a number of different causes. The treatment is not always satisfactory but nevertheless there are a number of modalities that can be tried. Assessment and treatment should always be multidisciplinary.

REFERENCES

Agnew, D. D. and Goldberg, V. D. (1976). A brief trial of phenytoin therapy for thalamic pain. *Bull Los Angeles Neurol Soc* **41**: 9–12.

Ancliffe, J. (1992). Strapping the shoulder in patients following a cerebrovascular accident: a pilot study. *Aust J Physiother* **38**: 37–41.

Andersen, G., Vestergaard, K., and Ingeman-Nielsen, T. S. (1995). Incidence of central post-stroke pain: *Pain* **61**: 187–193.

Ansreddine, Z. S. and Saver, J. L. (1997). Pain after thalamic stroke: right diencephalic predominance and clinical features in 180 patients. *Neurology* **48**: 1196–1999.

Ashworth, B. (1964). Preliminary trail of carisoprodol in multiple sclerosis. *Practitioner* **192**: 540–542.

Attal, N., Brasseur, L., Parker, F., *et al.* (1998). Effects of gabapentin on the different components of peripheral and central neuropathic pain syndromes: a pilot study. *Eur Neurol* **40**: 191–200.

Aymard, C., Katz, R., Lafitte, C., *et al.* (2000). Presynaptic inhibition and homosynaptic depression: a comparison between lower and upper limbs in normal subjects and patients with hemiplegia. *Brain* **123**: 1688–1702.

Bainton, T., Fox, M., Bowsher, D., and Wells, C. (1992). A double blind trial of noloxone in central pain post-stroke pain. *Pain* **48**: 159–162.

Bakheit, A. M. O., Badwan, D. H. A., and McLellan, D. L. (1996). The effectiveness of chemical neurolysis in the treatment of lower limb muscle spasticity. *Clin Rehabil* **10**: 40–43.

Bakheit, A. M., Thilmann, A. F., Ward, A. B., *et al.* (2000). A randomized, double-blind, placebo-controlled, dose-ranging study to compare the efficacy and safety of three doses of botulinum toxin type A (Dysport) with placebo in upper limb spasticity after stroke. *Stroke* **31**: 2402–2406.

Barnes, M. P. and Johnson, G. R. (2001). *Upper Motor Neurone Syndrome and Spasticity*. Cambridge, UK: Cambridge University Press.

Bas, B., Weinshenker, B., Rice, G. P. A., *et al.* (1988). Tizanidine versus baclofen in the treatment of spasticity in patients with multiple sclerosis. *Can J Neurol Sci* **15**: 15–19.

Basmajan, J. V. (1975). Lioresal (baclofen) treatment of spasticity in multiple sclerosis. *Am J Phys Med* **54**: 175–177.

Bastings, E. P. and Malapira, A. (2002). Baclofen. In *Clinical Evaluation and Management of Spasticity*, ed. D. Gelber and D. Jeffery. Totowa, NJ: Humana Press, pp. 103–124.

Becker, R., Alberti, O., and Bauer, B. L. (1997). Continuous intrathecal baclofen infusion in severe spasticity after traumatic or hypoxic brain injury. *J Neurol* **244**: 160–166.

Benson, H., Pomeranz, B., and Kutz, I. (1989). The relaxation response and pain. In: *A Textbook of Pain*, 2nd edn. ed. P. Wall and R. Melzack. Edinburgh: Churchill Livingstone, pp. 817–922.

Bes, A., Eyssette, M., Pierrot-Deseilligny, E., Rohmer, T., and Warter, J. M. (1988). A multicentre, double-blind trial of tizanidine as an antispastic agent, in spasticity associated with hemiplegia. *Curr Med Res Opin* **10**: 709–718.

Bobath, B. (1990). *Adult Hemiplegia: Evaluation and Treatment*, 3rd edn. Oxford: Butterworth-Heinemann.

Bohannon, R. W. and Smith, M. B. (1987). Inter-rater reliability of a modified Ashworth scale of muscle spasticity. *Phys Ther* **67**: 206–207.

Borodic, G. E., Ferrante, R., Wiegner, A. W., and Young, R. R. (1992). Treatment of spasticity with botulinum toxin. *Ann Neurol* **31**: 113.

Bowery, N. (1989). GABA-B receptors and their significance in mammalian pharmacology. *Trends Pharmacol Sci* **10**: 401–407.

Bowsher, D. (1996). Central pain: clinical and physiological characteristics. *J Neurol Neurosurg Psychiatry* **61**: 62–69.

Braun, R. M., Hoffer, M. M., Mooney, V., McKeever, J., and Roper, B. (1973). Phenol nerve block in the treatment of acquired spastic hemiplegia in the upper limb. *J Bone Joint Surg* **55**: 580–585.

Braus, D. F., Krauss, J. K., and Strobel, J. (1994). The shoulder hand syndrome after stroke. A prospective clinical trial. *Ann Neurol* **36**: 728–733.

Brown, P. (1994). Pathophysiology of spasticity. *J Neurol Neurosurg Psychiatry* **57**: 773–777.

Brunnstrom, S. (1970). *Movement Therapy in Hemiplegia*. New York: Harper and Row.

Budd, K. and Follows, O. J. (1987). The use of naloxone in the treatment of chronic pain of central original. *Pain* **4**(Suppl.): S252.

Burbaud, P., Wiart, L., Dubos, J. L., *et al.* (1996). A randomized, double blind, placebo controlled trial of botulinum toxin in the treatment of spastic foot in hemiparetic patients. *J Neurol Neurosurg Psychiatry* **61**: 265–269.

Burgen, A. S. V., Dickens, F., and Zatman, L. J. (1949). The action of botulinum toxin on the neuromuscular junction. *J Physiol* **109**: 10–24.

Carr, J. H. and Shepherd, R. B. (1982). *A Motor Relearning program for Stroke*, 2nd edn. Oxford: Butterworth-Heinemann.

Cendrowski, W. and Sobczyk, W. (1977). Clonazepam, baclofen and placebo in the treatment of spasticity. *Eur Neurol* **16**: 257–262.

Chantraine, A., Baribeault, A., Uebelhart, D., *et al.* (1999). Shoulder pain and dysfunction in hemiplegia. Effects of functional electrical stimulation. *Arch Phys Med Rehabil* **80**: 328–331.

Charait, S. E. (1968). A comparison of volar and dorsal splinting of the hemiplegic hand. *Am J Occup Ther* **22**: 319–321.

Chyatte, S. B. and Bergman, B. A. (1971). The effects of dantrolene sodium on spasticity and motor performance in hemiplegia. *South Med J* **64**: 180–185.

Cobbel, B. S. (1986). Amitriptyline in the treatment of thalamic pain. *South Med J* **79**: 759–761.

Cocchiarella, A., Downey, J. A., and Darling, R. C. (1967). Evaluation of the effect of diazepam on spasticity. *Arch Phys Med Rehabil* **49**: 393–396.

Craig, A. D. and Bushnell, M. C. (1994). The thermal grill illusion: unmasking the burn of cold pain. *Science* **265**: 252–255.

Craig, A. D., Reiman, E. M., Evans, A., *et al.* (1996). Functional imaging of an illusion of pain. *Nature* **384**: 258–260.

Davidoff, R. A. (1985). Antispasticity drugs: mechanisms of action. *Ann Neurol* **17**: 107–116.

Davidoff, G., Roth, E., Guarracini, M., Sliwa, J., and Yarkony, G. (1987). Function-limiting dysesthetic pain syndrome among traumatic spinal cord injury patients: a cross-sectional study. *Pain* **29**: 39–48.

Davis, E. C. and Barnes, M. P. (2000). Botulinum toxin and spasticity. *J Neurol Neurosurg Psychiatry* **69**: 143–147.

Dejerine, J. and Roussy, G. (1906). Le syndrome thalamique. *Rev Neurol* **14**: 521–532.

Dekker, J. H. M., Wagenaar, R. C., Lankhorst, G. J., and De Jong, B. A. (1997). The painful hemiplegic shoulder. Effects of intra-articular triamcinolone acetomide. *Am J Phys Med Rehabil* **76**: 43–48.

Delwaide, P. J., Martinelli, P., and Crenna, P. (1980). Clinical neurophysiological measurement of spinal reflex activity. In *Spasticity: Disordered Motor Control*, ed. R. Feldman, R. Young and W. Koella., Chicago, IL: Year Book Medical, pp. 345–371.

Dengler, R., Neyer, U., Wohlfarth, K., Bettig, U., and Janzik, H. H. (1992). Local botulinum toxin in the treatment of spastic foot drop. *J Neurol* **239**: 375–378.

Dietz, V., Quintern, J., and Berger, W. (1981). Electrophysiological studies of gait in spasticity and rigidity. *Brain* **104**: 431–449.

Dressnandt, J., Carola, A., and Conrad, B. (1995). Influence of baclofen upon the alpha-motoneuron in spasticity by means of F-wave analysis. *Muscle and Nerve* **18**: 103–107.

Duncan, G. W., Shamani, B. T., and Young, R. R. (1976). An evaluation of baclofen treatment for certain symptoms in patients with spinal cord lesions. *Neurology* **26**: 441–443.

Dunne, J. W., Heye, N., and Dunne, S. L. (1995). Treatment of chronic limb spasticity with botulinum toxin A. *J Neurol Neurosurg Psychiatry* **58**: 232–235.

Edwards, S. (1996). Analysis of normal movement. In *Neurological Physiotherapy: A Problem-solving Approach*, ed. S. Edwards. London: Churchill Livingstone, pp. 15–40.

Edwards, S. and Charlton, P. T. (1996). Splinting and use of orthoses in the management of patients with neurological dysfunction. In *Neurological Physiotherapy: A Problem-solving Approach*, ed. S. Edwards. London: Churchill Livingstone, p. 161.

Eyssette, M., Rohmer, F., Serratrice, G., *et al.* (1988). Multicentre, double-blind trial of a novel antispastic agent, tizanidine, in spasticity associated with multiple sclerosis. *Curr Med Res Opin* **10**: 699–708.

Faist, M., Mazevet, D., Dietz, V., and Pierrot-Deseilligny, E. (1994). A quantitative assessment of presynaptic inhibition of Ia afferents in spastics. Differences in hemiplegics and paraplegics. *Brain* **117**: 1449–1455.

Feldman, R. G., Young, R. R., and Koella, W. P. (1980). *Spasticity: Disordered Motor Control.* Chicago: Year Book Medical.

Fellows, S. J. and Thilmann, A. F. (1994). Voluntary movement at the elbow in spastic hemiparesis. *Ann Neurol* **36**: 397–407.

Francisco, L. (2002). Longitudinal evaluation of the effects of intrathecal baclofen on function and quality of life survivors with spastic hypertonia. In *Proceedings of the Third World Congress on Neurological Rehabilitation,* Venice, (ed. B. Bragante, A. Leone, and T. Battistin), p. 194.

Gelber, D. A., Good, D. C., Dromerick, A., Sergay, S., and Richardson, M. (2001). An open-label dose-titration safety and efficacy of Zanaflex (tizanidine HCl) in the treatment of spasticity associated with chronic stroke. *Stroke* **32**: 1841–1846.

Glass, A. and Hannah, A. (1974). A comparison of dantrolene sodium and diazepam in the treatment of spasticity. *Paraplegia* **12**: 170–174.

Goff, B. (1976). Grading of spasticity and its effects on voluntary movement. *Physiotherapy* **62**: 358–361.

Goldspink, G. and Williams, P. E. (1990). Muscle fiber and connective tissue changes associated with use and disuse. In *Topics in Neurological Physiotherapy,* ed. A. Ada and C. Canning. London: Heinemann, pp. 197–218.

Gonzales, G. R. and Casey, K. L. (2003). Central pain syndromes. In *Clinical Pain Management: Chronic Pain,* ed. T. S. Jensen, P. R. Wilson and A. S. C. Rice. Arnold: London, p. 407.

Hammond, D. (1991). Do opioids relieve central pain? In *Pain and Central Nervous System Disease: The Central Pain Syndromes,* ed. K. L. Casey. New York: Raven Press.

Harbison, J., Dennehy, F., and Keating, D. (1997). Lamotrigine for pain with hyperalgesia. *I R Med J* **90**: 56.

Hattab, J. R. (1980). Review of European clinical trials with baclofen. In *Spasticity: Disordered Motor Control,* ed. R. G. Feldman, R. R. Young and W. P. Koella. Chicago: Year Book Medical, pp. 71–85.

Herman, R., Freedman, W., and Meeks, S. (1973). Physiological aspects of hemiplegic and paraplegic spasticity. In *New Developments in Electromyography and Clinical Neurophysiology: Human Reflexes, Pathophysiology of Motor Systems, Methodology of Human Reflexes,* ed. J. Desmedt. Basel: Karger, pp. 579–589.

Hesse, S., Friedrich, H., Domasch, C., and Mauritz, K. H. (1992). Botulinum toxin therapy for upper limb flexor spasticity: preliminary results. *J Rehabil Sci* **5**: 98–101.

Hesse, S., Lucke, D., Malezic, M., *et al.* (1994). Botulinum toxin treatment for lower limb extensor spasticity in chronic hemiparetic patients. *J Neurol Neurosurg Psychiatry* **57**: 1321–1324.

Hesse, S., Reiter, F., Konrad, M., and Jahnke, M. T. (1998). Botulinum toxin type A and short term electrical stimulation in the treatment of upper limb flexor spasticity after stroke: a randomized, double blind, placebo controlled trial. *Clin Rehab* **12**: 381–388.

Hufschmidt, A. and Mauritz, K. H. (1985). Chronic transformation of muscle in spasticity: a peripheral contribution to increased tone. *J Neurol Neurosurg Psychiatry* **48**: 676–685.

Hylton, N. and Allan, C. (1997). The development and use SPIO Lycra compression bracing in children with neuromotor deficits. *Paediatr Rehabil* **1**: 109–116.

Hysey, M. S. and Keenan, M. A. E. (1999). Orthopaedic management of upper extremity dysfunction following stroke or brain injury. In *Operative Hand Surgery*, 4th edn., ed. D. Green, R. Hotchkiss, W. Pederson. London: Churchill Livingstone, pp. 287–337.

Johnson, G. R. (2001). Measurement of spasticity. In *Upper Motor Syndrome and Spasticity: Clinical Management and Neurophysiology,* ed. M. P. Barnes and G. R. Johnson. Cambridge: Cambridge University Press, pp. 79–95.

Justins, D., Paes, M., and Richardson, P. (2003). Pain relief in neurological rehabilitation. In: *Handbook of Neurological Rehabilitation*, 2nd edn., ed. R. J. Greenwood, M. P. Barnes, T. M. McMillan and C. D. Ward. Hove, UK: Psychology Press, p. 261.

Kaplan, N. (1962). Effects of splinting on reflex inhibition and sensorimotor stimulation in treatment of spasticity. *Arch Phys Med* **43**: 565–569.

Katrak, P. H., Cole, A., Poulos, C. J., and McCauley, J. C. K. (1992). Objective assessment of spasticity, strength and function with early exhibition of dantrolene sodium after cerebro-vascular accident: a randomised double-blind study. *Arch Phys Med Rehabil* **73**: 4–9.

Katz, R. T. (1988). Management of spasticity. *Am J Phys Med Rehab* **67**: 108–116.

Keenan, M. A. (1987). The orthopedic management of spasticity. *J Head Trauma Rehabil* **2**: 62–71.

Kendall, H. P. (1964). The use of diazepam in hemiplegia. *Ann Phys Med* **7**: 225–228.

Kerns, R. D., Turk, D. C., Holzman, A. D., and Rudy. T. E. (1986). Comparison of cognitive–behavioral and behavioral approaches to the outpatient treatment of chronic pain. *Clin J P* **1**: 195–203.

Khalili, A. A. and Betts, H. B. (1967). Peripheral nerve block with phenol in the management of spasticity. *JAMA* **200**: 1155–1157.

Knott, M. T. and Voss, D. E. (1968). *Proprioceptive Neuromuscular Facilitation.* New York: Harper and Row.

Kottke, F. J., Pauley, D. L., and Ptak, R. A. (1966). Rationale for prolonged stretching for correction shortening of connective tissue. *Arch Phys Med Rehabil* **47**: 345–352.

Kumral, E., Kocaer, T., Ertubey, N., *et al.* (1995). Thalamic hemorrhage. A prospective study of 100 patients. *Stroke* **26**: 964–970.

Lance, J. W. (1980). Symposium synopsis. In *Spasticity: Disordered Motor Control*, ed. R. Feldman, R. Young and W. Koella. Chicago: Year Book Medical, pp. 485–494.
    (1984). Pyramidal and extrapyramidal disorders. In *Electromyography in CNS Disorders: Central EMG*, ed. D. Shahani. Boston: Butterworth, pp. 1–19.

Landau, W. M. (1974). Spasticity: the fable of a neurological demon and the emperor's new therapy. *Arch Neurol* **31**: 217–219.

Lataste, X., Emre, M., Davis, C., and Groves, L. (1994). Comparative profile of tizanidine in the management of spasticity. *Neurology* **44**(Suppl. 9): S53–S59.

Leandri, M., Parodi, C. I., Corrieri, N., and Rigard, S. (1990). Comparison of TENS treatment in hemiplegic shoulder pain. *Scand J Rehab Med* **22**: 69–72.

Leijon, G. and Boivie, J. (1989a). Central post-stroke pain: controlled trial of amitriptyline and carbamazepine. *Pain* **38**: 27–36.

(1989b). Central post-stroke pain: the effect of high and low frequency TENS. *Pain* **38**: 187–192.

(1996). Central post-stroke pain (CPSP): a long term follow-up. In *Proceedings of the 8th World Congress of the International Association for the Study of Pain*, p. 380.

Losseff, N. and Thompson, A. J. (1995). The medical management of increased tone. *Physiotherapy* **81**: 480–484.

Margolis, L. H. and Gianascol, A. J. (1956). Chlorpromazine in thalamic pain syndrome. *Neurology* **6**: 302–304.

Mayer, N. H., Esquenazi, A., and Childers, M. K. (1997). Common patterns of clinical motor dysfunction. *Muscle and Nerve*, **20**(Suppl. 6): S21–S35.

McCollough, N. C. (1985). Biomechanical analysis systems for orthotic prescription. In *Atlas of Orthotics: Biomechanical Principles and Application*, 2nd edn., ed. American Academy of Orthopaedic Surgeons. St Louis: Mosby CV, pp. 35–75.

McLellan, D. L. (1977). Co-contraction and stretch reflexes in spasticity during treatment with baclofen. *J Neurol Neurosurg Psychiatry* **40**: 30–38.

McPherson, J. J., Becker, A. H., and Franszczak, N. (1985). Dynamic splint to reduce the passive component of hypertonicity. *Arch Phys Med Rehabil* **66**: 249–252.

Mémin, B., Pollak, P., Hommel, M., and Perret, J. (1992). Effets de la toxine botulique sur la spasticité. *Rev Neurol* **148**: 212–214.

Merskey, H. and Bogduk, N. (1994). *Classification of Chronic Pain: Description of Chronic Pain Syndromes and Definitions of Pain Terms*, 2nd edn. Seattle: IASP Press.

Mertens, P. and Sindou, M. (2001). The surgical management of spasticity. In *Upper Motor Neurone Syndrome and Spasticity: Clinical Management and Neurophysiology*, eds. M. P. Barnes and G. R. Johnson. Cambridge: Cambridge University Press, pp. 239–265.

Meythaler, J. M., DeVivo, M. J., and Hadley, M. (1996). Prospective study on the use of bolus intrathecal baclofen for spastic hypertonia due to acquired brain injury. *Arch Phys Med Rehabil* **77**: 461–466.

Milanov, I. G. (1992). Mechanisms of baclofen action on spasticity. *Acta Neurol Scand* **85**: 305–310.

Moskowitz, E. and Porter, J. I. (1963). Peripheral nerve lesions in the upper extremity in hemiplegic patients. *New Engl J Med* **269**: 776–778.

Neuhaus, B. E., Ascher, E. R., Coullon, B. A., *et al.* (1981). A survey of rationales for and against hand splinting in hemiplegia. *Am J Occup Ther* **35**: 83–90.

Newman, P. M., Nogues, M., Newman, P. K., Weightman, D., and Hudgson, P. (1982). Tizanidine in the treatment of spasticity. *Eur J Clin Pharmacol* **23**: 31–35.

Nogen, A. G. (1976). Medical treatment for spasticity in children with cerebral palsy. *Child's Brain* **2**: 304–308.

Norkin, C. C. and White, D. J. (1995). *Measurement of Joint Range. A Guide to Goniometry*, 2nd edn. Philadelphia: FA Davies.

O'Dwyer, N. J. and Ada, L. (1996). Reflex hyperexcitability and muscle contractures in relation to spastic hypertonia. *Curr Opin Neurol* **9**: 451–455.

O'Dwyer, N. J., Ada, L., and Neilson, P. D. (1996). Spasticity and muscle contractures following stroke. *Brain* **119**: 1737–1749.

Pandyan, A. D., Johnson, G. R., Price, C. I. M., *et al.* (1999). A review of the properties and limitations of the Ashworth and modified Ashworth Scale as measures of spasticity. *Clin Rehabil* **13**: 373–383.

Park, D. M. (1995). Spasticity in adults. In *Handbook of Botulinum Toxin*, ed. P. Moore. Oxford: Blackwell Science, pp. 209–221.

Pedersen, E., Arlien-Soborg, P., Grynderup, V., and Henriksen, O. (1970). GABA derivative in spasticity. *Acta Neurol Scand* **46**: 257–266.

Pedersen, E., Arlien-Soborg, P., and Mai, J. (1974). The mode of action of the GABA derivative baclofen in human spasticity. *Acta Neurol Scand* **50**: 665–680.

Pérennou, D., Bussel, B., and Pélissier, J. (2001). *La spasticité*. Paris: Masson.

Perfetti, C., Briganti, S., Noccioli, V., and Cecconello, R. (2001). *L'exercice thérapeutique cognitif pour la rééducation du patient hémiplégique*. Paris: Masson.

Perry, J. (1980). Rehabilitation of spasticity. In *Spasticity: Disordered Motor Control*, ed. R. Feldman, R. Young and W. Koella. Chicago: Year Book Medical.

Peyron, R., Garcia-Larrea, L., Gregoire, MC., *et al.* (1999). Haemodynamic brain responses to acute pain in humans: sensory and attentional networks. *Brain* **122**: 1765–1780.

Pierrot-Deseilligny, E. (1990). Electrophysiological assessment of the spinal mechanisms underlying spasticity. *Electroencephalogr Clin Neurophysiol Suppl* **41**: 264–273.

Pinder, R. M., Brogden, R. N., Speight, T. M., and Avery, G. S. (1977). Dantrolene sodium: a review of its pharmacological properties and therapeutic efficacy in spasticity. *Drugs* **13**: 3–23.

Pope, P. (1992). Management of the physical condition in patients with chronic and severe neurological pathologies. *Physiotherapy* **78**: 896–903.

(1996). Postural management and special seating. In *Neurological Physiotherapy: A Problem-Solving approach*, ed. S. Edwards. London: Churchill Livingstone, pp. 135–160.

Randall, L. O. (1982). Discovery of benzodiazepines. In *Pharmacology of Benzodiazepines*, ed. E. Usdin, P. Skolnick and J. Thallman. London: Macmillan Press, pp. 15–22.

Randall, L. O., Heise, G. A., Schallek, W., *et al.* (1961). Pharmacological and clinical studies on valium, a new psychotherapeutic agent of the benzodiazepine class. *Curr Ther Res* **3**: 405–421.

Reiter, F., Danni, M., Ceravolo, M. G., and Provinciali, L. (1996). Disability changes after treatment of upper limb spasticity with botulinum toxin. *J Neurol Rehab* **10**: 47–52.

Reiter, F., Lagalla, G., Ceravolo, G., and Provinciali, L. (1998). Low dose botulinum toxin with taping for the treatment of spastic equinovarus foot after stroke. *Arch Phys Med Rehab* **79**: 532–535.

Rice, G. P. (1987). Pharmacotherapy of spasticity: some theoretical and practical considerations. *Can J Neurol Sci* **14**: 510–512.

Richardson, D., Sheean, G., Werring, D., *et al.* (2000). Evaluating the role of botulinum toxin in the management of focal hypertonia in adults. *J Neurol Neurosurg Psychiatry* **69**: 499–506.

Rifici, C., Kofler, M., Kronenberg, M., *et al.* (1994). Intrathecal baclofen application in patients with supraspinal spasticity secondary to severe traumatic brain injury. *Funct Neurol* **9**: 29–34.

Rodda, J. and Graham, H. K. (2001). Classification of gait patterns in spastic hemiplegia and spastic diplegia: a basis for a management algorithm. *Eur J Neurol* **8**(Suppl. 5): S98–S108.

Rood, M. (1956). Neurophysiological mechanisms utilized in the treatment of neuromuscular dysfunction. *Am J Occup Ther* **10**: 220.

Rosales, R., Arimura, K., Takenaga, S., and Osame, M. (1996). Extrafusal and intrafusal muscle effects in experimental botulinum toxin A injection. *Muscle and Nerve* **19**: 488–496.

Rosenstiel, A. K. and Keefe, F. J. (1983). The use of coping strategies in chronic low back pain patients: relationship of patient characteristics to current adjustment. *Pain* **17**: 33–44.

Roussan, M., Terrence, C., and Fromm, G. (1987). Baclofen versus diazepam for the treatment of spasticity and long-term follow-up of baclofen therapy. *Pharmatherapeutica* **4**: 278–284.

Rousseaux, M., Dubrulle, B., Kozlowski, O., *et al.* (2002a). Intérêt de la méthode Perfetti dans la rééducation du membre supérieur de l'hémiplégique vasculaire. In *Préhension et hémiplégie vasculaire*, ed. J. Pélissier, C. Bénaïm C and M. Enjalbert. Paris: Masson, pp. 78–88.

Rousseaux, M., Kozlowski, O., and Froger, J. (2002b). Efficacy of botulinum toxin A in upper limb function of hemiplegic patients. *J Neurol* **249**: 76–84.

Sahrmann, S. A. and Norton, B. J. (1977). The relationship of voluntary movement to spasticity in the upper motor neuron syndrome. *Ann Neurol* **2**: 460–465.

Saltuari, L., Kronenberg, M., Marosi, M. J., *et al.* (1992). Long-term intrathecal baclofen treatment in supraspinal spasticity. *Acta Neurol Napoli* **14**: 195–207.

Sampaio, C., Ferreira, J. J., Pinto, A. A., *et al.* (1997). Botulinum toxin type A for the treatment of arm and hand spasticity in stroke patients. *Clin Rehabil* **11**: 3–7.

Sandroni, P., Dotson, R., and Low, P. A. (2003). Complex regional pain syndromes. In *Clinical Pain Management: Chronic Pain*, ed. T. S. Jensen, P. R. Wilson, S. C. Rice. London: Arnold, pp. 383–402.

Schmidt, R. T., Lee, R. H., and Spehlman, R. (1976). Comparison of dantrolene sodium and diazepam in the treatment of spasticity. *J Neurol Neurosurg Psychiatry* **39**: 350–356.

Schwartzmann, R. J., Grothusen, J., Kiefer, T. R., *et al.* (2001). Neuropathic central pain: epidemiology, etiology and treatment options. *Arch Neurol* **58**: 1547–1550.

Sheean, G. L. (2001a). Neurophysiology of spasticity. In *Upper Motor Neurone Syndrome and Spasticity: Clinical Management and Neurophysiology*, ed. M. P. Barnes and G. R. Johnson. Cambridge, UK: Cambridge University Press, pp. 12–78.

(2001b). Botulinum treatment of spasticity: why is it difficult to show a functional benefit? *Curr Opin Neurol* **14**: 771–776.

Sherrington, C. (1947). *The Integrative Action of the Nervous System.* Cambridge, UK: Cambridge University Press.

Simpson, D. M., Alexander, D. N., O'Brien, C. F., *et al.* (1996). Botulinum toxin type A in the treatment of upper extremity spasticity: a randomized double-blind, placebo-controlled trial. *Neurology* **46**: 1306–1310.

Sindou, M., Abbott, R., and Ketravel, Y. (1991). *Neurosurgery for Spasticity: A Multidisciplinary Approach.* New York: Springer-Verlag.

Sjolund, B. (1991). Role of TENS, CNS stimulation and ablative procedures in the central pain syndromes. In: *Pain and Central Nervous System Disease: The Central Pain Syndromes*, ed. K. L. Casey. New York: Raven Press.

Skeil, D. A. and Barnes, M. P. (1994). The local treatment of spasticity. *Clin Rehab* **8**: 240–246.

Smith, S. J., Ellis, E., White, S., and Moore, A. P. (2000). A double-blind placebo-controlled study of botulinum toxin in upper limb spasticity after stroke or head injury. *Clin Rehabil* **14**: 5–13.

Spasticity Study Group (1997). Spasticity: etiology, evaluation, management, and the role of Botulinum toxin type A. *Muscle and Nerve* **6**(Suppl.): S208–S220.

Stein, R., Nordal, H. J., Oftedal, S. I., and Slettebo, M. (1987). The treatment of spasticity in multiple sclerosis: a double-blind clinical trial of a new anti-spasticity drug tizanidine compared with baclofen. *Acta Neurol Scand* **75**: 190–194.

Swerdlow, M. and Cundill, J. G. (1981). Anticonvulsant drugs used in the treatment of lancinating pain: a comparison. *Anaesthesia* **36**: 1129.

Tabary, J. C., Tabary, C., Tardieu, C., Tardieu, G., and Goldspink, G. (1972). Physiologic and structural changes in cat's soleus muscle due to immobilzation at different lengths by plaster casts. *J Physiol* **224**: 231–244.

Tardieu, G., Rondot, P., Dalloz, J., Mensch-Dechenne, J., and Monfraix, C. (1959). The stretch reflex in man: a study of electromyography and dynamometry (strain gauge) contribution to classification of the various types of hypertonus. *Cereb Palsy Bull* **7**: 14–17.

van den Pol, A. N. (1997). Reversal of GABA actions by neuronal trauma. *Neuro Scientist* **3**: 281–286.

van der Heijden, J. M. G., van der Windt, D. A. W. M., and de Vinter, A. F. (1997). Physiotherapy for patients with soft tissue shoulder disorders: a systematic review of randomised clinical trials. *BMJ* **315**: 25–30.

van Hemert, J. C. J. (1980). A double-blind comparison of baclofen and placebo in patients with spasticity of cerebral origin. In *Spasticity: Disordered Motor Control*, ed. R. Feldman, R. Young and W. Koella. Chicago: Year Book Medical, pp. 41–49.

Vauagnat, H. and Chantraine, A. (2003). Shoulder pain and hemiplegia revisited: contribution of functional electrical stimulation and other therapies. *Rehab Med* **35**: 49–56.

Wallace, J. D. (1994). Summary of combined clinical analysis of controlled clinical trials with tizanidine. *Neurology* **44**(Suppl. 9): S60–S69.

Ward, A. B. and Ko, C. K. (2001). Pharmacological management of spasticity. In *Upper Motor Neurone Syndrome and Spasticity*, ed. M. Barnes and G. Johnson. Cambridge, UK: Cambridge University Press, pp. 165–187.

Ward, A., Chaffman, M. O., and Sorkin, E. M. (1986). Dantrolene. A review of its pharmacodynamic and pharmacokinetic properties and therapeutic use in malignant hyperthermia, the neuromalignant syndrome and an update of its use in muscle spasticity. *Drugs* **32**: 130–168.

Wiegand, H., Erdmann, G., and Wellhoner, H. H. (1976). I-Labelled botulinum A neurotoxin: pharmacokinetics in cats after intramuscular injection. *Arch Pharmacol* **292**: 161–165.

Winters, T. F., Gage, J. R., and Hicks, R. (1987). Gait patterns in spastic hemiplegia in children and young adults. *J Bone Joint Surg* **69**: 437–441.

Working Party of the Pain Society (1997). *Desirable Characteristics for Pain Management Programs*. London: The Pain Society.

Young, R. R. (1994). Spasticity: a review. *Neurology* **44**(Suppl. 9): S12–20.

Young, R. R. and Delwaide, P. J. (1981). Drug therapy: spasticity. *N Engl J Med* **304**: 96–99.

Zorowitz, R. D., Hughes, M. B., Idank, D., et al. (1996). Shoulder pain and subluxation after stroke: correlational coincidence? *Am J Occup Ther* **50**: 194–201.

13

Balance disorders and vertigo after stroke: assessment and rehabilitation

Dominque A. Pérennou

Centre Hospitalier-Universitaire de Rééducation, Dijon, France

Adolfo M. Bronstein

Imperial College, Charing Cross Hospital, London, UK

Introduction

Postural control is a complex function that involves most brain areas (Horak and MacPherson, 1996). Many brain lesions may cause a perturbation of postural control, and postural disorders represent one of the most frequent disabilities after stroke. Their nature and their severity depend on the ability of undamaged brain areas to compensate, therefore on age (Pérennou et al., 1999) and premorbid status, as well as on lesion size (Pérennou et al., 1999, 2000) and location (Viallet et al., 1992; Dichgans and Fetter, 1993; Brandt and Dieterich, 1994; Palmer et al., 1996; Ioffe, 1997; Miyai et al., 1997; Karnath et al., 2000a; Pérennou et al., 2000).

After a stroke, the ability to maintain or to change a position can be altered in the three basic postures: lying, sitting, and standing. Consequently, assessment of these critical postures is often standardized for clinical follow-up in terms of the ability to roll from supine to side lateral and vice versa; the ability to maintain an independent sitting posture without any extension of support (buttocks on a bed or a physiotherapy couch and feet on the floor); the ability to rise up from a chair; and the ability to stand unaided. The assessment of gait ability require other specific tools that are beyond the topic of this chapter.

One week after stroke, about 40% of patients are not able to roll from supine to side lateral (Partridge and Edwards, 1988). On day 30 after stroke, only 60–70% of patients can perform this change of posture without any help (Benaim et al., 1999); 20–25% can do so with help (Benaim et al., 1999), and the other 10–15% are still not able to do so, always with more difficulty toward the non-affect side (Partridge and Edwards, 1988; Benaim et al., 1999). The restoration of an independent sitting posture is a key point for patient autonomy and so the sitting posture has long been one of the most frequently postures analyzed after stroke. Up to 75–80% of patients keep or recover the ability to maintain an independent sitting posture for

Recovery after Stroke, ed. Michael P. Barnes, Bruce H. Dobkin and Julien Bogousslavsky. Published by Cambridge University Press. © Cambridge University Press 2005.

several minutes within the first month (Perrigot *et al.*, 1980; Sandin and Smith, 1990; Benaim *et al.*, 1999). The median time to recover the ability to sit independently for one minute covaries with the size and site of the lesion: from 0 days for a lacunar or a posterior circulation infarct to 11 days (25–75th percentile, 7–19.3 days) for a total anterior circulation infarct (Smith and Baer, 1999). In stroke patients undergoing rehabilitation, the mean time to achieve independent sitting from admission is approximately 11 days (Mayo *et al.*, 1991). This recovery is better or shorter in patients with a left lesion than in those with a right lesion (Wade *et al.*, 1984, 1985; Bohannon *et al.*, 1986a; Pérennou *et al.*, 1999), especially in those displaying spatial neglect (Bohannon *et al.*, 1986b; Taylor *et al.*, 1994; Pérennou *et al.*, 1999). We will return to this point later in the chapter. One month after stroke onset, 40% of patients undergoing rehabilitation are able to stand independently for one minute; 40% are not able to stand at all, and the other 20% can stand with help (Benaim *et al.*, 1999). The median time to recover the ability to stand for 10 seconds covaries with the size and site of the lesion: 0 days for a lacunar infarct, 4 days for a posterior circulation infarct, and 44 days (25–75th percentile, 38–57 days) for a total anterior circulation infarct (Smith and Baer, 1999).

These landmarks show how postural disorders constitute a primary disability in stroke patients, leading to a loss of autonomy and exposing patients to a risk of falling. The risk of falling is so high in the first weeks after stroke onset that it must be considered as a significant problem in stroke rehabilitation. The incidence rate is about 1–2 falls per 100 patient-day approximately of hospitalization (Nyberg and Gustafson, 1995; Tutuarima *et al.*, 1997). Falls occur mainly during transfers (active changes of posture) (Nyberg and Gustafson, 1995; Hyndman *et al.*, 2002), and they are more frequent with increasing age and depression (Ugur *et al.*, 2000). Their risk is not linearly related to the number of impairments: individuals with heavy deficits being less mobile and, therefore, less exposed to hazardous activities than more independent patients (Yates *et al.*, 2002). After discharge in non-institutionalized individuals with long-standing stroke, the risk of falling is more than twice as high for patients with stroke than for elderly controls (Forster and Young, 1995; Jorgensen *et al.*, 2002).

Assessing balance in stroke patients

In stroke patients, assessing balance responds to several needs: severity estimation and follow-up, analysis of the nature of postural impairments to orientate physiotherapy and care in the rehabilitation ward, and to support research. Although the universal tool suitable for all these criteria does not exist, clinicians and researchers have now many validated tools at their disposal, each bringing relevant information in relation to a given query. In addition to the more qualitative clinical examination, there are schematically two types of complementary tools for measuring postural abilities: ordinal scales and instrumentation. Both are broadly used in stroke patients. Balance ordinal scales are clinical scales that are scored 0, 1, 2, etc., depending on the deficit, to perform a given task. They can be applied to all patients, irrespective of the severity of their postural impairment. They are favored in epidemiological studies but yield limited information on the cause of the postural disability. The instrumental assessment is based on the measurement of the performance and/or strategies for a given postural task. It contributes more to disease understanding than balance ordinal scales and is also generally more sensitive to changes. The instrumental assessment has some disadvantages. It requires technical equipment; can be time consuming; requires normalization between laboratories or clinical units, which is not easily achieved; and, above all, is limited to patients who are able to perform the postural task considered (patients with the poorest postural ability cannot be assessed).

Qualitative clinical examination

Changes in a patient's perception of verticality can lead to abnormal alignment of body parts with respect to each other and to the base of support. The patient's alignment with respect to vertical and with respect to adjacent body segments needs to be observed in sitting and standing. A plumbline in conjunction with a grid can be used to quantify alignment at the head, shoulders, trunk, pelvis, hips, knees, and ankle, photographed or videotaped if necessary. Therapists can assess a patient's internal sense of vertical by passively moving them off vertical in stance or sitting and asking them to voluntarily realign to vertical. Both surface orientation and visual information can be analyzed in this assessment.

Controlling body position for the purpose of balance and orientation requires motor coordination processes that organize muscles throughout the body into coordinated movement strategies. The three main postural response strategies used to recover stance balance in both the anterior/posterior and lateral directions are an ankle strategy, a hip strategy, and a stepping strategy. (Nashner, 1976, 1977) (Fig. 13.1). Although many injuries to the central nervous system (CNS), such as stroke, head injury, and cerebral palsy, result in improperly timed postural synergies, patients with peripheral vestibular pathology usually show normally coordinated muscle activation in the legs and trunk (Nashner *et al.*, 1983; Di Fabio and Badke, 1990; Horak *et al.*, 1994; Allum *et al.*, 2001; Carpenter *et al.*, 2001a). However, even in peripheral vestibular disease, postural responses can be hypo- or hypermetric and the neck and trunk often exhibit abnormal co-contraction that stiffens joints. A coordinated adult responds to a small perturbation in the anterior/posterior direction by using sway principally about the ankles and in the lateral direction by

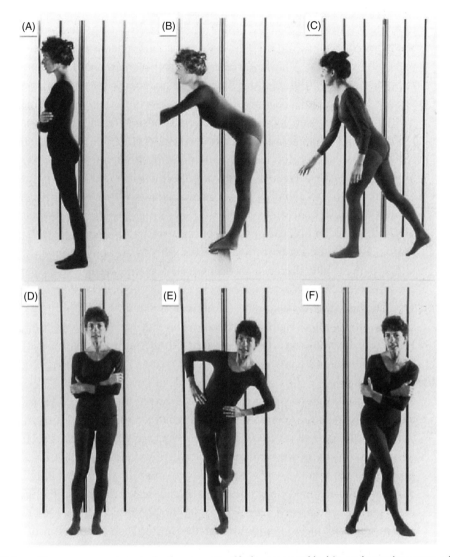

Fig. 13.1   Three movement strategies for recovery of balance: an ankle, hip, and stepping strategy for the anterior/posterior direction (A–C) and for the lateral direction (D–F). (A, D) In an ankle strategy, a vertical orientation of the trunk is preserved. (B, E) In a hip strategy, vertical orientation of the trunk is compromised while the hips or lumbothoracic spine actively moves the center of mass. (C, F) In a stepping strategy, the base of support moves under the falling center of body mass. (Reprinted with permission from Shumway-Cook and Horak, 1989.)

using hip abduction/adduction. A therapist should carefully observe the ankle joints to determine if the tibialis anterior muscles are active in both legs in response to backward body sway. If knee and hip motion are minimal during these compensatory ankle sway movements, this indicates that the appropriate proximal muscle synergists have been activated in addition to the ankle muscles. Larger displacements to stance posture with the feet planted on the surface cause greater amounts of hip and trunk responses, a hip strategy, as the subject attempts to maintain the center of mass within the base of support. Displacements that are large or fast may result in a stepping response. Although this hierarchy of responses does not always manifest as a series of sequential responses (e.g. ankle, then hip), then step normal subjects naturally stepping in response to small perturbations can maintain balance without initiating a step if asked (Maki and McIlroy, 1997). Runge *et al.* (1998) reported that all subjects with and without vestibular loss respond to large, forward sway displacements with a step at least once although they had been instructed to try to avoid stepping. Many patients with CNS deficits will show uniquely uncoordinated movement strategies for postural control, which cannot be classified as an ankle, hip, or stepping strategy, for example excessive knee flexion, asymmetric leg movements, excessive trunk or arm movements.

The patient with dizziness or vertigo may require formal vestibular testing. However, vestibular function can be assessed at the bedside by examination of spontaneous, gaze-evoked, and positional nystagmus and head thrust tests (Bronstein, 2003). (Vestibular aspects will be discussed later in the chapter.) How critical vision is to a patient's balance is assessed with the Romberg test.

Clinical balance scales

Postural assessment of stroke patients has evolved in the last few years. Postural disability *per se* is now assessed and distinguished from the assessment of other functions such as walking and the assessment of basic impairments such as range of motion, muscle power, and sensory loss. This evolution in the assessment of stroke patients is associated with an improvement in the practical, quantitative properties of functional scales, including balance scales. By practical properties, we mean good feasibility and specific meaning for the clinical team. Quantitative or metric properties include validity, reliability, internal consistency, lack of ceiling or floor effects, and ability to discriminate changes. Numerous clinical scales may be used to assess postural abilities of stroke patients. These can be classified as motor scales dedicated to stroke patients but not specifically to assess balance disorders (*composite motor scales*), scales focused on the assessment of balance disorders but not especially in stroke patients (*non-categorical balance scales*), and postural scales especially dedicated for stroke patients (*specific scales*). The last ones are used increasingly more often in clinics and in research.

Composite motor scales

Many composite motor scales used in stroke patients include a balance section (Fugl-Meyer *et al.*, 1975; Ashburn, 1982; Carr *et al.*, 1985; Lindmark and Hamrin,

1988; Collen *et al.*, 1990; Gowland *et al.*, 1993). One of the first composite motor scales dedicated to stroke patients, the Fugl-Meyer assessment (Fugl-Meyer *et al.*, 1975; Fugl-Meyer, 1980) gives information on various impairments and incapacities, which usually covary with the recovery. Despite using a mixture of impairments and incapacities, this scale has often proved to be a valid and reliable tool, both as a whole and particularly with regard to the mobility and balance sections, which assess postural abilities (Sanford *et al.*, 1993). The major drawback of the this scale is that most items (including the mobility and balance items) have only three levels of assessment; consequently, many hemiplegic patients score the intermediate level and remain at this stage for quite a long time. More recent scales designed for assessing postural disorders of stroke patients now respond to these psychometric properties required for ordinal scoring.

Non-categorical balance scales

The Berg Balance Scale (BBS) was probably one of the most popular non-specific balance scales in the 1990s. It was initially designed to help to determine change in functional standing balance over time in the elderly (Berg *et al.*, 1992). The BBS is a 56-point scale that grades one sitting and 13 standing tasks from 0 to 4. It has been shown to have strong internal consistency and high inter-rater reliability in patients with acute stroke (Berg *et al.*, 1995). The main drawbacks are its inability to assess rolling in a lying position, a crucial problem at an early stage after stroke, and insufficiently accurate assessment of the sitting ability. This results in a "floor effect," limiting the relevance of this scale in the first weeks after stroke onset (Mao *et al.*, 2002). For this reason, the BBS seems more suited to assess balance of patients who are not too severely affected or who are at a chronic stage, even if a ceiling effect after three months may occur (Mao *et al.*, 2002). The use of balance scales originally designed for assessing balance in the elderly for assessments in stroke is hampered by both floor or ceiling effects. The Get-up and Go test (Mathias *et al.*, 1986) and the Tinetti (1986) assessment are both affected in this way. The former requires the subject to stand up from a chair, walk 3 m, turn around, and return. Performance is judged subjectively and graded using the following scale: 1, normal; 2, very slightly abnormal; 3, mildly abnormal; 4, moderately abnormal; and 5, severely abnormal. Older adults who scored 3 or higher on this test had an increased risk for falls (Mathias *et al.*, 1986). In the Functional Reach test (Duncan *et al.*, 1990), patients are asked to stand with feet shoulder width apart, and with the arm raised to 90 degrees to the front. The person is asked to reach as far forward as possible while still maintaining stability. The distance that can be reached is predictive of falls in the elderly. The Dynamic Gait Index (Shumway-Cook and Woollacott, 2001) assesses an individual's ability to modify gait according to changing task demands, such as walking at varying gait speeds, while performing head movements or pivot turns. Performance is rated on a 4 point scale. The test has been shown to be a valid predictor of falls in both the elderly population (Shumway-Cook *et al.*, 1997) and patients with vestibular disorders (Whitney *et al.*, 2000).

Postural scales for stroke patients

There are several balance scales specifically designed for stroke patients. They can be classified as short or full scales. Short tests may be useful to describe and quantify a given behavior such as the inability to maintain a sitting or standing posture (Sandin and Smith, 1990; Bohannon *et al.*, 1993; Brun *et al.*, 1993), to analyze a crucial point such as trunk control (Collin and Wade, 1990), or to document "pusher" behavior (Karnath *et al.*, 2000b). Sitting balance or trunk control have also been assessed by the corresponding subscales of more extensive assessments (Feigin *et al.*, 1996; Hsieh *et al.*, 2002). These short tests usually take a couple of minutes to be completed and do not require any equipment. They can be useful at the acute stage and are sometimes considered as "bedside tests." They can also serve as a preliminary evaluation of the patient on admission to rehabilitation, giving a first impression about prognosis. For instance, trunk control can easily be assessed by examining the ability to roll from a supine position to the weak side and to the strong side, the ability to sit up from a lying-down position, and the sitting balance (Collin and Wade, 1990; Franchignoni *et al.*, 1997; Hsieh *et al.*, 2002). The Postural Assessment Scale for Stroke (PASS) is the first and so far the only full balance scale specifically dedicated for stroke patients. The PASS was developed to be applicable to all stroke patients, even those with very poor postural abilities (Pérennou *et al.*, 1998a; Benaim *et al.*, 1999). It contains 12 items, each scored between 0 and 3 (Table 13.1), that grade postural abilities of increasing difficulty in lying, sitting, or standing posture (total score from 0 to 36). Two postural domains are scanned: the ability to maintain a given posture and the ability to ensure equilibrium in changing positions. With concrete postural tasks and a precise guideline for scoring, assessing balance of a stroke patient with the PASS takes no more than 10 minutes. The metric properties of the PASS are satisfactory, especially in the first three months after stroke (Benaim *et al.*, 1999; Mao *et al.*, 2002). Interestingly, a recent paper (Mao *et al.*, 2002) has compared three balance scales used in stroke patients: the balance subsection of the Fugl-Meyer assessment, the BBS, and the PASS. While the first two have significant floor effects 14 days after stroke, the PASS does not, implying that the PASS is best suited to detect postural changes in the first few months after stroke. This property has been used to detect differences in postural capacities between patients with right and left strokes (Pérennou *et al.*, 1999).

Table 13.1 The Postural Assessment Scale for Stroke (PASS)

Grade	Ability
Maintaining a posture	
1 Sitting without support (sitting on the edge of an 50 cm height examination table – a Bobath plane for instance – with the feet touching the floor)	0: Cannot sit 1: Can sit with slight support, for example by one hand 2: Can sit for more than 10 seconds without support 3: Can sit for 5 minutes without support
2 Standing with support (feet position free, no other constraints)	0: Cannot stand even with support 1: Can stand with strong support of two persons 2: Can stand with moderate support of one person 3: Can stand with only one support of one hand
3 Standing without support (feet position free, no other constraints)	0: Cannot stand without support 1: Can stand without support for 10 seconds or leans heavily on one leg 2: Can stand without support for 1 minute or stands slightly asymmetrically 3: Can stand without support for more than 1 minute and at the same time perform arm movements above the shoulder level
4 Standing on non-paretic leg (no other constraints)	0: Cannot stand on non-paretic leg 1: Can stand on non-paretic leg for a few seconds 2: Can stand on non-paretic leg for more than 5 seconds 3: Can stand on non-paretic leg for more than 10 seconds
5 Standing on paretic leg (no other constraints)	0: Cannot stand on paretic leg 1: Can stand on paretic leg for a few seconds 2: Can stand on paretic leg for more than 5 seconds 3: Can stand on paretic leg for more than 10 seconds
Changing posture	
Items 6 to 9 are performed with a 50 cm height examination table)	0: Cannot perform the activity 1: Can perform the activity with a lot of help 2: Can perform the activity with only a little help 3: Can perform the activity without help
6 Supine to affected side lateral 7 Supine to non-affected side lateral 8 Supine to sitting up on the edge of the bed	

Table 13.1 (*cont.*)

Grade	Ability
9 Sitting on the edge of the bed to supine	
Items 10–12 performed without any support (no other constraints)	0: Cannot perform the activity
	1: Can perform the activity with a lot of help
	2: Can perform the activity with only a little help
	3: Can perform the activity without help
10 Sitting to standing up	
11 Standing up to sitting down	
12 Standing, picking up a pencil from the floor	

From: Benaim *et al.* (1999).

Chronometric assessment

Many ordinal balance scales check if a given patient is able to maintain a given posture during a given time. The results are then converted into item levels. Chronometric measurements of postural abilities can also be used, especially for assessing the ability to maintain standing posture, possibly with increasing difficulties according to the variation of the base of support (feet apart or together, sharpened Romberg or tandem stance, heel-to-toe, eventually single limb stance) and the sensory availability (at least eyes open and closed). Although often used as a predictor of falls in the elderly, these tests are often too difficult for hemiplegics and are not used for routine assessment of their balance disorders. However, they can be useful for detecting impairments in patients who appear clinically to have adequate postural control (Collen, 1995). As already mentioned, timed balance tests allow analysis of the sensory contribution to postural control, especially in erect stance. The Sensory Organization Balance Test is a posturography-based test that evaluates somatosensory, visual, and vestibular contribution to the maintenance of upright posture (Shumway-Cook and Horak, 1986; Di Fabio and Badke, 1990). Using a clinical variant of this test (the "foam and dome" test; see Fig. 13.7). Di Fabio and Badke (1991) analyzed the stance duration of hemiplegics. They found that visual deprivation or visual conflict conditions did not decrease the duration of the task when stance was performed on a stable surface, whereas stance duration was lower when patients stood on a compliant surface. Visual compensation was evident during the compliant-surface condition because stance duration showed the greatest reductions with eyes closed and with the visual dome. Di Fabio and Badke (1991) concluded that the ability of stroke patients to integrate somatosensory information from the lower extremities is compromised.

The subjective verticals

Several sources of information about verticality can be distinguished. First, the direction of gravity constitutes the physical vertical and is the only absolute coordinate. Most living organisms exert responses against this force. The nature of these responses characterizes the antigravitational behavior of species. The orientation of the body relative to the ambient gravito-inertial force constitutes the *behavioral vertical* (Luyat *et al.*, 1997; Pérennou *et al.*, 2002a), which is the expression of an implicit representation of verticality used to control balance. In upright humans, the behavioral vertical usually corresponds to the direction of the longitudinal body axis. It can be measured by movement analysis systems. It is also possible to estimate the direction of the longitudinal body axis by means of a force platform, allowing an indirect assessment of body orientation in a standing subject (Hlavacka *et al.*, 1996; Zatsiorsky and King, 1998). However, body orientation with respect to gravity can be estimated by the projection of the center of mass onto the ground only when the body is aligned along the gravitational force. This is not the case when subjects must ensure a dynamic balance, or when there is an obvious asymmetry of weightbearing as in hemiplegics. This is why it has been suggested that the behavioral vertical could be estimated using a rocking-chair paradigm (Figs. 13.2 and 13.3). With this paradigm, it is possible to measure the mean orientation of the supporting surface and so estimate the direction of the trunk in the roll plane (Pérennou *et al.*, 1998b, 2002a). The relevance of this type of measurement is limited by the possible covariation between postural orientation and stability (which can only be dissociated in microgravity conditions), and also by the fact that the most severely impaired patients are not able to perform the task. The behavioral vertical must be distinguished from the explicit perceptions of verticality, namely the visual vertical, the haptic (tactile) vertical, and the postural vertical. These modality-related perceptions of verticality usually provide convenient and complementary ways of drawing inferences about the sense of verticality in a given individual. To assess the visual vertical, the subject in darkness is asked to adjust a luminous rod visually to the estimated vertical direction. This assessment is normally very precise with errors of less than 1 degree (Mann *et al.*, 1949). To assess the haptic vertical, the subject in darkness is asked to set a rotating bar to vertical using tactile sense. Again this adjustment is precise, although subject to a possible directional hand–side effect (Bauermeister *et al.*, 1964). For the assessment of the postural vertical, the subject is seated on a tilting chair in darkness and asked to set the body to vertical (Witkin and Asch, 1948). Normally with practice, this body adjustment is remarkably accurate (Witkin and Asch, 1948; Mann *et al.*,

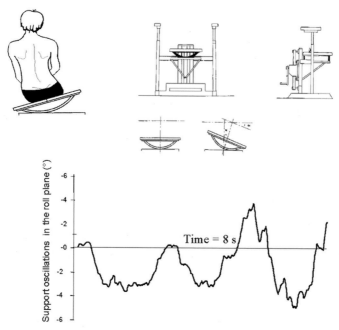

Fig. 13.2   The rockingly impaired-platform (chair) paradigm adapted for analyzing dynamic lateral balance of neurological patients in a sitting posture. Patients sit on a rigid plane support mounted on a seesaw, allowing lateral oscillations. They are asked to maintain an upright sitting posture as still as possible while looking straight ahead and fixing a target for eight seconds. During the trials, their hands are crossed, resting on the thighs. Safety armrests at the sides prevent falls. The height of the sitting support is adjustable so that the subject's legs hang freely. The movement of the seesaw associate rotation and translation. Kinematics of body movements in roll can be analyzed by means of an automatic optical television image processor. The control of body tilt is termed "orientation." The control of the oscillations is termed "stabilization." The raw data show both a left tilt and large oscillations at the support level compared with head and lumbar angular variation.

1949; Solley, 1956; Clark and Graybiel, 1963). The subjective visual vertical has widely been assessed in stroke patients (Bender and Teuber, 1948; Teuber and Mishkin, 1954; Bruell *et al.*, 1956; Birch *et al.*, 1960; De Renzi *et al.*, 1971; Dieterich and Brandt, 1992; Brandt *et al.*, 1994; Kerkhoff and Zoelch, 1998; Anastasopoulos and Bronstein, 1999; Tilikete *et al.*, 2001a; Yelnik *et al.*, 2002). Although only recently applied in stroke patients, the measurement of the subjective haptic vertical (Kerkhoff, 1999; Bronstein *et al.*, 2003) and the subjective postural vertical (Pérennou *et al.*, 1998b, 2002a; Anastasopoulos *et al.*, 1999; Karnath *et al.*, 2000b) are promising. Indeed, correlation between the visual vertical and postural abilities in daily life are not as strong as expected (Kerkhoff, 1999; Pérennou *et al.*, 2002b). Since this is a poorer predictor of postural abilities than the haptic or postural

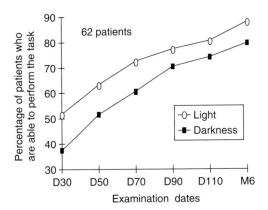

Fig. 13.3   Feasibility study of the rocking-chair paradigm in non-selected patients admitted for neurorehabilitation after a first hemisphere stroke. Most of patients were able to perform this dynamic postural task within two or three months of stroke onset. D, day; M, month. (From Perennou *et al.*, 2000.)

verticals (Pérennou *et al.*, 2002b), and because dissociation can occur between the visual vertical and the haptic/postural verticals (Bisdorff *et al.*, 1996; Karnath *et al.*, 2000b; Pérennou *et al.*, 2001a; Bronstein *et al.*, 2003), the visual vertical cannot be used in isolation as a guide to rehabilitation in stroke patients (Pérennou *et al.*, 2002b). Consequently, there is an increasing demand for routine measurement of the postural vertical in a neurorehabilitation context. The fly simulators or motorized gimbal used in research laboratories are not suited for stroke patients so a device has been designed that is suited for the measurement of the postural vertical in stroke patients (Pérennou *et al.*, 2001a, 2002b). Patients are strapped into a sitting position in a framework within a wheel (Fig. 13.4), with the head, trunk, and lower limbs aligned in an upright position. In order to determine the postural vertical, the subject is tilted to a given position to either side of the vertical. The wheel is then rolled towards the other side until the patient reports reaching an upright position. The wheel is manually turned as gently and steadily as possible at an approximate velocity of 1.5 degrees per second. Twenty unpredictable trials are performed, 10 from left to right, and 10 from right to left, the mean value yielding the postural vertical. Only patients who display a supramodal bias in the perception of vertical (tilt in vertical, haptic, and postural vertical) are suspected to have a high-order disruption in the construction of the vertical: a tilted representation of the vertical (Pérennou *et al.*, 2001a, 2002b). One can assume that these patients actively adjust their erect sitting or standing posture to this tilted subjective vertical. According to this view, disorders of balance encountered by stroke patients should be partly caused by a bias in the

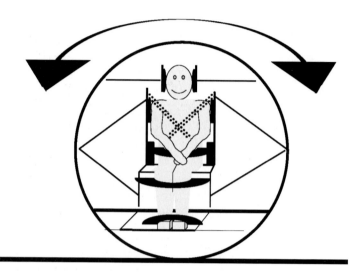

Fig. 13.4   Schematic view of the apparatus for measuring the subjective postural vertical in a clinical context (Perennou *et al.*, 2001a, 2002b).

representation of the verticality, severe bias being incompatible with the maintenance of an autonomous erect posture. Most often these patients have a hemisphere lesion; patients with brainstem lesion having a net visual vertical tilt, with postural and haptic verticals being normal or slightly tilted.

Posturography

Posturography (stabilometry) is a measurement of postural body sway (Fig. 13.5). It is usually recorded by force platform(s), measuring the successive positions of the center of foot pressure inside the base of support during a given period of time. The center of pressure is also the application point of the resultant upward force exerted by the support surface on the feet in reaction to gravity. Although many postures can be quantified using posturography (in particular the ability to maintain a short single-limb stance), clinical posturography usually serves to characterize and quantify bipedal erect stance. In standing still, the body is normally kept upright and the center of mass projects over the base of support provided by the two feet. In the sagittal axis, the base of support is determined by foot length. In the lateral axis, the base of support is defined by the distance between the outside edges of the feet. Posturographic assessment can be made by one or two force platforms. The use of a single force platform yields information about positions and displacements of the center of pressure (metric data) together with information about rhythmic aspects of postural sways. To evaluate postural instability, one can compute the length of the sway path (in millimeters), the stabilogram area (in square millimeters), or the dispersion of the center of pressure

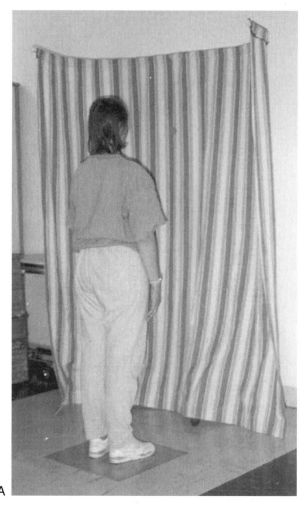

A

Fig. 13.5   Posturographic assessment can be made by one or two force platforms. (A) The use of a single force platform (here integrated in the ground to facilitate assessments in disabled people) yields information about positions and displacements of the center of pressure (metric data) together with information about rhythmic aspects of postural sways. (B) The use of two force platforms yields direct information about the symmetry of weight bearing, expressed in percentage of body weight loaded on each foot. This is especially relevant in hemiplegics.

coordinates on the lateral and sagittal axes during a given time. If the instruction is to stand still, one assumes that the more the body sways, the less stable the person is. The use of two force platforms yields direct information about the symmetry of weight bearing, expressed in percentage of body weight loaded on each foot. This is especially relevant in hemiplegics. The term "static posturography" refers to the ability to maintain balance on a fixed platform; "dynamic posturography"

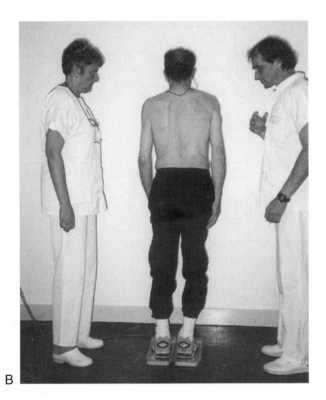

B

measures postural reactions in response to a translation/rotation of the support. This latter technique may be of value for analyzing postural reflexes (Nashner, 1976), dizzy patients (Bronstein, 2003), or for specific retraining purposes, but only static posturography will be considered in this section.

Static posturography is now often used in stroke patients. Three main patterns may be observed (Fig. 13.6).

- *Weight-bearing asymmetry*: More weight is borne on the non-paretic leg. With a single platform, a lateral shift of the center of pressure toward the non-paretic leg is observed. This behavior is caused by biomechanical and cognitive impairments and is partly the result of a compensatory strategy.
- *Increased center of pressure displacement*: An increase of the centre of pressure both in sagittal and lateral axes. This gives rise to large body sways, reflecting postural instability, which may result from orthopedic, sensorimotor and cognitive impairments.
- *Decreased limit of stability*: Beyond this, the center of pressure cannot move further without exposing the person to a loss of balance. This represents the inability to control a stressed equilibrium system or an impaired coordination between posture and movement (Massion and Woollacott, 1996).

CP mean position and oscillations

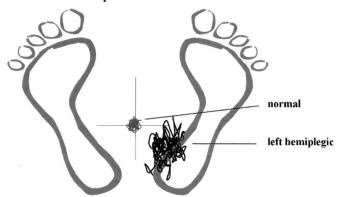

normal

left hemiplegic

Fig. 13.6   Static posturography in a patient with left hemiplegia showing a rightward shift of the centre of pressure (CP) and big postural oscillations.

Asymmetrical weight bearing

It has long been know that the majority of stroke patients bear less weight on the paretic limb than on the non-paretic one. This asymmetrical weight bearing was first reported in quiet stance (Arcan *et al.*, 1977; Seliktar *et al.*, 1978; Dickstein *et al.*, 1984; Bohannon and Larkin, 1985; Caldwell *et al.*, 1986; Dettmann *et al.*, 1987; Shumway-Cook *et al.*, 1988; Mizrahi *et al.*, 1989; Winstein *et al.*, 1989; Sackley, 1990), then in more dynamic motor tasks such as rising from or stepping on a chair (Engardt *et al.*, 1993; Hesse *et al.*, 1994; Cheng *et al.*, 1998; Laufer *et al.*, 2000). The non-paretic leg supports an average 65% of the body weight (Shumway-Cook *et al.*, 1988; Sackley, 1990), the load on the paretic leg being mainly distributed around the forefoot (Geurts *et al.*, 2001; Nardone *et al.*, 2001). The degree of weight-bearing asymmetry during quiet stance is correlated with motor function, level of self-care independence, and length of hospital stay after stroke (Sackley, 1990, 1991). It is also indicative of walking performance (Dettmann *et al.*, 1987; Gruendel, 1992; Goldie *et al.*, 1996a; Cheng *et al.*, 1998), although even functionally ambulant hemiplegics demonstrate marked limitations in weight shifting (Turnbull *et al.*, 1996). Many commercial devices are now available to measure (Eng and Chu, 2002) and follow the course of this asymmetrical weight bearing in stroke rehabilitation, many of them also including a feedback training package.

Although asymmetrical weight bearing is a major focus in stroke rehabilitation, the basis of this abnormality remains poorly understood. Engardt (1994a) speculated that the patients may favor the non-paretic leg for safety and speed reasons, thus resulting in "disuse" of the paretic limb. Weakness certainly plays a role, as well as cognitive disorders observed in lesions of the right hemisphere (Rode *et al.*, 1997). Further studies will be needed to extend our understanding of this behavior, and especially to clarify why some patients with left hemiplegia display a left bias in the subjective vertical but a rightwards shift of their center of pressure. The contralesional tilt of the subjective vertical should mechanically overload the paretic leg, but this is not the case. It is possible that they are trying to compensate: to reconcile the tilt of the subjective vertical toward their paretic side with the inability of their paretic leg to support body weight? Finally, how does this asymmetry in weight bearing correlate with the asymmetry in the dynamic aspects of postural stabilization (Geurts et al., 2001)?

Increased center of pressure

Compared with healthy subjects, hemiplegics display larger postural sway (Shumway-Cook et al., 1988; Pélissier et al., 1990; Dickstein and Dvir, 1993), especially on the lateral axis (Shumway-Cook et al., 1988; Pélissier et al., 1990). When the postural sway is recorded separately for each lower limb, it is noted that the paretic leg sways more than the non-paretic leg (Dickstein and Abulaffio, 2000; Geurts et al., 2001). A regular reduction of body sway is the rule in patients who recover, and posturography is a very sensitive tool that is able to detect stability improvement within a week once the patient is able to stand independently.

Limits of stability

In patients who are recovering successfully, it may be useful to measure the ability to perform movements while standing. For instance, dynamic aspects of standing balance can be assessed by asking patients to lean the body as far as possible in specific directions. Hemiplegics usually show a reduction in their stability limit (Goldie et al., 1996b).

Other assessment tools

Many paradigms have been proposed for analyzing balance performance and/or strategies of stroke patients. Some paradigms have been proposed to investigate the ability to withstand external forces applied mechanically to the hip in the frontal plane (Gauthier et al., 1992; Wing et al., 1993a). These paradigms are useful for analyzing and quantifying the coordinated generation of ipsilesional and contralesional lateral torque, either in sitting (Gauthier et al., 1992) or in standing (Wing et al., 1993a).

The rocking-chair paradigm has been especially designed for analyzing the sitting posture of stroke patients (Pérennou et al., 1998b, 2002a). Subjects maintain balance while sitting on a freely rocking support, which implies an active orientation of the body with respect to gravity, and also the stabilization of this mean body position in space (Fig. 13.2). This task presents four advantages. First, since the sitting posture is often preserved, or is the first to be restored, this paradigm is suited to an analysis of balance shortly after a stroke. Hence the observed postural behavior deals more with the consequences of the lesion than with possible compensation mechanisms. In addition, there is no influence of orthopedic problems while sitting (such as equinus foot deformity), making this task only sensorimotor. Second, dynamic balance tasks in which balance control is challenged, as in this paradigm, are more appropriate than static balance tasks for revealing impairments. Third, since this task allows some degree of body tilt compatible with the maintenance of an erect posture, it is useful to assess the natural strategies of body orientation with respect to both gravity (mean body position) (Pérennou et al., 1998b, 2002a) and stabilization (amount of sway) (Pérennou et al., 2001b).

In order to determine how sensory information from visual, somatosensory, and vestibular systems is utilized to maintain a vertical orientation, Shumway-Cook and Horak (1986) designed the Clinical Test of Sensory Interaction for Balance (Fig. 13.7), modeled after Nashner's dynamic posturography, sensory organization protocol (Nashner, 1982; Peterka and Black, 1990). Body sway is measured while the subject stands quietly for 20 seconds under six different conditions. Eye closure, blindfolds, and a modified Japanese lantern are used to alter visual information, and a hard floor and a compliant foam surface are used to alter somatosensory inputs for postural orientation (the "foam and dome" test). Patients are tested in an identical posture for all six conditions, for example, feet together with hands placed on hips. Using condition one as a baseline reference, the patient is observed for changes in the amount and direction of sway over the subsequent five conditions. If the patient is unable to stand for 20 seconds, a second trial is given (Horak, 1987). Differences in amount of body sway in the various conditions are used to determine a subject's ability to organize and select appropriate sensory information for postural control. A single fall, regardless of the condition, is not considered abnormal (Di Fabio and Badke, 1990; Cohen et al., 1993). However, two or more falls are indicative of difficulties adapting sensory information for postural control. Neurologically intact young adults are able to maintain balance for 20–30 seconds on all conditions with minimal amounts of body sway. The results obtained with this test are similar but not identical with those from computed dynamic posturography (Shepard et al., 1993; El-Kashlan et al., 1998). Dynamic posturography produces perturbations in the pitch (sagittal) plane but real-life situations provoke destabilizing forces in multiple directions. Furthermore, the postural responses required to stand on an uneven surface are different to those for walking or performing a reaching task on the same surface and cannot be assessed accurately by a single test. Therefore, posturography results should only be considered as an adjunctive contribution to the complex task of assessing a patient's functional disabilities and sensory deficits (Cass et al., 1996;

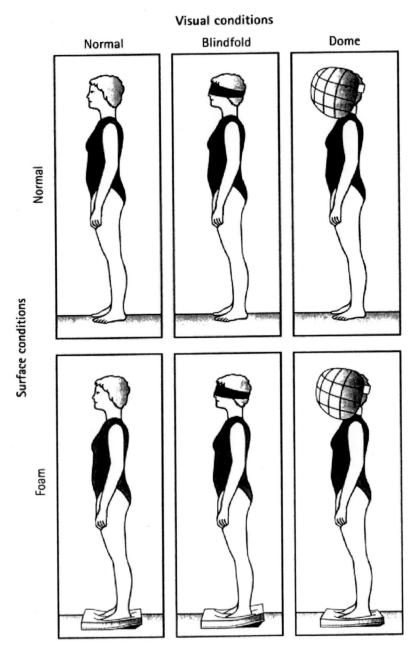

Fig. 13.7   A rehabilitation approach for testing the ability to maintain stance balance under altered sensory conditions: the Clinical Test for Sensory Interaction in Balance. (Adapted from Shumway-Cook, A. and Horak, F, 1986.)

Gill-Body *et al.*, 2000). Little information is available on the practical use of posturography in CNS disease but it would seem not to add significantly to clinical assessment (Jackson *et al.*, 1995; Nelson *et al.*, 1995).

Predicting recovery in an early postural assessment

Trunk control is required to perform activities of daily living, and numerous studies have shown that trunk control or sitting balance at an early stage after stroke could predict outcome for activities of daily living at a late stage (Wade *et al.*, 1983; Loewen and Anderson, 1990; Sandin and Smith, 1990; Franchignoni *et al.*, 1997; Hsieh *et al.*, 2002). The Trunk Control Test (ch. 6) at admission is a very good predictor of length of sway, gait velocity, walking distance, BBS, and the motor component of the Functional Independence Measure (motFIM) at discharge (Franchignoni *et al.*, 1997; Duarte *et al.*, 2002). The Trunk Control Test at admission also predicts motFIM at discharge even better than motFIM itself at admission (Franchignoni *et al.*, 1997). A recent survey of 169 stroke patients has shown that the trunk-control-related items of the PASS (PASS-TC) at 14 days after stroke were the strongest predictors of the comprehensive activities of daily living at 6 months (Hsieh *et al.*, 2002). In this study, the PASS-TC alone (made up by the five items of the PASS related to trunk control) accounted for 45% of the variance in predicting comprehensive activities of daily living function, and the power of the PASS-TC for this prediction was better than that of the Barthel Index. These two studies demonstrated that trunk control is a key point for recovery prediction in stroke patients and that the severity of the initial postural impairment is a good indicator of the recovery potential. There is no consensus about the right time to perform this clinical assessment with a view to predicting long-term disability. At the acute stages, medical problems are multiple and patients are usually bedridden, sometimes in intensive-care units. An extensive postural evaluation would be difficult to perform, and the postural potential of many patients may be masked by medical problems. At this stage, we suggest using short tests such as the PASS-TC or the Trunk Control Test. More complete tests can refine the walking prognosis as soon as the patient is medically stable. Based on routine use of a PASS in clinics for six years (Pérennou *et al.*, 1998a; Benaim *et al.*, 1999) and a systematic survey of more than 200 stroke patients (Pérennou *et al.*, 2002a,b), it appears that, without any other medical problem, a patient with a PASS score of <10 (maximum, 36) on day 30 after stroke onset has little chance to recover an independent gait, whereas a patient with a PASS score of <20 generally recovers independent gait (with a walking aid such a stick or a crutch if necessary). It has also been emphasized that measuring the BBS scores of patients upon admission to an acute stroke rehabilitation unit may assist in approximating length of stay and predicting eventual discharge destination (Wee *et al.*, 1999).

Understanding balance disorders in stroke patients

Postural control is organized to build up and update the body orientation (posture) and stabilize body segments (Massion, 1994). The existence of two separate mechanisms, one for the control of body orientation with respect to gravity and one for its stabilization, is an emerging concept (Horak and MacPherson, 1996) that allows a better understanding of postural disorders after a stroke. Indeed, it would seem that, after a stroke, the postural disability can be caused by misrepresentation of verticality (Brandt *et al.*, 1994; Pérennou *et al.*, 1998b; Kerkhoff, 1999), by pronounced postural instability (Pérennou *et al.*, 2000), or by a combination of these two impairments (Pérennou and Amblard, 2004). We will consider impairments in postural orientation first and then discuss and stabilization.

Postural misorientation

On Earth, gravity is an absolute reference and perception of body verticality is normally very accurate. A subjective vertical is built up in the parieto-insular cortex (Brandt *et al.*, 1994), mainly in the right hemisphere (Kerkhoff and Zoelch, 1998; Pérennou *et al.*, 1998b). Vestibular, somesthetic, and visceral graviceptors contribute to the updating of the subjective vertical (Bisdorff *et al.*, 1996; Mittelsteadt, 1992). Golgi tendon organs may monitor the forces exerted by the muscles to compete against gravity (Dietz *et al.*, 1992). Any lesion of the brain overlapping an area involved in the integration of the vestibular or somesthetic graviceptive information should give rise to a perturbation in the construction of the subjective vertical. A lesion of otolithic and vertical canal vestibular pathways will give an ocular torsion and subsequently a tilt of the visual perception of the vertical, whereas a lesion in the somesthetic graviceptive pathways will give a tilt bearing on the postural perception of the vertical (Clark and Graybiel, 1963; Bisdorff *et al.*, 1996; Pérennou *et al.*, 1998b, 2002a; Anastasopoulos and Bronstein, 1999).

It has long been known that, after a stroke, patients can show a bias in the subjective vertical (Bender and Teuber, 1948; Teuber and Mishkin, 1954; Bruell *et al.*, 1956; Birch *et al.*, 1960; Carmon and Benton, 1969; De Renzi *et al.*, 1971; Benton *et al.*, 1975). More recent and systematic studies of patients with hemisphere lesions have shown that this bias holds for the visual perception of the vertical (Brandt *et al.*, 1994; Kerkhoff and Zoelch, 1998; Yelnik *et al.*, 2002), for the tactile perception of the vertical (Kerkhoff, 1999), and also for the postural perception of the vertical (Pérennou *et al.*, 1998b, 2001a; Anastasopoulos and

Bronstein, 1999; Karnath *et al.*, 2000b). The mechanism and the direction of the subjective vertical tilt depend on lesion location. Schematically, if the lesion is located in the brainstem, especially involving a vestibular nucleus as it is the case in Wallenberg syndrome, the tilt of the subjective vertical is mainly a result of ocular torsion. It concerns the subjective visual vertical and is ipsilesional. In the acute stage of the stroke, tilts in subjective visual vertical may reach 15–20 degrees then decrease in parallel with the reduction of the ocular torsion (Brandt and Dieterich, 1992). If the lesion is located in one cerebral hemisphere, the tilt is mostly contralesional, concerns one, two, or the three modalities of the subjective vertical (visual, haptic, postural), with a continuum between normality, mild, and severe bias (Pérennou *et al.*, 2002b). The tilt is not caused by ocular torsion or skew deviation (Brandt *et al.*, 1994; Kerkhoff, 1999), it is mainly induced by lesions involving the parieto-insular cortex (Brandt *et al.*, 1994), and is proportional to the severity of spatial neglect (Kerkhoff, 1999).

Pusher behavior might be the most dramatic clinical manifestation of an extreme bias in the construction of the vertical. As defined by Davies (1985), pushers push themselves away actively from the non-paralyzed side. Typically in the sitting position, they lean to the side opposite the lesion and resist any attempt to make them more upright. The more they are pushed, the more they push. This puzzling motor behavior is not frequent, observed in 5% of stroke patients (Pedersen *et al.*, 1996), not always obvious, and, therefore, not always easy to diagnose. It usually affects the more severely impaired patients and has a negative impact on the period of recovery (Pedersen *et al.*, 1996). Few studies have attempted to understand the mechanisms underlying pusher behavior. It is clear that the bias crucially affects the whole-body (postural) perception of the vertical (Karnath *et al.*, 2000b; Pérennou *et al.*, 2002b), suggesting that the trouble might partly result from an impaired integration of somesthetic graviceptive information (Karnath *et al.*, 2000b; Pérennou *et al.*, 2002b). This might be a form of graviceptive extinction or graviceptive neglect (Pérennou *et al.*, 2002a). It is also clear that the bias in the postural vertical is more important in darkness than in light (Karnath *et al.*, 2000b; Pérennou *et al.*, 2002a), indicating that pushers use vision to compensate and improve their active body orientation with respect to gravity. This could be an interesting starting point to develop further rehabilitation techniques.

Some other important points in the pushing behavior need to be clarified. According to Karnath *et al.* (2000b), pusher behavior could result from a conflict between a severe ipsilesional bias in the postural vertical and a normal visual vertical. According to this view, the conflict induces an idiosyncratic postural response: pushing. These findings were not confirmed by Pérennou *et al.* (2002b), who found a severe contralesional bias in any modalities of the subjective vertical. This transmodality would suggest that pushers have a strong disruption in the representation of verticality. This high-order disruption in the construction of the vertical would explain why pushers are not aware of their trouble, in contrast to patients with Wallenberg syndrome, who display a more mechanical lateropulsion (vestibulospinal tone asymmetry). The direction of the tilt, opposite to that reported by Karnath *et al.* (2000b) but congruent with that observed many times in brain-damaged patients (see above), would suggest that pushing could be the most dramatic clinical manifestation of a bias in the construction of the subjective vertical. Because these apparent discrepancies could result through different methodologies, further studies are needed to explain pusher behavior.

Stabilization impairment

Many stroke patients show difficulties in responding to postural perturbations. These perturbations can be studied while subjects are standing on a moveable platform and subjected to a translation or to a rotation of the platform. Electromyographic recordings show that, after an unexpected perturbation, the latency of postural muscle activation as well as the amplitude of the muscle response patterns are altered in stroke patients (Badke and Duncan, 1983; Di Fabio, 1987; Di Fabio and Badke, 1988; Fung *et al.*, 2003), especially in the paretic limb (Di Fabio *et al.*, 1986; Di Fabio, 1987). However, the latency of reactive balance responses in stroke patients can be as rapid as that measured in healthy persons when the perturbation can be anticipated (Di Fabio, 1987). This could be interesting from a rehabilitation point of view. Deficits in the timing of agonist versus antagonist muscle discharge have also been observed, with a trend to inefficient muscle coactivations (Di Fabio, 1987; Fung *et al.*, 2003). Postural stabilization involves regulating various body segment positions with respect to each other, to external support, and/or to absolute space. In standing, hemiplegic patients show a low temporal synchronization between sway of the legs and the pelvis, as well as between the two legs (Dickstein and Abulaffio, 2000). It has been suggested that impairment in the ability to stabilize the distal segments of the lower extremity on the paretic side, rather than in stabilization of the pelvis, could underlie their postural instability in stance (Dickstein and Abulaffio, 2000). More generally, the postural instability of stroke patients depends on mechanical, motor, sensory, and cognitive factors, which we will consider next.

Spasticity

Equinovarus is the most common complication of spastic legs. This modifies both the nature and the area of the base of support in erect stance, thus altering body stability. At the midstance phase of gait, equinovarus can also induce a biomechanical foot instability, resulting in a postural instability. These mechanical factors of instability can become crucial in the presence of severe paresis or sensory loss. Apart from this induced foot deformity, spasticity does not seem to influence crucially body stabilization in response to a postural perturbation (Berger *et al.*, 1984; Di Fabio, 1987; Nardone *et al.*, 2001), nor in daily life (Pérennou *et al.*, 1999). Furthermore, it is accepted that mild spasticity can help in maintaining a static standing posture, counterbalancing the negative effects of weakness on uprightness. However, spasticity perturbs the execution of dynamic postural tasks that require good multijoint coordination (Dietz and Berger, 1984; Diener *et al.*, 1993) or a precise coordination between posture and movement (Rogers *et al.*, 1993).

Weakness

Since minimum muscle power is required to support body weight, there is a correlation between weakness severity and degree of imbalance in stroke patients (Bohannon, 1989; Pérennou *et al.*, 1999). This link is far more important in standing (Bohannon, 1989) than in sitting (Pérennou *et al.*, 2001b), and in dynamic balance tasks than in static balance. This is attested by the very small percentage of patients who are able to stand on a single leg, even for some seconds only (Benaim *et al.*, 1999).

Sensory deficits

As for the control of postural orientation, the sensory control of postural stabilization also requires the integration of information from multiple channels, including somatosensory, vestibular, and visual systems. Each sensory system conveys specific information and has different threshold and properties (Horak and MacPherson, 1996), and a close correlation between sensory disturbance and postural instability has been observed in stroke. In particular, the ability to integrate somatosensory information from the lower extremities (Di Fabio and Badke, 1991) and the degree of sensory loss closely relate to postural instability (Benaim *et al.*, 1999; Pérennou *et al.*, 2001b). Patients with proprioception deficits also show impaired postural learning (Ioffe *et al.*, 2001). It has been demonstrated that the existence of a visual field defect decreases the visual contribution to postural stabilization (Pérennou and Amblard, 2004) and increases postural body sway (Rondot *et al.*, 1992; Pérennou and Amblard, 2004). However a study based on the Equitest has suggested that stroke patients may be abnormally dependent on visual information in the presence of sensory conflict (Bonan *et al.*, 1996). The importance of vestibular information is indicated by the significant postural disorder that directly results from vestibular nuclear lesions (e.g. Wallenberg syndrome) and that dysfunction of the vestibulo-ocular reflex is associated with postural instability (Catz *et al.*, 1994). All these sources of sensory information are centrally integrated and participate in the generation of multi-sensory motor responses. In addition, they are the foundation of spatial cognition and, for this reason, some strokes interfere with postural control via disorders of sensory integration and spatial cognition.

Impaired spatial cognition

The "postural body scheme" plays a crucial role in postural stabilization (Gurfinkel and Levik, 1991). This concept incorporates body geometry, orientation of the interface between bodily and non-bodily spaces, and body dynamics (Massion, 1994). Spatial neglect, often associated with a disruption of, or failure to attend to, the body scheme, represents an interesting way to analyze cognitive aspects of postural control. Currently, rather than a concept of a unitary representation of egocentric space, the concept of multiple representations of space appears more convenient to account for numerous disorders involving spatial cognition. Stabilizing the body consists of regulating the position of body segments, with respect to each other, to external support, or to absolute space. One may assume that this function relies on multisegmental body representations (for instance eye–head, head–shoulders, shoulders–pelvis, pelvis–lower legs, feet-supporting surface). The transformation of the coordinates of these multisegmental body representations is vulnerable in patients with neglect (Pizzamiglio *et al.*, 1997); therfore, the postural instability in patients with spatial neglect could partly result from difficulty in the multisegmental postural coordination process (Pérennou *et al.*, 2001b). This concept could explain why such patients display postural instability whatever the postural task considered (Pérennou *et al.*, 1999). In the patients suffering from spatial neglect usually display a bias in the construction of their subjective vertical. In addition their stabilization capacities are also impaired. These two mechanisms explain why such patients show such a dramatic postural imbalance compared with other stroke patients (Gottlieb and Levine, 1992; Pérennou and Amblard, 2004).

The view that the right hemisphere may be dominant for postural control is another emerging concept, congruent with right hemisphere dominance for spatial attention and representation. This view is supported by numerous clinical studies showing worse postural recovery after right hemispheric strokes than after left hemispheric strokes. This concerns the standing posture (Sackley, 1991; Hesse *et al.*, 1994; Rode *et al.*, 1997; Pérennou *et al.*, 1999), the sitting posture (Wade *et al.*, 1984; Bohannon *et al.*, 1986a; Pérennou *et al.*, 1999), and the lying posture (Pérennou *et al.*, 1999). There is also a delay of autonomous gait (Held *et al.*, 1997; Cassvan *et al.*, 1976) and other motor tasks involving postural control (Denes *et al.*, 1982; Bernspång and Fisher, 1995) in left hemiplegics.

Lesion location

Studies in stroke patients have indicated that the cerebral cortex plays a key role in postural control. Many cortical lesions alter postural stabilization. The premotor and motor cortices generate anticipatory and associated postural adjustments. In the "barman" paradigm, a flexed forearm is loaded (Bennis et al., 1996) or unloaded (Viallet et al., 1992), either voluntarily in a bimanual task or by an imposed event. In the self-induced perturbation, the anticipatory postural adjustments of the elbow are impaired in patients with a contralateral cerebral lesion (Viallet et al., 1992; Bennis et al., 1996), particularly in patients with a lesion extending to the supplementary area region or the motor cortex (Viallet et al., 1992; Bennis et al., 1996). Associated postural adjustments normally observed in the contralateral latissimus dorsi during a ballistic abduction of one arm are also impaired in patients with a large single lesion involving the motor cortex (Palmer et al., 1996). The polymodal sensory cortex and especially the temporoparietal junction is thought to be a nodal point of the networks underlying the properties of internal models: resolving sensory ambiguities, synthesizing information from disparate sensory modalities, and combining efferent and afferent information (Merfeld et al., 1999). This is why, compared with other hemispheric stroke locations, strokes that overlap the temporoparietal junction have been found have more effect on dynamic postural stabilization both sitting (Pérennou et al., 2000) and standing (Miyai et al., 1997). Anterior lobe cerebellar lesions are characterized by ataxia with a 3 Hz postural oscillation (Dichgans and Fetter, 1993; Hayashi et al., 1997) and an impaired coordination of posture and voluntary movements (Diener et al., 1992; Dichgans and Fetter, 1993). The concordance between lesion location and posturokinetic activities has been studied less for infratentorial lesions.

Coordination between posture and movement

Appropriate postural orientation and stabilization are necessary but not sufficient for a good autonomy in daily life: the coordination between posture and movement (Massion, 1994) must also be preserved. The coordination between posture and movement in stroke patients has been analyzed in motor tasks such as weight transfer in standing (Diener et al., 1993; Rogers et al., 1993; Pai et al., 1994), rising from a chair (Ada et al., 1993), stepping (Kirker et al., 2000; Laufer et al., 2000), pedalling (Brown et al., 1997), walking (Said et al., 1999; Lamontagne et al., 2001), and moving or lifting the upper limb (Horak et al., 1984; Palmer et al., 1996; Garland et al., 1997). Basically, these studies have shown that: the postural preparatory phase of the movement may be altered, both in spatial and temporal terms; the brain takes into account the new mechanical constraints imposed by the paretic leg; an upright stance exacerbates the movement deficit of the paretic leg; additional voluntary movements may be detrimental to body stabilization; and the coordination between posture and movement may be improved by training.

Recognizing adaptive postural behaviors

Individual patients with poor balance after stroke may utilize adaptive motor behaviors, voluntary or involuntarily, to compensate or substitute the function(s) impaired. Carr and Shepherd (1998) suggested that the most commonly observed adaptive behaviors are widening the base of support, shifting onto the non-paretic leg, stiffening of the body, and avoiding threats to balance. In analyzing postural behavior in order to plan appropriate interventions, it is critical to distinguish primary problems affecting balance from these secondary adaptive behaviors. In order to widen the base of support, patients can place the legs apart with the feet externally rotated, or even use the hand as an additional support in erect stance. The shift of the body weight toward the non-paretic leg was discussed above. Stiffening the body is achieved by using multisegmental co-contractions. This is a common adaptation observed in individuals for whom postural challenges are perceived as beyond their postural abilities. This behavior seems frequent in stroke patients. In addition, fear of falling drastically limits postural and daily activities.

Vertigo

Vertigo, defined as a sensation that oneself or the environment is rotating, indicates involvement of the angular motion detection system (rotational vertigo). This comprises the semicircular canals and their central projections. Less frequently, sensations of tilt, fall, or linear motion can also occur; they may indicate involvement of the peripheral and central otolith system (linear vertigo) (Gresty et al., 1992). Ischemic and hemorrhagic stroke can cause vertigo by involvement of the vestibular system all the way from the labyrinth to the cortex. In addition, the acute symptoms of some common vestibular disorders, such as vestibular neuritis or benign paroxysmal positional vertigo (BPPV), can be initially confused with a posterior fossa stroke. The incidence of vertigo in unselected stroke patients is low (2.1%), not only when compared with common symptoms such as limb pareses (81.6%) but also when compared with other cerebellar or brainstem symptoms such as gait disturbance (10.8%) or diplopia (5.5%) (Rathore et al., 2002). In other series, a fall can be the presenting symptom (21.2%), but the proportion of patients or relatives reporting vertigo is still low (5.6%) (Handschu et al., 2003). This is related to the fact that less than 20% of strokes occur in the vertebrobasilar territory, because the incidence of vertigo rises sharply to approximately 70% when cerebellar and brainstem strokes are considered separately (Caplan, 1996).

Syndromes with vertigo

Here we will briefly discuss syndromes that can either have a vascular etiology or be confused with stroke. The reader is referred to general references for more details (Brandt, 1999; Solomon, 2000; Baloh and Honrubia, 2001).

Types of vertigo

Peripheral disorders

Vestibular neuritis (neuronitis, neurolabyrinthitis) is a name given to the clinical picture of acute vertigo, nausea, and imbalance caused by sudden, peripheral, unilateral vestibular failure. The etiology of the disorder is not entirely clear but it is thought to be caused by viral infection or reactivation (herpes simplex virus 1; Strupp and Arbusow, 2001) of the vestibular nerve. In older patients either with atypical features (e.g. additional ipsilateral auditory involvement) or increased vascular risk factors, an ischemic origin is suspected (labyrinthine stroke).

A similar view is taken of the condition called idiopathic sudden deafness. When unilateral deafness is the only symptom this is also believed to be caused by a virus; however, vascular mechanisms are thought to be more likely causes for more severe cases with additional vestibular features. Indeed, complete and irreversible cochleovestibular loss should raise the suspicion that the patient had a labyrinthine hemorrhagic stroke; this can be detected as increased T^1 signal in unenhanced magnetic resonance imaging (MRI) scans (Shinohara $et\ al.$, 2000).

The typical findings in vestibular neuritis and in labyrinthine stroke are spontaneous, fixed direction nystagmus (horizontal with a minor torsional component added) and a tendency to fall with eyes closed in the direction of the hypoactive labyrinth (i.e. in the direction of the $slow$ phase of the nystagmus). Rapid head (nose) turns towards the hypoactive labyrinth while the patient fixates an object straight ahead will demonstrate hypoactive vestibulo-ocular reflex. This is denoted by one or more catch-up saccades towards the target (head thrust test) (Halmagyi and Curthoys, 1988). Alternatively, caloric irrigation of the suspected ear will fail to modify the vertigo or nystagmus.

In the differential diagnosis, it should be borne in mind that vascular lesions in the root entry zone of the vestibular nerve are capable of producing a very similar picture to that of vestibular neuritis. For this reason, a careful neurological and eye movement examination is mandatory; if any central signs are detected (broken pursuit, dysmetric saccades) an MRI should be arranged. Inferior cerebellar infarcts can also mimic vestibular neuritis and care must be exercised as these infarcts can become "pseudotumoral" and require emergency neurosurgery (Lehrich *et al.*, 1970; Duncan *et al.*, 1975). Affected patients usually have severe walking difficulties and central eye movement disorders such as vertical, torsional, or direction-changing nystagmus, abnormalities of pursuit or saccades, ocular pulsion, or strabismus. Caloric or head thrust testing of the vestibulo-ocular reflex should be essentially preserved in cerebellar lesions but absent in vestibular neuritis. Finally, it should be remembered that posterior circulation ischemia can affect both the labyrinth and CNS structures simultaneously, with combined peripheral and central vestibular, auditory, and ocular signs. As a consolidated stroke this is typical of the anterior cerebellar artery syndrome, with ipsilateral caloric canal paresis, deafness, and cerebellar signs (Caplan, 1996; Solomon, 2000).

Positional or cervical vertigo?

A word of caution is required for the poorly defined syndrome of "cervical vertigo," for which two mechanisms, vascular or proprioceptive, have been proposed. The cervical vertebrae carry the vertebral arteries and, in theory, movements of the neck might cause intermittent arterial compression. This mechanism would be unlikely to cause vertigo in isolation but, if other brainstem symptoms are present, it should be investigated with angiograms or magnetic resonance angiography. The proprioceptive hypothesis for cervical vertigo is based on the fact that neck stimuli cooperate with vestibular and visual inputs in the control of posture and eye movements (Brandt and Bronstein, 2001). Neck conditions such as ostheoarthritis could then give rise to vertiginous sensations during head–neck motion. However, local anesthetics injected in neck structures fail to elicit motor or postural response (Dieterich *et al.*, 1993). So far, no single test has validated the existence of the syndrome of cervical vertigo.

In contrast, clinical experience indicates that symptoms of vertigo and imbalance related to head–neck movements are usually explained by a vestibular disorder. Any vestibular disorder, central or peripheral, is aggravated by head movements, but the one that should be in all physicians' minds is beingn paroxysmal positional vertigo (BPPV). While a full review is not appropriate here, we should like to emphasize that BPPV can only be diagnosed with the Hallpike positional maneuver, or variants (Bronstein, 2003). Treatment with repositioning maneuvers (Epley or Semont) is easy, extremely effective, and can be conducted by any doctor or physiotherapist. One still sees many patients with BPPV, referred by general practitioners and specialists alike, with a possible diagnosis of cervical vertigo or vertebrobasilar disease and without a Hallpike test ever having been done.

As a result of a vestibular disorder, patients do stiffen up the neck as a subconscious defence against vestibular symptoms induced by head movements. Further, cervical arthritis may also coexist in a patient with a vestibular disorder. For these reasons, physiotherapy can be added to the specific treatment for the underlying vestibular disorder. The subjective improvement in symptoms that usually follows, however, cannot be taken as evidence that the cause of the problem was cervical vertigo; however, this seems to be an academic rather than a practical clinical problem.

Central disorders

Neurologists and physicians in stroke or rehabilitation units will be familiar with ischemic and hemorrhagic posterior fossa strokes, and with the fact that vertigo is a prominent symptom in the acute stages. The presence of brainstem/cerebellar symptoms and signs makes confusion with a peripheral vestibular disorder unlikely, and the exceptions to this rule have been discussed above. For these reasons we will not discuss the individual vascular brainstem syndromes in detail.

In vertebrobasilar stroke, vertigo is prominent, and the anterior inferior cerebellar artery syndrome includes sudden deafness and ipsilateral canal paresis caused by labyrinthine infarction (Lee *et al.*, 2002). Pontine tegmental strokes also have eye movement and vestibular features (Kumral *et al.*, 2002). Regardless of the specific syndrome, the clinician should bear in mind that vertigo and brainstem symptoms, with head or neck pain, may indicate vertebral artery dissection (Saeed *et al.*, 2000).

Examination and impact of vertigo in stroke patients

Little work has been carried out on the impact of dizziness or vertigo in the recovery and rehabilitation of stroke. Clinical experience both with peripheral and central lesions shows that the natural reaction to dizziness and vertigo is to avoid head movements. This tendency, in turn, interferes with patient cooperation and motivation and, therefore, with the rehabilitation process. Consequently, it is essential to establish which factors may be contributing to this chain reaction. Factors likely to produce dizziness or intolerance to motion and upright posture can be of vestibular, oculomotor, and vasculo-orthostatic origin. It is important to identify these in order to obtain patients' full cooperation during rehabilitation.

Vestibular aspects

Lesions of the vestibular receptors, nerves, and nuclei, and their numerous connections, create an asymmetric ascending vestibular input, interpreted centrally (cortex) as vertigo. However, vertigo in brainstem stroke disappears gradually so a compensatory process must be at work. It is tempting to speculate that supra-vestibulonuclear structures (thalamus, cortex) are capable of redressing this nuclear asymmetry, probably in a similar way to the role of vestibular nuclei in peripheral vestibular lesions. However, head movements or unusual head positions will provoke vestibular symptoms. Vestibularly mediated intolerance to movement can be investigated clinically with the head thrust test, the head shaking test (shaking the head 20 times and observing whether nystagmus appears, usually conducted with Frenzel's glasses) and the more established positional tests (e.g. the Hallpike maneuver).

Both cerebellar and brainstem lesions produce severe and varied types of (central) positional vertigo and nystagmus. Although, at least in the chronic phase, central vertigo tends to be less severe than that in BPPV, patients with cerebellar–brainstem stroke do report vertigo, dizziness, and oscillopsia in certain head positions. Indeed, many patients adopt counteractive head positions, for instance when trying to read or to watch television; in these compensatory positions patients usually have less nystagmus. The positional maneuver is useful to make sure that the cause of the patient's vertigo is not conventional BPPV. Ischemia of the labyrinth, lack of mobility, head trauma, and awkward head positions in bed are known to predispose to BPPV, and patients with stroke are often exposed to many of these. If BPPV is found, treatment with the Semont or Epley maneuver is warranted (see below).

Oculomotor aspects

Following vertebrobasilar stroke, patients may be impeded in their rehabilitation by diplopia and/or oscillopsia. The double vision can be caused by nuclear or infra-nuclear (intrabrainstem fascicles) lesion of cranial nerves III, IV, or VI, or by internuclear and supranuclear lesions. The syndrome of internuclear ophthalmo-plegia is a disconnection syndrome of cranial nerve VI to III caused by lesion of the medial longitudinal fasciculus. The ipsilesional eye is unable to adduct and the abducting eye may move normally or excessively (with additional abducting or "ataxic" nystagmus); horizontal diplopia is reported but not by all patients. Skew eye deviation is the name given to a supranuclear vertical strabismus caused by asymmetry in torsional vestibulo-ocular pathways (Bronstein, 2002). Affected patients report vertical (or skew) double vision usually in all positions of gaze, as the strabismus is largely a result of concomitant ocular misalignment (i.e. little or no change during examination in the six cardinal positions of gaze). Skew deviations are part of the ocular tilt reaction and are common in patients with lateropulsion, as in Wallenberg syndrome or other posterior fossa strokes.

In patients with strabismus and diplopia of ischemic origin, the spontaneous prognosis is good, with resolution of diplopia in primary gaze in two to three months. Larger lesions and additional neurological symptoms are associated with a worse prognosis (Eggenberger et al., 2002). Management for the first few months should be conservative, with ocular occlusion or prisms, but the problem should be addressed in order to obtain full patient cooperation in the wider rehabilitation process. Later, extraocular injections of botulinum toxin or corrective surgery may be considered either for cosmetic or visual reasons, but doctors and patients alike should be aware that these two indications can counteract each other (e.g. the diplopia in a large squint might be centrally suppressed but not in a small-angle squint).

Oscillopsia can also be a debilitating visual symptom in patients with posterior fossa strokes. The more troublesome oscillopsia is caused by pendular nystagmus. The name pendular implies that the nystagmus does not have the typical slow and fast phases seen in "jerk" nystagmus; it is a slow phase, quasisinusoidal eye oscillation. It is often associated with palatal myoclonus. Pendular nystagmus results from deafferentation of the inferior olive by lesions interrupting the central tegmental tract carrying rubro-olivary fibers (the tremorgenic triangle of Mollaret) (Lopez *et al.*, 1996). The nystagmus and oscillopsia develop weeks or months after the brainstem stroke, presumably as the inferior olive develops an autonomous oscillatory discharge pattern. Patients have great difficulty in reading and watching television, but also in walking as the visual oscillation interferes with foot placement and obstacle avoidance. The treatment of pendular nystagmus (and other central nystagmus) is empirical and not very successful. Some patients report benefit with gabapentin, clonazepam, valproate, biperiden, memantine (Averbuch-Heller, 1999), alcohol (Mossman *et al.*, 1993), or cannabis (Schon *et al.*, 1999; Dell'Osso, 2000).

In contrast to pendular nystagmus, which invariably develops weeks after the stroke, jerk nystagmus is maximum in the acute phase and then often decays or disappear. If present in primary gaze (up-, downbeat, and torsional nystagmus), it is more troublesome than if it appears on gaze deviation (e.g. gaze-evoked nystagmus or abducting nystagmus of internuclear ophthalmoplegia). For these reasons, it is advisable to wait a few weeks before treating the oscillopsia pharmacologically, particularly as these drugs cause drowsiness and gait ataxia, which interfere with balance and rehabilitation. Some patients with brainstem strokes develop paroxysmal nystagmus (Lawden *et al.*, 1995) and skew deviations (Bentley *et al.*, 1998), causing troublesome attacks of diplopia, oscillopsia, and imbalance. These symptoms can respond well to carbamazepine and, at the dosage usually needed (200–400 mg daily), drowsiness and ataxia are not prominent.

Cardiovascular orthostatic mechanisms

Postural or orthostatic vertigo may be vestibular, caused by vasomotor reflex involvement by the stroke (Kihara *et al.*, 2001; Brozman *et al.*, 2002), associated autonomic system dysfunction (e.g. diabetes mellitus), prolonged bed-rest, medications, or combinations of these. In distinguishing between vestibular and vascular–orthostatic dizziness, one should remember that vestibular positional vertigo is equally (or more) likely to be triggered by lying down as by standing up. Indeed, vertigo on turning over in bed is typical of BPPV. More vague dizziness on standing up is more likely to be orthostatic. Orthostatic hypotension is diagnosed when there is a postural drop of >20 mmHg in systolic blood pressure within three minutes. Some patients may need formal autonomic function assessment but in many, measurements of blood pressure and pulse rate lying and standing up (initially and at three minutes) is enough.

Another factor that may interfere with the rehabilitation process is the occurrence of a cautious gait. After any stroke, but particularly after brainstem strokes with vertigo and imbalance, patients may develop a cautious gait strategy and fear of falling. It is sometimes difficult to distinguish the latter from the gait disorder present in leukoaraiosis (diffuse white matter vascular disease). Elderly patients with peripheral vestibular disorders can also develop this walking pattern. These patients appear to have an increased reaction to a vague sense of impending fall and move their feet as if they were walking on ice. The risk of falls, as assessed with the Dynamic Gait Index (eight items), is slightly increased in uni- or bilateral peripheral vestibular disorder. Of note, rehabilitation brings these patients back into the non-risk band (Herdman *et al.*, 2001). We will not discuss gait rehabilitation in this chapter but vestibular rehabilitation will be addressed in a specific section.

Treating vertigo

The discussions of the treatment of vertigo and vestibular rehabilitation that follow are based on Pavlou *et al.* (2004). Since the early 1980s, significant research efforts have been devoted to the mechanisms and usefulness of vestibular rehabilitation. Such rehabilitation is effective in peripheral vestibular disorders. Clinical trials typically report improvement in symptoms in over 80% of those participating, but with complete elimination of vertigo in less than a third (Norre and de Weerdt, 1980; Cohen, 1992; Shepard *et al.*, 1993). Unfortunately, almost no research has been conducted in central or combined peripheral–central vestibular disorders. Head trauma can compromise labyrinthine and central mechanisms and it would seem that central neural injury affects a patient's ability to recover (Shumway-Cook, 2000). A study by Gurr and Moffat (2001) showed that vestibular rehabilitation is effective in head injury, but patients with serious CNS lesions were excluded. Therefore, management of vertigo in stroke or other structural lesions relies on an eclectic approach combining vestibular suppressants (anticholinergic, benzodiazepines, antiemetics) and physical therapy (Hain and Uddin, 2003).

A key aspect to rehabilitation of balance disorders is the understanding that the control of posture and balance emerges from an interaction of many sensorimotor systems. These systems are organized in accordance with the stability requirements inherent in the task performed and constrained by the environment. Since lesions of peripheral and central vestibular structures vary in their type and severity, patients show a wide range of functional limitations, which must be assessed independently of one another (Shumway-Cook and Horak, 1989, 1990). Vestibular deficits affect stance, gait, and eye–head coordination and provoke various vertiginous symptoms. Recovery depends on the nature and extent of the deficits and the individual's capacity to compensate for the pathology. Treatment involves an individualized program of exercises and activities aimed at remediating direct and indirect impairments, maximizing function, and facilitating the natural compensatory process.

Physiological rationale

The purpose of a rehabilitation approach for vestibular problems is to facilitate the ability of the CNS to compensate for vestibular deficits and to seek resolution of the underlying pathological mechanisms when possible. Studies have shown that the neural basis for compensation is distributed throughout the nervous system such that lesions in, or pharmacological depression of, the cerebellum, cortex, spinal cord, brainstem, or sensory systems can prevent or reduce the capacity for compensation. Inactivity, whether from bed rest, fear, anxiety, or neurolocomotor limitations, has been demonstrated to delay and impair complete compensation (Lacour and Xerri, 1981). Stroke patients present many such factors but formal outcome comparisons between patients with central and peripheral disorders have not been published.

Several physiological mechanisms have been proposed to account for functional changes associated with CNS compensation, including central sensory substitution, rebalancing of tonic activity in central pathways (reviewed by Curthoys and Halmagyi, 1995), and physiological habituation.

1. *Central sensory substitution mechanisms.* These are the basis by which vision and somatosensory information can partially substitute for missing vestibular information for the purpose of dynamic and static orientation (Pfaltz and Karnath, 1983; Marchand and Amblard, 1984). Studies have shown an increased reliance on visual information (Bles *et al.*, 1983) or an increased responsiveness to somatosensory-triggered equilibrium responses following the absence of vestibular inputs (Horak *et al.*, 1994).

2. *Rebalancing central tonic neural activity.* Such rebalancing has been shown to accompany behavioral signs of recovery of function following vestibular injury. As recovery of symmetric tonic activity in vestibular nuclei occurs, abnormal eye movements and asymmetrical postures resolve. Compensatory processes that reestablish symmetry of tonic vestibular nuclei activity include cerebellar disinhibition, increased sensitivity to visual and somatosensory input, and active sensorimotor activity (McCabe, 1970; Lacour and Xerri, 1981; Curthoys and Halmagyi, 1995).

Table 13.2 Impairments commonly associated with vestibular pathology

	Components
Balance	
Musculoskeletal	Neck/back muscle tension
	Limited range of joint motion
	Pain (headache, neck/back pain, etc.)
Sensory	Visual dependence/visual vertigo
	Somatosensory dependence
	Poor use of vestibular information
	Inflexible sensory strategy
Motor	Poor alignment
	Excessive hip strategy
	Lack of hip strategy
	Lack of stepping strategy
	Inefficient, inflexible movement strategy
	Asymmetry
Eye–head coordination	Poor gaze stabilization
	Poor head stabilization
Abnormal perception of stability and motion	
Vertigo	Positional
	Movement related
Internal representation of posture	Poor sense of vertical
	Inaccurate sense of stability limits

3. *Physiological habituation.* This is a decrease in response magnitude to repetitive sensory stimulation. Habituation of vertigo by systematically repeating the symptom provoking head movements or positions has been known for many years (Cawthorne, 1945) and probably has its effects through multiple physiologic mechanisms.

Impairments associated with vestibular pathologies

Unilateral vestibular loss

Primary and secondary impairments in patients with unilateral vestibular loss can involve all the components listed in Table 13.2. Immediately after unilateral vestibular loss of acute onset, patients have constant vertigo, lean their head and trunks, and show spontaneous nystagmus to the side of the lesion. They may have a positive Romberg test for a few days. Postural and locomotor ataxia is usually a result of left/right asymmetries and unsteadiness associated with head movements. Eye–head coordination during both voluntary and passive head movements is usually disturbed. The perception of verticality and their stability limits may be skewed to one side.

Patients with unilateral loss of vestibular function often compensate, with few long-term symptoms. In general, recovery of tonic impairments such as postural instability in quiet stance is faster and greater than that of dynamic impairments such as gait ataxia when patients move their heads. At the clinical level, well-compensated patients with complete unilateral vestibular loss show either no spontaneous nystagmus or only some in the dark. The Romberg test is normal but some patients continue to report transient vertigo, oscillopsia during fast head movements, and reduced postural balance during a demanding task.

Acute disruption of vestibular input, as in vestibular neuronitis, labyrinthitis, labyrinthine stroke, accidents, or surgical trauma, cause sudden, severe balance deficits. The intense initial symptoms resolve quickly over a few weeks but the presence of protracted, unresolved balance and dizziness symptoms is well known to clinicians.

Central vestibular disorders

Patients who complain of dizziness following a vascular event or head injury may have a combination of central and peripheral vestibular deficits as well as neck injury (Furman and Whitney, 2000). As mentioned above, only a few studies (Fitzgerald, 1995; Burton, 1996; Gill-Body *et al.*, 1997; Godbout, 1997) have applied rehabilitation protocols in central vestibular disorders and none of these studies included a control group.

Studies including a heterogeneous population with peripheral, central, and multiple deficits have provided varying results, with some reporting poor outcome for the last two groups (Konrad *et al.*, 1992; Shepard *et al.*, 1993) and others reporting a similar degree of improvement as in patients with stable peripheral vestibular disorders (Cass *et al.*, 1996; Cowand *et al.*, 1998). Overall though, patients with central vestibular disorders are expected to require a longer time period for improvement and have worse outcomes in rehabilitation than patients with peripheral vestibular disorders (Konrad *et al.*, 1992; Shepard *et al.*, 1993). These results may depend on the location and extent of the central deficit and the additional complications that result, including cognitive and neuromuscular impairments.

Fluctuating vestibular deficits

Many patients have incomplete damage, fluctuating function (as in labyrinthine hydrops, e.g. Meniere's disease), positional symptoms (peripheral BPPV or central positional nystagmus), and additional CNS, medical, or psychological complications. It is much more difficult for the CNS to compensate for a fluctuating vestibular deficit or for multiple deficits than for a steady loss of any kind (Hahn *et al.*, 2001). In general, these patients are more difficult to treat with an exercise approach than those with a steady loss of function, except for specific repositioning treatment for BPPV (see below). The dizziness is often associated with cognitive complaints such as inability to concentrate or poor memory, especially during dynamic balancing tasks such as walking while moving their heads.

Visual vertigo

A subgroup of patients with balance disorders complain that their symptoms are precipitated or exacerbated by complex visual surroundings (Jacob *et al.*, 1993; Bronstein, 1995). These include situations with repetitive or unstable visual patterns such as those encountered while walking down supermarket aisles, in crowds, or viewing moving scenes; these symptoms can be seen in patients with peripheral, central, or combined vestibular disorders including brainstem stroke (Bronstein, 1995). Symptoms may also be precipitated by driving, particularly in certain conditions such as going over the brow of a hill or around bends: what is known as motorist disorientation syndrome (Page and Gresty, 1985). These patients rely more on visual cues for postural stability, showing greater postural sway in response to moving visual scenes than normal controls (Bles *et al.*, 1983; Redfern and Furman, 1994; Bronstein, 1995; Guerraz *et al.*, 2001). Rehabilitation with optokinetic stimulation provides a significant improvement in postural stability (Vitte *et al.*, 1994; Tsuzuku *et al.*, 1995); however, comparable results are also obtained with a customized vestibular exercise program (Pavlou *et al.*, 2004b). A rehabilitation program incorporating repeated progressive exposure to visual–vestibular stimulation during therapy provides substantially greater improvement in symptoms associated with visual vertigo than does therapy with vestibular exercises alone (Pavlou *et al.*, 2004b).

Cervical vertigo

As discussed above, this topic is surrounded by controversy (Brandt and Bronstein, 2001). Oculomotor and vestibular testing is usually normal following experimental cervical injury (Dieterich *et al.*, 1993). Increased postural sway has been reported with posturography testing (Alund *et al.*, 1993; Karlberg *et al.*, 1996) but this may be caused by symptoms of dizziness, neck pain, headache, and decreased cervical motion, which are observed in most vestibular disorders. Cervical vertigo is a diagnosis contemplated only after extracervical causes (vestibular in particular) have been excluded and if there is a close association between neck pain and dizziness (Biesinger, 1988; Wrisley *et al.*, 2000). Despite the ambiguity surrounding the diagnosis, it seems logical to suggest that a patient presenting with cervical pain and imbalance should be assessed by the therapist for both conditions and treated accordingly.

Vestibular rehabilitation

Vestibular rehabilitation is an exercise approach to treating primary and secondary symptoms associated with vestibular pathology. The purpose is to stimulate central compensation and to provide a structured opportunity for recovery of sensorimotor coordination over a wide range of orientations and movements. It was first employed as a method of speeding neurophysiological habituation following surgically induced unilateral vestibular loss (Cooksey, 1945). The treatment protocol used in this initial rehabilitation program came to be known as the Cawthorne–Cooksey exercises. The patient was asked to perform repeatedly a generic progressive sequence of eye, head, and body movements in order to stimulate the vestibular system and enhance the natural process of central compensation for the asymmetry in the peripheral vestibular input. These exercises continue to remain popular today for many reasons. These include cost and time efficiency, since patients are educated in the exercises on a single visit, either in an individual or group setting, and then instructed to continue them in their home environment often with no further supervision or follow-up. Table 13.3 include a sample of the type of symptom-provoking exercises that are usually included in VR programs and are based on the initial Cawthorne–Cooksey exercises.

Individualized therapy incorporating a combination of habituation, adaptation exercises, and balance and mobility exercises are becoming more common, particularly in light of recent studies showing that a customized therapy program results in greater improvement than a generic one (Szturm et al., 1994; Shepard and Telian, 1995). In customized VR programs, the exercises the patient is asked to perform are specific to those eye, head, or body positions and movements that provoke vertigo. For example, if a patient complains of dizziness every time they reach up into a cupboard, that particular movement should be given as a specific exercise. In addition, VR includes exercises and activities customized to improve the particular balance and mobility problems associated with vestibular pathology. Vestibular rehabilitation begins with a comprehensive rehabilitation assessment, which is then used to develop a customized treatment program.

Rehabilitation assessment

Assessment of the patient with vestibular pathology focuses on three main areas: balance and postural control underlying mobility skills, eye–head coordination and gaze stabilization, and vertigo (Shumway-Cook and Horak, 1989, 1990).

Table 13.3 Range of movements typically included in vestibular rehabilitation programs

Exercise type	Movements
Head exercises (performed with eyes open and eyes closed)	Bend head backwards and forwards
	Turn head from side to side
	Tilt head from one shoulder to the other
Fixation exercises	Move eyes up and down, side to side
	Perform head exercises while fixating stationary target
	Perform head exercises while fixating moving target
Positioning exercises (performed with eyes open and closed)	While seated, bend down to touch the floor
	While seated, turn to look over shoulder both to left and right
	Bend down with head twisted first to one side and then the other
	Lying down, roll from one side to the other
	Sit up from lying on the back and on each side
	Repeat with head turned to each side
Postural exercises (performed eyes open; eyes closed under supervision)	Practice static stance with feet as close together as possible
	Practice standing on one leg, and heel to toe
	Repeat head and fixation exercises while standing and then walking
	Practice walking in circles, pivot turns, up slopes, stairs, around obstacles
	Standing and walking in environments with altered surface and/or visual conditions with and without head and fixation exercises
	Aerobic exercises including alternative touching the fingers to the toes, trunk bends and twists, etc.

During VR, the therapist must constantly evaluate and monitor the changing constellation of impairments affecting each patient and adjust the treatment program accordingly.

Assessing posture and balance control

In this section assessments are only discussed if they are often used in the context of vertigo or vestibular disorders and may be useful additions to the examination of balance described earlier. The rehabilitation assessment of balance control is directed at evaluating a patient's ability to perform functional balance tasks, to use and adapt strategies appropriately for changing task conditions, and to see whether dizziness/vertigo develops during such tasks. If functional performance is suboptimal, assessment aims to identify the sensory, motor, and cognitive impairments responsible and to decide whether therapy will be able to improve functional task performance despite the existing impairments. If therapy is judged to be beneficial, the information gained through assessment is used to develop a comprehensive list of problems, establish short- and long-term goals, and formulate a plan of care for retraining posture control and decreasing symptoms.

In patients with vestibular pathology, complaints of vertigo and oscillopsia often lead to compensatory strategies that restrict head and trunk movement (Bronstein and Hood, 1987; Shumway-Cook and Horak, 1990). This can lead to secondary musculoskeletal impairments, including muscle tension, fatigue, and pain in the cervical and, sometimes, thoracolumbar regions. Assessment of the musculoskeletal system includes evaluation of range of motion, flexibility, and alignment in as functional a situation as possible (Magee, 1987; Saunders, 1991). Lower limb muscle strength and coordination must also be examined, particularly in patients with stroke-related vertigo.

Assessing gaze control and head–eye coordination

Adequate head and gaze stability is required for complex tasks such as balancing on a beam or walking, although it may not be critical for postural stability in quiet stance (Berthoz and Melvill Jones, 1985; Shuppert et al., 1994). During head movement, stability of the eyes in space depends on the vestibulo-ocular reflex, which rotates the eyes in the opposite direction to the head. Several aspects of eye–head coordination essential to the ability to stabilize gaze are evaluated to develop a customized VR program. Eye movements used to locate targets presented within both the central and the peripheral visual fields are assessed first without any head movements. The patient is asked to keep the head still and move only the eyes. The separate oculomotor subsystems are examined: smooth pursuit to slowly moving targets, saccades to different objects, fixation stability, and binocular convergence. For rehabilitation assessment purposes, eye movements may be graded subjectively as intact, impaired, or unable; additionally, any subjective complaints related to blurred or unstable vision are recorded. Nystagmus and strabismus (and their consequences, oscillopsia and diplopia, respectively) are major complicating factors in the rehabilitation of patients with posterior fossa stroke.

It is also important to evaluate the patient's ability to stabilize gaze on an earth-fixed target (e.g. stationary object in the room) and on a target moving in phase with the head (e.g. walking and simultaneously reading a newspaper you are holding) during head movements. Task performance depends on the intactness of the vestibulo-ocular reflex and visual suppression of the vestibulo-ocular response respectively.

Eye–head coordination is assessed in sitting, standing, and walking. For example, the patient is asked to look to the right or left and up or down while walking a straight path. The impact of head movements on stability is reported. For example, head movements during gait often cause the patient to deviate from a straight path and in severe cases stagger and lose balance. Finally, the patient's ability to make eye/head/trunk movements necessary to locate targets oriented in the far periphery is tested.

Assessing perceptions of stability and motion

Dizziness and vertigo

Neural and labyrinthine lesions can profoundly affect a patient's sense of self-motion or environmental motion. When dizziness is provoked, it is often a contributor to unsteadiness and loss of balance. It is critical to evaluate the particular environments, conditions, head movements, and positions that provoke vertigo in order to design appropriate exercises and to counsel patients about how to control their symptoms. Assessment of dizziness begins with a careful history to determine the patient's perceptions of whether dizziness is constant or provoked, and the situations or conditions that stimulate dizziness. Grouped questionnaires can be employed to provide a quantitative measure of the frequency, severity, and triggers of symptoms, their effect on daily activities, and any associated psychological correlates (e.g. Guerraz *et al.*, 2001). Norre (1984) examined the intensity of dizziness on a scale of 0 to 10 (no dizziness to most severe possible) and its duration in response to movement and positional changes of the head and body (Table 13.4). A dizziness index was calculated by multiplying the intensity by the duration and summing all the numbers (Norre, 1987).

Internal representation of posture

Patients' subconscious internal representations of their stability limits and of their sensory and biomechanical capabilities may be distorted by CNS lesions. When internal representation of stability limits is smaller than actual, patients minimize body sway and center of mass movements using excessive movement strategies for equilibrium; when it is larger than actual, patients easily exceed their limits of stability and fall without taking appropriate action. The consistency between the patient's perceived versus actual stability limits is subjectively assessed for both the sitting and standing position using self-initiated postural movements. Alternatively, patients are asked to reach for an object held at the outer edge of

Table 13.4 Vertigo positions and movement test

Test	Imbalance (yes/no)	Intensity (0–10)	Duration (seconds)
1. Baseline : seated (eyes open)			
2. Position provoked : look right			
3. Position provoked : look left			
4. Movement provoked : side to side			
5. Position provoked : look up			
6. Position provoked : look down			
7. Movement provoked : up and down			
8. Sit to supine			
9. Rolling to right			
10. Rolling to left			
11. Supine to sit			
12. Sit to stand			
13. Passive head/trunk rotation			
14. Passive trunk rotation : head still			
15. Bend to floor			
16. Standing : look over right shoulder			
17. Standing : look over left shoulder			
18. Walking : horizontal head turns			
19. Walking : vertical head turns			
20. Walking : change speed			
21. Walking : quick stop			
22. Walking : pivot turn			
23. Hallpike right			
24. Hallpike left			
25. Other:			

their stability limits. The therapist observes the extent to which the patient is willing to move the center of mass and makes a subjective judgement regarding whether the patient is moving to the full stability limits in all directions. We have already discussed the internal sense of gravitional vertical (p. 329).

Specific components of vestibular rehabilitation

Treating musculoskeletal impairments

Musculoskeletal problems, including limited range of motion, decreased flexibility, and muscle weakness, whether primary or caused by inactivity can be improved or completely remediated using traditional physical therapy techniques, including modalities such as heat, passive manipulation, massage, stretching exercises, casting, biofeedback, and strengthening exercises. Musculoskeletal problems can also include problems in postural alignment. The goal when retraining alignment is to help the patient to develop an initial position that is appropriate for the task, is efficient with respect to gravity, and maximizes stability (i.e. places the center of mass well within the patient's stability limits). There are a number of approaches that can be used to help patients to develop a symmetrically vertical posture; these must be tailored to the patient's condition. Verbal and manual cues are often used to assist a patient in finding and maintaining an appropriate vertical posture. Patients practice with eyes open and closed and on firm or compliant surfaces, learning to maintain a vertical position in the absence of visual and/or somatosensory cues. Mirrors can also be used to provide patients with visual feedback about their position in space. Another approach to retraining vertical posture involves having patients stand (or sit) with their back against the wall, which provides enhanced somatosensory feedback about their position in space. This feedback can be further increased by placing a small protruding object vertically on the wall (e.g. yardstick or a rolled-up towel) and having the patient lean against it. Somatosensory feedback can be made intermittent by having the patient lean away from the wall, only occasionally leaning back to get knowledge of results. Kinetic or force feedback devices are often used to provide patients with information about postural alignment and weight-bearing status. Kinetic feedback can be provided with devices as simple as bathroom scales or through load limb monitors (Herman, 1973), or force-plate biofeedback systems (Shumway-Cook *et al.*, 1988).

Retraining sensory and movement strategies

The goal when retraining movement strategies involves helping the patient to develop coordinated movements effective in meeting the demands for posture and balance in sitting and in standing, essentially keeping the center of mass within the base of support. This includes strategies that move the center of mass relative to a stationary base of support, for example an ankle or hip strategy in standing and strategies for changing the base of support, for example a stepping strategy in standing or a protective reach in sitting.

Developing a coordinated ankle strategy

When retraining the use of an ankle strategy during self-initiated sway, patients are asked to practice swaying back and forth, and side to side, within small ranges, keeping the body straight and not bending at the hips or knees. Knowledge of results regarding how far the center of mass is moving during self-initiated sway can be facilitated using static force-plate retraining systems (Shumway-Cook et al., 1988), which can effectively be used to retrain scaling problems (Shumway-Cook and Horak, 1992). Patients are asked to move the center of mass voluntarily to different targets displayed on a screen. Targets are made progressively smaller and are placed closed together, requiring greater precision in force control. However, balance rehabilitation in stroke patients seems no better with a commercial device based on these principles (Balance master; Geiger et al., 2001). Patients may also practice amplitude scaling by responding to perturbations of various amplitudes applied at the hips or shoulders. Small perturbations, such as a small pull or push at the hips or shoulders, are used to practice the use of an ankle strategy to recover equilibrium. Feedback regarding the appropriateness of their response is provided by the clinician. Finally, patients are asked to carry out a variety of manipulation tasks, such as reaching, lifting, and throwing; these help patients to develop strategies for anticipatory postural control. The magnitude of anticipatory postural activity is directly related to the potential for instability inherent in a task: small when a patient who is externally supported by the therapist is asked to lift a light load slowly, or large in an unsupported patient who must lift a heavy load quickly.

Developing a coordinated hip strategy

A hip strategy can be facilitated by asking the patient to maintain balance without taking a step and using faster and larger displacements than those used for an ankle strategy. Use of a hip strategy can also be facilitated by restricting force control at the ankle joints by standing across a narrow beam, standing heel to toe or in a single limb stance. Patients practice both voluntary sway and response to external perturbations on altered surfaces to relearn how to control a hip strategy. Attempts to stabilize the head and eyes in space by focusing on a visual target can also help to improve control of a hip strategy.

Developing a coordinated step strategy

Learning to step in response to a large perturbation is an essential part of balance retraining (Shumway-Cook and Horak, 1992; Shumway-Cook and Woollacott, 2001). Both the preparatory postural adjustment toward the stance leg and the step itself can be practiced independently prior to putting them together. Stepping can be practiced by passively shifting the patient's weight to one side and then quickly bringing the center of mass back towards the unweighted leg, or by initiating a response to large backward or forward perturbations. If needed, manual assistance at the ankle can be used to facilitate a stepping response. In order to increase the size of a compensatory step, subjects can also practice stepping over a visual target or obstacle in response to the external perturbations.

When providing balance exercises, the environment must be modified to allow a patient to practice the exercises safely and without the continual supervision of a therapist. Patients who are very unsteady or fearful of falling can practice movements while wearing a harness connected to the ceiling, in the parallel bars, standing close to a wall or corner, or with a chair or table in front of them.

Improving perception of orientation and movement

The goal when retraining perception of postural orientation in space is to help the patient learn to integrate sensory information effectively in a variety of altered environments. This necessitates correctly interpreting the body's position and movements in space. Treatment strategies generally require the patient to maintain balance during progressively more difficult static and dynamic movement tasks while the clinician systematically varies the availability and accuracy of sources of sensory information for orientation. Patients are asked to perform tasks while sitting or standing on surfaces with disrupted somatosensory cues for orientation, such as carpets, compliant foam, and moving surfaces (e.g. a tilt or wobble board).

Patients who are visually dependent are prescribed a variety of balance tasks when visual cues are absent (eyes closed or blindfolded) or reduced (blinders or diminished lighting). Visual cues can also be made inaccurate for orientation through the use of glasses smeared with petroleum jelly, prisms, vision-reversing goggles (Yardley et al., 1992), or complex moving visual scenes (Fig. 13.8) such as exposure to optokinetic stimuli by means of real motion, projected moving scenes, or head-mounted virtual reality systems (Shumway-Cook and Horak, 1989, 1990; Vitte et al., 1994; Pavlou et al., 2001). Exposure to optokinetic stimuli in the home environment may be accomplished by having the patient watch videos with conflicting visual scenes such as high-speed car chases or "busy" screen savers on a computer. Exposure to any complex visual stimulation should be gradual and involve varying distances from the visual scene while conducting exercises in sitting, standing, and during walking, first alone and then in combination with voluntary head movements. Finally, in order to enhance the patient's ability to use remaining vestibular information for postural stability, exercises are given that ask the patient to balance while both visual and somatosensory are simultaneously reduced (e.g. blindfolded or eyes closed while standing on foam).

Learning to adapt strategies to changing contexts

Developing adaptive capacities in the patient is also a critical part of retraining balance. A hierarchy of tasks can be used, beginning with tasks that have relatively few stability demands and moving to those that place heavy demands on the postural control system. For example, postural demands involved in maintaining an upright seated posture while in a semi-supported seated position are relatively

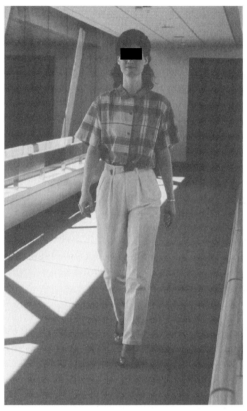

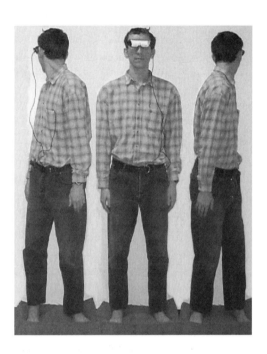

A   B

Fig. 13.8   Examples of exercises to reduce visual motion sensitivity. (A) Walking across a windowed
bridge with complex visual orientation information from shadow and traffic in the street
below; (B) using a head-mounted display (Eye-Trek FMD-200, Olympus Optical Co. Ltd) for
image projection. Patients may watch a video showing visually conflicting stimuli while
performing head and body movements in sitting, standing, and walking. (From Pavlou *et al.*,
2004.)

few. In contrast, sitting on a moving tilt board while holding a cup of water has
fairly rigorous stability requirements, reflecting the changing and unpredictable
nature of the task. Therefore, as the patient improves, more difficult and demanding tasks can be introduced using varying speeds of movement. During balance
retraining, patients practice a wide collection of functional tasks in a variety of
contexts, including maintaining balance with a reduced base of support, maintaining balance while changing the orientation of the head and trunk, and maintaining balance while performing a variety of upper extremity tasks.

Eye and head exercises

Adaptation exercises incorporating gaze fixation during head movements as well as eye movements and postural exercises are also prescribed to promote the recovery of normal vestibulo-ocular and vestibulospinal reflex function. Gaze fixation exercises are performed at varying distances from the target and with increasing frequency of head oscillation (Herdman, 1997).

Relaxation exercises

There are a variety of reasons why particular patients with vertigo may benefit from being taught relaxation techniques (Beyts, 1987; Odkvist and Odkvist, 1988), particularly when dizziness is associated with stress, neck tension, hyperventilation, or jaw-clenching or grinding. For significant cervical problems, a formal course of physical therapy and anti-inflammatory drugs may be needed, but simple techniques for reducing neck tension that can be performed before commencing exercises for vertigo are shoulder shrugging, shoulder/arm rotation (backwards and forwards), and gentle stretching exercises specific for the neck region. Relaxation training has also been suggested as a means of increasing tolerance of the symptoms provoked by exercise-based therapy (Leduc and Decloedt, 1989).

The presence of hyperventilation has to be identified as it interferes with basic vestibular compensatory processes (Sakellari and Bronstein, 1997; Sakellari *et al.*, 1997). Therapies that have been used successfully to enable the patient to control arousal, hyperventilation, and autonomic symptoms include various relaxation techniques, education in respiration control, and biofeedback. One of the simplest and most widely used methods of relaxation is known as "progressive relaxation." This involves focusing on one set of muscles at a time, first deliberately clenching them and then relaxing them. A training program known as "applied relaxation" (Ost, 1987) can be used to teach the patient how to implement relaxation techniques in progressively more stressful situations.

Slow, diaphragmatic breathing is a vital component of relaxation. The aim is to establish a breathing pattern of 10–14 breaths a minute, by monitoring and then deliberately slowing the respiratory cycle. By placing one hand on the chest and the other on the stomach the patient can monitor whether their breathing is thoracic or diaphragmatic; if thoracic, they may need to be taught to draw in and expel air by deliberately inflating and compressing the stomach, while keeping the chest flat and motionless.

Biofeedback is a more elaborate technique whereby the patient's physiological state is monitored (e.g. muscle tension, heart or respiratory rate). A feedback signal, such as a light or tone, is provided to inform the patient when they are progressing towards the relaxed state. Although biofeedback requires more resources than other relaxation training programs, the technological aspect of the technique can help to motivate patients who are sceptical of the value of "soft" therapies such as relaxation.

General aspects of vestibular rehabilitation

General characteristics of every exercise program include specificity, repetition, and progression. The patient is only given exercises that specifically provoke their symptoms. Norré and de Weerdt (1980) found that the symptoms of patients who performed exercises *not* provoking symptoms resulted in unchanged vertigo, but after the same patients had practiced performing disorienting movements, their symptoms improved. The prescribed exercises are performed for at least 10–20 minutes, twice a day. Pacing of the exercises is crucial. Unless they are performed slowly at first, exercises may induce an unacceptable degree of vertigo and nausea. As symptoms abate, the patient gradually increases the pace and difficulty of the exercises. As patients become more accustomed to the exercises and their tolerance increases, they are advised to expose themselves gradually once again to everyday situations that they have come to avoid over time, such as supermarket aisles, crowds, and shopping malls. Once all the exercises can be performed without dizziness, it is important that patients maintain a high degree of physical activity (e.g. ball games or dancing) in order to sustain compensation.

An essential part of VR involves educating the patient regarding the dynamic nature of vestibular compensation. This understanding is critical to forming positive but realistic expectations. For example, patients are warned that their symptoms may at first worsen, and that improvement may be uneven: they will probably experience good days and bad days. In addition, patients are cautioned that even after compensation is achieved and symptoms have largely resolved, periods of stress, fatigue, or illnesses may result in a temporary reoccurrence of symptoms.

Vestibular sedatives are often needed in the management of acute vestibular disorders, both peripheral and central. However, prolonged use of these drugs is believed to delay long-term vestibular compensation. Therefore, they should be gradually suppressed as early as possible although they may be needed at some point during rehabilitation to facilitate patient compliance with the exercise program.

Therapies for benign paroxysmal positional vertigo

BPPV is one of the most common vestibular disorders. It arises as a result of the accumulation of debris (dislodged otoconia) in the posterior semicircular canal, although recent evidence has shown that anterior and horizontal canal involvement may also occur to a much lesser extent (McClure, 1985; Herdman and Tusa, 1996; Fife, 1998; Bertholon *et al.*, 2002). The debris is usually freely moving in the canal (canal lithiasis) and, during reorientation of the head with respect to gravity, creates endolymphatic currents and cupular displacement. Patients complain of intense but brief vertigo on looking up, bending over, and, typically, on turning over in bed. Spontaneous remissions may occur but new physical treatments cure 70 to 90% of patients in one or two sessions, respectively (Epley, 1992; Wolf *et al.*, 1999; Nunez *et al.*, 2000). Positive diagnosis can only be established by observing the typical nystagmus during the Hallpike maneuver. For the most common form, the posterior canal type, the nystagmus is torsional, beating towards the under-most ear, lasting for 5–20 seconds, and usually accompanied by intense vertigo.

There are essentially two treatment procedures, often called "repositioning" man-euvers because they relocate the debris particles from the semicircular canal back into the vestibule: the Semont maneuver and the Epley maneuver (Semont *et al.*, 1988; Epley, 1992). There is no advantage in using one or the other technique, nor in using whole-body rotators to promote particle migration (Lempert *et al.*, 1997). The clinician should be familiar with at least one procedure. In the Semont technique, a variant Hallpike maneuver is used to identify the position provoking BPPV (Fig. 13.9), which is maintained for at least 30 seconds (to allow all particles to sink down the canal). The therapist then moves the patient quickly from this position, in a single movement, to the opposite side of the couch. The movement required is oblique,

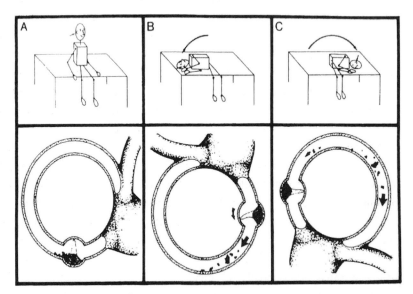

Fig. 13.9   In the Semont technique, a variant Hallpike maneuver is used to identify the position provoking benign paroxysmal positional vertigo(Aland B), in this case the right side. The treatment consists of a rapid movement of the patient from the right-ear-down position to the opposite-eye-down position (C). The lower panels illustrate the movement of the intracanalicular deloris. (From Braudt, 1999, with permission).

according to the anatomical orientation of the posterior canal. It is easily remembered: from an ear-side-down the patient should land on the opposite-eye-down (say from right ear down to left eye down; Fig. 13.9). In overweight, elderly, or neurologically impaired patients, an assistant is often required for the Semont maneuver as it is important that the movement be fast. Recommendations that patients must try to keep their head vertical for 48 hours are now considered not to be necessary. Other physical treatments like the Epley (1992) and self-positioning maneuvers (Brandt and Daroff, 1980; Radtke et al., 1999) can be found in reviews (Furman and Cass, 1999) and references quoted therein.

Balance rehabilitation in stroke patients

Preventing falls

The prevention of falls involves most members of the rehabilitation team, particularly medical doctors, physiotherapists, occupational therapists, nurses, and nursing auxiliaries. The risk of falling, its possible consequences, and prevention strategies must be explained to patients themselves as well as to the families. The "no fall" objective must above all be defined with the patient and the family. Particular attention must be paid to patients with anosodiaphoria, who minimize their impairment and are not aware of their risk of falling (usually large right hemisphere lesions at the acute or subacute stage). Beds must be equipped with barriers, and these measures must be maintained for a long time in patients with spatial misrepresentation. At the early stages of rehabilitation, it is important to strap the patient to the wheelchair to avoid attempts to stand up by patients who are not able to do so. Patients who do not recover the ability to sit may need to be strapped for long periods (weeks or month). Transfers (specially from wheelchair to bed and vice versa) must be initially performed with a carer or under surveillance. This measure must be maintained until the patient is clearly able to stand up and walk independently (with a crutch or a stick if necessary). This measure is not popular and must be explained and discussed many times with patients and families on the basis of objective assessments (postural performances, verticality perception, spatial neglect, and anosodiaphoria). Depending on the country, a rehabilitation team could face legal procedures in the event of a fall with severe complications if these preventive measures have not been correctly applied. Falls occurring during balance retraining programs are rare because trained physiotherapists will adjust the difficulty of exercises to patients' capabilities and fatigue and will also react promptly to any imbalance. Although these preventive measures are considered to be necessary and efficient, it must be stressed that their actual benefit remains to be quantified. In contrast, oriented balance retraining (Cheng *et al.*, 2001) and a long time elapsed since the stroke (El Fatimi *et al.*, 2001) have been shown to decrease the risk of falling.

Retraining balance

For patients who have suffered a stroke, improving balance is often a key point to reduce the degree of dependence in activities of daily living. The time is probably past when truly randomized prospective studies of stroke rehabilitation versus no stroke rehabilitation can be done. This is especially true for balance retraining, which still relies on empirical views. The general principles of balance retraining are similar to those of other functional retraining schemes in stroke patients. First, all elementary deficits and impairments must be identified and specifically treated (orthopedic problems, spasticity, muscular weakness, attention disorders, spatial cognition, depression, etc.). Second, motor retraining favors brain plasticity, hence the functional recovery (see corresponding chapters in this book). Third, programs of focused stroke rehabilitation improve functional performance (Ottenbacher and Jannell, 1993). Fourth, the training must be regularly adjusted to patients' capabilities. At early stages, postural retraining requires a support, either by the hand of the therapist or, preferably, by a harness. As the patient recovers, the exercises are performed without holding on but under close supervision, and finally only with intermittent supervision. Finally, recovery appears related to early initiation of treatment (Ottenbacher and Jannell, 1993) and to the intensity of the training (Kwakkel *et al.*, 1999).

Historically, one can consider two stages in balance retraining after stroke. Supported by vague "neurophysiological" views, the first approaches proposed by Bobath or Brunnstrom in the 1960s were mainly elaborated from observation and practice. Although widely applied today, they remain empirical since their efficiency has not really been tested, particularly regarding balance impairment. From the 1980s, stroke rehabilitation became less reflexive and more sensorimotor, or even cognitive, supported by new emerging ideas concerning brain plasticity. Several techniques were proposed to facilitate balance recovery, with their clinical relevance usually tested. Schematically these techniques are postural biofeedback; space exploration, which can be an implicit way to train postural control; sensory stimulations; and task-specific postural retraining. In order to change the body weight distribution in standing, some plantar orthoses have also been proposed. "Classical" or modern, all these techniques have as objectives to modulate postural tone (Bobath, Brunnstrom), to improve righting reflexes and other postural reflexes (many old and new techniques), to even out weight bearing as symmetrically as possible (postural biofeedback, use of ortheses), to improve body stability and especially trunk control (exercises based on postural reactions, postural biofeedback, space exploration combined with a postural task), to improve body representation in space (many techniques), to recalibrate postural coordinate systems (sensory stimulations), to facilitate the appropriate reweighing of sensory cues contributing to postural control (multisensory or vestibular rehabilitation), and to condition patients to execute specific postural tasks (task-related training). Some other substitutive measures are also useful, such as the extension of the base of support by the hand while sitting and by placing the legs apart or using a walking aid in standing. It is noteworthy that little attention has been paid up to now to the rehabilitation of verticality disorders and this is an important challenge for the future. The various techniques are complementary rather than incompatible, and clinicians have to select those that are the most appropriate for a given patient at a given time of the rehabilitation course. This is why the objectives of balance retraining must be regularly determined for a given stroke patient and updated according to severity and evolution of the disease. As a corollary, clinicians need to extend their practice to a large number of validated techniques.

Classical approaches to stroke rehabilitation (Bobath, Brunnstrom, etc.) have influenced physiotherapy practice worldwide (Ashburn, 1995; Lennon, 1996). The two best known concepts of neurorehabilitation (rather than proper techniques) were proposed by Bobath and by Brunnstrom. According to Bertha and Karel Bobath, increased tone and increased reflex activity emerge as a result of lack of inhibition from a damaged postural reflex mechanism, and movement is abnormal if it stems from a background of abnormal tone (Bobath, 1978). They proposed an approach that aimed to control the responses resulting from what they called "the damaged postural reflex mechanism." In particular, they claimed that direct handling of the body at key points such as the trunk was able to control afferent input and facilitate normal postural reactions. According to this concept, postures must be used to inhibit spasticity and tonic neck reflexes and to facilitate righting and equilibrium reactions (Lennon, 1996). In contrast to Bobath, Brunnstrom (1970) suggested the use of primitive reflexes to initiate movement. Tactile, proprioceptive, visual, and auditory stimuli are employed, along with asymmetrical tonic neck reflex, tonic lumbar and tonic labyrinthine reflexes, for facilitating movements. Brunnstrom's approach does not aim to normalize tone or inhibit the expression of primitive movement (Ashburn, 1995). Regarding the recovery of postural control after a cerebral lesion, both approaches have probably overestimated the role of archaic postural reflexes (labyrinthine and neck reflexes). They neglected the crucial role played by spatial cognition and never refer to neuroplasticity and motor relearning mechanisms. Their principal merit has been to emphasize the importance of trunk control both in sitting and standing, and to draw attention to leg positioning in standing. Some authors (e.g. Davies, 1985) have clearly acknowledged the incorporation of this legacy in their "step by step" training program for adult hemiplegics. Such a program retrains trunk control by asking the patient to maintain or to change posture in lying, sitting, and standing positions. Righting reactions are evoked by making the patient balance passively while lying or sitting on a rocking support (in the frontal or saggital planes). To this aim, devices have been designed to allow the assessment and rehabilitation of the sitting posture (Avery, 1979; Pérennou *et al.*, 2002a). The benefit of this training, however, remains to be investigated.

The ability to respond to external postural perturbations is also trained in conventional balance retraining programs. Studies of automatic responses to external surface perturbation have identified quick, coordinated, multisegmental strategies responsible for maintaining equilibrium. These strategies are organized to control a variety of postural objectives and are adapted to particular conditions, behavioral goals, and environmental contexts. What is important from a rehabilitation point of view is that these strategies become more efficient with practice (Horak *et al.*, 1997). In stroke patients, postural perturbations are applied in sitting or standing depending on patients' abilities, often manually delivered by the physiotherapist. More rarely, the patient is exposed to a quantified perturbation. Hocherman *et al.* (1984) showed that when stroke patients were trained to stand on a movable platform (15 sessions of 10 minutes over three weeks) they recovered better postural characteristics than those trained conventionally. Surprisingly, no attempt has been made to replicate this interesting work. One would expect hemiplegic patients to encounter difficulties in mastering the high-frequency postural oscillations elicited by sudden postural perturbations. Wing *et al.* (1993b) believe that the relative paucity of research in training stroke patients' balance by means of destabilizing situations relates to the need to protect patients from falling.

Task-related training

Since the early 1990s, a large number of studies conducted in stroke patients and in experimental animal models have suggested that the cerebral cortex undergoes significant and functional plasticity for weeks to months following injury. There is also evidence that intensive task-specific practice involving the impaired limb has a modulatory effect on cortical plasticity (Nudo and Friel, 1999). The cerebral cortex seems also involved in the reorganization of postural coordination after a cerebral lesion (Ioffe, 1997). It is now agreed that specific postural training can influence adaptive reorganizational mechanisms in the intact cerebral cortex and, thus, promote functional recovery. Dean and Shepherd (1997) performed the first randomized placebo-controlled study to test the effect of intensive task-related postural training. They trained patients chronically affected by stroke to increase the distance manually reached while seated and to increase the contribution of the affected lower leg to support and balance. At the end of a two week program, subjects were able to reach faster and further, increased the load through the affected foot, and increased activation of affected leg muscles compared with the control group. The experimental group also improved in sit-to-stand movement whereas the control group did not improve in reaching or in sit-to-stand maneuvers. Neither group, however, improved in walking. This study provided strong evidence of the efficacy of task-related motor training in improving the ability to balance during seated reaching activities after stroke. Rising from a chair is the type of complex movement that requires a good coordination between postural control and movement control. This task is difficult to perform by stroke patients, exposing them to a risk of falling (Cheng et al., 1998). If stroke patients were given repetitive sit-to-stand training associated with a biofeedback on their weight bearing during the task, they showed a substantial decrease in their risk of falling in daily life (Cheng et al., 2001). It seems that even a home-based exercise protocol focused on sit-to-stand training associated with additional exercises to strengthen lower limb extensor can improve performance of sit to stand and increase walking speed more than a year after stroke (Monger et al., 2002). Neurorehabilitation in general, and postural retraining of stroke patients in particular, offer many examples of task-related training. Indeed, such training is exactly what physiotherapists have done for years: for example when anticipating the need to maintain erect standing (orthosis-assisted erect stance), when repeating turn-around exercises, when conditioning the patient to perform safely sit-to-stand and stand-to-sit maneuvers, or when asking patients repeatedly to pick up objects from the floor. The repetitive practice of complex gait cycles on a treadmill (Visintin and Barbeau, 1989; Malouin et al., 1992) or with an electromechanical gait trainer (Hesse, 2001) with body weight partly supported represents one of the most promising example of task-related training in neurorehabilitation. One cannot exclude that this conditioning also partly involves postural control required for walking.

Postural biofeedback has been being one of the most investigated balance retraining techniques in stroke patients. The biofeedback may be visual (Shumway-Cook et al., 1988; Winstein et al., 1989; Sackley and Lincoln, 1997; Geiger et al., 2001), auditory (Pélissier et al., 1990; Engardt, 1994b; Pedersen et al., 1996; Batavia et al., 1997), or may combine visual and auditory information (Dursun et al., 1996; Lee et al., 1996). The feedback is used either to correct the sitting posture (Bjork and Wetzel, 1983; Dursun et al., 1996) or, more often, to correct the standing posture (Wannstedt and Herman, 1978; Shumway-Cook et al., 1988; Winstein et al., 1989; Engardt, 1994b; Lee et al., 1996; Petersen et al., 1996; Batavia et al., 1997; Sackley and Lincoln, 1997; Wong et al., 1997; Simmons et al., 1998; Geiger et al., 2001). In standing, the feedback information is used either to make weight bearing as symmetrical as possible (Wannstedt and

Herman, 1978; Shumway-Cook *et al.*, 1988; Winstein *et al.*, 1989; Lee *et al.*, 1996; Batavia *et al.*, 1997; Sackley and Lincoln, 1997; Wong *et al.*, 1997; Cheng *et al.*, 2001; Mudie *et al.*, 2002), to minimize postural sway (assuming that this improves body stability) (Shumway-Cook *et al.*, 1988; Winstein *et al.*, 1989) or to drive voluntary movements off the center of foot pressure by reaching or following a visual target (Di Fabio *et al.*, 1990; Hamman *et al.*, 1992; Sackley and Baguley, 1993). Techniques that consist of making weight bearing more symmetrical can be applied in static erect stance or in more dynamic task such as rising from a chair (Engardt *et al.*, 1993). It is said that it is possible to modify posturographic characteristics of stroke patients using intensive biofeedback training (Nilsson *et al.*, 2001). However, it is not proven that this apparent improvement still holds when the final assessment uses not posturography but rather a functional assessment including gait assessment, or when the experimental group is compared with a control group matched for age, delay from stroke onset, and elementary deficits. Whether there is a transference of effects to daily life or not is, therefore, the key question that will have to be definitively addressed in the next few years. What is the most relevant target: to reduce postural sway, to make weight bearing more symmetrical, or to enlarge the limit of stability? This is the second point that requires further investigations. It seems that training techniques that aim to reduce the amount of sway give inconsistent results. This can be interpreted in the light of new trends in the field, which do not consider any longer that a decrease in body sway necessarily means a good stability (Carpenter *et al.*, 2001b). Techniques that aim to make weight bearing symmetrical are confronted by the fact that we still do not know what this asymmetry represents. If this is partly a compensatory strategy as discussed above, it must be relatively considered as a compromise between orientation bias and impaired stabilization. It might be more relevant to work on the rehabilitation of orientation, using specific biofeedback devices, and to work on postural instability, using biofeedback techniques in dynamic postural tasks. Finally, although postural biofeedback training is widely used in stroke rehabilitation, and appreciated by patients and caregivers alike, further studies are required to clarify how this technique facilitates postural recovery.

Implicit balance training

Asking a patient to put load on the paretic leg, eventually with the help of a biofeedback, is typically an explicit way to retrain postural control. A motor skill can also be learned implicitly, without awareness of what is being learned. For instance, asking a patient to reach a target can be an implicit a way to retrain postural control. Because different cortical regions seem to be involved in implicit and explicit motor learning (Stadler, 1994; Honda *et al.*, 1998), it seems relevant to associate both explicit and implicit postural relearning in stroke rehabilitation.

When Carr and Shepherd (1998) proposed a set of reaching tasks in sitting, they did not refer only to task-related training but also to an implicit training of dynamic postural control, more especially of the coordination mechanisms between postural control and movement control. Initially, the target to reach, or the object to pick up, can be placed just beyond arm's length. Then it can be moved further and further away so that the person is 'pushed' near his (her) own limits of stability. The task appears easier for the patient since the goal is concrete (to reach a target instead of retraining balance). de Sèze et al. (2001) have proposed a combination of such an implicit postural training with spatial exploration exercises, the principle being to orientate the trunk voluntary by rotation and flexion movements. In practice, the patient wears a light trunk orthosis that supports a posterior mast on which a 150 cm horizontal rod projecting over the head is fixed. A pointer is fixed at the end of this rod, directed toward the targets. The physiotherapist illuminates a given target that the patient must touch. Exercises can be performed in sitting or in standing. Targets placed far on the contralesional side attract patient attention toward this possibly neglected space while the patient must implicitly control postural stabilization. Compared with conventional rehabilitation, such a technique could facilitate postural restoration (de Sèze et al., 2001). Because of an overlap in the right hemisphere between neural networks engaged in spatial cognition and those engaged in postural control (Pérennou et al., 1999), it could be that the recruitment of networks underlying spatial cognition may induce postural improvement and vice versa. Further studies will be required to increase out understanding of the role of trunk control in this technique. Other simple devices, such as a rod fixed on to the head, could also give promising results by combining space exploration and whole-body postural engagement in standing patients.

Sensory stimulations

Most manifestations of spatial neglect may be temporarily reduced by appropriate sensory manipulation. Such effects have been obtained with vestibular, visual, or somatosensory stimulation (reviewed by Vallar et al., 1997; Kerkhoff, 2003). Their efficiency in reducing neglect is usually temporary and may be the result of recruiting intact systems to produce the observed result, rather than specific boosting of the impaired representational systems. Similar effects could be also beneficial in postural disorders of stroke patients (Pérennou et al., 1998b, 2001b; Rode et al., 1998; Tilikete et al., 2001a). Caloric vestibular stimulation (Rode et al., 1998), transcutaneous electrical stimulation (Pérennou et al., 1998a,b, 2001b), and also visuomanual adaptation to prisms (Tilikete et al., 2001a) can modify the postural behavior of stroke patients. The weight-bearing asymmetry can be reduced by cold irrigation of the contralesional ear (Rode et al., 1998) and after a visuomanual prism adaptation inducing an ipsilesional optical deviation (Tilikete *et al.*, 2001a). In addition, low-intensity electrical stimulation applied on the contralesional neck side (below the contraction threshold) can improve active body orientation with respect to gravity (Pérennou *et al.*, 1998b) and body stabilization (Pérennou *et al.*, 2001b). It is important to note that all these reported effects have been obtained in the frontal plane. Although transient, improvements are dramatic in patients with a right hemisphere lesion (Rode *et al.*, 1998; Tilikete *et al.*, 2001a), particularly those with spatial neglect (Pérennou *et al.*, 1998b, 2001b). These effects may be interpreted in terms of recalibration of the body scheme involved in postural control (weight bearing, postural stabilization), and also in terms of recalibration of the subjective vertical (behavioral vertical). This cognitive approach to postural rehabilitation in stroke patients is very promising and it is likely that many other studies will investigate this avenue further in the next few years. The possible value of these sensory stimulation or manipulation procedures for restoring body balance will need to be confirmed by studies on large groups of patients, investigated in a clinical context. Apparatus portability and the possibility of inducing prolonged or repetitive stimulation should also be taken into account in planning these future clinical studies.

The optimization of attentional resources required for balance control

In traumatic or vascular brain injuries, the attentional demand required for motor control is high and the interference between cognitive tasks and motor control activities such as postural control and gait may represent a problem (Geurts *et al.*, 1999; Haggard *et al.*, 2000). In stroke patients, this can even concern static postural tasks such as sitting (Brown *et al.*, 2002). Performing a verbal cognitive task while walking has been shown to affect adversely balance and gait velocity (Bowen *et al.*, 2001). The interference between cognitive and motor tasks may progressively decrease with rehabilitation (Cockburn *et al.*, 2003). These findings suggest that multiple tasks, including dual cognitive and balance tasks, could be incorporated in stroke rehabilitation programs, with a view to optimizing attentional resources required for balance control. Gait exercises based on avoiding and crossing obstacles (Said *et al.*, 2001) could also be helpful to promote interactions between balance control and spatial attention.

Adjusting the level of confidence to actual postural abilities

Balance confidence modifies postural control (Adkin *et al.*, 2000). We have already pointed out that stiffening of the body by multisegmental co-contractions is relatively frequent in people who perceive a postural threat that they feel unable to handle. This is a common adaptation process that mainly concerns elderly or disabled people as stroke patients, particularly those who experience fear of falling. It results in them not being able to perform activities that minimally challenge their balance, drastically limiting their activities of daily living. It is, therefore, important for some patients to enhance confidence in their new postural abilities. Conversely, some patients with anosodiaphoria do not realize the severity of their postural impairment and expose themselves to a high risk of falling. In such cases, it is important to make these patients aware of their actual postural abilities. They may have to learn to take a step when looking around or reaching out for an object, or to avoid performing a given movement required to reach an object in one go but rather decompose the hazardous postural tasks in several phases. In any case, an effort must be made to adjust patients' level of confidence to their actual postural abilities, and vice versa.

The use of a postural support

Many stroke patients walk better and faster with a stick held by the non-paretic hand. This is because the walking aid increases postural stability in erect stance. It has been recently shown that a four-point cane increases stability of moderately severe hemiparetic patients during stance more than a one-point cane, and that the shift of weight toward the walking aid does not adversely affect weight bearing on the paretic limb (Laufer, 2002). Regarding gait, there is an inverse relationship between severity of hemiplegia and the percentage of body weight taken through the aid, between aid contact time and severity of hemiplegia, and between aid contact time and walking ability (Tyson, 1998). The use of a walking frame is less common in hemiplegics.

Summary

Many brain lesions interfere with postural control. Postural disorders constitute a primary disability in stroke patients, leading to a loss of autonomy and exposing patients to a risk of falling.

In stroke patients, balance assessment has several goals: severity estimation, analysis of the nature of postural impairments to orientate physiotherapy, follow-up, and recovery prediction. Postural assessment of stroke patients is evolving and clinicians have now at their disposal short or full postural scales specially devised for stroke patients. Short tests may be useful to describe and quantify a given behavior, such as the inability to maintain a sitting or standing posture, and to analyze a crucial point such as trunk control. They usually take a couple of minutes to be completed without any equipment and are considered as bedside tests. The PASS is the first full balance scale specifically dedicated for stroke patients and can be applied even to those with very poor postural abilities. The perception of vertical is now often assessed in stroke patients, with the idea that a biased subjective vertical may cause postural disorders. This assessment should be done keeping in mind that the postural vertical (and not the visual vertical) is the most relevant information to predict postural disability. Static posturography is becoming a routine assessment tool for stroke patients. Three main patterns may be observed: a weight-bearing asymmetry, with more weight on the non-paretic leg; an increase in body sway; and a small limit of stability beyond which the center of pressure cannot move further without exposing the person to a loss of balance.

After a stroke, the postural disability can be caused by misrepresentation of verticality, by pronounced postural instability, or by a combination of these two impairments. The nature and the severity of postural disorders depend on the ability of undamaged brain areas to compensate. Biases in the subjective vertical can involve one or all of the visual vertical, haptic (tactile) vertical and postural (whole-body) vertical modalities. The mechanism and the direction of the subjective vertical tilt depend on lesion location. In brainstem lesions involving vestibular nuclei, as in Wallenberg syndrome, the tilt of the subjective vertical is mainly a result of ocular torsion, which induces an ipsilateral tilt of the subjective visual vertical. If the lesion is located in one cerebral hemisphere, the tilt is mostly contralesional; concerns one, two, or the three modalities of the subjective vertical (visual, haptic, postural); and has a continuum between no, mild, and severe bias. It is induced by lesions involving the parietoinsular cortex and is proportional to the severity of spatial neglect. Pusher behavior seems to be the most dramatic clinical manifestation of an extreme bias in the construction of the vertical but further studies need to be carried out in order to explain this puzzling behavior.

Many stroke patients show difficulties in responding to postural perturbations. This postural instability depends on mechanical, motor, sensory, and also cognitive factors. Weakness, sensory loss, and spatial neglect seems to be the most detrimental factors to postural stabilization. Many cortical lesions alter postural stabilization. Appropriate postural orientation and stabilization are necessary but not sufficient for a good autonomy in daily life; the coordination between posture and movement must also be preserved. This coordination may often be lost in stroke patients for a number of reasons: the postural preparatory phase of the movement may be altered; the brain adjusts to the new mechanical constraints imposed by the paretic leg; upright stance exacerbates the movement deficit of the paretic leg; and additional voluntary movements may be detrimental to body stabilization. However, after a stroke, the coordination between posture and movement may be improved by training.

Ischemic and hemorrhagic stroke can cause vertigo by involvement of the vestibular system all the way from the labyrinth to the cortex. The acute symptoms of posterior fossa stroke can be initially confused with some common vestibular disorders, such as vestibular neuritis or BPPV. It should be borne in mind that vascular lesions in the root entry zone of the vestibular nerve are capable of producing a very similar picture to that in vestibular neuritis. For this reason, a careful neurological and eye movement examination is mandatory and if any central signs are detected a magnetic resonance image should be arranged. The incidence of vertigo in unselected stroke patients is, however, low (2.1%). In vertebrobasilar stroke, vertigo, nystagmus, and eye movement disorders are prominent. In turn, vertigo, diplopia, oscillopsia, and orthostatic intolerance can significantly interfere with the rehabilitation process, so these factors have to be specifically addressed if present in stroke patients.

Balance rehabilitation in stroke patients include fall prevention programs, postural retraining programs, and the learning of walking with an aid. In addition to historical approaches to stroke rehabilitation (Bobath, Brunnstrom), balance retraining programs may now rely on various techniques, including responses to external perturbation, task-related training, postural biofeedback, implicit balance training, sensory stimulations, the optimization of attentional resources required for balance control, and adjusting the level of confidence to actual postural abilities. The general principles of balance retraining include: all elementary deficits and impairments must be identified and specifically treated; postural retraining favors brain plasticity, hence functional recovery; programs of focused stroke rehabilitation improve functional performance; the training must be regularly adjusted to patients' capabilities; the recovery appears related to early initiation of treatment and to the intensity of the training; and right strokes generally need more postural retraining than left strokes.

The presence of vertigo requires additional vestibular rehabilitation therapy, based on the principle of gradual exposure to symptoms in order to promote habituation and vestibular compensation. The efficacy of vestibular rehabilitation in central vestibular disorders is, however, not yet proven. Patients with stroke have many predisposing risk factors for peripheral BPPV. Therefore, the presence of positional vertigo has to be assessed with a Hallpike maneuver, and, if BPPV is present, the physician or physiotherapist should proceed to treatment with a particle-repositioning maneuver (Epley or Semont).

REFERENCES

Ada, L., O'Dwyer, J., and Neilson, P. D. (1993). Improvement in kinematic characteristics and coordination following stroke quantified by linear systems analysis. *Hum Mov Sci* **12**: 137–153.

Adkin, A. L., Frank, J. S., Carpenter, M. G., and Peysar, G. W. (2000). Postural control is scaled to level of postural threat. *Gait Posture* **12**: 87–93.

Allum, J. H., Bloem, B. R., Carpenter, M. G., and Honegger, F. (2001). Differential diagnosis of proprioceptive and vestibular deficits using dynamic support-surface posturography. *Gait Post* **14**: 217–226.

Alund, M., Ledin, T., Odkvist, L., and Larsson, S. E. (1993). Dynamic posturography among patients with common neck disorders. A study of 15 cases with suspected cervical vertigo. *J Vestib Res* **3**: 383–389.

Anastasopoulos, D. and Bronstein, A. M. (1999). A case of thalamic syndrome: somatosensory influences on visual orientation. *J Neurol Neurosurg Psychiatry* **67**: 390–394.

Anastasopoulos, D., Bronstein, A., Haslwanter, T., Fetter, M., and Dichgans, J. (1999). The role of somatosensory input for the perception of verticality. *Ann N Y Acad Sci* **871**: 379–383.

Arcan, M., Brull, M., Najenson, T., and Solzi, P. (1977). FGP assessment of postural disorders during process of rehabilitation. *Scand J Rehabil Med* **9**: 165–168.

Ashburn, A. (1982). A physical asssessment for stroke patients. *Phys Ther* **68**: 109–113.

 (1995). A review of current physiotherapy in the management of stroke. In: *Physiotherapy in Stroke Management*, ed. M. Harrisson and R. Rustad. London: Churchill Livingstone, pp. 3–22.

Averbuch-Heller, L. (1999). Acquired nystagmus. *Curr Treat Options Neurol* **1**: 68–73.

Avery, S. (1979). Modified rocking chair. *Phys Ther* **59**: 427.

Badke, M. B. and Duncan, P. W. (1983). Patterns of rapid motor responses during postural adjustments when standing in healthy subjects and hemiplegic patients. *Phys Ther* **63**: 13–20.

Baloh, R. and Honrubia V. (2001). *Clinical Neurophysiology of the Vestibular System*. Oxford: Oxford University Press.

Batavia, M., Gianutsos, J. G., and Kambouris, M. (1997). An augmented auditory feedback device. *Arch Phys Med Rehabil* **78**: 1389–1392.

Bauermeister, M., Werner, H., and Wapner, S. (1964). The effect of body tilt on tactual-kinesthetic perception of verticality. *Am J Psychol* **77**: 451–456.

Benaim, C., Pérennou, D. A., Villy, J., Rousseaux, M., and Pélissier, J. (1999). Validation of a standardized assessment of postural control in stroke patient: the PASS. *Stroke* **30**: 1862–1868.

Bender, B. and Teuber, H. L. (1948). Spatial organization of visual perception following injury to the brain. *Arch Neurol Psych* **58**: 721–739.

Bennis, N., Roby-Brami, A., Dufosse, M., and Bussel, B. (1996). Anticipatory responses to a self-applied load in normal subjects and hemiparetic patients. *J Physiol* (Paris) **1990**: 27–42.

Bentley, C., Bronstein, A., Faldon, M., *et al.* (1998). Fast eye movement initiation of ocular torsion in mesodiencephalic lesions. *Ann Neurol* **43**: 729–737.

Benton, A., Hannay, H., and Varney, N. (1975). Visual perception of line direction in patients with unilateral brain disease. *Neurology* **25**: 907–910.

Berg, K. O., Wood-Dauphinee, S. L., Williams, J. I., and Maki, B. (1992). Measuring balance in the elderly: validation of an instrument. *Can J Public Health* **83**(Suppl. 2): S7–S11.

Berg, K. O., Wood-Dauphinee, S., and Williams, J. I. (1995). The balance scale: reliability assessment with elderly residents and patients with an acute stroke. *Scand J Rehabil Med* **27**: 27–36.

Berger, W., Horstmann, G., and Dietz, V. (1984). Tension development and muscle activation in the leg during gait in spastic hemiparesis: independence of muscle hypertonia and exaggerated stretch reflexes. *J Neurol Neurosurg Psychiatry* **47**: 1029–1033.

Bernspång, B. and Fisher, A. G. (1995). Differences between persons with right or left cerebral vascular accident on the assessment of motor and process skills. *Arch Phys Med Rehabil* **76**: 1144–1151.

Bertholon, P., Bronstein, A. M., Davies, R. A., Rudge, P., and Thilo, K. V. (2002). Positional down beating nystagmus in 50 patients: cerebellar disorders and possible anterior semi-circular canalithiasis. *J Neurol Neurosurg Psychiatry* **72**: 366–372.

Berthoz, A. and Melvill Jones, G. (1985). *Adaptive Mechanisms in Gaze Control*. New York: Elsevier Science.

Beyts, J. (1987). Vestibular rehabilitation. In: *Adult Audiology*, Scott-Brown's Otolaryngology, ed. D. Stephens. London: Butterworth.

Biesinger, E. (1988). Vertigo caused by disorders of the cervical vertebral column. Diagnosis and treatment. *Adv Otorhinolaryngol* **39**: 44–51.

Birch, H., Proctor, F., Bortner, M., and Lowenthal, M. (1960). Perception in hemiplegia. I. Judgment of vertical and horizontal by hemiplegic patients. *Arch Phys Med Rehabil* **41**: 19–27.

Bisdorff, A. R., Wolsley, C. J., Anastasopoulos, D., Bronstein, A. M., and Gresty, M. A. (1996). The perception of body verticality (subjective postural vertical) in peripheral and central vestibular disorders. *Brain* **119**: 1523–1534.

Bjork, L. and Wetzel, A. (1983). A positional biofeedback device for sitting balance. *Phys Ther* **63**: 1460–1461.

Bles, W., Vianney de Jong, J. M., and de Wit, G. (1983). Compensation for labyrinthine defects examined by use of a tilting room. *Acta Otolaryngol* **95**: 576–579.

Bobath B. (1978). *Adult Hemiplegia: Evaluation and Treatment*. London: Heinemann Medical.

Bohannon, R. (1989). Selected determinants of ambulatory capacity in patients with hemiplegia. *Clin Rehabil* **3**: 47–53.

Bohannon, R. W. and Larkin, P. A. (1985). Lower extremity weight bearing under various standing conditions in independently ambulatory patients with hemiparesis. *Phys Ther* **65**: 1323–1325.

Bohannon, R. W., Smith, M. B., and Larkin, P. A. (1986a). Relationship between independent sitting balance and side of hemiparesis. *Phys Ther* **66**: 944–5.

Bohannon, R., Cook, A., Larkin, P. *et al.* (1986b). The listing phenomenon of hemiplegic patients. *Neurol Rep* **10**: 43–44.

Bohannon, R., Walsh, S., and Joseph, M. (1993). Ordinal and timed balance measurements: reliability and validity in patients with stroke. *Clin Rehabil* **7**: 9–13.

Bonan, I., Yelnik, A., Laffont, I., Vitte, E., and Freyss, G. (1996). Selection of sensory information in postural control of hemiplegics after unique stroke. *Ann Readapt Med Phys* **39**: 157–163.

Bowen, A., Wenman, R., Mickelborough, J. *et al.* (2001). Dual-task effects of talking while walking on velocity and balance following a stroke. *Age Aging* **30**: 319–323.

Brandt T. (1999). *Vertigo (Its Multisensory Syndromes)*. London: Springer Verlag.

Brandt, T. and Bronstein, A. (2001). Cervical vertigo. *J Neurol Neurosurg Psychiatry* **71**: 8–12.

Brandt, T. and Daroff, R. B. (1980). Physical therapy for benign paroxysmal positional vertigo. *Arch Otolaryngol* **106**: 484–485.

Brandt, T. and Dieterich, M. (1992). Cyclorotation of the eyes and subjective visual vertical in vestibular brain stem lesions. *Ann N Y Acad Sci* **656**: 537–549.

(1994). Vestibular syndromes in the roll plane: topographic diagnosis from brainstem to cortex. *Ann Neurol* **36**: 337–347.

Brandt, T., Dieterich, M., and Danek, A. (1994). Vestibular cortex lesions affect the perception of verticality. *Ann Neurol* **35**: 403–412.

Bronstein, A. M. (1995). The visual vertigo syndrome. *Acta Otolaryngol Suppl* **520**: 45–48.

(2002). Under-rated neuro-otological symptoms: Hoffman and Brookler 1978 revisited. *Br Med Bull* **63**: 213–221.

(2003). Vestibular reflexes and positional maneuvers. *J Neurol Neurosurg Psychiatry* **74**: 289–293.

Bronstein, A. M. and Hood, J. D. (1987). Oscillopsia of peripheral vestibular origin. Central and cervical compensatory mechanisms. Acta Otolaryngol **104**: 307–314.

Bronstein, A. M., Pérennou, D., Guerraz, M., Playford, D., and Rudge, P. (2003). Dissociation of visual and haptic vertical in two patients with vestibular nuclear lesions. *Neurology* **61**: 1172–1173.

Brown, D. A., Kautz, S. A., and Dairaghi, C. A. (1997). Muscle activity adapts to anti-gravity posture during pedalling in persons with post-stroke hemiplegia. *Brain* **120**: 825–837.

Brown, L. A., Sleik, R. J., and Winder, T. R. (2002). Attentional demands for static postural control after stroke. *Arch Phys Med Rehabil* **83**: 1732–1735.

Brozman, B., Romano, J. G., Tusa, R. J., and Forteza, A. M. (2002). Postural vertigo and impaired vasoreflexes caused by a posterior inferior cerebellar artery infarct. *Neurology* **59**: 1469–1470.

Bruell, J. H., Peszcznski, M., and Albee, G. W. (1956). Disturbance of perception of verticality in patients with hemiplegia. *A preliminary report. Arch Phys Med Rehabil* **37**: 677–679.

Brun, V., Dhoms, G., Henrion, G., *et al.* (1993). L'équilibre postural de l'hémiplégique par accident vasculaire cérébral: méthodologie d'évaluation et étude corrélative. *Ann Réadapt Méd Phys* **36**: 166–177.

Brunnstrom, S. (1970). *Movement Therapy in Hemiplegia: a Neurophysiological Approach.* Hagerstown, MD: Harper and Row.

Burton, J. (1996). Physical therapy management of a patient with central vestibular dysfunction: a case report. *Neurol Rep* **20**: 61–62.

Caldwell, C., Macdonald, D., Macneil, K. *et al.* (1986). Symmetry of weight distribution in normals and stroke patients using digital weigh scales. *Physiother Pract* **2**: 109–116.

Caplan L. (1996). Migraine and posterior circularion stroke. In *Posterior Circulation Disease: Clinical Findings, Diagnosis, and Management*, ed. L. Caplan. Cambridge, MA: Blackwell Science, pp. 544–568.

Carmon, A., and Benton, A. (1969). Tactile perception of direction and number in patients with unilateral cerebral disease. *Neurology* **19**: 525–532.

Carpenter, M. G., Allum, J. H., and Honegger, F. (2001a). Vestibular influences on human postural control in combinations of pitch and roll planes reveal differences in spatiotemporal processing. *Exp Brain Res* **140**: 95–111.

Carpenter, M. G., Frank, J. S., Silcher, C. P., and Peysar, G. W. (2001b). The influence of postural threat on the control of upright stance. *Exp Brain Res* **138**: 210–218.

Carr J. and Shepherd R. (1998). *Neurological Rehabilitation: Optimizing Motor Performance.* Melbourne: Butterworth and Heinemann.

Carr, J., Shepherd, R., Lynne, D., and Nordholm, L. (1985). Investigation of a new motor assessment scale for stroke patients. *Phys Ther* **65**: 175–180.

Cass, S. P., Borello-France, D., and Furman, J. M. (1996). Functional outcome of vestibular rehabilitation in patients with abnormal sensory-organization testing. *Am J Otol* **17**: 581–594.

Cassvan, A., Ross, P. L., Dyer, P. R., and Zane, L. (1976). Lateralization in stroke syndromes as a factor in ambulation. *Arch Phys Med Rehabil* **57**: 583–587.

Catz, A., Ron, S., Solzi, P., and Korczyn, A. (1994). The vestibulo-ocular reflex and dysequilibrium after hemispheric stroke. *Am J Phys Med Rehabil* **73**: 36–39.

Cawthorne, T. (1945). Vestibular injuries. *Proc R Soc Med* **39**: 270–273.

Cheng, P. T., Liaw, M. Y., Wong, M. K. *et al.* (1998). The sit-to-stand movement in stroke patients and its correlation with falling. *Arch Phys Med Rehabil* **79**: 1043–1046.

Cheng, P. T., Wu, S. H., Liaw, M. Y., Wong, A. M., and Tang, F. T. (2001). Symmetrical body-weight distribution training in stroke patients and its effect on fall prevention. *Arch Phys Med Rehabil* **82**: 1650–1654.

Clark, B. and Graybiel, A. (1963). Perception of the postural vertical in normals and subjects with labyrinthine defects. *J Exp Psychol* **65**: 490–494.

Cockburn, J., Haggard, P., Cock, J., and Fordham, C. (2003). Changing patterns of cognitive-motor interference (CMI) over time during recovery from stroke. *Clin Rehabil* **17**: 167–173.

Cohen, H. (1992). Vestibular rehabilitation reduces functional disability. *Otolaryngol Head Neck Surg* **107**: 638–643.

Cohen, H., Blatchly, C. A., and Gombash, L. L. (1993). A study of the clinical test of sensory interaction and balance. *Phys Ther* **73**: 346–351.

Collen, F. M. (1995). The measurement of standing balance after stroke. *Physiother Theory Pract* **11**: 109–118.

Collen, F. M., Wade, D. T., and Bradshaw, C. M. (1990). Mobility after stroke: reliability of measures of impairment and disability. *Int Disabil Stud* **12**: 6–9.

Collin, C. and Wade, D. (1990). Assessing motor impairment after stroke: a pilot reliability study. *J Neurol Neurosurg Psychiatry* **53**: 576–579.

Cooksey, F. (1945). Rehabilitation in vestibular injuries. *Proc R Soc Med* **39**: 273–278.

Cowand, J. L., Wrisley, D. M., Walker, M., Strasnick, B., and Jacobson, J. T. (1998). Efficacy of vestibular rehabilitation. *Otolaryngol Head Neck Surg* **118**: 49–54.

Curthoys, I. S. and Halmagyi, G. M (1995). Vestibular compensation: a review of the oculomotor, neural, and clinical consequences of unilateral vestibular loss. *J Vestib Res* **5**: 67–107.

Davies P. (1985). *Step to Follow: a Guide to the Treatment of Adult Hemiplegia*. New York: Springer Verlag.

Dean, C. M. and Shepherd, R. B. (1997). Task-related training improves performance of seated reaching tasks after stroke. A randomized controlled trial. *Stroke* **28**: 722–728.

Dell'Osso, L. (2000). Supression of pendular nystagmus by smoking cannabis in a patient with multiple sclerosis. *Neurology* **54**: 2190–2191.

Denes, G., Semenza, C., Stoppa, E., and Lis, A. (1982). Unilateral spatial neglect and recovery from hemiplegia: a follow-up study. *Brain* **105**: 543–552.

De Renzi, E., Faglioni, P., and Scotti, G. (1971). Judgement of spatial orientation in patients with focal brain damage. *J Neurol Neurosurg Psychiatry* **34**: 489–495.

de Sèze, M., Wiart, L., Bon-Saint-Come, A., *et al.* (2001). Rehabilitation of postural disturbances of hemiplegic patients by using trunk control retraining during exploratory exercises. *Arch Phys Med Rehabil* **82**: 793–800.

Dettmann, M. A., Linder, M. T., and Sepic, S. B. (1987). Relationships among walking performance, postural stability, and functional assessments of the hemiplegic patient. *Am J Phys Med* **66**: 77–90.

Di Fabio, R. and Badke, M. (1990). Relationship of sensory organization to balance function in patients with hemiplegia. *Phys Ther* **70**: 542–548.

(1991). Stance duration under sensory conflict conditions in patients with hemiplegia. *Arch Phys Med Rehabil* **72**: 292–295.

Di Fabio, R. P. (1987). Lower extremity antagonist muscle response following standing perturbation in subjects with cerebrovascular disease. *Brain Res* **406**: 43–51.

Di Fabio, R. P. and Badke, M. B. (1988). Influence of cerebrovascular accident on elongated and passively shortened muscle responses after forward sway. *Phys Ther* **68**: 1215–1220.

Di Fabio, R. P., Badke, M. B., and Duncan, P. W. (1986). Adapting human postural reflexes following localized cerebrovascular lesion: analysis of bilateral long latency responses. *Brain Res* **363**: 257–264.

Di Fabio, R. P., Badke, M. B., McEvoy, A., and Ogden, E. (1990). Kinematic properties of voluntary postural sway in patients with unilateral primary hemispheric lesions. *Brain Res* **513**: 248–254.

Dichgans, J. and Fetter, M. (1993). Compartmentalized cerebellar functions upon the stabilization of body posture. *Rev Neurol (Paris)* **149**: 654–664.

Dickstein, R. and Abulaffio, N. (2000). Postural sway of the affected and nonaffected pelvis and leg in stance of hemiparetic patients. *Arch Phys Med Rehabil* **81**: 364–367.

Dickstein, R. and Dvir, Z. (1993). Quantitative evaluation of stance balance performance in the clinic using a novel measurement device. *Physiother Can* **45**: 102–108.

Dickstein, R., Nissan, M., Pillar, T., and Scheer, D. (1984). Foot-ground pressure pattern of standing hemiplegic patients. Major characteristics and patterns of improvement. *Phys Ther* **64**: 19–23.

Diener, H. C., Dichgans, J., Guschlbauer, B., *et al.* (1992). The coordination of posture and voluntary movement in patients with cerebellar dysfunction. *Mov Disord* **7**: 14–22.

Diener, H. C., Bacher, M., Guschlbauer, B., Thomas, C., and Dichgans, J. (1993). The coordination of posture and voluntary movement in patients with hemiparesis. *J Neurol* **240**: 161–167.

Dieterich, M. and Brandt, T. (1992). Wallenberg's syndrome: lateropulsion, cyclorotation, and subjective visual vertical in thirty-six patients. *Ann Neurol* **31**: 399–408.

Dieterich, M., Pollmann, W., and Pfaffenrath, V. (1993). Cervicogenic headache: electronystagmography perception or verticality and posturography in patients before and after C2-blockade. *Cephalalgia* **13**: 285–288.

Dietz, V. and Berger, W. (1984). Interlimb coordination of posture in patients with spastic paresis. Impaired function of spinal reflexes. *Brain* **107**: 965–978.

Dietz, V., Gollhofer, A., Kleiber, M., and Trippel, M. (1992). Regulation of bipedal stance: dependency on "load receptors". *Exp Brain Res* **89**: 229–231.

Duarte, E., Marco, E., Muniesa, J. M., *et al.* (2002). Trunk control test as a functional predictor in stroke patients. *J Rehabil Med* **34**: 267–272.

Duncan, G. W., Parker, S. W., and Fisher, C. M. (1975). Acute cerebellar infarction in the PICA territory. *Arch Neurol* **32**: 364–368.

Duncan, P. W., Weiner, D. K., Chandler, J., and Studenski, S. (1990). Functional reach: a new clinical measure of balance. *J Gerontol* **45**: M192–M197.

Dursun, E., Hamamci, N., Donmez, S., Tuzunalp, O., and Cakci, A. (1996). Angular biofeedback device for sitting balance of stroke patients. *Stroke* **27**: 1354–1357.

Eggenberger, E., Golnik, K., Lee, A., *et al.* (2002). Prognosis of ischemic internuclear ophthalmoplegia. *Ophthalmology* **109**: 1676–1678.

El Fatimi, A., Masmoudi, M., Loigerot, M., *et al.* (2001). Prévalence et circonstances des chutes chez l'hémiplégique vasculaire: étude prospective sur quatre ans dans une unité de rééducation neurologique. *Ann Réadapt Méd Phys* **44**: 462.

El-Kashlan, H. K., Shepard, N. T., Asher, A. M., Smith-Wheelock, M., and Telian, S. A. (1998). Evaluation of clinical measures of equilibrium. *Laryngoscope* **108**: 311–319.

Eng, J. and Chu, K. (2002). Reliability and comparison of weight-bearing ability during standing tasks for individuals with chronic stroke. *Arch Phys Med Rehabil* **83**: 1138–1144.

Engardt, M. (1994a). Rising and sitting down in stroke patients. Auditory feedback and dynamic strength training to enhance symmetrical body weight distribution. *Scand J Rehabil Med Suppl* **31**: 1–57.

(1994b). Long-term effects of auditory feedback training on relearned symmetrical body weight distribution in stroke patients. A follow-up study. *Scand J Rehabil Med* **26**: 65–69.

Engardt, M., Ribbe, T., and Olsson, E. (1993). Vertical ground reaction force feedback to enhance stroke patients' symmetrical body-weight distribution while rising/sitting down. *Scand J Rehab Med* **25**: 41–48.

Epley, J. M. (1992). The canalith repositioning procedure: for treatment of benign paroxysmal positional vertigo. *Otolaryngol Head Neck Surg* **107**: 399–404.

Feigin, L., Sharon, B., Czaczkes, B., and Rosin, A. J. (1996). Sitting equilibrium 2 weeks after a stroke can predict the walking ability after 6 months. *Gerontology* **42**: 348–353.

Fife, T. D. (1998). Recognition and management of horizontal canal benign positional vertigo. *Am J Otol* **19**: 345–351.

Fitzgerald, D. C. (1995). Persistent dizziness following head trauma and perilymphatic fistula. *Arch Phys Med Rehabil* **76**: 1017–1020.

Forster, A. and Young, J. (1995). Incidence and consequences of falls due to stroke: a systematic inquiry. *BMJ* **311**: 83–86.

Franchignoni, F. P., Tesio, L., Ricupero, C., and Martino, M. T. (1997). Trunk control test as an early predictor of stroke rehabilitation outcome. *Stroke* **28**: 1382–1385.

Fugl-Meyer, A. R. (1980). Post-stroke hemiplegia: assessment of physical properties. *Scand J Rehabil Med Suppl* **7**: 85–93.

Fugl-Meyer, A. R., Jääskö, L., Leyman, I., Olsson, S., and Seglind, S. (1975). The post-stroke hemiplegic patient. I A method for evaluation of physical performance. *Scand J Rehab Med* **7**: 13–31.

Fung J, Boonsinsukh R, and Rapagna M. (2003). Effects of CNS lesions on balance during standing and walking. In *Proceedings of the XVIth Conference of the International Society for Postural and Gait Research (ISPGR)*, Sydney, ed. S.Lord and H. Menz, p. 82.

Furman, J. M. and Cass, S. P. (1999) Benign paroxysmal positional vertigo. *N Engl J Med* **341**: 1590–1596.

Furman, J. M. and Whitney, S. L. (2000). Central causes of dizziness. *Phys Ther* **80**: 179–187.

Garland, S. J., Stevenson, T. J., and Ivanova, T. (1997). Postural responses to unilateral arm perturbation in young, elderly, and hemiplegic subjects. *Arch Phys Med Rehabil* **78**: 1072–1077.

Gauthier, J., Bourbonnais, D., Filiatrault, J., Gravel, D., and Arsenault, A. B. (1992). Characterization of contralateral torques during static hip efforts in healthy subjects and subjects with hemiparesis. *Brain* **115**: 1193–1207.

Geiger, R. A., Allen, J. B. and O'Keefe, J., and Hicks, R. R. (2001). Balance and mobility following stroke: effects of physical therapy interventions with and without biofeedback/forceplate training. *Phys Ther* **81**: 995–1005.

Geurts, A. C., Knoop, J. A. and van Limbeek J. (1999). Is postural control associated with mental functioning in the persistent postconcussion syndrome? *Arch Phys Med Rehabil* **80**: 144–149.

Geurts, A., de Haart, M., van Nes, I., Fasotti, L., and van Limbeek, J. (2001). Restoration of postural symmetry following stroke. In *Proceedings of the Symposium of the International Society for Postural and Gait Research*, Maastricht, ed. J. Dyusens, B. Smits-Engelsman, and H. Kingma, pp. 637–640.

Gill-Body, K. M., Popat, R. A., Parker, S. W., and Krebs, D. E. (1997). Rehabilitation of balance in two patients with cerebellar dysfunction. *Phys Ther* **77**: 534–552.

Gill-Body, K. M., Beninato, M., and Krebs, D. E. (2000). Relationship among balance impairments, functional performance, and disability in people with peripheral vestibular hypofunction. *Phys Ther* **80**: 748–758.

Godbout, A. (1997). Structured habituation training for movement provoked vertigo after severe traumatic brain injury: a single-case experiment. *Brain Inj* **11**: 629–641.

Goldie, P., Evans, O., and Matyas, T. (1996a) Performance in the stability limits test during rehabilitation following stroke. *Gait Posture* **4**: 315–322.

Goldie, P. A., Matyas, T. A., and Evans, O. M. (1996b). Deficit and change in gait velocity during rehabilitation after stroke. *Arch Phys Med Rehabil* **77**: 1074–1082.

Gottlieb, D. and Levine, D. (1992). Unilateral neglect influences the postural adjustments after stroke. *J Neuro Rehab* **6**: 35–41.

Gowland, C., Stratford, P., Ward, M., *et al.* (1993). Measuring physical impairment and disability with the Chedoke-McMaster Stroke Assessment. *Stroke* **24**: 58–63.

Gresty, M. A., Bronstein, A. M., Brandt, T., and Dieterich, M. (1992). Neurology of otolith function. Peripheral and central disorders. *Brain* **115**: 647–673.

Gruendel, T. (1992). Relationship between weight-bearing characteristics in standing and ambulatory independence in hemiplegics. *Physiother Can* **44**: 16–17.

Guerraz, M., Yardley, L., Bertholon, P., *et al.* (2001). Visual vertigo: symptom assessment, spatial orientation and postural control. *Brain* **124**: 1646–1656.

Gurfinkel V and Levik Y. (1991). Perceptual and automatic aspects of the postural body scheme. In, *Brain and Space*, ed. J. Paillard. Oxford: Oxford Science Publications, pp. 147–162.

Gurr, B. and Moffat, N. (2001). Psychological consequences of vertigo and the effectiveness of vestibular rehabilitation for brain injury patients. *Brain Inj* **15**: 387–400.

Haggard, P., Cockburn, J., Cock, J., Fordham, C., and Wade, D. (2000). Interference between gait and cognitive tasks in a rehabilitating neurological population. *J Neurol Neurosurg Psychiatry* **69**: 479–486.

Hahn, A., Sejna, I., Stolbova, K., and Cocek, A. (2001). Visuo-vestibular biofeedback in patients with peripheral vestibular disorders. *Acta Otolaryngol Suppl* **545**: 88–91.

Hain, T. C. and Uddin, M. (2003). Pharmacological treatment of vertigo. *CNS Drugs* **17**: 85–100.

Halmagyi, G. and Curthoys, I. (1988). A clinical sign of canal paresis. *Arch Neurol* **45**: 737–739.

Hamman, R., Mekjavic, I., Mallinson, A., and Longridge, N. (1992). Training effects during repeated therapy sessions of balance training using visual feedback. *Arch Phys Med Rehabil* **73**: 738–744.

Handschu, R., Poppe, R., Rauss, J., Neundorfer, B., and Erbguth, F. (2003). Emergency calls in acute stroke. *Stroke* **34**: 1005–1009.

Hayashi, R., Tako, K., Tokuda, T., and Yanagisawa, N. (1997). Three-Hertz postural oscillation in patients with brain stem or cerebellar lesions. *Electromyogr Clin Neurophysiol* **37**: 431–434.

Held, J., Pierrot-Desselligny, E., Bussel, B., Perrigot, M., and Mahler, M. (1997). Devenir des hémiplégies vasculaires par atteinte sylvienne en fonction du côté de la lésion. *Ann Réadaptation Méd Phys* **18**: 592–604.

Herdman, S. J. (1997). Advances in the treatment of vestibular disorders. *Phys Ther* **77**: 602–618.

Herdman, S. J. and Tusa, R. J. (1996). Complications of the canalith repositioning procedure. *Arch Otolaryngol Head Neck Surg* **122**: 281–286.

Herdman, S. J., Schubert, M., and Tusa, R. (2001). Strategies for balance rehabilitation: fall risk and treatment. *Ann N Y Acad Sci* **942**: 394–412.

Herman S. (1973). Augmented sensory feedback in control of limb movement. In *Neural Organization and its Relevance to Prosthetics.*, ed. W. Fields. New York: Intercontinental Medical Book

Hesse, S. (2001)Locomotor therapy in neurorehabilitation. *NeuroRehabilitation* **16**: 133–139.

Hesse, S., Schauer, M., Malezic, M., Jahnke, M., and Mauritz, K. H. (1994). Quantitative analysis of rising from a chair in healthy and hemiparetic subjects. *Scand J Rehabil Med* **26**: 161–166.

Hlavacka, F., Mergner, T., and Krizkova, M. (1996). Control of the body vertical by vestibular and proprioceptive inputs. *Brain Res Bull* **40**: 431–434.

Hocherman, S. and Dickstein, R. (1984). Platform training and postural stability in hemiplegia. *Arch Phys Med Rehabil* **65**: 588–592.

Honda, M., Deiber, M. P., Ibanez, V., *et al.* (1998). Dynamic cortical involvement in implicit and explicit motor sequence learning. A PET study. *Brain* **121** 2159–2173.

Horak, F. (1987). Clinical measurement of postural control in adults. *Phys Ther* **67**: 1881–1885.

Horak, F. and MacPherson, J. (1996). Postural orientation and equilibrium. In *Handbook of Physiology*, ed. L. B. Rowell and J. T. Sheperd. New York: Oxford University Press, pp. 255–292.

Horak, F. B., Esselman, P., Anderson, M. E., and Lynch, M. K. (1984). The effects of movement velocity, mass displaced, and task certainty on associated postural adjustments made by normal and hemiplegic individuals. *J Neurol Neurosurg Psychiatry* **47**: 1020–1028.

Horak, F. B., Shupert, C. L., Dietz, V., and Horstmann, G. (1994). Vestibular and somatosensory contributions to responses to head and body displacements in stance. *Exp Brain Res* **100**: 93–106.

Horak, F. B., Henry, S. M., and Shumway Cook, A. (1997). Postural perturbations: new insights for treatment of balance disorders. *Phys Ther* **77**: 517–533.

Hsieh, C. L., Sheu, C. F., Hsueh, I. P., and Wang, C. H. (2002). Trunk control as an early predictor of comprehensive activities of daily living function in stroke patients. *Stroke* **33**: 2626–2630.

Hyndman, D., Ashburn, A., and Stack, E. (2002). Fall events among people with stroke living in the community: circumstances of falls and characteristics of fallers. *Arch Phys Med Rehabil* **83**: 165–170.

Ioffe, M. (1997). On the functions of the motor cortex in reorganization of postural coordinations. *J High Nerv Act* **47**: 86–92.

Ioffe, M. E., Ustinova, K. I., Chernikova, L. A., and Sliva, S. S. (2001). Deficit of learning voluntary control of posture in stroke patients with different cortical lesions. In *Control of Posture and Gait*, ed. J. Duysens, B. Smits-Engelman, and H. Kingma. Maastricht: International Society for Postural and Gait Research, pp. 656–659.

Jackson, R. T., Epstein, C. M., and De l'Aune, W. R. (1995). Abnormalities in posturography and estimations of visual vertical and horizontal in multiple sclerosis. *Am J Otol* **16**: 88–93.

Jacob, R., Woody, S., Clark, D., *et al.*, (1993). Discomfort with space and motion: a possible marker of vestibular dysfunction assessed by the situational characteristics questionnaire. *J Psychopathol Behav Ass* **15**: 299–324.

Jorgensen, L., Engstad, T., and Jacobsen, B. K. (2002). Higher incidence of falls in long-term stroke survivors than in population controls: depressive symptoms predict falls after stroke. *Stroke* **33**: 542–547.

Karlberg, M., Magnusson, M., Malmstrom, E. M., Melander, A., and Moritz, U. (1996). Postural and symptomatic improvement after physiotherapy in patients with dizziness of suspected cervical origin. *Arch Phys Med Rehabil* **77**: 874–882.

Karnath, H. O., Ferber, S., and Dichgans, J. (2000a). The neural representation of postural control in humans. *Proc Natl Acad Sci USA* **97**: 13931–13936.

(2000b). The origin of contraversive pushing: evidence for a second graviceptive system in humans. *Neurology* **55**: 1298–1304.

Kerkhoff, G. (1999). Multimodal spatial orientation deficits in left-sided visual neglect. *Neuropsychologia* **37**: 1387–1405.

Kerkhoff, G. (2003). Modulation and rehabilitation of spatial neglect by sensory stimulation. In *Progress in Brain Research,* ed. C. Prablanc, D. Pélisson, and V. Rossetti. Elsevier, 257–271.

Kerkhoff, G. and Zoelch, C. (1998). Disorders of visuospatial orientation in the frontal plane in patients with visual neglect following right or left parietal lesions. *Exp Brain Res* **122**: 108–120.

Kihara, M., Nishikawa, S., Nakasaka, Y., Tanaka, H., and Takahashi, M. (2001). Autonomic consequences of brainstem infarction. *Auton Neurosci* **14**: 202–207.

Kirker, S. G., Simpson, D. S., Jenner, J. R., and Wing, A. M. (2000) Stepping before standing: hip muscle function in stepping and standing balance after stroke. *J Neurol Neurosurg Psychiatry* **68**: 458–464.

Konrad, H. R., Tomlinson, D., Stockwell, C. W., *et al.* (1992). Rehabilitation therapy for patients with disequilibrium and balance disorders. *Otolaryngol Head Neck Surg* **107**: 105–108.

Kumral, E., Afsar, N., Kirbas, D., Balkir, K., and Ozdemirkiran, T. (2002). Spectrum of medial medullary infarction: clinical and magnetic resonance imaging findings. *J Neurol* **249**: 85–93.

Kwakkel, G., Wagenaar, R. C., Twisk, J. W., Lankhorst, G. J., and Koetsier, J. C. (1999). Intensity of leg and arm training after primary middle-cerebral-artery stroke: a randomised trial. *Lancet* **354**: 191–196.

Lacour, M. and Xerri C. (1981). Vestibular compensation: new perspective. In *Lesion Induced Neuronal Plasticity in Sensorimotor Systems*, ed. H. Flohr and W. Precht. New York: Springer Verlag

Lamontagne, A., Kairy, D., Paquet, N., and Fung J. (2001). Postural adjustments to voluntary head turns during walking in hemiparetic subjects. In *Control of Posture and Gait*, ed. J. Duysens, B. Smits-Engelman, and H. Kingma. Symposium of the International Society for Postural and Gait Research, Maastricht, pp. 660–665.

Laufer, Y. (2002). Effects of one-point and four-point canes on balance and weight distribution in patients with hemiparesis. *Clin Rehabil* **16**: 141–148.

Laufer, Y., Dickstein, R., Resnik, S., and Marcovitz, E. (2000). Weight-bearing shifts of hemiparetic and healthy adults upon stepping on stairs of various heights. *Clin Rehabil* **14**: 125–129.

Lawden, M., Bronstein, A., and Kennard, C. (1995). Repetitive paroxysmal nystagmus and vertigo. *Neurology* **45**: 276–280.

Leduc, A. and Decloedt, V. (1989). La kinésithérapie en ORL. *Acta Otorhinolaryngo Belg* **43**: 381–390.

Lee, H., Sohn, S. I., Jung, D. K., *et al.* (2002). Sudden deafness and anterior inferior cerebellar artery infarction. *Stroke* **33**: 2807–2812.

Lee, M. Y., Wong, M. K., and Tang, F. T. (1996). Clinical evaluation of a new biofeedback standing balance training device. *J Med Eng Technol* **20**: 60–66.

Lehrich, J. R., Winkler, G. F., and Ojemann, R. G. (1970). Cerebellar infarction with brain stem compression. Diagnosis and surgical treatment. *Arch Neurol* **22**: 490–498.

Lempert, T., Wolsley, C., Davies, R., Gresty, M. A., and Bronstein, A. M. (1997). Three hundred sixty-degree rotation of the posterior semicircular canal for treatment of benign positional vertigo: a placebo-controlled trial. *Neurology* **49**: 729–733.

Lennon, S. (1996). The Bobath concept: a critical review of the theoritical assumptions that guide physiotherapy practice in stroke rehabilitation. *Phys Ther Rev* **1**: 35–45.

Lindmark, B. and Hamrin, E. (1988). Evaluation of functional capacity after stroke as a basis for active intervention. Presentation of a modified chart for motor capacity assessment and its reliability. *Scand J Rehabil Med* **20**: 103–109.

Loewen, S. and Anderson, B. (1990). Predictors of stroke outcome using objective measurement scales. *Stroke* **21**: 78–81.

Lopez, L., Bronstein, A., Gresty, M., DuBoulay, E., and Rudge, P. (1996). Clinical and MRI correlates in 27 patients with acquired pendular nystagmus. *Brain* **119**: 465–472.

Luyat, M., Ohlmann, T., and Barraud, P. A. (1997). Subjective vertical and postural activity. *Acta Psychol Amst* **95**: 181–193.

Magee D. (1987). *Orthopedic Physical Assessment*. Philadelphia: Saunders.

Maki, B. E. and McIlroy, W. E. (1997). The role of limb movements in maintaining upright stance: the "change-in-support" strategy. *Phys Ther* **77**: 488–507.

Malouin, F., Potvin, M., Prevost, J., Richards, C. L., and Wood-Dauphinee, S. (1992). Use of an intensive task-oriented gait training program in a series of patients with acute cerebrovascular accidents. *Phys Ther* **72**: 781–793.

Mann, C., Berthelot-Berry, N., and Dauterive, H. (1949). The perception of the vertical: I. Visual and non-labyrinthine cues. *J Exp Psychol* **39**: 538–547.

Mao, H. F., Hsueh, I. P., Tang, P. F., Sheu, C. F., and Hsieh, C. L. (2002) Analysis and comparison of the psychometric properties of three balance measures for stroke patients. *Stroke* **33**: 1022–1027.

Marchand, A. R., and Amblard, B. (1984). Locomotion in adult cats with early vestibular deprivation: visual cue substitution. *Exp Brain Res* **54**: 395–405.

Massion, J. (1994). Postural control system. *Curr Opin Neurobiol* **4**: 877–887.

Massion, J. and Woollacott M. (1996). Posture and equilibrium. In *Clinical Disorders of Balance Posture and Gait*, ed, A. M. Bronstein, T. Brandt, and M. Woollacott. London: Arnold pp. 1–8.

Mathias, S., Nayak, U. S., and Isaacs, B. (1986). Balance in elderly patients: the "get-up and go" test. *Arch Phys Med Rehabil* **67**: 387–389.

Mayo, N. E., Korner-Bitensky, N. A., and Becker, R. (1991). Recovery time of independent function post-stroke. *Am J Phys Med Rehabil* **70**: 5–12.

McCabe, B. F. (1970). Labyrinthine exercises in the treatment of diseases characterized by vertigo: their physiologic basis and methodology. *Laryngoscope* **80**: 1429–1433.

McClure, J. A. (1985). Horizontal canal BPV. *J Otolaryngol* **14**: 30–35.

Merfeld, D., Zupan, L., and Peterka, R. (1999). Humans use internal models to estimate gravity and linear acceleration. *Nature* **398**: 615–618.

Mittelsteadt, H. (1992). Somatic versus vestibular gravity reception in man. *Ann N Y Acad Sci* **656**: 124–139.

Miyai, I., Mauricio, R. L. R., and Reding, M. J. (1997). Parietal-insular strokes are associated with impaired standing balance as assessed by computerized dynamic posturography. *J Neurol Rehabil* **11**: 35–40.

Mizrahi, J., Solzi, P., Ring, H., and Nisell, R. (1989). Postural stability in stroke patients: vectorial expression of asymmetry, sway activity and relative sequence of reactive forces. *Med Biol Eng Comput* **27**: 181–190.

Monger, C., Carr, J. H., and Fowler, V. (2002). Evaluation of a home-based exercise and training program to improve sit-to-stand in patients with chronic stroke. *Clin Rehabil* **16**: 361–367.

Mossman, S., Bronstein, A., Rudge, P., and Gresty, M. (1993). Acquired pendular nystagmus supressed by alcohol. *Neuro-ophthalmology* **13**: 99–106.

Mudie, M. H., Winzeler-Mercay, U., Radwan, S., and Lee, L. (2002). Training symmetry of weight distribution after stroke: a randomized controlled pilot study comparing task-related reach, Bobath and feedback training approaches. *Clin Rehabil* **16**: 582–592.

Nardone, A., Galante, M., Lucas, B., and Schieppati, M. (2001). Stance control is not affected by paresis and reflex hyperexcitability: the case of spastic patients. *J Neurol Neurosurg Psychiatry* **70**: 635–643.

Nashner, L. (1976). Adaptating reflexes controlling human posture. *Exp Brain Res* **26**: 59–72.

(1977). Fixed patterns of rapid postural responses among leg muscles during stance. *Exp Brain Res* **26**: 59–72.

(1982). Adaptation of human movement to altered environments. *Trends in Neuroscience* **5**: 358–361.

Nashner, L. M., Shumway-Cook, A., and Marin, O. (1983). Stance posture control in select groups of children with cerebral palsy: deficits in sensory organization and muscular coordination. *Exp Brain Res* **49**: 393–409.

Nelson, S. R., Di Fabio, R. P., and Anderson, J. H. (1995). Vestibular and sensory interaction deficits assessed by dynamic platform posturography in patients with multiple sclerosis. *Ann Otol Rhinol Laryngol* **104**: 62–68.

Nilsson, L., Carlsson, J., Danielsson, A., *et al.* (2001). Walking training of patients with hemiparesis at an early stage after stroke: a comparison of walking training on a treadmill with body weight support and walking training on the ground. *Clin Rehabil* **15**: 515–527.

Norre M. (1984). Treatment of unilateral vestibular hypofunction. In *Otoneurology*, ed. W. Osterveld. New York: Wiley, pp. 23–29.

(1987). Rationale of rehabilitation treatment for vertigo. *Am J Otolaryngol* **8**: 31–35.

Norre, M. E. and de Weerdt, W. (1980). Treatment of vertigo based on habituation. 2. Technique and results of habituation training. *J Laryngol Otol* **94**: 971–977.

Nudo, R. J. and Friel, K. M. (1999). Cortical plasticity after stroke: implications for rehabilitation. *Rev Neurol (Paris)* **155**: 713–717.

Nunez, R. A., Cass, S. P., and Furman, J. M. (2000). Short- and long-term outcomes of canalith repositioning for benign paroxysmal positional vertigo. *Otolaryngol Head Neck Surg* **122**: 647–652.

Nyberg, L. and Gustafson, Y. (1995). Patient falls in stroke rehabilitation. A challenge to rehabilitation strategies. *Stroke* **26**: 838–842.

Odkvist, I. and Odkvist, L. M. (1988). Physiotherapy in vertigo. *Acta Otolaryngologica (Stockholm)* **455**(suppl.): 74–76.

Ost, L. G. (1987). Applied relaxation: description of a coping technique and review of controlled studies. *Behav Res Ther* **25**: 397–409.

Ottenbacher, K. J. and Jannell, S. (1993). The results of clinical trials in stroke rehabilitation research. *Arch Neurol* **50**: 37–44.

Page, N. G. and Gresty, M. A. (1985). Motorist's vestibular disorientation syndrome. *J Neurol Neurosurg Psychiatry* **48**: 729–735.

Pai, Y. C., Rogers, M. W., Hedman, L. D., and Hanke, T. A. (1994). Alterations in weight-transfer capabilities in adults with hemiparesis. *Phys Ther* **74**: 647–657.

Palmer, E., Downes, L., and Ashby, P. (1996). Associated postural adjustments are impaired by a lesion of the cortex. *Neurology* **46**: 471–475.

Partridge, C. and Edwards, S. (1988). Recovery curves as a basis for evaluation. *Physiotherapy* **74**: 141–143.

Pavlou, M., Lingeswaran, A., Davies, R., Gresty, M. A., and Bronstein, A. M. (2001). Machine-based vs. customised rehabilitation for the treatment of chronic vestibular patients. *Proceedings of the ISPG Symposium*, Maastricht.

Pavlou, M., Shumway-Cook, A., Horak, F. B., Yardley, L., and Bronstein, A. M. (2004). Rehabilitation of balance disorders in the patient with vestibular pathology. In *Clinical Disorders of Balance Posture and Gait*, ed. A. M. Bronstein, T. Brandt, M. H. Woollacott and J. G. Nutt. London: Arnold, pp. 317–343.

Pavlou, M., Lingeswaran, A., Davies, R. A., Gresty, M. A., and Bronstein, A. M. (2004). Simulator based rehabilitation in refractory dizziness. *J Neurol* **251**: 983–95.

Pedersen, P. M., Wandel, A., Jorgensen, H. S., *et al.* (1996). Ipsilateral pushing in stroke: incidence, relation to neuropsychological symptoms, and impact on rehabilitation. The Copenhagen Stroke Study. *Arch Phys Med Rehabil* **77**: 25–28.

Pélissier, J., Pérennou, D., Dupeyron, G., *et al.* (1990). Hémiplégie ictale et cécité: problèmes spécifiques de rééducation. *Ann Réadaptation Méd Phys* **33**: 309–314.

Pérennou, D. A. and Amblard, B. (2004). Man against gravity: the control of orientation and that of stabilisation are dissociated. *Exp Brain Res*, in press.

Pérennou, D. A., Amblard, B., Leblond, C., *et al.* (1998a). Posture, équilibre et syndromes de négligence spatiale. In *Les Syndromes de Négligence Spatiale*, ed. D. Pérennou, V. Brun, and J. Pélissier. Paris: Masson pp. 144–155.

Pérennou, D. A., Amblard, B., Leblond, C., and Pélissier, J. (1998b). Biased postural vertical in humans with hemispheric lesions. *Neurosci Lett* **252**: 75–78.

Pérennou, D., Benaim, C., Rouget, E., *et al.* (1999). Postural balance following stroke: towards a disadvantage of the right brain-damaged hemisphere. *Rev Neurol* **155**: 281–290.

Pérennou, D., Leblond, C., Amblard, B., *et al.* (2000). The polymodal sensory cortex is crucial for controlling lateral postural stability: evidence from stroke patients. *Brain Res Bul* **53**: 359–365.

Pérennou, D., Playford, D., Guerraz, M., *et al.* (2001a). Dissociation in the verticality perception after a stroke. In *Proceedings of the International Society for Postural and Gait Research*, ed. H. Kingma and J. Duysens.

Pérennou, D., Leblond, D., Amblard, B., *et al.* (2001b). Transcutaneous electric nerve stimulation reduces neglect-related postural instability after stroke. *Arch Phys Med Rehabil* **82**: 440–448.

Pérennou, D. A., Amblard, B., Laassel, el M., *et al* . (2002a). Understanding the pusher behavior of some stroke patients with spatial deficits: a pilot study. *Arch Phys Med Rehabil* **83**: 570–575.

Pérennou, D. A., Mazibrada, G., Playford, D., *et al.* (2002b). Verticality perception in pusher patients: ipsi or contralesional bias? In *Proceedings of the Third World Forum of Neurorehabilitation*, Venice.

Perrigot, M., Bergeco, C., Fakacs, C., Bastard, J., and Held, J. (1980). Hémiplégie vasculaire. Bilan et éléments du pronostic de la rééducation. *Ann Réadaptation Méd Phys* **23**: 229–241.

Peterka, R. J. and Black, F. O. (1990). Age-related changes in human posture control: sensory organization tests. *J Vestib Res* **1**: 73–85.

Petersen, H., Magnusson, M., Johansson, R., and Fransson, P. A. (1996). Auditory feedback regulation of perturbed stance in stroke patients. *Scand J Rehabil Med* **28**: 217–223.

Pfaltz, C. R. and Karnath, R. (1983). Central compensation of vestibular dysfunction: Peripheral lesions. *Adv Otorhinolaryngol* **30**: 355.

Pizzamiglio, L., Vallar, G., and Doricchi, F. (1997). Gravitational inputs modulate visuospatial neglect. *Exp Brain Res* **117**: 341–345.

Radtke, A., Neuhauser, H., von Brevern, M., and Lempert, T. (1999). A modified Epley's procedure for self-treatment of benign paroxysmal positional vertigo. *Neurology* **53**: 1358–1360.

Rathore, S. S., Hinn, A. R., Cooper, L. S., Tyroler, H. A., and Rosamond, W. D. (2002). Characterization of incident stroke signs and symptoms: findings from the atherosclerosis risk in communities study. *Stroke* **33**: 2718–2721.

Redfern, M. S. and Furman, J. M. (1994). Postural sway of patients with vestibular disorders during optic flow. *J Vestib Res* **4**: 221–230.

Rode, G., Tiliket, C., and Boisson, D. (1997). Predominance of postural imbalance in left hemiparetic patients. *Scand J Rehab Med* **29**: 11–16.

Rode, G., Tiliket, C., Charlopain, P., and Boisson, D. (1998). Postural asymmetry reduction by vestibular caloric stimulation in left hemiparetic patients. *Scand J Rehabil Med* **30**: 9–14.

Rogers, M., Hedman, L., and Pai, Y. (1993). Kinetic analysis of dynamic transitions in stance support accompanying voluntary leg flexion movements in hemiparetic adults. *Arch Phys Med Rehabil* **74**: 19–25.

Rondot, P., Odier, F., and Valade, D. (1992). Postural disturbances due to homonymous hemianopic visual ataxia. *Brain* **115**: 179–188.

Runge, C. F., Shupert, C. L., Horak, F. B., and Zajac, F. E. (1998). Role of vestibular information in initiation of rapid postural responses. *Exp Brain Res* **122**: 403–412.

Sackley, C. M. (1990). The relationship between weight bearing asymmetry after stroke, motor function and activities of daily living. *Physiother Theory Pract* **6**: 179–185.

(1991). Falls, sway, and symmetry of weight-bearing after stroke. *Int Disabil Stud* **13**: 1–4.

Sackley, C. and Baguley, B. (1993). Visual feedback after stroke with the balance performance monitor: two single-case studies. *Clin Rehabil* **7**: 189–195.

Sackley, C. M. and Lincoln, N. B. (1997). Single blind randomized controlled trial of visual feedback after stroke: effects on stance symmetry and function. *Disabil Rehabil* **19**: 536–546.

Saeed, A. B., Shuaib, A., Al-Sulaiti, G., and Emery, D. (2000). Vertebral artery dissection: warning symptoms, clinical features and prognosis in 26 patients. *Can J Neurol Sci* **27**: 292–296.

Said, C. M., Goldie, P. A., Patla, A. E., Sparrow, W. A., and Martin, K. E. (1999). Obstacle crossing in subjects with stroke. *Arch Phys Med Rehabil* **80**: 1054–1059.

Said, C. M., Goldie, P. A., Patla, A. E., and Sparrow, W. A. (2001). Effect of stroke on step characteristics of obstacle crossing. *Arch Phys Med Rehabil* **82**: 1712–1719.

Sakellari, V., and Bronstein, A. M. (1997). Hyperventilation effect on postural sway. *Arch Phys Med Rehabil* **78**: 730–736.

Sakellari, V., Bronstein, A. M., Corna, S., *et al.* (1997). The effects of hyperventilation on postural control mechanisms. *Brain* **120**: 1659–1673.

Sandin, K. J., and Smith, B. S. (1990). The measure of balance in sitting in stroke rehabilitation prognosis. *Stroke* **21**: 82–86.

Sanford, J., Moreland, J., Swanson, L., Stratford, P., and Gowlang, C. (1993). Reliability of the Fugl-Meyer Assessment for testing motor performance in patients following stroke. *Phys Ther* **73**: 447–454.

Saunders D. (1991). *Evaluation, Treatment and Prevention of Musculoskeletal Disorders.* Minneapolis, MN: Viking Press.

Schon, F., Hart, P., Hodgson, T., *et al.* (1999). Suppression of pendular nystagmus by smoking cannabis in a patients with multiple sclerosis. *Neurology* **53**: 2209–2210.

Seliktar, R., Susak, Z., Najenson, T., and Solzi, P. (1978). Dynamic features of standing and their correlation with neurological disorders. *Scand J Rehab Med* **10**: 59–64.

Semont, A., Freyss, G., and Vitte, E. (1988). Curing the BPPV with a liberatory maneuver. *Adv Otorhinolaryngol* **42**: 290–293.

Shepard, N. T. and Telian, S. A. (1995). Programmatic vestibular rehabilitation. *Otolaryngol Head Neck Surg* **112**: 173–182.

Shepard, N. T., Telian, S. A., Smith-Wheelock, M., and Raj, A. (1993). Vestibular and balance rehabilitation therapy. *Ann Otol Rhinol Laryngol* **102**: 198–205.

Shinohara, S., Yamamoto, E., Saiwai, S., *et al.* (2000). Clinical features of sudden hearing loss associated with a high signal in the labyrinth on unenhanced T1-weighted MRI. *Eur Arch Otorhinolaryngol* **257**: 480–484.

Shumway-Cook A. (2000). Vestibular rehabilitation in traumatic brain injury. In *Vestibular Rehabilitation*, ed. S. Herdman. Philadelphia: FA Davis, pp. 476–493.

Shumway-Cook, A. and Horak, F. B. (1986). Assessing the influence of sensory interaction of balance. *Phys Ther* **66**: 1548–1550.

(1989). Vestibular rehabilitation: an exercise approach to managing symptoms of vestibular dysfunction. *Semin Hear* **10**: 196–205.

(1990). Rehabilitation strategies for patients with vestibular deficits. *Neurol Clin* **8**: 441–457.

(1992). *Balance Rehabilitation in the Neurological Patient.* Seattle: NERA.

Shumway-Cook, A. and Woollacott, M. (2001). *Motor Control: Theory and Practical Applications.* Philadelphia: Lippincott, Williams and Wilkens.

Shumway-Cook, A., Anson, D., and Haller, S. (1988). Postural sway biofeedback: its effect on reestablishing stance stability in hemiplegic patients. *Arch Phys Med Rehabil* **69**: 395–400.

Shumway-Cook, A., Woollacott, M., Kerns, K. A., and Baldwin, M. (1997). The effects of two types of cognitive tasks on postural stability in older adults with and without a history of falls. *J Gerontol A Biol Sci Med Sci* **52**: M232–M240.

Shuppert, C., Horak, F., and Black, F. (1994). Hip sway associated with vestibulopathy. *J Vestib Res* **4**: 231–244.

Simmons, R. W., Smith, K., Erez, E., Burke, J. P., and Pozos, R. E. (1998). Balance retraining in a hemiparetic patient using center of gravity biofeedback: a single-case study. *Percept Mot Skills* **87**: 603–609.

Smith, M. T. and Baer, G. D. (1999). Achievement of simple mobility milestones after stroke. *Arch Phys Med Rehabil* **80**: 442–447.

Solley, C. (1956). Reduction of error with practice in perception of the postural vertical. *J Exp Psychol* **52**: 329–333.

Solomon, D. (2000). Distinguishing and testing causes of central vertigo. In *Practical Issues in the Management of Dizzy and Balance Disorder Patient*, ed. N. T. Shepard and D. Solomon. London: WB Saunders.

Stadler, M. A. (1994). Explicit and implicit learning and maps of cortical motor output. *Science* **265**: 1600–1601.

Strupp, M. and Arbusow, V. (2001). Acute vestibulopathy. *Curr Opin Neurol* **14**: 11–20.

Szturm, T., Ireland, D., and Lessing-Turner, M. (1994). Comparison of different exercise programs in the rehabilitation of patients with chronic peripheral vestibular dysfunction. *J Vestib Res* **4**: 461–479.

Taylor, D., Ashurn, A., and Ward, C. (1994). Asymmetrical trunk posture,unilateral neglect and motor performance following stroke. *Clin Rehabil* **8**: 48–53.

Teuber, H. and Mishkin, M. (1954). Judgement of visual and postural vertical after brain injury. *J Psychol* **38**: 161–175.

Tilikete, C., Rode, G., Rossetti, Y., *et al.* (2001a). Prism adaptation to rightward optical deviation improves postural imbalance in left-hemiparetic patients. *Curr Biol* **11**: 524–528.

Tilikete, C., Rode, G., Nighoghossian, N., Boisson, D., and Vighetto, A. (2001b). Otolith manifestations in Wallenberg syndrome. *Rev Neurol (Paris)* **157**: 198–208.

Tinetti, M. E. (1986). Performance-oriented assessment of mobility problems in elderly patients. *J Am Geriatr Soc* **34**: 119–126.

Tsuzuku, T., Vitte, E., Semont, A., and Berthoz, A. (1995). Modification of parameters in vertical optokinetic nystagmus after repeated vertical optokinetic stimulation in patients with vestibular lesions. *Acta Otolaryngol Suppl* **520**: 419–422.

Turnbull, G. I., Charteris, J., and Wall, J. C. (1996). Deficiencies in standing weight shifts by ambulant hemiplegic subjects. *Arch Phys Med Rehabil* **77**: 356–362.

Tutuarima, J. A., van der Meulen, J. H., de Haan, R. J., van Straten, A., and Limburg, M. (1997). Risk factors for falls of hospitalized stroke patients. *Stroke* **28**: 297–301.

Tyson, S. F. (1998). The support taken through walking aids during hemiplegic gait. *Clin Rehabil* **12**: 395–401.

Ugur, C., Gucuyener, D., Uzuner, N., Ozkan, S., and Ozdemir, G. (2000). Characteristics of falling in patients with stroke. *J Neurol Neurosurg Psychiatry* **69**: 649–651.

Vallar, G., Guariglia, C., and Rusconi, M.L. (1997). Modulation of the neglect syndrome by sensory stimulation. In *Parietal Lobe Contribution to Orientation in 3D Space.*, ed. P. Thier and H. O. Karnath. Heidelberg: Springer-Verlag.

Viallet, F., Massion, J., Massarino, R., and Khalil, R. (1992). Coordination between posture and movement in a bimanual load lifting task: putative role of a medial frontal region including the supplementary motor area. *Exp Brain Res* **88**: 674–684.

Visintin, M. and Barbeau, H. (1989). The effects of body weight support on the locomotor pattern of spastic paretic patients. *Can J Neurol Sci* **16**: 315–325.

Vitte, E., Semont, A., and Berthoz, A. (1994). Repeated optokinetic stimulation in conditions of active standing facilitates recovery from vestibular deficits. *Exp Brain Res* **102**: 141–148.

Wade, D., Skilbeck, C., and Langton Hewer, R. (1983). Predicting Barthel ADL score at 6 month after an acute stroke. *Arch Phys Med Rehabil* **64**: 24–28.

Wade, D., Langton, Hewer R., and Wood, V. (1984). Stroke: influence of patient's sex and side of weakness on outcome. *Arch Phys Med Rehabil* **65**: 513–516.

Wade, D., Wood, V., and Langton Hewer, R. (1985). Recovery after stroke: the first 3 months. *J Neurol Neurosurg Psychiatry* **48**: 7–13.

Wannstedt, G. and Herman, R. (1978). Use of augmented sensory feedback to achieve symmetrical standing. Phys Ther **58**: 533–559.

Wee, J. Y, Bagg, S. D, and Palepu, A. (1999). The Berg balance scale as a predictor of length of stay and discharge destination in an acute stroke rehabilitation setting. *Arch Phys Med Rehabil* **80**: 448–452.

Whitney, S. L, Hudak, M. T, and Marchetti, G. F. (2000). The dynamic gait index relates to self-reported fall history in individuals with vestibular dysfunction. *J Vestib Res* **10**: 99–105.

Wing, A. M, Goodrich, S., VirjiBabul, N., Jenner, J. R., and Clapp, S. (1993a). Balance evaluation in hemiparetic stroke patients using lateral forces applied to the hip. *Arch Phys Med Rehabil* **74**: 292–299.

Wing, A. M, Allison, S., and Jenner, J. R. (1993b). Retaining and retraining balance after stroke. *Bailliéres Clin Neurol* **2**: 87–120.

Winstein, C. J., Gardner, E. R., McNeal, D. R., Barto, P. S., and Nicholson, D. E. (1989). Standing balance training: effect on balance and locomotion in hemiparetic adults. *Arch Phys Med Rehabil* **70**: 755–762.

Witkin, H. A. and Asch, S. E. (1948). Studies in space orientation. III. Perception of the upright in the absence of a visual field. *J Exp Psychol* **38**: 603–614.

Wolf, M., Hertanu, T., Novikov, I., and Kronenberg, J. (1999). Epley's maneuver for benign paroxysmal positional vertigo: a prospective study. *Clin Otolaryngol* **24**: 43–46.

Wong, A. M., Lee, M. Y., Kuo, J. K., and Tang., F. T. (1997). The development and clinical evaluation of a standing biofeedback trainer. *J Rehabil Res Dev* **34**: 322–327.

Wrisley, D. M., Sparto, P. J., Whitney, S. L., and Furman, J. M. (2000). Cervicogenic dizziness: a review of diagnosis and treatment. *J Orthop Sports Phys Ther* (2000)**30**: 755–766.

Yardley, L., Lerwill, H., Hall, M., and Gresty, M. (1992). Visual destabilisation of posture in normal subjects. *Acta Otolaryngol* **112**: 14–21.

Yates, J. S., Lai, S. M., Duncan, P. W., and Studenski, S. (2002). Falls in community-dwelling stroke survivors: an accumulated impairments model. *J Rehabil Res Dev* **39**: 385–394.

Yelnik, A. P., Lebreton, F. O., Bonan, I. V., *et al.* (2002). Perception of verticality after recent cerebral hemispheric stroke. *Stroke* **33**: 2247–2253.

Zatsiorsky, V. M. and King, D. L. (1998). An algorithm for determining gravity line location from posturographic recordings. *J Biomech* **31**: 161–164.

14

Management of dysphagia after stroke

Jeri A. Logemann

Northwestern University, Evanston, IL, USA

Introduction

This chapter will review the nature of swallowing disorders after stroke, the process of evaluation and treatment of dysphagia in stroke patients, and research needs in the area.

Dysphagia is a frequent effect of stroke. It can be short or longterm, mild or severe. Dysphagia can, in turn, cause aspiration and ultimately a costly pneumonia in addition to dehydration and malnutrition. As a result, a great deal of research has, and continues to, examine various aspects of dysphagia post-stroke including methods for its evaluation and treatment.

Swallow disorders by site of lesion

The body of knowledge on swallow abnormalities resulting from stroke at specific sites in the central nervous system is still evolving (Meadows, 1973; Wade and Hewer, 1987; Delgado, 1988; Barer, 1989; Celifarco et al., 1990; Logemann and Kahrilas, 1990; Smith and Dodd, 1990). However, there is adequate information to begin to understand the types of swallow disorder exhibited by patients with isolated lesions in the brainstem, subcortical regions, and left and right hemispheres of the cerebral cortex. The discussion below is based on data from our studies of patients at three weeks post-stroke who have suffered a single infarct with no prior history of stroke or other neurological disorders or damage to the head and neck, and who have been otherwise apparently healthy until their stroke. Medical complications, preexisting medical problems and medications can affect the severity of swallowing problems post-stroke.

There has also been the suggestion in the literature that each individual may have a dominant hemisphere for swallowing, thus explaining the variability in reports of site of lesions causing dysphagia (Hamdy et al., 1996, 1997, 1998a,b, 2000, 2001; Hamdy and Rothwell, 1998; Fraser et al., 2002). This research group

Recovery after Stroke, ed. Michael P. Barnes, Bruce H. Dobkin and Julien Bogousslavsky. Published by Cambridge University Press. © Cambridge University Press 2005.

has reported that "dysphagia after unilateral hemispheric stroke is related to the management of pharyngeal motor representation in the unaffected hemisphere" (Hamdy *et al.*, 1996).

Effects of lesions in the brainstem

Lesions in the lower brainstem (medullary region) generally result in significant oropharyngeal swallow impairment because of the location of the major swallow centers (nucleus tractus solitarius and nucleus ambiguous) within the medulla (Jean and Car, 1979; Miller, 1982). Patients with unilateral medullary lesions typically exhibit functional or near normal oral control with significantly impaired triggering and neuromotor control of the pharyngeal swallow. Specifically, these patients often exhibit what appears to be an absent pharyngeal swallow in the first week post-ictus. As the pharyngeal swallow begins to appear (usually in the second week post-stroke), there is a significant delay in triggering the pharyngeal swallow (often 10 to 15 seconds or more). When the pharyngeal swallow triggers, these patients exhibit (a) reduced laryngeal elevation and anterior motion, which contributes to reduced opening of the cricopharyngeal region, with the symptom of residual food collecting in the pyriform sinuses, particularly on one side; and (b) unilateral pharyngeal weakness, which further contributes to the residual food remaining in the pyriform sinus on one side. Some patients also exhibit unilateral adductor vocal fold paresis. While these patients often exhibit significant dysphagia necessitating no oral intake at one to two weeks post-stroke, by three weeks their swallow has often recovered sufficiently to be functional and allow full oral intake. In general, the more severe the swallow abnormalities at two to three weeks post-ictus, and the more medical complications present, the longer the swallow recovery period. After medullary stroke, some patients will not recover functional swallowing for four to six months and a very few will remain permanently unable to support any oral intake.

Pharyngeal swallow measures at 12 and 24 weeks post-stroke in patients after medullary stroke whose swallow was functional at three weeks post-ictus has revealed that, although their swallow is functional (i.e. they are eating a full, normal diet orally with no aspiration and only small amounts of residue in the pyriform sinuses), their measures of pharyngeal movement during swallow are just outside the normal range.

Effects of subcortical stroke

Subcortical lesions may affect motor as well as sensory pathways to and from the cortex. Subcortical stroke usually results in mild delays in oral transit times (three to five seconds), mild delays in triggering the pharyngeal swallow (three to five seconds), and mild-to-moderate impairments in timing of the neuromuscular components of the pharyngeal swallow. A small number of these patients exhibit aspiration as a result of the pharyngeal swallow delay. Their recovery of full oral intake after stroke may take three to six weeks if no medical complications are present and longer if medical problems, such as diabetes or pneumonia, are present.

Effects of stroke in the cerebral cortex

Patients with lesions in the left or right hemisphere of the cerebral cortex display differences in swallow function, as described below. To date, swallow disorders characteristic of various areas within each hemisphere have not been well examined.

Stroke within the left hemisphere of the cerebral cortex can result in apraxia for swallow, which can range from mild to severe and usually accompanies some degree of oral apraxia. Apraxia of swallow is characterized by delay in initiating the oral swallow, with no tongue motion in response to presentation of a bolus in the mouth, or by mild-to-severe searching motions of the tongue prior to initiating the swallow. Generally, patients with swallow apraxia exhibit better swallow function when eating automatically without any verbal commands to swallow. Patients who have suffered left cortical stroke also usually exhibit mild oral transit delays (three to five seconds) and mild delays in triggering the pharyngeal swallow (two to three seconds). Usually, motor aspects of the pharyngeal swallow itself are normal in these patients.

In contrast, the patient who has suffered a stroke in the right hemisphere exhibits mild oral transit delays (two to three seconds) and slightly longer pharyngeal delays (three to five seconds). When the pharyngeal swallow triggers in these patients, laryngeal elevation may be slightly delayed, contributing to aspiration before or as the pharyngeal swallow is triggering. Despite both verbal and physical prompting, the patient with a right hemisphere stroke often has difficulty integrating therapy or compensatory strategies into their oral feeding, including postural compensations such as the chin-down head position, because of their cognitive disorders and relative inattention. For this reason, patients suffering a right cortical stroke may be later in returning to oral intake.

Effects of multiple strokes

Patients who have suffered multiple strokes often exhibit more significant swallowing abnormalities. Their oral function may be slower, with many repetitive tongue movements and oral transit times greater than five seconds. Delay in triggering the pharyngeal swallow is also usually more severe (five or more seconds). When the pharyngeal swallow triggers, these patients may exhibit reduced laryngeal elevation and reduced closure of the laryngeal vestibule/

entryway, resulting in penetration of food into the laryngeal entrance, plus uni-lateral weakness of the pharyngeal wall, resulting in residual food remaining on the pharyngeal wall and in the pyriform sinus on the affected side. Often their attention is affected and their ability to utilize therapy strategies and to focus on the task of eating and swallowing is also impaired.

Recovery of swallow post-stroke

Few data exist on recovery of swallow after stroke affecting specific locations in the brainstem or cortex (Wade and Hewer, 1987; Barer, 1989). A study of recovery in first-time stroke patients completed at Northwestern University and the Rehabilitation Institute of Chicago indicated that in these patients with non-complicated stroke, recovery is steady, vigorous, and rapid. All subjects to date (85 patients) have returned to full oral intake by six weeks post-ictus, regardless of site of lesion. However, even when these patients return to full oral intake, their temporal measures of swallow physiology, such as duration of airway closure and cricopharyngeal opening, and the temporal relationship between these actions do not return entirely to the normal values seen in age-matched controls. This would indicate that the swallow mechanism is never quite the same post-stroke, and it may help to explain why swallow function is more severely affected when/if the patient later suffers a second or third stroke.

Recovery is most rapid in the first three weeks post-stroke, indicating the need to evaluate the stroke patient's swallow function in the first week, and reevaluate at three to four weeks post-stroke. This is particularly important if a non-oral feeding system is instituted in the first few days post-stroke. The patient may no longer need this nutritional support three to four weeks later.

Because the criteria for entry to the study of recovery at Northwestern University and the Rehabilitation Institute of Chicago were very narrow, excluding patients with a history of any factors that might affect swallow function, as outlined in the next section, the population of stroke patients studied represents only approximately 10% of the total stroke admissions to the two institutions in any one year. However, the resulting data represent (as much as possible) only the effect of the infarct on the patients' swallow function. The preliminary data from this study indicate that the patient's prior medical history and any complications that arise in the patient's post-stroke care are more important contributors to the patient's post-stroke swallow function and recovery than previously acknowledged.

Other factors affecting swallowing function and recovery post-stroke

A number of other factors in the patient's medical history or medical management can affect their swallow ability post-stroke (Wright, 1985). Tracheostomy during the acute stroke phase may worsen the patient's swallowing problem, particularly if the tracheostomy cuff is kept inflated (Leder and Ross, 2000). Inflating the tracheostomy cuff for long periods of time can create tracheal irritation, but it also produces a greater friction on the tracheal wall as the larynx tries to elevate, potentially reducing laryngeal elevation more than a tracheostomy tube with the cuff deflated (Buckwalter and Sasaki, 1984; Nash, 1988). Particularly in older patients (over 80 years), tracheostomy may contribute to reducing laryngeal elevation and closure during the swallow. Studies of oropharyngeal swallow physiology in normal male subjects over 80 years of age have indicated a significant reduction in the range of hyoid and laryngeal movement compared with that in young men aged 21 to 30 years (Logemann et al., 2000, 2002). These changes may further exacerbate the negative effects of a tracheostomy. Long-term tracheostomy (more than six months) can contribute to reduced closure of the airway during the swallow, since the sensory receptors under the vocal folds are not stimulated by airflow. In addition, an open tracheostomy tube does not permit the build-up of subglottic pressure during swallow, which is thought to facilitate airway closure. Patients with tracheotomies should be taught to lightly cover the external end of the tracheostomy during the swallow to facilitate more normal vocal fold closure and airway protection.

Some medications given to the stroke patient may worsen any post-stroke swallowing disorders. Antidepressant medications, in particular, may slow swallow coordination and increase the severity of swallow disorders. The interaction of medications may cause xerostomia (dry mouth), which makes swallowing more difficult (Hughes et al., 1987).

Other concurrent medical problems, such as long-standing diabetes mellitus, can increase the severity of swallowing dysfunction or prolong the recovery time because of the potential for myopathies and neuropathies, which may affect pharyngeal muscle coordination and range of motion. Any prior history of transient ischemic attacks, prior strokes, or other neurological damage may increase the stroke patient's chances for significant swallow problems or worsen their severity. It is important that the speech–language pathologist investigates the patient's medical history carefully from chart review and family/patient interview to identify factors that may pertain to the patient's dysphagia and recovery. In this way, patient/family counselling regarding recovery can be more realistic.

Evaluation of swallow post-stroke

The process of evaluation of swallowing post-stroke begins with screening followed by diagnostic evaluation and treatment. Optimally, oropharyngeal swallow post-stroke should be evaluated first at the bedside with a clinical assessment and then radiographically (Simmons, 1986; Soren *et al.*, 1988; Chen *et al.*, 1990; Dodds *et al.*, 1990a,b, Gresham 1990; Logemann, 1993, 1998). The purpose of the swallow evaluation is to define the patient's swallow abnormalities and the effects of treatment strategies and not just to determine whether or not the patient aspirates.

Bedside/clinical examination

The initial bedside examination can be conducted as soon as 24 hours after a stroke, as long as the patient is alert, awake, and medically stable. The bedside clinical examination is designed to define the patient's medical history; oromotor function, including oral and pharyngeal anatomy; saliva management; and normalcy of oral and pharyngeal reflexes, laryngeal function, and cognitive and behavioral characteristics. All these may affect safe and efficient swallowing and successful eating. In addition, the need for further in-depth physiological testing, such as radiographic studies, is evaluated. The patient's behavioral characteristics are assessed at the bedside in order to determine the patient's ability to maintain adequate oral intake, as well as to cooperate with the radiographic study and utilize various compensatory and therapy strategies. A patient whose attention wanders and who cannot focus on the task of eating may have difficulty getting adequate nutrition, despite normal or near normal swallow physiology.

Designed as the protective mechanism for vomit and reflux (both foreign bodies when brought up to the pharynx from the stomach), the gag reflex cannot be used to predict the presence or normalcy of a swallow (Leder, 1996). There has been no neurophysiological relationship established between presence of a gag reflex and presence of a normal oropharyngeal swallow. In fact, many normal individuals have no gag reflex, or have a variable gag reflex.

At the end of the bedside/clinical examination, the clinician should have a good understanding of the patient's ability to focus on task and follow directions, as well as of the patient's level of alertness, cooperation, and orosensory and oromotor characteristics as applied to eating and swallowing. What is missing from this assessment is information on the patient's pharyngeal swallow physiology. The radiographic study is designed to define pharyngeal anatomy and swallow physiology, thereby determining the efficiency of the swallow, the etiology for any aspiration that may occur, and the efficacy of treatment strategies. If the clinician feels that the stroke patient's swallowing disorder is solely oral, with no pharyngeal involvement, then a radiographic study is not necessary. However, if any pharyngeal dysfunction is suspected, a radiographic study should be completed.

A relatively new test for the laryngeal cough reflex, which has not been completely validated, uses nebulized tartaric acid to evaluate the laryngeal cough reflex and the risk for development of aspiration pneumonia in stroke patients (Addington *et al.*, 1999a,b). This is not a swallowing test but will be an ancillary test to be completed by speech–language pathologists in the bedside assessment when the test becomes available nationally.

Radiographic evaluation

The radiographic evaluation of the dysphagic stroke patient has three purposes: to define the nature of the anatomy and physiology of the oropharyngeal swallow, to examine the effects of treatment strategies on the safety and efficiency of the swallow, and to recommend strategies for optimal management of the dysphagia (Logemann, 1993). The radiographic study is not done to determine if the patient aspirates but rather to define the abnormality in anatomy or physiology that causes food or liquid to enter the airway below the vocal folds (Martin-Harris et al., 2000).

Optimally, during the radiographic study, the patient should be seated upright in a normal eating position and viewed radiographically in the lateral plane. The patient's posture should be a comfortable one, enabling view of the oral cavity and pharynx from the soft palate superiorly to the bottom of the cervical esophagus inferiorly, and from the lips anteriorly to the posterior pharyngeal wall. If the oral cavity and pharynx cannot be viewed simultaneously, the pharynx should be examined first, since the oral cavity and its function can be examined at bedside. The foods to be given to the dysphagic stroke patient should be standardized in terms of volume and viscosity. Our typical protocol includes two swallows each of 1, 3, 5, and 10 ml of thin liquids, cup drinking of thin liquids, 1 ml of chocolate pudding mixed with barium in a 2:1 ratio (Esophatrast), and one-quarter of a "Lorna Doone cookie" coated with the barium pudding for contrast.

If the patient aspirates at any time during the radiographic study, or if the patient exhibits a highly inefficient swallow without aspiration, treatment strategies should be introduced to improve swallow efficiency or eliminate the aspiration. Such strategies include (a) postural techniques that redirect food flow or change pharyngeal dimension; (b) increased sensory input; (c) swallow maneuvers that apply voluntary control to selected aspects of swallow physiology; or (d) changes in bolus viscosity thick liquids, purees, etc. Generally, postural techniques and swallow maneuvers are both attempted before a particular food consistency (such as thin liquid) is eliminated from the patient's diet, since the goal of the radiographic study is to identify conditions under which the patient can retain oral intake on all food consistencies, rather than eliminating a particular food, such as thin liquids, from the diet.

Table 14.1 presents the various available postural strategies and their effects on swallow disorders. In general, postural techniques change the direction of food flow and/or change the dimensions of the pharynx.

Table 14.1 Postural techniques appropriate for each swallow disorder and the effect of the posture on pharyngeal dimensions or bolus flow

Disorder observed on fluoroscopy	Posture applied	Effect of posture
Inefficient oral transit (reduced posterior propulsion of bolus by tongue)	Head back	Utilizes gravity to clear oral cavity
Delay in triggering the pharyngeal swallow (bolus past ramus of mandible but pharyngeal swallow is not triggered)	Head down	Widens valleculae to prevent bolus entering airway and narrows airway entrance
Reduced tongue base retraction (residue in valleculae)	Head down	Pushes tongue base backward toward pharyngeal wall
Unilateral laryngeal dysfunction (aspiration during swallow)	Head down	Places epiglottis in more posterior, protective position
Reduced laryngeal closure (aspiration during the swallow)	Head rotated to damaged side	Increases vocal fold closure by applying extrinsic pressure; narrows laryngeal entrance
Reduced pharyngeal contraction (residue spread throughout pharynx)	Lying down on one side	Eliminates gravitational effect on pharyngeal residue
Unilateral pharyngeal paresis (residue on one side of pharynx)	Head rotated to damaged side	Eliminates damaged side from bolus path
Cricopharyngeal dysfunction (residue in pyriform sinuses)	Head rotated	Pulls cricoid cartilage away from posterior pharyngeal wall, reducing resting pressure in cricopharyngeal sphincter

Table 14.2 Bolus consistencies and the swallow problems for which they are most appropriate

Food consistencies	Disorders for which these foods are most appropriate
Thin liquids	Reduced tongue base retraction; reduced pharyngeal wall contraction; reduced laryngeal elevation; reduced cricopharyngeal opening
Thickened liquids	Oral tongue dysfunction
Purees and thick foods, including thickened liquids	Delayed pharyngeal swallow; reduced laryngeal closure at the entrance; reduced laryngeal closure throughout

Additional bolus types may be introduced in the radiographic study to define the patient's ability to swallow varying food consistencies (Table 14.2). It is suggested that a patient's swallows of thickened liquids be evaluated radiographically to be sure that these can be managed successfully before they are added to the diet. Any number of foods and liquids can be given during the radiographic study by mixing them with barium. Usually, the patient's radiographic exposure time should be limited to approximately five minutes. Ordinarily, 25 to 30 swallows can be examined during a five minute assessment.

The clinician participating in the videofluoroscopic study of oropharyngeal swallow should receive minimal radiation exposure as long as radiation precautions are used. These include wearing a lead apron, a lead collar to cover the thyroid, a badge to register the amount of radiation exposure, and, if desired, lead goggles.

Other assessment techniques

A number of other instrumental assessment techniques are available to evaluate various aspects of oral or pharyngeal swallow physiology in the stroke patient. Some of these techniques offer the opportunity for biofeedback during therapy. Each procedure answers specific clinical questions regarding the patient's swallowing function. None of these procedures provides all of the information generated from videofluoroscopy.

Ultrasound

Ultrasound is a non-invasive imaging procedure (using high-frequency sound waves) that enables visualization of the oral cavity, particularly the tongue, during swallow (Shawker, *et al.*, 1984; Stone and Shawker, 1986). Ultrasound enables the clinician to visualize tongue movements over time and to provide the patient with biofeedback during therapy. Because ultrasound is non-invasive, it can be utilized over a long period of time and repeatedly.

Fiberoptic endoscopy

Fiberoptic endoscopic examination of swallow involves placement of a 3.5 mm fiberoptic bundle transnasally so that the pharynx is viewed from above (Langmore *et al.*, 1988). This superior view of the pharynx enables the clinician to visualize the bolus coming over the back of the tongue and entering the pharynx prior to the triggering of the pharyngeal swallow. Prior to the swallow, as the bolus comes into view over the base of the tongue, the clinician can determine the presence of a pharyngeal delay and the duration of that delay. Oral function during the oral stage of swallow cannot be seen. During the pharyngeal swallow, the image disappears; consequently, the actual pharyngeal swallow cannot be assessed. After the swallow, as the pharynx and larynx lower and relax, the larynx and pharynx return to view, and the clinician can identify residual food remaining in the valleculae or pyriform sinuses, as well as any aspiration of this residue after the swallow. Aspiration of saliva before or after the swallow can also be visualized. The fiberoptic bundle can be lowered to contact the laryngeal vestibule so that laryngeal sensation can be tested directly.

Fiberoptic examination can also be utilized to provide biofeedback to the patient learning airway-closure techniques, as the vocal folds can be visualized from above during breath-hold maneuvers, prior to the swallow. The patient will be able to visualize vocal fold position. The technique has the disadvantage of requiring nasal placement of a tube, which is not possible in all stroke patients because of behavioral factors or nasal obstruction.

Pharyngeal manometry

Pharyngeal manometry also involves placement of a tube transnasally. In the case of manometry, this tube contains several pressure sensors (usually 1 cm long) at spaced intervals (Dodds *et al.*, 1987; McConnel *et al.*, 1988). When the tube is in place, the sensors will register pressure changes as the bolus passes each of them, or as any pharyngeal structure contacts them. Unfortunately, without simultaneous videofluoroscopy, manometry in the pharynx is difficult to interpret, since without X-ray the position of the manometric sensors cannot be identified in relation to pharyngeal structures. In addition, manometry alone does not define movement patterns of the pharynx to enable identification of pharyngeal movement abnormalities, nor does it define the presence or timing of aspiration. Manometry does provide information about the pressure generated within the pharynx and transmitted to the bolus itself during the pharyngeal swallow.

Surface electromyography

Surface electromyography can be used to identify the presence of a swallow but cannot be used to identify swallowing abnormalities in the oral or pharyngeal stage of deglutition.

Treatment procedures

The treatment plan for the dysphagic stroke patient should be developed after the patient's swallow physiology has been carefully studied and abnormalities identified. The key to effective swallowing rehabilitation is directing therapy management to the abnormal components of the oropharyngeal swallow (Logemann 1986, 1993, 1998).

Swallowing therapy can be direct or indirect. Direct therapy involves the presentation of food during attempts to swallow, using various strategies. Indirect therapy involves muscle exercises to improve the range of motion, coordination, and strength of movements involved in swallowing, or it utilizes swallow practice on specific techniques without giving food (i.e. using saliva). In general, indirect therapy is utilized when it is unsafe for the patient to swallow food of any consistency.

Swallowing therapy can also be divided into compensatory management or therapy strategies. In general, compensatory management is under the control of the clinician and requires minimal cognition or direction following on the part of the patient. In contrast, therapy strategies are designed to change swallow physiology and involve sensory stimulation, exercise programs, and swallow maneuvers.

Compensatory management

Compensatory management utilizes techniques that affect the symptoms of the swallow disorders without, necessarily, changing the actual swallow physiology. Compensatory strategies include changes in posture, changes in bolus volume or viscosity, as well as changes in feeding procedures (Logemann 1998; Logemann et al., 1989; Shanahan et al., 1993; Welch et al., 1993). Each of these postures is successful in improving swallow efficiency or safety in particular swallow disorders. These postures and their effects on pharyngeal dimensions or bolus flow are presented in Table 14.1. Postural techniques can be highly effective strategies in eliminating aspiration or improving the efficiency of the swallow (Rasley et al., 1993). Horner et al. (1988) reported elimination of aspiration 80% of the time with the use of postural techniques in stroke patients.

Changing bolus volume can improve swallow physiology in some stroke patients (Lazarus et al., 1993; Bisch et al., 1994). Many stroke patients exhibit significant difficulty swallowing small bolus volumes, such as saliva (1–3 ml), or swallowing large bolus volumes (10–20 ml), as in cup drinking. Providing a variety of bolus volumes during the radiographic study will enable the clinician to identify the bolus volume most effective for each patient.

Changes in bolus viscosity will also change the speed of bolus flow (normal transit times are slower on thicker foods); therefore, some viscosities are more easily swallowed in the presence of particular swallow abnormalities. For example, the patient with a delay in triggering the pharyngeal swallow typically exhibits greater difficulty, as evidenced by coughing, on thin liquids than on thick liquids and purees. Patients with other swallow disorders may find purees more difficult. For example, the patient with a cricopharyngeal dysfunction has greater difficulty with thick foods, such as purees, and is more easily able to handle thin liquids. Table 14.2 presents a list of food consistencies and the swallow disorders for which they are most effective.

The manner in which stroke patients are fed can increase efficiency or safety of oral intake, or decrease intake and increase the danger of aspiration, particularly in patients who have suffered several strokes or who have dementia. In general, patients who are easily distracted should be positioned in a quiet room with no auditory or visual distractions during meals. Giving the patient several seconds to become acclimated to the food smells can increase appetite and the desire to eat and swallow. The feeder should observe the patient's neck for laryngeal elevation to ensure that the patient has completed a swallow before presenting a new bolus. In some cases, several dry swallows should be encouraged to clear the pharynx. Feeding staff should be trained to stop feeding the patient if the patient exhibits any abnormal behaviors or difficulty swallowing, including coughing or breathing difficulties and to immediately contact the swallowing therapist. The swallowing therapist's role is to train and supervise the feeding staff.

Therapy strategies

Therapy strategies fall into one of three categories: sensory stimulation, exercise programs, and swallow maneuvers (Heimlich, et al., 1983; Selley, 1985; Lazzara et al., 1986; Logemann and Kahrilas, 1990; Kahrilas et al., 1991).

Sensory stimulation

Sensory stimulation is generally appropriate for the patient with swallow apraxia or with generally reduced oral sensation. Increasing sensory stimulation may be accomplished by presentation of a cold or warm bolus, by increasing the downward pressure of the spoon on the patient's tongue as the food is being presented, or by presenting foods with strong flavors or textures (Logemann et al., 1995). These techniques usually improve the oral onset of the swallow and may improve the speed of triggering of the pharyngeal swallow. For some patients, presentation of a bolus requiring chewing will also facilitate faster oral onset and increased oral motion. For other patients, self-feeding is the key to initiation of the oral activity for swallowing.

For some stroke patients, chewing provides the additional oral sensation required to reduce the pharyngeal delay. These patients exhibit less pharyngeal delay on boluses involving chewing, and also present less delay when asked to chew liquids than when swallowing liquids without the chewing behavior.

Exercises

Exercise programs may be provided to improve the range of lip, tongue, and jaw motion after stroke; to improve the coordination of lip and tongue motion; to improve vocal fold adduction; and to improve laryngeal elevation and tongue base retraction and cricopharyngeal opening. Range of motion exercises for the lips, tongue, hyoid, larynx, and/or jaw can be presented for unilateral or bilateral weakness (Shaker et al., 1997a,b, 2002). All range-of-motion exercises involve moving the target structure as far as possible in the desired direction, holding the structure extended in that direction for several seconds, and then relaxing.

Resistance exercises, using a tongue blade between the lips or against the tongue, can also be used to improve range of motion.

Swallow maneuvers

Swallow maneuvers, another category of swallow therapy, involve the application of voluntary control to specific components of the pharyngeal swallow. The **supraglottic swallow** involves voluntary closure of the vocal folds before and during the swallow. The **super supraglottic swallow** creates closure of the entrance to the airway (between the arytenoids and base of epiglottis) before and during the swallow. The **Mendelsohn maneuver** utilizes information on the role of hyolaryngeal anterior–superior motion in the normal opening of the upper esophageal sphincter to gain volitional control over the duration of cricopharyngeal opening by teaching the patient to prolong maximal elevation of the larynx during the swallow. The **effortful swallow** is designed to increase posterior tongue-base motion and tongue pressure during the pharyngeal swallow and to improve clearance of the bolus from the valleculae. For the most part, patients requiring these maneuvers are most often those with brainstem strokes with the cognitive ability to learn and implement the maneuvers. Swallow maneuvers in general require more effort and will fatigue the patient faster than techniques such as changes in head or body posture.

Multidisciplinary team

Management of dysphagia in the patient post-stroke requires multidisciplinary input from assessment through treatment.

Assessment

A variety of assessment techniques may be utilized in the stroke patient as discussed above, requiring the joint involvement of the speech–language pathologist with the otolaryngologist (endoscopy), gastroenterologist (manometry), or radiologist (videofluoroscopy).

Dietary/nutritional management

In the management of the patient's nutritional needs, the dietician is essential. When recommendations are needed regarding non-oral feeding during the initial recovery stages in dysphagia after stroke, the dietician and the patient's attending physician will discuss the various alternatives for nutritional intake, taking into account the patient's medical status, gastrointestinal function, finances, and behavior. Throughout the patient's recovery, the various members of the dysphagia rehabilitation team will interact in decision making regarding swallowing treatment and return to oral intake.

Non-oral feeding plays an important role in dysphagia rehabilitation. It provides the patient with adequate calories and hydration to support their recovery and rehabilitation. Nutrition should never be compromised in the process of management of a swallowing disorder. Rather, nutritional support should be provided to facilitate the patient's recovery and rehabilitation back to full oral intake. When presenting the need for non-oral feeding or supplements to the patient and family, it is important to stress the value of both nutrition and hydration, and the temporary nature of all of these methods. Oral and non-oral feedings can coexist as the patient recovers. Any non-oral feeding can be discontinued as soon as the patient is ready to resume full oral intake.

Physical and occupational therapy

Physical and occupational therapy is important in providing seating devices and positioning appropriate for the patient's swallowing disorders and to provide assistive devices to facilitate hand-to-mouth coordination in those patients able to feed themselves.

Medical and surgical management

Medical and surgical intervention for dysphagia is generally not needed in the stroke patient unless the swallowing problems fail to recover with therapy (Butcher, 1982; Blitzer et al., 1988). Surgical management may be needed for patients who are chronically aspirating their own secretions, despite significant and aggressive therapy over a prolonged period. There are techniques available for airway diversion, vocal fold suturing or epiglottic pulldown; these can, in some cases, eliminate chronic aspiration by preventing material from entering the airway. The ultimate solution for chronic aspiration leading to repeated pneumonia is total laryngectomy. These procedures are used only infrequently in stroke-induced dysphagia and only after prolonged therapy has been found to be unsuccessful and when the patient's general health is compromised by the chronic aspiration.

Patient/family counselling and follow-up

Teaching the patient and family about normal swallow physiology and the nature of the stroke patient's dysphagia is critical to their support of and their participation in a therapy program. Involvement of the family in management of the patient can often be helpful. At the very least, enlisting the family's support for the patient as he or she progresses through therapy is often critical to continued high motivation. Families can participate in therapy, by providing encouragement for repeating exercises or by actually participating in direct therapy, such as providing thermal/tactile stimulation. If the dysphagic patient has a slower recovery, reevaluation by radiography or other instrumental techniques is usually needed to document recovery and move the patient to more normal diet. Usually, this follow-up occurs approximately three to four weeks after the initial assessment, but it may be as much as two to three months later. If a patient's progress is extremely slow or the patient's function plateaus, exhibiting no improvement for at least one month, the clinician may decide to dismiss the patient from direct therapy and to reassess their function in three to six months. Because there are significant gaps in our knowledge base regarding recovery rates for specific neural damage, it is impossible to say that a patient will never recover swallow ability. Rather, the clinician should schedule the patient for a reevaluation after a period of time without therapy to determine any improvement in status. Many stroke patients will recover 3 to 12 months after their stroke.

Research approaches

There are many questions about recovery of swallow post-stroke that deserve attention. Recently, the Agency for Healthcare Research and Quality completed an analysis of the available evidence on the diagnosis and treatment of dysphagia in preventing pneumonia (Doggett *et al.*, 2001, 2002). These authors concluded that implementation of dysphagia programs is accompanied by substantial reduction in pneumonia rates. They indicated that more research is needed.

ACKNOWLEDGEMENTS

This research was funded by NIH grants R01-NS28525 and NIH R01 DC 00550.

REFERENCES

Addington, W. R., Stephens, R. E., and Gilliland, K. A. (1999a). Assessing the laryngeal cough reflex and the risk of developing pneumonia after stroke: an interhospital comparison. *Stroke* **30**: 1203–1207.

Addington, W. R., Stephens, R. E., Gilliland, R. E., and Rodriguez, M. (1999b). Assessing the laryngeal cough reflex and the risk of developing pneumonia after stroke. *Arch Phys Med Rehabil* **80**: 150–154.

Barer, D. H. (1989). The natural history and functional consequences of dysphagia after hemispheric stroke. *J Neurol Neurosurg Psychiatry* **52**: 236–241.

Bisch, E. M., Logemann, J. A., Rademaker, A. W., Kahrilas, P. J., and Lazarus, C. L. (1994). Pharyngeal effects of bolus volume, viscosity and temperature in patients with dysphagia resulting from neurologic impairment and in normal subjects. *J Speech Hear Res*, **37**: 1041–1049.

Blitzer, A., Krespi, Y., Oppenheimer, R., and Levine, T. (1988). Surgical management of aspiration. *Otolaryngol Clin North Am* **21**: 743–750.

Buckwalter, J. A. and Sasaki, C. T. (1984). Effect of tracheostomy on laryngeal function. *Otolaryngol Clin North Am* **17**: 41–48.

Butcher, R. (1982). Treatment of chronic aspiration as a complication of cerebrovascular accident. *Laryngoscope* **92**: 681–685.

Celifarco, A., Gerard, G., Faegenburg, D., and Burakoff, R. (1990). Dysphagia as the sole manifestation of bilateral strokes. *Am J Gastroenterol* **85**: 610–613.

Chen, M., Ott, D., Peele, V., and Gelfand, D. (1990). Oropharynx in patients with cerebrovascular disease: evaluation and videofluoroscopy. *Radiology* **176**: 641–643.

Delgado, J. J. (1988). Paralysis, dysphagia and balance problems associated with stroke. *J Neurosci Nurs* **20**: 260.

Dodds, W. J., Kahrilas, P. J., Dent, J., and Hogan, W. J. (1987). Considerations about pharyngeal manometry. *Dysphagia* **1**: 209–214.

Dodds, W. J., Logemann, J. A., and Stewart, E. T. (1990a). Radiological assessment of abnormal oral and pharyngeal phases of swallowing. *Am J Roentgenol* **154**: 965–974.

Dodds, W. J., Stewart, E. T., and Logemann, J. A. (1990b). Physiology and radiology of the normal oral and pharyngeal phases of swallowing. *Am J Roentgenol* **154**: 953–965.

Doggett, D. L., Tappe, K. A., Mitchell, M. D., *et al.* (2001). Prevention of pneumonia in elderly stroke patients by a systematic diagnosis and treatment of dysphagia: an evidence-based comprehensive analysis of the literature. *Dysphagia* **16**: 279–295.

Doggett, D. L., Turkelson, C. M., and Coates, V. (2002). Recent developments in diagnosis and intervention for aspiration and dysphagia in stroke and other neuromuscular disorders. *Curr Atheroscl Rep* **44**: 311– 318.

Fraser, C., Power, M., Hamdy, S., *et al.* (2002). Driving plasticity in human adult motor cortex is associated with improved motor function after brain injury. *Neuron* **34**: 831–840.

Gresham, S. L. (1990). Clinical assessment and management of swallowing difficulties after stroke. *Med J Aust* **153**: 397–399.

Hamdy, S. and Rothwell, J. C. (1998). Gut feelings about recovery after stroke: the organization and reorganization of human swallowing motor cortex. *Trends Neurosci* **21**: 278–282.

Hamdy, S., Aziz, Q., Rothwell, J. C., *et al.* (1996). The cortical topography of human swallowing musculature in health and disease. *Nat Med* **2**: 1217–1224; [Comment in: *Nat Med* (1996). **2**. 1190–1191.]

Hamdy, S., Aziz, Q., and Rothwell, J. C. (1997). Explaining oropharyngeal dysphagia after unilateral hemispheric stroke. *Lancet* **350**: 686–692.

(1998a). Recovery of swallowing after dysphagic stroke relates to functional reorganization in the intact motor cortex. *Gastroenterology* **115**: 1104–1112.

Hamdy, S., Rothwell, J. C., Aziz, Q., Singh, K. D., and Thompson, D. G. (1998b). Long-term reorganization of human motor cortex driven by short-term sensory stimulation. *Nat Neurosci* **1**: 64–68.

Hamdy, S, Rothwell, J. C., Aziz, Q., and Thompson, D. G. (2000). Organization and reorganization of human swallowing motor cortex: implications for recovery after stroke. *Clin Sci* **99**: 151–157.

Hamdy, S., Aziz, Q., Thompson, D. G., and Rothwell, J. C. (2001). Physiology and pathophysiology of the swallowing area of human motor cortex. *Neur Plast*, **8**: 91–97.

Heimlich, H. (1983). Rehabilitation of swallowing after stroke. *Ann Otol Rhinol Laryngol* **92**: 357–359.

Horner, J., Massey, E., Riski, J., Lathrop, D., and Chase, K. (1988). Aspiration following stroke: clinical correlates and outcomes. *Neurology* **38**: 1359–1362.

Hughes, C. V., Baum, B. J., Fox, P. C., *et al.* (1987). Oral–pharyngeal dysphagia: a common sequelae of salivary gland dysfunction. *Dysphagia* **1**: 173–177.

Jean, A. and Car, A. (1979). Inputs to the swallowing medullary neurons from the peripheral afferent fibers and the swallowing cortical area. *Brain Res* **178**: 567–572.

Kahrilas, P. J., Logemann, J. A., Krugler, C., and Flanagan, E. (1991). Volitional augmentation of upper esophageal sphincter opening during swallowing. *Am J Physiology* **260**: G450–9456.

Kahrilas, P. J., Logemann, J. A., and Gibbons, P. (1992). Food intake by maneuver: an extreme compensation for impaired swallowing. *Dysphagia* **7**: 155–159.

Langmore, S. E., Schatz, K., and Olsen, N. (1988). Fiberoptic endoscopic examination of swallowing safety: a new procedure. *Dysphagia* **2**: 216–219.

Lazarus, C. L., Logemann, J. A., Rademaker, A. W., *et al.* (1993). Effects of bolus volume, viscosity and repeated swallows in non-stroke subjects and stroke patients. *Arch Phys Med Rehabil* **74**: 1066–1070.

Lazzara, G., Lazarus, C., and Logemann, J. A. (1986). Impact of thermal stimulation on the triggering of the swallowing reflex. *Dysphagia* **1**: 73–77.

Leder, S. B. (1996). Gag reflex and dysphagia. *Head Neck* **18**: 138–141.

Leder, S. B. and Ross, D. A. (2000). Investigation of the causal relationship between tracheotomy and aspiration in the acute care setting. *Laryngoscope* **110**: 641–646.

Logemann, J. A. (1986). Treatment of aspiration related to dysphagia: an overview. *Dysphagia* **1**: 34–38.

(1993). *Manual for Videofluoroscopic Evaluation of Swallowing*, 2nd edn. Austin, TX: Pro-Ed.

(1998). *Evaluation and Treatment of Swallowing Disorders*, 2nd edn. Austin, Tx: Pro-Ed.

Logemann, J. A. and Kahrilas, P. J. (1990). Relearning to swallow post CVA: application of maneuvers and indirect biofeedback – a case study. *Neurology* **40**: 1136–1138.

Logemann, J., Kahrilas, P., Kobara, M., and Vakil, N. (1989). The benefit of head rotation on pharyngoesophageal dysphagia. *Arch Phys Med Rehabil* **70**: 767–771.

Logemann, J. A., Pauloski, B. R., Colangelo, L., *et al.* (1995). Effects of a sour bolus on oropharyngeal swallowing measures in patients with neurogenic dysphagia. *J Speech Hear Res* **38**: 556–563.

Logemann, J. A., Pauloski, B. R., Rademaker, A. W., *et al.* (2000). Temporal and biomechanical characteristics of oropharyngeal swallow in younger and older men. *J Speech Lang Hear Res* **43**: 1264–1274.

Logemann, J. A., Pauloski, B. R., Rademaker, A. W., and Kahrilas, P. J. (2002). Oropharyngeal swallow in younger and older women: videofluoroscopic analysis. *J Speech Lang Hear Res* **45**: 434–444.

Martin-Harris, B., Logemann, J. A., McMahon, S., Schleicher, M., and Sandidge, J. (2000). Clinical utility of the modified barium swallow. *Dysphagia* **15**: 136–141.

McConnel, F. M. S., Cerenko, D., and Mendelsohn, M. (1988). Manofluorographic analyses of swallowing. *Otolaryngol Clin North Am* **21**: 625–635.

Meadows, J. (1973). Dysphagia in unilateral cerebral lesions. *J Neurol Neurosurg Psychiatry* **36**: 853–860.

Miller, A. (1982). Deglutition. *Physiol Rev* **62**: 129–184.

Nash, M. (1988). Swallowing problems in the tracheotomized patient. *Otolaryngol Clin North Am* **21**: 701–709.

Rasley, A., Logemann, J. A., Kahrilas, P. J., *et al.* (1993). Prevention of barium aspiration during videofluoroscopic swallowing studies: value of change in posture. *Am J Roentgenol* **160**: 1005–1009.

Selley, W. G. (1985). Swallowing difficulties in stroke patients: a new treatment. *Age Aging* **14**: 361–365.

Shaker, R., Kern, M., Bardan, E., Arndorfer, R. C., and Hofmann, C. (1997a). Effect of isotonic/isometric head lift exercise on hypopharyngeal intrabolus pressure. *Dysphagia* **12**: 107, 1997.

Shaker, R., Kern, M., Bardan, E., *et al.* (1997b). Augmentation of deglutitive upper esophageal sphincter opening in the elderly by exercise. *Am J Physiol* **272**: G1518–G1522.

Shaker, R., Kern, M., *et al.* (2002). Rehabilitation of swallowing by exercise in tube fed patients with pharyngeal dysphagia secondary to abnormal UES opening. *Gastroenterology* **122**: 1314–1321.

Shanahan, T. K., Logemann, J. A., Rademaker, A. W., Pauloski, B. R., and Kahrilas, P. J. (1993). Chin-down posture effect on aspiration in dysphagic patients. *Arch Phys Med Rehabil* **74**: 736–739.

Shawker, T. H., Sonies, P. C., and Stone, M. (1984). Sonography of speech and swallowing. In *Ultrasound Annual*, ed. R. Sanders and M. Hill. New York: Raven, pp. 237–260.

Simmons, K. (1986). Dysphagia management means diagnosis, exercise, reeducation. *JAMA* **255**: 3209–3212.

Smith, D. S. and Dodd, B. A. (1990). Swallowing disorders in stroke. *Med J Aust* **153**: 372–373.

Soren, R., Somers, S., Austin, W., and Bester, S. (1988). The influence of videofluoroscopy on the management of the dysphagic patient. *Dysphagia* **2**: 127–135.

Stone, M. and Shawker, T. H. (1986). An ultrasound examination of tongue movement during swallowing. *Dysphagia* **1**: 78–83.

Wade, D. and Hewer, R. (1987). Motor loss and swallowing difficulty after stroke: frequency, recovery, and prognosis. *Acta Neurol Scand* **76**: 50–54.

Welch, M. W., Logemann, J. A., Rademaker, A. W., and Kahrilas, P. J. (1993). Changes in pharyngeal dimensions effected by chin tuck. *Arch Phys Med Rehabil* **74**: 178–181.

Wright, A. (1985). An unusual but easily treatable cause of dysphagia and dysarthria complicating stroke. *B M J* **291**: 1412–1413.

15

Continence and stroke

Barbara J. Chandler

Hunters Moor Regional Neurorehabilitation Centre, Newcastle upon Tynpe, UK

Introduction

In early childhood, the achievement of continence is a major goal and attracts great reward when it is successfully mastered. Following this, continence is forgotten – it is simply assumed to exist. The occurrence of *in*continence in adult life is associated with shock, embarrassment, and often fear. It may have far-reaching effects on lifestyle. Patients have described becoming housebound because of fear of incontinence. Fecal incontinence may be even more distressing and have a profound effect upon rehabilitation and reintegration into social and family life. It has been termed the "unvoiced symptom" (Leigh and Turnberg, 1982). In a study amongst 115 patients with spinal cord injury, bowel dysfunction was considered to be one of the most distressing of their disabilities (Glickman and Kamm, 1996).

Daily urinary incontinence is not uncommon, affecting at least 1 in 20 of those under 65 years and increasing with age (Brittain, 1998). There may be a reticence about disclosing the problem even to a health professional. People may have too low an expectation of benefit from treatment and yet there is much that can be offered to alleviate symptoms (Yarnell *et al.*, 1981; Jarvis, 1993).

Urinary incontinence

Urinary incontinence is defined as the involuntary leakage of urine that is a social or hygienic problem and is objectively demonstrable (Anon., 1990).

Prevalence

A survey by MORI involving interviews with 4000 people aged 30 years and over, in their own homes, revealed that 14% of women and 6.6% of men had experienced urinary incontinence. The definition of urinary incontinence used in the study was a positive reply to the question, "Have you suffered from bladder problems, for example leaking, wet pants, damp pants?" (Brocklehurst, 1993). Half of those with incontinence had seen their general practitioner. An earlier

Recovery after Stroke, ed. Michael P. Barnes, Bruce H. Dobkin and Julien Bogousslavsky. Published by Cambridge University Press. © Cambridge University Press 2005.

study involving a postal questionnaire sent to 22 430 people used a definition of regular urinary incontinence as "involuntary excretion or leakage of urine in inappropriate places or at inappropriate times twice or more a month." This study revealed a prevalence of urinary incontinence of 8.5% in women and 1.6% in males aged 15–64 years. These figures rose to 11.6% of women and 6.9% of males aged 65 and over (Thomas *et al.*, 1980).

Problems with continence increase with advancing age; for example, bladder outflow obstruction secondary to benign prostatic hypertrophy in men and stress incontinence resulting from incompetence of the urethral sphincter mechanism in women are common causes. Other morbidities such as diabetes mellitus, cardiovascular and peripheral vascular disease, the postmenopausal hormonal changes, and age-related bladder instability may all affect continence (Marincov and Badlani, 2001).

Physiology

The urinary bladder

The bladder has two functions: storage and voiding. Normal control of the bladder depends upon intact connections between the sacral spinal cord and the pontine micturition center. The latter receives input from higher centers especially the medial aspects of the frontal lobes.

Storage

During bladder filling, the high wall compliance keeps the intravesical pressure low (less than $10\,cm\,H_2O$). There is also inhibition of parasympathetic activity. The first sensation of an urge to void may occur at approximately 300 ml. At this time, the urge to void can be suppressed via supraspinal, spinal, and peripheral mechanisms, which suppress unwanted detrusor contractions whilst maintaining a closed urethra until an appropriate time and place for voiding is found.

Storage problems occur when unwanted detrusor contractions cannot be suppressed; this may occur in spinal cord pathology and also in some people with suprapontine pathology. For example, it appears that the basal ganglia may have an inhibitory effect on the micturition reflex in health. In Parkinson's disease, the cell loss in the substantia nigra is thought to reduce this inhibitory effect, resulting in detrusor hyperreflexia (Sakakibara and Fowler, 1999). Patients will complain of *urgency, frequency,* and *urge incontinence.*

Voiding

The first event in voiding is cessation of the tonically active striated external urethral sphincter followed by detrusor contraction. This coordinated activity depends upon intact connections between the sacral cord and the pontine micturition center. Voiding dysfunction occurs particularly in spinal cord pathology, where loss of the sequential activity results in detrusor sphincter dyssynergia (simultaneous contraction of the external urethral sphincter and the detrusor during volume-determined detrusor hyperreflexia (Fowler and Chandiramani, 2000). Dysfunctions may also occur with suprapontine pathology such as stroke, frontal lobe disorders and Parkinson's disease. Patients may complain of *difficulty with micturition, hesitancy, interrupted stream* and *incomplete emptying*. More than 50% of people with a neurological cause of voiding difficulty may be unaware that they have incomplete emptying (Fowler and Chandiramani, 2000).

Electromyographic (EMG) studies in the majority of patients with suprapontine lesions reveal uninhibited relaxation of the external sphincter during or preceding detrusor contractions. There is, in general, an absence of true detrusor sphincter dyssynergia in the majority of post-stroke patients. This gives a quite different picture than that found in patients with disease affecting the spinal cord, for example multiple sclerosis, where detrusor sphincter dyssynergia is one of the most common findings. Pseudodyssynergia may occur post-stroke; this is characterized by voluntary contraction of the external sphincter during an involuntary detrusor contraction (Burney *et al.*, 1996).

Supraspinal centers

Frontal lobes

Prior to the advent of dynamic scanning techniques, studies were undertaken using careful observation and recording of symptoms from patients with various cerebral pathologies and on whom surgery had been performed. The relationship of urinary incontinence to frontal tumors associated with the "frontal lobe syndrome," manifesting as indifference, altered affect, self-neglect, and intellectual deterioration, has been well recognized. Andrew and Nathan (1964) published a description of patients with frontal lobe lesions and disorders of micturition. It was shown that there was a relationship between the control of micturition and also defecation and the superomedial part of the frontal lobe. Their patients were all aware and distressed by their symptoms. Micturition occurred normally, but the patient experienced frequency, extreme urgency when awake, and incontinence when asleep. There was impaired awareness of the increasing fullness of the bladder and the sensation that micturition was imminent. The patient, therefore, could experience either extreme urgency or sudden incontinence. If the symptoms were less severe, the patient might be able to inhibit micturition, despite a sense of urgency. Ten years later, Maurice-Williams (1974) in a study of 100 consecutive patients with intracranial tumor, identified a symptom cluster of frequency of micturition, urgency, and incontinence in the absence of signs of intellectual deterioration in patients with frontal lobe lesions. Seven (14%) patients out of 50 with frontal lobe tumors had this syndrome.

Pons

Sakakibara *et al.* (1996a, b) studied 39 patients with brainstem stroke (32 infarction and seven hemorrhage). Magnetic resonance imaging was used to locate the lesion. Within three months after the onset of stroke, 19 (49%) subjects had urinary symptoms. The most common problem was nocturnal frequency and voiding difficulty (11 patients). Eight experienced urinary retention, but subsequently five of these achieved independent voiding. Three patients experienced urgency and incontinence. Cystometrography (CMG) was carried out in 11 patients and the most common finding was of detrusor hyperreflexia. Most of the symptomatic patients had lesions of the pontine tegmentum and dorsal medulla. Sakakibara *et al.* (1996a, b) concluded that their findings supported the idea of a pontine micturition center in humans, similar to that found in animal studies.

Blok *et al.* (1998) used positron emission tomographic scanning to study brain activation during micturition. Their initial studies used male volunteers. They then repeated their work amongst 18 right-handed female volunteers. There was activation of a distinct area in the dorsal pontine tegmentum and, as with the studies of Sakakibara *et al.* (1996a, b), this was felt to support the idea of a pontine micturition center. They also found activation of the right inferior frontal gyrus in their male and female subjects. They comment that this area, in addition to the dorsolateral prefrontal cortex, is involved in attention mechanisms and response selection. They postulated, that, with regard to micturition, this area might have a role in deciding whether or not micturition can take place.

Methods of investigation

Urodynamics

Cystometry allows measurement of bladder pressure and volume. A catheter in the bladder measures pressure and allows bladder filling while a rectal catheter measures intra-abdominal pressure, which can be subtracted from the bladder pressure reading to give a true detrusor pressure, (Figs. 15.1 and 15.2). Flow rate is recorded as the patient voids. Visualization of the bladder during the study is possible using radio-opaque contrast and X rays. Ambulatory monitoring is also now available.

Ultrasound

Ultrasound is used to measure residual urine and does not require the skill of a radiographer. Precision is not required, just an estimate of whether the residual is greater or less than 100 ml (Fowler, 1996). Assessment of the post-void residual is critical in planning the management of a continence disorder. For examination of the upper tracts, skilled ultrasound assessment is the test of choice. Other techniques such as intravenous urography and isotope scanning may be used.

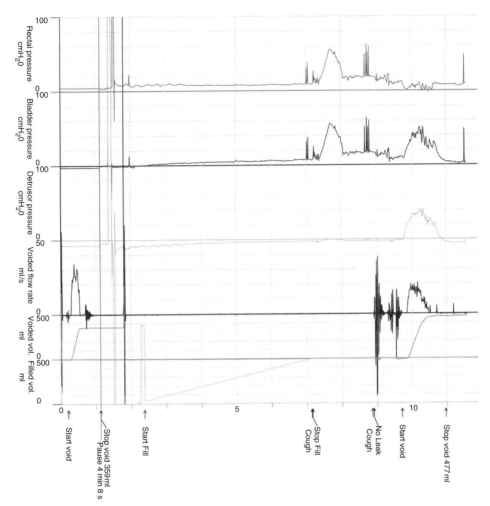

Fig. 15.1   Cystometrogram showing normal filling and voiding phases. The filling phase shows a stable detrusor. The intra-abdominal pressure is increased during coughing, but the detrusor pressure is unchanged and there is no leakage. As voluntary voiding is initiated, the detrusor pressure increases and complete bladder emptying is achieved with a detrusor pressure of <40 cmH$_2$O and a maximum flow rate of 20 ml/s. (Cystometrograms kindly provided by Mr R. Pickard, Consultant Urologist, Freeman Hospital, Newcastle upon Tyne, UK.)

Neurophysiology

Detailed studies involving tests such as EMG and evoked potentials are useful but lie within the province of specialist uroneurology (Fowler 1996).

Prevalence of urinary incontinence after stroke

Brocklehurst *et al.* (1985), in a study of 135 consecutive stroke patients over a six-month period, found that 51% had urinary incontinence at some stage during the

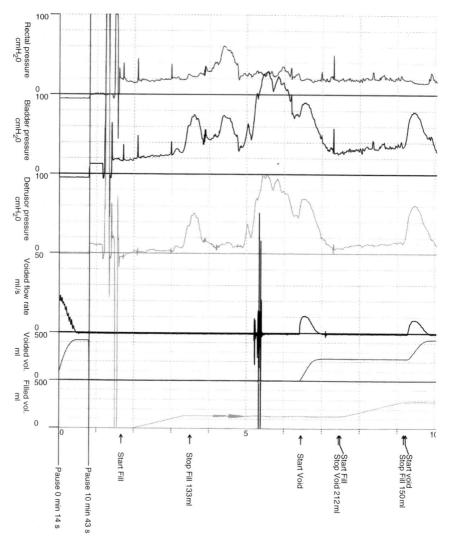

Fig. 15.2   Cystometrogram showing detrusor instability. Involuntary contractions of the detrusor are evident. High pressures are generated both by the involuntary and voluntary contractions. The filling phase was curtailed because of the involuntary contractions and associated voiding. (Cystometrogram kindly provided by Mr R. Pickard, Consultant Urologist, Freeman Hospital, Newcastle upon Tyne, UK.)

first year following the stroke. In 75% of these, the onset was within the first two weeks and in 41% it resolved within that time. At the end of 12 months, 20% remained incontinent of urine. The authors proposed that although incontinence was common it was largely transient and was related to impairment of consciousness, immobility, and dependency, rather than to impairment of neurological pathways.

In a study of 935 patients with acute strokes over a 19-month period, Nakayama *et al.* (1997) found that 36% (309) had "full urinary incontinence on admission" and 11% had partial incontinence (occasional accidents). This had decreased to 15% and 13%, respectively, at discharge and to 8% and 11%, respectively, at six months. Overall, 81% of stroke survivors were continent.

Given the frequency of urinary problems in the population at large, it is not surprising that some stroke patients may have had preexisting problems. Badlani *et al.* (1987) undertook a prospective study of continence post-stroke with assessment at 1, 4, and 12 weeks. At these times, they identified 60%, 42% and 29%, respectively, of survivors with incontinence. There was pre-existing incontinence in 17%, but with appropriate investigation and management, seven of these survivors regained continence, although it was noted that in each the neurological deficit was mild.

In the immediate post-stroke phase, acute urinary retention may occur as a result of detrusor areflexia. This phase has been termed "cerebral shock" and is likened to "spinal shock," but the precise physiological explanation is uncertain (Burney *et al.* (1996). Other factors, such as altered consciousness, inability to communicate, or detrusor failure owing to overdistension, may also contribute. Preexisting medication, particularly anticholinergic agents, may also contribute to this phase of urinary retention, as may constipation. With time, the most common symptoms to emerge are frequency, urgency, and urge incontinence secondary to detrusor hyperreflexia.

Risk factors for incontinence post-stroke

Nakayama *et al.*, 1997 identified risk factors for incontinence following stroke:
- age
- lesion diameter
- diabetes
- hypertension
- other disabling diseases
- initial score on the Scandinavian Stroke Scale (assessing functional ability).

Patients with initial urinary incontinence were significantly older, female, and more likely to have diabetes mellitus and comorbidity of other disabling diseases. On computed tomography (CT), the lesions in those patients with urinary incontinence were significantly more frequently a hemorrhage or larger in size and more often involved the cerebral cortex than in those patients without incontinence.

Incontinence as a predictor of disability

Wade and Langton Hewer (1985) examined the place of urinary incontinence as a predictor for survival and recovery amongst 532 patients seen within seven days of their stroke. Both a depressed level of consciousness and incontinence in conscious patients were associated with a more severe stroke. These patients were more likely to be unable to transfer from bed to chair or to be able to communicate and to have severe initial disability as measured by the Barthel Index. Of these two predictors, urinary incontinence had a better specificity and predictive value. Of those with urinary incontinence within one week of the stroke, 50% had died by six months. They concluded that the presence of urinary incontinence in the first seven days post-stroke separated patients who had a poor prognosis for survival and eventual functional independence from those who had a good prognosis.

Taub *et al.* (1994) examined outcome predictors following first stroke in patients under the age of 75 years. Assessments were undertaking using the Barthel Index at the time of maximum impairment immediately post-stroke and at 3 and 12 months. Four predictors present within the first 72 hours were identified:

- coma
- paralysis
- speech and swallowing problems
- urinary incontinence (patients with a urinary catheter in place during this time were classed as incontinent).

Little change was identified in the disability state between 3 and 12 months; therefore, the predictors could be applied to the 12-month assessment.

It is clearly not the urinary incontinence itself that has this marked effect on prognosis, but what it implies. Incontinence does highlight a group of stroke patients with special needs. Khan *et al.* (1981), commented that "aphasia and decreased motor power of the upper limb must be considered when evaluating management of the urinary tract in rehabilitation." Additional factors linking incontinence to outcome are its effect on morale (Brittain, 1998) and its association with related severe disabilities such as dysphasia (Badlani *et al.*, 1987).

Investigations after stroke

Measuring residual urine

Garrett *et al.* (1989) examined the incidence of urinary retention amongst 85 patients admitted to a rehabilitation center. Measurements were taken by inter-mittent catheterization and those with an admission post-void residual volume volume of more than 50 ml underwent a further three measurements of post-void residual volume. They identified an initial group of 48 patients with retention defined as a post-void residual volume of >50ml. This number decreased to 22 patients by the time of discharge, of whom seven were incontinent. A significantly higher rate of urinary tract infections occurred amongst those retaining >50 ml.

Other contributory factors such as prostatic hypertrophy were not discussed nor whether the urinary tract infections were symptomatic or identified on routine screening.

Cystometrograms

Khan *et al.* (1981) studied 20 patients (9 males and 11 females) referred for urological assessment following a stroke confirmed by CT scan. Assessments took place between 3 and 24 months following stroke. Patients with basal ganglia or frontoparietal cortical lesions both showed uninhibited detrusor contractions and reflex inhibition of the external sphincter during detrusor contraction. The clinical result of this was urge incontinence. Lesions in the frontal lobe predominantly affected bladder stability without affecting sphincter function, resulting in urgency rather than incontinence. All the patients with basal ganglial lesions and six out of the eight with frontoparietal lesions had dominant hemisphere lesions. By contrast, Kuroiwa *et al.* (1987) studied 134 patients 12 months post-stroke, 68 with left cerebral lesions and 66 with right cerebral lesions. Frequency and urgency of micturition was found more commonly in patients with right hemisphere lesions.

Tsuchida *et al.* (1983) studied 39 patients with a hemiplegia following stroke: 26 complained of frequency or urge incontinence and 13 experienced dysuria or urinary retention. Out of 11 patients with frontal lobe and internal capsule lesions, 10 showed detrusor hyperreflexia and six had uninhibited sphincter relaxation. Of the 10 patients with putaminal lesions, nine had detrusor hyperreflexia, and normal sphincter activity was demonstrated in seven of these patients. Detrusor sphincter dyssynergia was uncommon. The results suggested that damage to the frontal lobe or the internal capsule results in an abnormality characterized by "hyperactive bladder with uninhibited sphincter relaxation" and that damage to the basal ganglia, especially the putamen, results in "detrusor hyperactivity, but rarely causes urethral dysfunction."

In 1990, Khan *et al.* carried out a study of 33 patients (15 males and 18 females) with voiding problems post-stroke. Twenty-six had involuntary detrusor contractions with the critical volume for involuntary contractions being approximately 200 ml. Seven patients had poor bladder contractions.

Unstable detrusor contractions are quite common with advancing age. Khan *et al.* (1990) emphasized that, "the finding of detrusor hyper-reflexia in a majority of elderly stroke patients may reflect the high prevalence of involuntary contractions in elderly patients in general. Such a patient may be continent, but following a stroke, the combination of impaired mobility and involuntary contraction may lead to urinary dysfunction." In the elderly, other morbidities that impact on bladder function become common (e.g. diabetes mellitus and Parkinson's disease).

Taking all this into account, "voiding dysfunctions as the result of cerebrovascular accident, when compounded with other possible pre-existing conditions in the elderly...can result in a challenging diagnostic and therapeutic dilemma" (Burney et al., 1996).

Summary of cystometrography studies

The most common finding is detrusor hyperreflexia with a coordinated response of the external sphincter. Urinary retention may occur and an areflexic detrusor has been identified especially in patients with cerebellar lesions (Burney et al., 1996).

Management of the patient with urinary incontinence

The aim of treatment is to restore urinary continence in a manner that is acceptable to the individual and will enable a restoration of lifestyle.

Adult incontinence can be intensely embarrassing and patients may choose not to volunteer a description of their symptoms. It is, therefore, extremely important that the healthcare professional *asks* about continence. In the acute rehabilitation phase, this will form part of the standard patient assessment. In an outpatient clinic, other symptoms may be more prominent and continence can be overlooked.

For the majority of patients, investigation and management can be completed within a nurse-led continence clinic with the option of referring patients to a specialist center if indicated. The holistic approach of rehabilitation staff allows full assessment of the multitude of factors that may affect continence:

- bladder function
- bowel function
- mobility
- upper limb function
- sensory neglect
- visuospatial problems or neglect
- dysphasia
- cognitive function
- type of clothing
- presence of a carer
- location of toilet
- ease of access to toilet.

History

The initial assessment phase involves establishing the pattern of voiding, associated problems, and fluid consumption (Table 15.1). Questions must be phrased in a manner that is clear and gives the patient a framework in which to describe their problems without embarrassment (Table 15.2).

Table 15.1 Guide to history taking in the continence assessment: these specific aspects of continence and associated factors must be clarified

Characteristic	Features
Urinary frequency	Day and night frequencies
Sense of urgency	
Leakage	Spontaneous with awareness; spontaneous without awareness; in response to coughing or straining
Hesitancy	
Dribbling	
Sensation of incomplete emptying	
Dysuria	
Discolored, smelly or cloudy urine	
Fluid intake	Volume, type
Bowel function	
Obstetric history	
Other morbidities	Prostatic disease, diabetes, previous pelvic surgery

Table 15.2 Examples of phrasing questions about continence and establishing the pattern of micturition

How often do you need to pass water during the day?

When you feel you have to pass water, do you have to get to the toilet quickly or are you able to hang on?

Do you ever have accidents where the water comes away before you can get to the toilet?

Do you sometimes find you are wet without having felt a need to pass water?

Do you ever pass water when you cough or laugh or stand up?

Are you able to start to pass water straight away when you are in the toilet, or do you sometimes have difficulty starting to pass water?

Once you have finished passing water, does the stream end completely or do you tend to dribble?

Once you have left the toilet, do you ever get the feeling that you have to go back to pass water again and, if so, do you actually pass a volume of water?

When you are passing water, do you apply any particular techniques? For example, do you have to strain or do you have to press the lower part of your tummy?

At night, do you have to get up to pass water? How many times?

The full assessment cannot be completed in one session. Patients will be asked to complete a fluid input and output chart at home over three or four consecutive days. Valuable information about the pattern and type of fluid consumption is obtained. Simple suggestions such as reducing evening fluids or avoiding caffeine

Time	DAY 1 Fluid	Urine	DAY 2 Fluid	Urine	DAY 3 Fluid	Urine	DAY 4 Fluid	Urine
6 am								
7 am								
8 am	200 coffee	120	200 coffee	180	Coffee 200	150	Coffee 200	120
9 am		50						50
10 am	150 water	50		100		80		80
11 am				50				
Noon	200 tea	80	250 juice		200 coffee	50	200 tea	
1 pm		80		50				100
2 pm	150 coke				150 juice	150	100 juice	50
3 pm		50	150 juice	80				
4 pm	200 tea					80		80
5 pm		120		50	250 tea		200 tea	
6 pm	250 tea	50	250 tea	100				
7 pm						100		50
8 pm		100		50	200 juice		200 tea	
9 pm						150		100
10 pm	250 hot choc	50	250 tea		250 hot choc		200 tea	
11 pm		150		100				125
12 pm		150				100		80
1 am				150				
2 am		100				80		
3 am		80						100
4 am				80		50		
5 am		50						

Fig. 15.3   Fluid input and output chart from a patient with urgency and frequency. This patient had reduced evening fluid intake but despite this had to pass urine three or four times during the night as well as hourly through the day. Measurement of a post-void residual urine will clarify whether this is primarily a voiding or a storage disorder.

may be sufficient to improve matters. Alternatively, it may be evident that the problem requires more detailed analysis and treatment (Fig. 15.3).

A sample of urine will be checked by urinalysis, microscopy, and culture. Hematuria in the absence of infection should be investigated further by referral to a urologist. Physical examination will document neurological status and include abdominal and genital examinations. The prostate must be assessed in men. A vaginal examination in women allows assessment of the pelvic floor musculature in addition to the pelvic viscera. It should be confirmed that women have been included in the cervical screening program within primary care.

Serum urea and electrolytes, full blood count, and serum glucose are measured as a baseline screen.

Considerable information has now been obtained, but the history and the evidence of charts still may be misleading. Urgency frequency and urge incontinence may be the presentation of both voiding and storage disorders. Ultrasound assessment of bladder emptying by measurement of post-void residual urine is essential to clarify the type of disorder.

The problem can now be categorized as a storage disorder or a voiding disorder. A post-void residual volume of greater than 100 ml is an indication that treatment of the voiding disorder is required (Fowler, 1996).

If patients continue to experience problems of leakage of small quantities of urine, there are a variety of continence pads available that will absorb these quantities of urine and are easy and comfortable to use. For men, it is possible to use a convene system and these will be most successful following expert assessment by the continence advisor.

Disorders of storage

Improvement can be effected by bladder retraining and pelvic floor exercises are effective where there is primarily stress incontinence (Jarvis and Millar, 1980; Jarvis, 1993). In neurological disorders, additional intervention is generally necessary and the mainstay of treatment is anticholinergic agents. Oxybutynin is probably the drug of first choice with a starting dose of 2.5 mg twice daily. Side-effects can be troublesome especially dry mouth and constipation. It is contraindicated in narrow-angle glaucoma. Dosage regimens can be adjusted and there is a slow-release preparation that some patients may find useful. Alternatives include tolterodine, propiverine and low-dose tricyclic drugs such as imipramine. It is essential to re-evaluate the patient after initiation of anticholinergic therapy. If symptoms have deteriorated, the post-void residual volume must be checked as anticholinergic agents may exacerbate a voiding disorder. If that is the case, then treatment must be added to deal with this problem (Fowler, 1996).

Disorders of voiding

There is no reliable drug treatment for a voiding disorder and so a physical means of assisting voiding is necessary. This generally involves catheterization, either indwelling or intermittent. Clean intermittent self-catheterization (CISC) can be taught by an experienced nurse in an outpatient setting (Lapides *et al.*, 1972). There is now a wide choice of catheters for CISC; a small gauge is recommended. CISC reduces the risk of infection associated with urinary retention and avoids the complications of a long-term indwelling catheter:

- bypassing of catheter
- small contracted bladder
- bladder calculi
- frequent infection

- blockage of catheter
- urethral damage
- allergic reaction of the skin.

Asymptomatic bacteriuria is not uncommon and is not an indication for antibiotic treatment. CISC does require manual dexterity and an understanding of what is required. An alternative that is effective in some patients with lesser degrees of retention is the Queen Square Bladder Stimulator (Dasgupta *et al.*, 1997). This is a hand-held vibratory device applied to the suprapubic region that triggers detrusor contraction. It has proved to be effective in patients with multiple sclerosis who are still ambulant and have normal suprapubic sensation. Some patients have found that application of the stimulus to the left iliac fossa can help to relieve constipation (Dasgupta *et al.*, 1997).

If CISC is not possible, then an indwelling urethral or suprapubic catheter is necessary. It is important that patients drink at least 2 litres of fluid per day. There are many anecdotal reports of the benefits of cranberry juice in reducing the risk of infection and people often like to take this although there has not been a large-scale randomized control trial of its effectiveness (Henig and Leahy, 2000; Kontiokari *et al.*, 2001). Patients with catheters must be reviewed regularly for the complications listed above. A common problem is bypassing of the catheter secondary to bladder spasm. This may be improved by a change of catheter, reducing the volume in the balloon, and, if necessary, by a small dose of oxybutynin to reduce involuntary detrusor contractions. If symptoms persist, then an ultrasound is required to exclude bladder calculi.

Generally every effort is made to avoid long-term catheterization, but frequent incontinence can be associated with damage to the skin and pressure sores, particularly in an immobile patient. The smell of stale urine is unpleasant and socially unacceptable. There is often a compromise regarding the use of drugs. Drugs that cause drowsiness may aggravate a continence problem yet may be an essential part of general management, for example antispasticity agents such as tizanidine or baclofen. The management of a more severely disabled patient, and particularly one with cognitive problems in addition to physical deficits, may ultimately be a compromise (Andrews, 1994).

Despite all these interventions, incontinence may persist; in which case further investigation and advice is required and referral should be made to a specialist urology department.

Fecal incontinence

Fecal incontinence has been described as having a devastating impact on patients and carers (Nelson *et al.*, 1995; Cooper and Rose, 2000). It is defined as the involuntary loss of stool at any time of life after toilet training.

Incontinence of feces occurring even episodically and rarely can have profound effects on self-confidence, self-image, and ability to participate in the community. It is a major burden for carers and is often associated with nursing home admission.

Prevalence

A community-based study in Wisconsin USA identified 153 out of 6959 individuals with fecal incontinence, giving a population prevalence of 2.2%; 30% of those with anal incontinence were over 65 years and 63% were women. Other associated factors were physical limitations and poor general health. The prevalence of anal incontinence in Wisconsin nursing homes was 39% (Cooper and Rose, 2000).

Neurophysiology

Acceptable bowel and bladder functioning requires integration of the central, peripheral, and autonomic nervous systems. The lower bowel (the colorectum) has an enteric nervous system that coordinates the smooth muscle activity and regulates secretion and absorption. This is a complex network with many different neurotransmitter pathways. It is subject to modulating influence of extrinsic nerves from the sympathetic and parasympathetic systems. The anorectum allows detection of the nature of its contents: whether solid, liquid, or gas. It can allow selective passage of gas and retrograde contractions can occur from rectum to colon for storage once the nature of the material has been determined. The smooth muscle of the internal anal sphincter is supplied by the enteric plexus and is responsible for the anorectal inhibitory reflex. There is also an external striated muscle sphincter that is functionally part of the pelvic floor and under voluntary control.

Herbst *et al.* (1997) undertook a study of ambulatory colonic motility in individuals with fecal incontinence and in healthy controls. They found that in health the left colon has approximately 14 high-pressure propagated waves in a 24-hour period. Most of these waves were associated with eating, waking from sleep, or defaecation, where the pressure wave continued into the rectum. The high-pressure waves did not differ in the patients with urge incontinence. It was postulated that the difference accounting for the incontinence rests in the anal pressure: that is, an inability to increase the anal pressure in response to the high rectal pressure.

Other studies have suggested that passive incontinence (passage of feces without awareness) is associated with internal sphincter dysfunction, and urge incontinence (incontinence despite efforts to postpone defaecation) is related to external sphincter dysfunction (Engel *et al.*, 1995).

Continence is influenced by stool consistency, colorectal activity, and the internal and external sphincters. A number of factors may contribute to bowel incontinence, including previously undetected damage to the sphincters (often secondary to childbirth), reduced rectal sensation, and impaired sacral reflex arcs, resulting in failure of external sphincter muscle recruitment during a rise in intra-abdominal pressure. The incidence of increased bowel frequency and loose bowel actions is also greater in patients with incontinence (Herbst *et al.*, 1997).

Defecation

For defecation to occur, there is a relaxation in the internal anal sphincter in response to a sensation of fullness in the rectum; stretching the anal wall causes reflex relaxation of the internal anal sphincter through the rectoanal inhibitory reflex. This can be overridden by voluntary control via the corticospinal tracts, resulting in contraction of the external sphincter. Maximum contraction of the anal sphincter can be maintained for approximately 60 seconds, but this is usually long enough for the rectal contractions to subside and the associated urge to abate (Craggs and Vaizey, 1999). This allows a postponement of defecation until a socially convenient time. If defecation is deemed appropriate, the external sphincter remains relaxed and the passage of feces occurs as the rectoanal inhibitory reflex allows opening of the anal canal, often assisted by a voluntary Valsalva maneuver. Disturbance of the rectoanal inhibitory reflex may result in obstructed defecation (Krogh *et al.*, 2001). A combination of poor abdominal musculature and failure of the sphincters to relax may occur in suprasacral lesions.

In the brain, the areas associated with defecation are thought to be similar to those involved in urinary continence: the medial prefrontal and the anterior cingulate gyrus. Andrew and Nathan (1964) reported defecation to be affected much less often than micturition in their patients.

Prevalence of fecal incontinence after stroke

In the Copenhagen Stroke Study, 296 (34%) of the 935 patients with stroke had fecal incontinence on admission and 51 had occasional accidents (Nakayama *et al.*, 1997). By the time of discharge, 82% of subjects were fully continent with regard to bowel function but 12% (84 individuals) still had fecal incontinence. At the six-month follow-up, this had reduced to 5% (24 individuals).

There was a large overlap of patients with urinary and fecal incontinence: 84% of those with initial urinary incontinence also had fecal incontinence and 98% of those with fecal incontinence had urinary incontinence.

Risk factors for incontinence post-stroke

Nakayama *et al.* (1997) found the risk factors for fecal incontinence post-stroke to be similar to those for urinary incontinence (p. 423).

Management of the patient with bowel incontinence

It is often easier to manipulate bowel control than bladder. Routine assessment of bowel function should be a standard part of rehabilitation assessment. Many problems are simple to sort out, but where there is ongoing difficulty referral to a continence specialist is helpful especially as bladder and bowel dysfunction often coexist. Table 15.3 lists useful questions for assessing bowel function. Symptoms suggestive of additional pathology such as passage of blood or a change to a stable pattern of bowel management should be referred to a colorectal specialist for further investigation as other pathologies such as colitis or a neoplasm may arise.

The commonest problem is undoubtedly constipation, not infrequently accompanied by episodes of fecal overflow (that is passage of liquid feces around a hard bolus) or urge incontinence.

The aim should be to regularize the bowel routine and achieve adequate evacuation. This may involve a combination of dietary manipulation, attention to fluid intake, use of laxatives and/or enemas or suppositories and housing adaptations to allow easier access to the toilet.

Laxatives

Bulk-forming laxatives

The bulk-forming laxatives soften stool, increase fecal mass and thereby stimulate peristalsis, but if peristalsis is impaired and there is inadequate fluid intake they can contribute to impaction. They may take several days to produce an effect when

Table 15.3 Assessment of bowel function

Has there been a change in bowel habit?
How frequently does defaecation occur?
Ability to distinguish flatus from stool
Ability to sense a full bowel and respond appropriately
Does anything trigger a bowel action, e.g. first thing in the morning, or a meal?
Is there any incontinence or soiling?
Is there urgency: is it possible to postpone even for a short period of time?
Is the individual aware of the need to defecate or of the process of defecation?
What volume of fecal material is passed?
What is the consistency of the faeces. (We have found it very helpful to show people a copy
    of the Bristol stool scale. This usually produces a laugh and facilitates the discussion
    that otherwise patients and carers often find extremely embarrassing and difficult.)
Is any blood or mucus passed?
How mobile is the patient?
What is the patient's manual dexterity like?
Where is the toilet: does accessing a toilet involve a lengthy procedure of hoisting,
    stairlift, and more transfers, by which time it is too late?

first started. Examples include bran and ispaghula husk (e.g. Fybogel). Before initiating treatment, it is worth ascertaining whether dietary manipulation is possible, i.e. increasing the fiber content of the diet.

Stimulation laxatives

Stimulation laxatives (e.g. senna or docusate sodium) increase intestinal motility and may cause intestinal cramp. Although they are generally not recommended for long-term use, people with neurological disease often find they are a valuable adjunct to bowel management once the effective dose has been found.

Osmotic laxatives

Osmotic laxatives retain fluid in the bowel. One of the commonest is lactulose and this can be useful in mild constipation; its main side-effect is flatulence. Polyethylene glycol has proved useful both in relieving chronic constipation and in maintaining regular bowel habit.

Suppositories/enemas

For more severe constipation and where there is difficulty evacuating the bowel, local stimulation of the rectum may be necessary. It may be possible to achieve a regular regimen of controlled defecation with a combination of an oral agent and a rectal preparation.

Constipating agents

If the problem is one of frequent and urgent passage of loose stool then it may be helped by an agent such as loperamide. It is always important to ensure that constipation does not ensue.

Further approaches

If continence cannot be achieved by these interventions, a more specialist assessment should be sought from a colorectal specialist. As with urinary incontinence, a considerable amount of help can be given within a rehabilitation department.

Summary

Promoting continence should be high priority in every rehabilitation unit. This can be assisted by an audit scheme (Brocklehurst, 1998). A nurse-led continence clinic provides an ideal service for patients and carers. The key message is that this distressing symptom, once identified, can be treated.

REFERENCES

Andrew, J. and Nathan, P. W. (1964). Lesions of the anterior frontal lobes and disturbances of micturition and defaecation. *Brain* **87**: 233–262.

Andrews K. (1994). Bladder disorders in brain damage. In *Handbook of Neuro-Urology*, Ch. 10, ed. D. N. Rushton. New York: Marcel Dekker.

Badlani, G. H., Forey, C. J., and Snyder, J. A. (1987). Evaluation of urinary dysfunction in the elderly. *Semin Urol* **5**: 87–93.

Anon. (1990). The standardization of terminology of lower urinary tract function. *Br J Obstet Gynaecol* suppl. **6**: 1–16.

Blok, B., Sturms, L., and Holstege, G. (1998). Brain activation during micturition in women. *Brain* **121**: 2033–2042.

Brittain, K. R., Peet, S. M., and Castleden, C. M. (1998). Stroke and incontinence. *Stroke* **29**: 524–528.

Brocklehurst, J. C. (1993). Urinary incontinence in the community: analysis of a MORI poll. *BMJ* **306**: 832–834.

(1998). Promoting continence. *In Clinical Audit Scheme for the Management of Urinary and Fecal Incontinence.* London: Royal College of Physicians.

Brocklehurst, J. C., Andrews, K., Richards, B., and Laycock, P. J. (1985). Incidence and correlates of incontinence in stroke patients. *J Am Geriatr Soc* **33**: 540–542.

Burney, T. L., Senapati, M. S., Desai, S., Choudhary, S. T., and Badlani, G. H. (1996). Effects of cerebrovascular accident on micturition. *Urol Clin North Am* **23**: 483–490.

Cooper, Z. R. and Rose, S. (2000). Fecal incontinence: a clinical approach. *Mt Sinai J Med* **67**: 96–105.

Craggs M. D. and Vaizey C. J. (1999). Neurophysiology of the bladder and bowel. In *Neurology of Bladder Bowel and Sexual Dysfunction*, ed. C. J. Fowler Woburn, MA: Butterworth Heinemann.

Dasgupta, P., Haslam, R., and Goodwin Fowler, C. J. (1997). The Queen Square bladder stimulator: a device for assisting emptying of the neurogenic bladder. *Br J Urol* **80**: 234–237.

Engel, A. F., Kamm, M. A., Bartram, C. I., and Nicholls, R. J. (1995). Relationship of symptoms in fecal incontinence to specific sphincter abnormalities. *Int J Colorectal Dis* **10**: 152–155.

Fowler, C. J. (1996). Investigation of the neurogenic bladder. *J Neurol Neurosurg Psychiat* **60**: 6–13.

Fowler, C. J. and Chandiramani, V. A. (2000). Neurological disturbances of bladder and bowel. *Medicine* **28**): 79–81.

Garrett, V., Scott, J., Costich, J., *et al.* (1989). Bladder emptying assessment in stroke patients. *Arch Phys Med Rehabil* **70**: 40–43.

Glickman, S. and Kamm, M. A. (1996). Bowel dysfunction in spinal cord injury patients. *Lancet* **347**: 1651–1653.

Henig, Y. S. and Leahy, M. M. (2000). Cranberry juice and urinary tract health: science supports folklore. *Nutrition* **16**: 684–687.

Herbst, F., Kamm, M. A., Morris, G P., *et al.* (1997). Gastro-intestinal transit and prolonged ambulatory colonic mobility in health and fecal incontinence. *Gut* **42**: 381–389.

Jarvis G. J. (1993). Urinary incontinence in the community. *BMJ* **306**: 809–810.

Jarvis G. J. and Millar, D. R. (1980). Controlled trial of bladder drill for detrusor instability. *BMJ* **281**: 1322–1323.

Khan, Z., Heranu, J., Yang, W., *et al.* (1981). Predictive correlation of urodynamic dysfunction and brain injury after cerebrovascular accident. *J Urol* **126**: 86–88.

Khan, Z., Starer, P., Yang, W., and Bhola, A. (1990). Analysis of voiding disorders in patients with cerebrovascular accident. *Urology* **35**: 263–270.

Kontiokari, T., Sundqvist, K., Nuuntinen, M., *et al.* (2001). Randomised trial of cranberry–ligonberry juice and *Lactobacillus* GC drink for the prevention of urinary tract infections in women. *B M J* **322**: 1–5

Krogh, K., Christensen, P., and Laurberg, S. (2001). Colorectal symptoms in patients with neurological diseases. *Acta Neurol Scand* **103**: 335–343.

Kuroiwa, Y., Tohgi, H., and Itoh, M. (1987). Frequency and urgency of micturition in hemiplegic patients: relationship to hemispheric laterality of lesions. *J Neurol* **234**: 100–102.

Lapides, J., Dolmo, C., Silber, S. J., and Lowe, B. S. (1972). Clean intermittent self catheterization in the treatment of urinary tract disease. *J Urol* **107**: 458–461.

Leigh, R. J. and Turnberg, L. A. (1982). Fecal incontinence: the unvoiced symptom. *Lancet*, **i**: 1349–1351.

Marincov, S. P. and Badlani, G. (2001). Voiding and sexual dysfunction after cerebrovascular accidents. *J Urol* **165**: 359–370.

Maurice-Williams, R. S. (1974). Micturition symptoms in frontal tumours. *J Neurol Neurosurg Psychiatry* **37**: 431–436.

Nakayama, H., Jorgensen, H. S., Pedersen, P. M., Raaschou, H. O., and Olsen, T. S. (1997). Prevalence and risk factors of incontinence after stroke. The Copenhagen Stroke Study. *Stroke* **28**: 58–62.

Nelson, R., Norton, N., Cautley, E., and Furner, S. (1995). Community-based prevalence of anal incontinence. *JAMA* **274**: 559–561.0

Sakakibara R. and Fowler C. J. (1999). Cerebral control of bladder, bowel and sexual function and effects of brain disease. In *Neurology of Bladder Bowel and Sexual Dysfunction*, ch. 14, ed. C. J. Fowler. Woburn, MA: Butterworth Heinemann.

Sakakibara, R., Haltori, T., Yasuda, K., and Yananishi, T. (1996a). Micturitional disturbance after acute hemispheric stroke: analysis of lesion site by CT and MRI. *J Neurol Sci* **137**: 47–56. (1996b). Micturitional disturbance and the pontine tegmental lesion: urodynamics and MRI analyses of vascular cases. *J Neurol Sci* **141**: 105–110.

Taub, N A., Wolfe, C .D., Richardson, E., and Burney, P. G. J. (1994). Predicting the disability of first-time stoke sufferers at 1 year. *Stroke* **25**: 352–357.

Thomas, T .M., Plymat, K .R., and Meade, T. W. (1980). Prevalence of urinary incontinence. *BMJ* **281**: 1243–1245.

Tsuchida, S., Noto, H., Yamaguchi, O., *et al.* (1983). Urodynamic studies on hemiplegic patients after cerebrovascular accident. *Urology* **21**: 315–318.

Wade, D. and Langton-Hewer, R. (1985). Outlook after an acute stroke: urinary incontinence and loss of consciousness compared in 532 patients. *Q J Med* **56**: 601–608.

Yarnell, J. W. G., Voyle, G. J., Richards, C. J., and Stephenson, T. P. (1981). The prevalence and severity of urinary incontinence in women. *J Epidemiol Community Health* **35**: 71–74.

16

Sex and relationships following stroke

Barbara J. Chandler

Hunters Moor Regional Neuorehabilitation Centre, Newcastle upon Tyne, UK

Introduction

Sexuality and the ability to form and sustain an intimate relationship is a fundamental aspect of human life. It results from a complex interplay of physical, psychological, and emotional functioning within a social and cultural context. This chapter reviews the prevalence of sexual problems in the general population, the population with neurological disability, and those specifically with stroke. Sexual development and the physiology of sexual responsiveness are discussed followed by a discussion of relationship functioning. Finally, approaches to dealing with sex and relationship problems are discussed.

Prevalence of sexual dysfunction

In the general population

Dunn *et al.*, (1998, 1999) carried out an anonymous postal questionnaire survey to examine the prevalence of sexual problems. From 4000 questionnaires, replies were received from 789 men and 979 women. The median age of the responders was 50 years, of whom 34% of the men and 41% of women reported a current sexual problem. The most common problems were erectile dysfunction and premature ejaculation in men and vaginal dryness and infrequent orgasm in women. Frequency of problems increased with age for men, but not women. Over half the responders reporting a sexual problem indicated they would like to receive professional help, but only 10% of these had received help.

Erectile dysfunction was most strongly associated with prostatic problems, but also with hypertension and diabetes mellitus. The most common associated factor with premature ejaculation was anxiety. In women, the most prominent association with arousal, orgasmic, and enjoyment problems was relationship difficulties, but anxiety and depression were also associated. The authors summarized that

Recovery after Stroke, ed. Michael P. Barnes, Bruce H. Dobkin and Julien Bogousslavsky. Published by Cambridge University Press. © Cambridge University Press 2005.

sexual problems clustered with self-reported physical problems in men whereas, in women, the association was with psychological and social problems.

A similar study in the USA amongst 1749 women and 1410 men, aged between 18 and 59 years, found sexual dysfunction amongst 43% of the female respondents and 31% of the male respondents. They described sexual dysfunction as being highly associated with negative experiences within sexual relationships and with overall well-being (Laumann *et al.*, 1999).

In neurological disability

Detailed studies of sexual functioning among various groups with neurological disability have disclosed a high prevalence of sexual dysfunction. For example in multiple sclerosis, almost two-thirds of men and over one-third of women described unsatisfactory sex lives (Lilius *et al.*, 1976). Commonly associated problems were muscle weakness, spasticity, loss of sexual drive, and relationship factors. One study amongst male survivors of traumatic brain injury identified a prevalence of sexual dysfunction of 50% (O'Carroll *et al.*, 1991). Kreuter *et al.* (1998) in a review of 92 men and women after a traumatic brain injury and found that at least one-third had erectile, ejaculatory, or orgasmic dysfunction, 47% had reduced frequency of intercourse, and 16% reduced sexual interest. The factors related to change in their sex lives included lack of an available partner (31% of the sample) and poor self-esteem. The impact of the cognitive and behavioral sequelae of brain injury on intimate relationships is high (Rosenbaum & Najenson, 1976; Oddy *et al.*, 1978, Elliott & Biever, 1996). In Parkinson's disease, a similar prevalence of sexual problems of 1 in 2 has been identified (Brown *et al.*, 1990).

A common theme emerging in many studies is the small number of people with sexual problems who seek help, and the lack of availability of such help – often caused by both a reluctance on the part of the patient to raise the issue and a reticence on the part of the health professional to be proactive in offering such help (Young, 1984; Finger *et al.*, 1992; Weston, 1993; Sawyer, 1996).

Szasz *et al.* (1984), in a study of people with multiple sclerosis, distinguished between the *presence* of a dysfunction and *concern* about the dysfunction. Approximately 50% of the study sample identified a change in sexual function. Using the same assessment scale, a study of a population with various neurological problems attending a neurological rehabilitation center revealed similar figures (Chandler & Brown 1998) (Fig. 16.1). Expression of concern could be interpreted as those who would wish for help with their problems, and this amounted to 25% of these outpatients. However, the figures cannot be viewed as true prevalence figures, as the response rate was low, with only 92 of 398 patients agreeing to take part in the study.

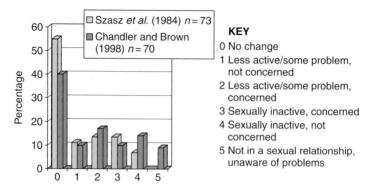

Fig. 16.1   Sexual problems in neurological disability assessed using the Szasz Sexual Function Scale
(Szasz *et al.*, 1984)

Nosek *et al.* (1996) undertook a review of existing research on sexuality in women with disabilities. The study was carried out by questionnaire, which was sent to 1150 women with physical disability and they were each asked to choose an able-bodied friend who also filled in a questionnaire. People with significant cognitive deficits were excluded. The age range was 18–65 years and 475 women responded with 425 able-bodied associates. Disabilities varied but included spinal cord injury, polio, muscular dystrophy, and cerebral palsy. There were significantly higher values for level of sexual activity, sexual response, and satisfaction for the able-bodied group. There was no significant difference in sexual desire between the two groups. Sexual desire was found to decrease with age, which is a well-recognized phenomenon. The strongest predictor of sexual activity was living with a "significant other." Women with disabilities who had a more positive sexual self-image, perceiving themselves to be "approachable by potential romantic partners," had higher levels of sexual activity. There was no association between level of sexual activity and severity of disability. Three hypotheses emerged from the study. First, there are significant differences in socio-sexual behavior of women who have physical disabilities compared with women who do not have disabilities. Second, sexual functioning in women with disabilities is significantly related to age at onset of disability; and, third, psychological factors explain more of the variance in sexual functioning of women with physical disabilities than do disability, social, and environmental factors. In summary, social status and psychological variables were found to be the best predictors of sexual satisfaction.

Hypersexuality

Although reduced sexual drive is the more common finding in disease or trauma affecting the brain, increased interest in sex can occur. In Parkinson's disease, hypersexuality has been associated with dopaminergic agents. Following brain injury, sexual disinhibition has been found more commonly in patients with frontal lobe damage (Elliot & Biever, 1996). Monga *et al.* (1986a, b) described three patients who displayed hypersexuality following stroke. All three had temporal lobe lesions and had experienced post-stroke seizures. The authors drew comparisons with the animal work of Kluver and Bucy (1937), who described a syndrome of increased sexual activity, changes in dietary habits, and antisocial behavior following bilateral temporal lobectomy.

After stroke

Bray *et al.* (1981) in a study of 35 patients pre- and post-stroke observed that no significant difference in sexual interest or desire was reported at either time, but there were significant levels of sexual dysfunction post-stroke. For example, over 50% of men had erectile dysfunction. In this study, over 70% of the subjects believed that sexual function was of importance to themselves.

Sjögren *et al.* (1983) examined the effect of antihypertensive medication and testosterone levels on sexual functioning. No association was identified. They concluded "sexual dysfunction in hemiplegics may rather be explained in terms of coping than by endocrine deficits or by anti-hypertensive treatment."

As part of a two-year follow-up study of patients who had sustained a stroke, Monga *et al.* (1986b) explored sexual functioning. A group of 78 men and 35 women were interviewed at 12 months following discharge from a rehabilitation unit; 63 of the men and 25 of the women were married. There was a reduction or deterioration in all parameters of sexual activity; for example, those reporting a "normal" sexual drive before stroke included 75% of the men and 60% of the women and this decreased to 21% of men and 34% of women post-stroke. Other parameters were erectile ability and vaginal lubrication, frequency of sexual intercourse, ability to ejaculate and achieve orgasm, enjoyment of sexual activity, and sexual satisfaction. Only 7% of the women identified having any sexual problems prior to stroke, and none of the men. However, 58% of men and 48% of women assessed themselves as having a problem following the stroke. The assessment of sexual problems pre-stroke was remarkably low and could possibly reflect a tendency to forget premorbid difficulties. The most commonly reported cause of sexual inactivity was fear of another stroke, together with a belief that sexual activity would adversely increase blood pressure.

Korpelainen *et al.* (1998) undertook a questionnaire study about pre- and post-stroke sexual function and habits amongst participants in a stroke adjustment course with 192 patients and 94 spouses participating. The majority of patients experienced a reduction in libido, coital frequency, sexual arousal (assessed by erectile function, orgasmic ability, vaginal lubrication), and sexual satisfaction. The most important factors associated with these reductions were general attitude towards sexuality, fear of erectile failure, inability to discuss sexuality and unwillingness to participate in sexual activity, and degree of functional disability. Spouses also described a significant decline in libido, sexual activity, and sexual satisfaction. From this study, it was apparent that sexual dysfunction post-stroke has a multifactorial etiology, including both organic and psychosocial factors.

Other studies have supported this hypothesis. For example, Boldrini *et al.* (1991) in a study of 86 patients following stroke concluded that "clinical factors do not seem to play a crucial role in determining these changes, which may be better explained in terms of maladjustment attributable to psychologic and inter-personal factors."

Kimura *et al.* (2001)undertook a prevalence study of sexual dysfunction following stroke involving 100 subjects (75 male, 25 female) with the intention of exploring the relationship between sexual dysfunction, neuropsychiatric impairment, and stroke characteristics. With regard to pre-stroke status, 21% of the males and 20% of the females reported experiencing dissatisfaction with sexual function and 10.6% males and 28% females reported experiencing reduced libido. Following stroke, the prevalence of these dysfunctions increased to 58.6% of males and 44% of females experiencing dissatisfaction with sexual function and 26.6% of males and 24% of females experiencing reduced libido. In the group as a whole, those with sexual dysfunction had significantly more depression; amongst the men, those with sexual dysfunction had significantly greater impairment of activities of daily living. Interestingly, based on logistic regression, predictors for sexual dysfunction following stroke included depression and left hemisphere lesions. The authors suggested that treatment of depression may have a beneficial effect on sexual function, but this is a hypothesis that requires further testing.

In summary, there is undoubtedly a decline in sexual activity following stroke and the reasons for this are multifactorial (Humphrey, 1985):

- disruption of the normal rhythm of married life
- side-effects of medication
- depression in either partner
- anxiety
- physical aversion
- the disabled partner's entrapment in a dependent role.

Sexual development

Sexuality encompasses a much broader concept than ability to have sexual intercourse. Feeling comfortable within a gender role and the ability to form and maintain intimate relationships are important aspects of sexual functioning. Anecdotal observation suggests that within a hospital or rehabilitation setting encouraging individuals to take an interest in their personal appearance can raise morale.

Sexual development begins *in utero* and depends on the genetic makeup of the individual and the hormonal environment. At birth, a gender is assigned and sexual development continues along three main strands (Bancroft 1989).

1 Sexual differentiation

2 Sexual responsiveness

3 Capacity to form intimate dyadic relationships.

With the onset of puberty, these separate developmental strands become integrated. Throughout life, the degree of integration may be challenged and disrupted by events in the domains of physical and mental health, emotional well-being, and social functioning. Identifying the determinants of sexual or relationship dysfunction will allow an appropriate therapeutic strategy to be planned. Bancroft (1989) described the many and varied functions of human sexual behavior, which extend beyond the biological function of reproduction and include maintenance of self-esteem, exertion of power, fostering intimacy and bonding a dyadic relationship, giving and receiving pleasure, reduction of tension, risk taking/excitement, and material gain.

Sexual response cycle and classification of dysfunction

Masters and Johnson (1966) categorized the sexual response cycle into four phases.

1 Excitement

2 Plateau

3 Orgasm

4 Resolution.

This allowed some categorization of disorders; for example erectile dysfunction, failure of vaginal lubrication, and dyspareunia are disorders of the excitement phase. Orgasmic and ejaculatory dysfunctions can be categorized in the orgasmic phase. This has remained a useful classification, particularly as a more detailed understanding of the neurophysiological basis of the sexual response has occurred. However, a very common disorder amongst women and amongst patients with neurological conditions is low sexual desire. Kaplan (1974) took account of this in a simplified three-phase cycle.

1 Desire

2 Excitement

3 Orgasm.

Figure 16.2 illustrates the relationship between sexual desire and sexual arousal.

Male disorders

The most common sexual dysfunction in men is erectile dysfunction (Bancroft & Coles, 1976). There is no doubt that treatment has been revolutionized by the advent of oral medication. The huge amount of media coverage has also given a

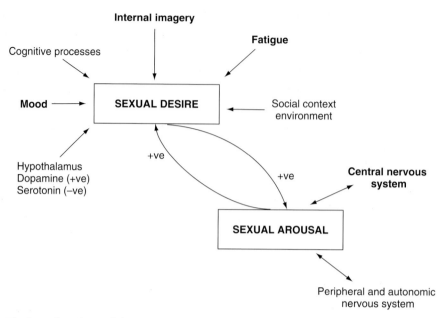

Fig. 16.2   The interplay of sexual desire and sexual arousal

positive message that erectile dysfunction is a valid concern to discuss with health professionals. Nevertheless, it is important that the advent of a simple pill does not obscure the need for holistic assessment. Medication may restore erectile ability but will not, on its own, cure a deep-seated psychosexual problem or a damaged relationship (Wise, 1999). Another common disorder is premature ejaculation, and this generally responds well to psychosexual intervention, especially in the context of a relationship with a supportive partner. Medication, such as the selective serotonin reuptake inhibitors, which are known to retard ejaculation, may help but can generally be avoided.

Options in "physical management" of erectile dysfunction include drugs such as oral sildenafil, sublingual apomorphine, perurethral alprostadil or intracavernosal alprostadil (Borg, 1998). Drugs may be contraindicated for various reasons; for example, sildenafil must not be used alongside nitrate therapy. In addition, some people prefer not to take medications. The vacuum constriction device, therefore, remains a useful and still popular treatment (Oakley and Moore, 1998).

For many patients with neurological disorders, a combination of psychological and physical treatment is necessary in the management of sexual dysfunction.

Female disorders

The classification of female sexual disorders has, until recently, attracted less attention and has reflected the lack of understanding of the basis of the disorders.

An international consensus development conference on female sexual disorders (Basson *et al.*, 2000) undertook the task of developing a classification. In their report, the authors stated that "female sexual dysfunction is a multi-causal and multi-dimensional problem combining biological, psychological and inter-personal determinants." The results were that the major categories of sexual dysfunction within the World Health Organization (WHO) ICD-10 (WHO, 1992) and the American Psychiatric Association DSM-IV (1994) classifications were preserved but were expanded to encompass fully the spectrum of female disorder. For example, the definition of hypoactive sexual desire was broadened to include "lack of receptivity to sexual activity" and this involved a persistent lack of desire and resulting personal distress. The aspect of personal distress was considered an essential element. For some women, low sexual desire would not be identified as a problem.

Physiology of sexual arousal

Biological mechanisms of sexual arousal and orgasm in women have been less extensively studied than male responses. Basson *et al.* (2000) commented that, "the neurophysiology of the female sexual response including the role of neurotransmitters and local vasoactive substances in determining vascular smooth muscle tone, vasodilatation and vaginal lubrication, has not been adequately studied. . . . the role of steroid hormones in the modulation of sexual desire and arousal in women is not well understood." By contrast, there is much greater understanding of the responses in men. For example, erection is a clear neurovascular event. The blood supply to the penis derives from paired pudendal arteries, which are terminal branches of the internal iliac arteries. The erectile tissue of the penis consists of three longitudinal structures known as the corpora, which consist of blood-filled spaces (sinusoids) and numerous anastomotic channels connecting the small arteries of the penis. The walls of the sinusoids contain smooth muscle and fibroelastic tissue. The corpora are surrounded by a layer of fibrous tissue, the tunica albuginea. The venous drainage is via small veins within the sinusoids, which coalesce to form emissary veins that pass through the tunica albuginea and drain into the deep dorsal vein of the penis.

In the flaccid state, the corporeal smooth muscle is contracted and the blood flow restricted. Stimulation of the erectile parasympathetic pathway releases neurotransmitters causing cavernous smooth muscle relaxation and blood flow into the sinusoidal spaces, with consequent expansion and compression of the veins deep to the tunica albuginea, thus obstructing venous outflow. Both reflex and psychogenic mechanisms of erection occur. Reflex erections arise in response to stimulation of the genitalia, with afferent impulses travelling in the somatic pudendal nerve (S_2, S_3, S_4); the efferent pathway is in the parasympathetic nerves (S_2, S_3, S_4). Psychogenic erections occur in response to audiovisual or olfactory stimuli or fantasy. The pathway involves long tracts connecting the cortex and spinal cord with the sympathetic nervous system. It has also been identified that sympathetic pathways are important for detumescence.

Studies of supraspinal pathways have been more difficult, and most of the information is from animal studies, although with the advent of dynamic scanning, there is greater potential for developing our understanding. Hypothalamic and limbic pathways are known to be important, and studies of neurotransmitters have been undertaken in animals. For example, dopamine in the hypothalamus is known to modulate erection (de Groat 1994). Single-photon emission computed tomography has shown an increase in activity in the right frontal lobe during ejaculation in healthy males but no focal activation in the somatosensory cortex of the genital projection area. This was interpreted to suggest that the right prefrontal cortex was important for the emotional responses of male sexuality (Sakakibara and Fowler, 1999).

Neurotransmitters and drugs

In humans, the effects of drugs that modulate neurotransmitters can be observed. There are a number of reports of increased sex drives in patients with Parkinson's disease following treatment with dopaminergic agents (Goodwin, 1971; Weinman and Ruskin, 1994) and apomorphine is now a recognized treatment for erectile dysfunction. The selective serotonin reuptake inhibitors, a group of antidepressants, may cause retarded ejaculation or anorgasmia, and serotonin is known to have an inhibitory effect on sexual desire.

It is known that human cavernous tissue can synthesize various prostaglandins, and prostaglandin E_1 can produce relaxation. The mechanism is possibly through increasing intracellular cyclic AMP, which inhibits calcium channels, thereby reducing intracellular calcium and causing relaxation. This is the basis of the use of alprostadil. Sildenafil is a selective phosphodiesterase 5 inhibitor. Sexual stimulation leads to a release of nitrous oxide from endothelial cells and non-adrenergic non-cholinergic nerve endings, which, in turn, stimulates cyclic GMP release. Sildenafil acts by raising levels of cyclic GMP. It is recognized that there are strong similarities in the neurophysiological basis of the sexual response in women and, therefore, the possibility that drugs such as sildenafil may affect certain disorders of female sexual functioning has been raised. It is important to note that, despite media speculation, the role of drugs such as sildenafil is to affect the final common pathway of erectile ability and not to affect the much earlier phase of the sexual response cycle, namely sexual drive or sexual desire.

Endocrine system

The hormonal environment also plays a part in sexual dysfunction. It is known that levels of oxytocin rise during sexual arousal in women. Sexual desire may vary with the menstrual cycle. Prolactin inhibits sexual drive and may be responsible for the reduced sexual responsiveness during lactation. In men, reduced testosterone level is associated with low sexual drive but has a less direct effect on erectile dysfunction. Some studies have suggested that hypothalamic hypogonadism may be a contributor to sexual problems in post-traumatic brain injury (Clark *et al.*, 1988).

Intimate relationships

The intimate relationship between two people is the context within which the greater part of sexual expression occurs. Other than in masturbation and fantasy, sex is experienced within a relationship (Neumann, 1979). As a relationship forms, the individual brings into it a number of functional parameters that contribute to the formation of the relationship. These parameters are given expression through thoughts, behaviors, and emotions. Each individual has a history in terms of upbringing and life events. They will have a number of assumptions, some of which may have little factual basis. Each individual has a set of needs, fears, expectations, and characteristic ways of behaving. A relationship can be challenged by disruption of any functional area, (Fig. 16.3). In order to understand the basis of a sexual dysfunction within a relationship, it is important to understand the wider aspects of that relationship and the context within which the relationship exists, including family and sociocultural environment (Spence, 1991).

The increased ease of access to treatment for erectile dysfunction has resulted in some challenges in the relationship domain. A not uncommon scenario is a patient with such dysfunction who describes his partner as very supportive and understanding. In practice, the erectile dysfunction may be a relief to a partner who has low sexual desire; so, in the context of an undemanding sexual partner, this does not create a problem. Once the erectile dysfunction has been treated, this may unmask the attitude of the partner towards sexual intercourse and produce an imbalance in the relationship. Conversely, where sexual intimacy is the only form of intimate communication, disruption in sexual function may have a substantial impact on the functioning of the relationship. Bancroft (1989) viewed the complex psychosomatic influences on sexual functioning as an interconnected circle of events. Each individual's sexual identity is unique and, therefore, the psychosomatic circle is also unique to each individual and, in turn, influences the functioning of the dyadic relationship (Fig. 16.4). Many factors influence sexual functioning at the cognitive and emotional points in the circle. Three examples are considered here.

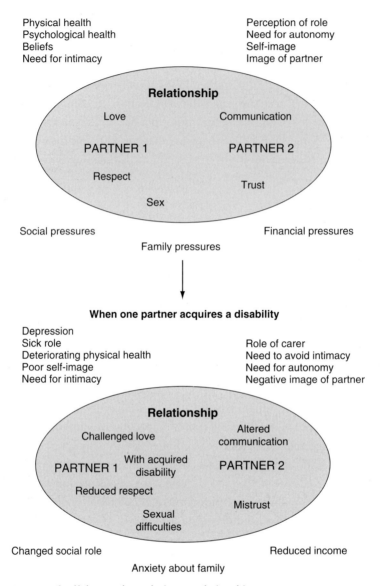

Physical health
Psychological health
Beliefs
Need for intimacy

Perception of role
Need for autonomy
Self-image
Image of partner

Relationship

Love

Communication

PARTNER 1

PARTNER 2

Respect

Trust

Sex

Social pressures

Financial pressures

Family pressures

When one partner acquires a disability

Depression
Sick role
Deteriorating physical health
Poor self-image
Need for intimacy

Role of carer
Need to avoid intimacy
Need for autonomy
Negative image of partner

Relationship

Challenged love

Altered
communication

PARTNER 1   With acquired
disability

PARTNER 2

Reduced respect

Mistrust

Sexual
difficulties

Changed social role

Reduced income

Anxiety about family

Fig. 16.3   Aspects of self that are brought into a relationship

Anxiety

Although anxiety does not inevitably impair sexual response and, in some situations, may enhance arousal (Bancroft, 1989), it is known to be a contributory factor to the development of some sexual dysfunctions, such as sexual aversion disorders, vaginismus, erectile dysfunction, and dyspareunia (Spence, 1991). Reducing anxiety will play a significant part in therapy (Kaplan, 1974; Masters and Johnson, 1996). Studies have shown that, following stroke, there is a very

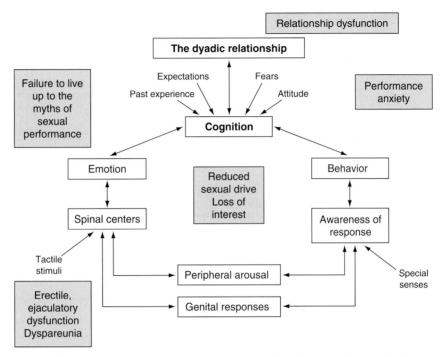

Fig. 16.4   The role of the nervous system in sexual experience. This illustrates the complex interplay within the nervous system that allows psychological and physical factors to interact. Pathology can arise at any point of the cycle. Dysfunctions are given in grey boxes. (Adapted from Bancroft, 1989)

specific fear of precipitating a further catastrophic event through sexual activity. Studies have shown that the cardiac changes associated with sexual activity are modest and similar to the changes that would occur on climbing two flights of stairs (Larson *et al.*, 1980; Muller, 1999). Education and reassurance is, therefore, possible.

Expectation

Unrealistic expectations of what represents a "successful" sex life can result in a cycle of failure. Stanley (1981a) described the concept of "normal sex" that couples present as their goal: "an erect penis entering a lubricated vagina, giving orgasm in both partners, preferably simultaneously is a typical picture. Anything short of this achievement is perceived as failure." The norm of sexual responsiveness within a dyadic relationship is probably unique to each couple, but their perception of the norm may enhance or detract from their sex life, depending on whether the reality of their experience is in accordance with their life expectations. One important aspect of working with individuals and couples is to explore their understanding of sexual expression and ascertain their goals. Many myths exist (Zilbergeld, 1978; DeLoache and Greer, 1981; Guirgius, 1991; Spence, 1991), such as:

- physical contact must always lead to sexual expression
- sexual activity should always involve sexual intercourse
- sexual activity involves a fixed path that should always end in simultaneous orgasm
- a man cannot be in love and fail to get an erection with his partner
- sex must be natural and spontaneous
- all couples have sexual intercourse several times per week
- if sex is not good, something must be wrong with the relationship.

A useful model to discuss with couples was proposed by Stanley (1981b), who described the sexual response cycle in terms of a ladder, beginning with no sexual thoughts and ascending through various levels of excitement to orgasm and resolution. Each individual has their own ladder and can ascend and descend to various levels as wished. Each level may be enjoyed in its own right.

Past experience

Studies have shown that one of the factors predicting resumption of a satisfactory sex life is satisfaction with premorbid sex life and relationship functioning (Bowers *et al.*, 1971, Miller *et al.*, 1981; Bancroft, 1993). Relationships formed prior to the onset of disease or disability may be more adversely affected than those formed subsequently because of the number of adjustments that must be made. Mona *et al.* (1994) found that sexual self-esteem was lower in individuals who acquired their disability later in life than in individuals who acquired their disability at a younger age. Traumatic events in childhood such as sexual or physical abuse may affect the ability of individuals to form intimate relationships and respond sexually (Jehu, 1989; Cotgrove and Kolvin, 1996).

The intimate relationship and neurological disability

The dynamics of a relationship are substantially altered by disease or disability, (Fig. 16.3). One of the greatest changes that may occur for a couple is the change from being *equal partners* to *carer* and *cared for*.

Some couples may experience a deepening and strengthening of their relationship in response to the change. Kreuter *et al.* (1994) in a study of 49 partners of patients with spinal cord injuries found that nearly half considered their current sex life to be as good as or better than their previous sex life. Some of the reasons cited were increased playfulness, prolonged foreplay, and feelings of sexual equality. The authors speculate that focusing on sensuality rather than achievement in sexual expression may have contributed to the feelings of sexual equality: moving away from performance goals (Stanley 1981b).

Changes in relationships may not always be directly the result of the disease or trauma. For example, Rodgers and Calder (1990) in a study of couples where one partner had multiple sclerosis found that of those participants who felt their relationship had deteriorated over the years all attributed the change to the disease. By comparison, those whose relationships had fluctuated attributed this to general stressful events rather than to the disease. Abrams (1981), in reviewing the literature on the impact of spinal injury on marital stability, found that low income and unemployment may be the most significant predictors of marital termination.

Treating a specific dysfunction such as erectile dysfunction may help to enhance the lowered self-esteem of the individual but may not always help the relationship if counselling is not available. A new basis for relationships may develop based on care and this new "brittle equilibrium" may be challenged by the newly acquired sexual potency of the partner (Vermote & Peuskins, 1996).

Intimate relationships and stroke

Williams (1993) undertook a retrospective study examining changes in marital satisfaction following stroke complicated by aphasia. The study was carried out amongst 40 spouses whose partners, following stroke, were classified as having mild, moderate, or severe aphasia. Amongst other parameters, the participants' knowledge of aphasia was assessed. A lower level of marital satisfaction was identified post-stroke. However, it was found that the more knowledge spouses had regarding aphasia, the less the negative impact the stroke had on marital satisfaction. This has implications for the provision of information to patients and partners.

In a qualitative study of sex and relationship functioning amongst people with neurological disability, a spouse whose partner had sustained a stroke commented "There's so much that you don't really understand about someone who's had a stroke...It's all very well them saying 'ask' but you don't know what to ask" (Brown, 1998).

Burgener and Logan (1989), in a review of sexuality post-stroke, commented that research showed that patients welcome frank and open discussion of sexuality and intimate relationships, although it seldom occurs. Research also suggests that changes in sexuality post-stroke are often a result of changes in role function because of the increased dependency of the partner who has sustained a stroke.

Sjögren (1983) in a study of 51 patients with stroke, looking particularly at sexual function and the intimate relationship, found a marked reduction in caressive behavior and this was followed by discontentment. Almost 50% of the subjects felt that their sexual relationship had deteriorated. There was reduced sexual satisfaction, which was significantly associated with an increase in sexual dysfunction, disturbed "partnership responsiveness" (i.e. relationship functioning), and reduced sexual fulfillment. They commented on the lack of sexual information and counselling available. Specific risk factors can be identified for relationships (Rosenbaum and Najenson, 1976; Woollett and Edelmann, 1988; Halvorson and Metz, 1992; Chandler and Brown, 1998):

- progressive conditions
- marriages begun before the onset
- sexual dysfunction
- cognitive and behavioral change.

Impact of acquired disability on the non-disabled partner

Masters and Johnson (1996) observed that there is no such thing as an "uninvolved partner." Hartman *et al.* (1983) identified a host of emotions that may be experienced by the partner: fear, anxiety, pity, shame, anger, helplessness, hopelessness, loneliness, depression, worry, and sadness. Some of these may, in turn, trigger further negative feelings in terms of guilt, confusion, and despair. Typical comments from partners (Chandler, 2002) include:

- He's not the person I knew before
- I still love him, but it's a motherly love
- He's not the man I married
- I just trail around from hospital to hospital with her; I've lost as well.

Unspoken pressures from family, society, and professionals may force the adoption of a role that is extremely difficult. Depression, anxiety, and physical ill-health may ensue.

Individuals without a sexual partner

There is a legitimacy about seeking help for sexual dysfunction in the context of a relationship. It may be much more difficult for those people not in relationships, and assumptions may easily be made by staff that sexuality is not an issue. Concerns may well exist about attractiveness, finding a partner, and sexual functioning. Restoration of erectile function may be important for self-esteem, masturbation, and reassurance that sexual intercourse remains a possibility if a relationship develops.

Management of sexual and relationship problems

A flexible approach that encompasses both sexual and relationship functioning is required to address those areas that are "malfunctioning." Elements that require consideration relate to the patient, the partner, and the relationship itself. The history and examination should include aspects of disability such as pain,

Table 16.1 Areas to cover in the history of a dysfunction with one or both partners

What has the individual's sex life been like?

What changes have occurred?

How do they feel about those changes?

How does the partner feel about the changes?

Classify the changes according to the sexual response model

Classify according to what is happening for the individual, the partner, and the relationship

Do they hold on to myths about sexual functioning?

Ascertain what the individual or the couple is hoping to achieve

Are their goals realistic?

spasticity, lack of sensation, poor mobility, depression, fatigue, and medication (Table 16.1). Some of these may be amenable to treatment (e.g. pain or spasticity); others may require adaptation by the individual or couple. For example, loss of sensation in the genital area can be approached by suggesting exploration of other areas of the body that may become responsive to sexual stimulation (Hooper, 1992). Many drugs impair sexual function and it may not always be possible to discontinue medication. Ability to achieve sexual intercourse may not always be restored, but sexual intimacy can be a realistic goal.

Use of P-LI-SS-IT in neurological disability

A useful model for approaching sex and relationship problems is P-LI-SS-IT (Annon, 1976), indicating permission (P), limited information (LI), specific suggestions (SS), and intensive therapy (IT). This is a hierarchical model that can be adapted depending on the skill and experience of the professional concerned.

Permission

Giving permission may involve recognizing unspoken questions or prompting through direct questions. Partners who are now in a caring role may need permission to express how they feel about the changes that have been imposed on them.

Limited information

Fears are powerful both in the individual with acquired disease and in the partner. Fear of causing pain, of triggering a catastrophic event, of agreeing to or refusing sexual contact can all have a powerfully negative effect on sexual arousal and relationship functioning. Simple factual information about the condition and medication can be of immense benefit. Patient organizations often produce information about sex and it can be useful to talk through such information with the patient and their partner.

Specific suggestions

Suggestions may include simple measures such as the timing of love-making to combat fatigue, use of medications, treatment of continence, and spasticity problems.

Intensive therapy

Intensive theraphy includes sex therapy or relationship counselling.

Summary

Sexual function and intimacy are not life or death issues but they are of immense importance in quality of life in the post-acute phase. Patients return to their partners and must adjust to the changes. This can be facilitated by appropriate support from health and social care professionals providing there is awareness and willingness to respond to this need.

REFERENCES

Abrams, K. S. (1981). The impact on marriages of adult onset paraplegia. *Paraplegia* **19**: 253–259.

American Psychiatric Association (1994). *DSM-IV: Diagnostic and Statistical Manual of Mental Disorders*, 4th edn. Washington, DC: American Psychiatric Press.

Annon, J. S. (1976). *The Behavioral Treatment of Sexual Problems: Brief Therapy*. New York: Harper and Row.

Bancroft, J. (1989). *Human Sexuality and its Problems*. Edinburgh: Churchill Livingstone.

(1993). Impact of environment, stress, occupational, and other hazards on sexuality and sexual behavior. *Environ Health Perspect* **101**(Suppl. 2): 101–107.

Bancroft, J. and Coles, L. (1976). Three years' experience in a sexual problem clinic. *BMJ*: 1575–1577.

Basson, R., Berman, J. Burnett, A. *et al.* (2000). Report on the international consensus development conference on female sexual dysfunction. *Urol* **163**: 888–893.

Boldrini, P., Basaglia, N. and Calanca, M.C. (1991). Sexual changes in hemiparetic patients. *Arch Phys Med Rehabil* **72**: 202–207.

Borg, G. (1998). The long term safety of alprostadil (prostaglandin-E^1) in patients with erectile dysfunction. *The International Alprostadil Study Group. J Urol* **82**: 538–543.

Bowers, M. B., Woert, M. V., and Davis, L. (1971). Sexual behavior during L-dopa treatment for parkinsonism. *Am J Psychiatry* **127**: 1691–1693.

Bray, G. P., de Frank, R. S., and Wolfe, T. L. (1981). Sexual functioning in stroke patients. *Arch Phys Med Rehabil* **62**: 286–288.

Brown, R. G., Jahanshahi, M., Quinn, N., and Marsden, C.D. (1990). Sexual function in patients with Parkinson's disease and their partners. *J Neurol Neurosurg Psychiatry* **53**: 480.

Brown S. J. (1998). Sexual and relationship difficulties in a clinical population of people with neurological disability. M Phil. Thesis, University of Newcastle Upon Tyne, UK.

Burgener, S. and Logan, G., (1989). Sexuality concerns of the post-stroke patient. *Rehabil Nurs* **14**: 178–181.

Chandler, B. J. (2003). The effect of disability on sexuality. *Update* **66**: 494–498.

Chandler, B. J. and Brown, S. (1998). Sex and relationship dysfunction in neurological disability. *J Neurol Neurosurg Psychiatry* **65**: 877–880.

Clark, J. D. A., Raggatt, P.R., and Edwards, O.M. (1988). Hypothalamic hypogonadism following major head injury. *Clin Endocrinol* **29**: 153–165.

Cotgrove, A. J. and Kolvin, I. (1996). Child sexual abuse. *Hosp Update* **22**: 401–406.

de Groat W. C. (1994). Neurophysiology of the pelvic organs. In *Handbook of Neuro-Urology*, Ch. 2 ed. D. N. Rushton. New York: Marcel Dekker.

DeLoach, C. and Greer, B. G. (1981). *Adjustment to Severe Physical Disability. A Metamorphosis*. New York: McGraw Hill.

Dunn, K. M., Croft, P. R., and Hackett, G. I. (1998). Sexual problems: a study of the prevalence and need for healthcare in the general population. *Fam Pract* **15**: 519–524.

(1999). Association of sexual problems with social psychological and physical problems in men and women: a cross sectional population survey. *J Epidemiol Community Health* **53**: 144–148.

Elliott., M. L. and Biever, L. S. (1996). Head injury and sexual dysfunction. *Brain Inj* **10**: 703–717.

Finger, W. W., Hall, E. S., and Peterson, F. L. (1992). Education in sexuality for nurses. *Sex Disabil* **10**: 81–89.

Goodwin, F. K. (1971). Behavioral effects of L-dopa in man. *Semin Psychiatry* **3** 477–491.

Guirgius, W. (1991). Sex therapy with couples. In *Couple Therapy. A Handbook*, Ch. 8, ed. D. Hooper and W. Dryden. Buckingham, UK: Open University Press.

Halvorson, J. G. and Metz, M. E. (1992). Sexual dysfunction, part 2: diagnosis, management and prognosis. *J Appl Board Family Pract* **5**: 177–192.

Hartman, C., MacIntosh, B., and Englehardt, B. (1983). The neglected and forgotton sexual partner of the physically disabled. *Soc Work* **28**: 370–374.

Hooper, M. (1992). *Spinal Cord Injured Men and Sexuality*. Milton Keynes, UK: Spinal Injuries Association.

Humphrey, M. (1985). Sexual consequences of cerebro-vascular accident. *J Roy Soc Med* **78**: 338–390.

Jehu, D. (1989). Sexual dysfunctions among women clients who were sexually abused in childhood. *Behav Psychother* **17**: 53–70.

Kaplan, H. S. (1974). *The New Sex Therapy*. London: Ballière Tindall.

Kimura, M., Murata, Y., Shimoda, K., and Robinson, R. G. (2001). Sexual dysfunction following stroke. *Comp Psychiatry* **42**: 217–222.

Kluver, H. and Bucy, P. C. (1937). Psychic blindness and other symptoms following bilateral temporal lobectomy in Rhesus monkeys. *Am J Physiol* **119**: 352–353.

Korpelainan, J. T., Kauhanen, M. L., Kemola, H., Malinen, U., and Myllyla,V. V. (1998). Sexual dysfunction in stroke patients. *Acta Neurol Scand* **98**: 400–405.

Kreuter, M., Sullivan, M., and Siosteen, A. (1994). Sexual adjustment after spinal cord injury (SCI) focusing on partner experiences. *Paraplegia* **32**: 225–235.

Kreuter, M., Dahllof, A. G., Gudjonsson, G., Sullivan, M., and Siosteen, A. (1998). Sexual adjustment and its predictors after traumatic brain injury. *Brain Inj* **12**: 349–368.

Larson, J. L., McNaughton, M. W., Wrad Kennedy, W., and Mansfield, L. W. (1980). Heart rate and blood pressure responses to sexual activity and a stair climbing test. *Heart Lung* **9**: 1025–1030.

Laumann, E. O., Paik, A., and Rosen, R. C. (1999). Sexual dysfunction in the United States: prevalence and predictors. *JAMA* **281**: 537–544. [Comment in: *JAMA* (1999) **282**: 1229.]

Lilius, H. G., Valtonen, E. J., and Wikstrom, J. (1976). Sexual problems in patients suffering from multiple sclerosis. *J Chronic Disease* 1976 **29**: 643–647.

Masters, W. H. and Johnson V. E. (1966). *Human Sexual Response*. London: J and A Churchill.

Miller, S., Szasz, G., and Anderson, L. (1981). Sexual health care clinician in an acute spinal cord injury unit. *Arch Phys Med Rehabil.* **62**: 315–320.

Mona, L. R., Gardos, P. S., and Brown, R. C. (1994). Sexual self views of women with disabilities: the relationship among age of onset, nature of disability and sexual self esteem. *Sex Disabil* **12**: 261–277.

Monga, T. N., Monga, M., Raina, M. S., and Hardjasudarma, M. (1986a). Hypersexuality in stroke. *Arch Phys Med Rehabil* **67**: 415–417.

Monga, T. N., Lawson, J. S., and Inglis, J. (1986b). Sexual dysfunction in stroke patients. *Arch Phys Med Rehabil* **67**: 19–22

Muller, J. E. (1999). Sexual activity as a trigger for cardiovascular events: what is the risk? *Am J Cardiol* **84**: 2N–5N.

Neumann, R. J. (1979). The forgotton other: women partners of spinal cord injured men, a preliminary report. *Sex Disabil* **2**: 287–292.

Nosek, M. A., Rintala, D. H., Young, M. A., *et al.* (1996). Sexual functioning among women with physical disabilities. *Arch Phys Med Rehabil* **77**: 107–115.

Oakley, N. and Moore, K. T. H. (1998). Vacuum devices in erectile dysfunction: indications and efficacy. *Br J Urol* **82**: 673–681.

O'Carroll, R. E., Woodrow, J., and Marouns, F. (1991). Psychosexual and psychosocial sequelae of closed head injury. *Brain Inj* **5**: 303–313.

Oddy, M., Humphrey, M., and Uttley, D. (1978). Stresses upon the relatives of brain injured patients. *Br J Psychiat* **133**: 507–513.

Rodgers, J. and Calder, P. (1990). Marital adjustment: a valuable resource for the emotional health of individuals with multiple sclerosis. *Rehabil Counsel Bull* **34**: 24–32.

Rosenbaum, M. and Najenson, T. (1976). Changes in life patterns and symptoms of low mood as reported by wives of severely brain injured soldiers. *J Consult Clin Psychol* **44**: 881–888.

Sakakibara, R. and Fowler, C. J. (1999). Cerebral control of bladder, bowel and sexual function and effects of brain disease. In *Neurology of Bladder Bowel and Sexual Dysfunction*, Ch. 14, ed. C. J. Fowler. Woburn, MA: Butterworth Heinemann.

Sawyer, S. M. (1996). Reproductive and sexual health in adolescents with cystic fibrosis. *BMJ* **313**: 1095–1096.

Sjörgen, K. (1983). Sexuality afer stroke with hemiplegia II. With special regard to partnership adjustment and to fulfilment. *Scand J Rehabil Med* **15**: 63–69.

Sjörgen, K., Damber, J. E., and Liliequist, B. (1983). Sexuality after stroke with hemiplegia I. Aspects of sexual functions. *Scand J Rehabil Med* **15**: 55–61.

Spence, S. (1991). *Psychosexual Therapy. A Cognitive Behavioral Approach.* London: Chapman & Hall.

Stanley, E. (1981a). Non organic causes of sexual problems. *BMJ* **282**: 1042–1044.

(1981b). Dealing with fear of failure. *BMJ* **282**: 1281–1283.

Szasz, G., Paty, D., Lawton-Speet, S., *et al.* (1984). A sexual function scale in multiple sclerosis. *Acta Neurol Scand* **101**: 37–43.

Vermote, R. and Peuskins, J. (1996). Sexual and micturition problems in multiple sclerosis patients: psychological issues. *Sex Disabil* **14**: 73–82.

Weston, A. (1993). Challenging assumptions. *Nurs Times* **89**: 26–31.

Weinman, E. and Ruskin, P. E. (1994). Levodopa dependence and hypersexuality in an older Parkinson's disease patient. *Am J Geriatr Psychiatry.* **3**: 81–83.

WHO (1992). *International Statistical Classification of Diseases and Related Health Problems.* Geneva: World Health Organization.

Williams, S. E. (1993). The impact of aphasia on marital satisfaction. *Arch Phys Med Rehabil* **74**: 361–367.

Wise, T. N. (1999). Psychosocial side effects of sildenafil therapy for erectile dysfunction. *J Sex Marital Ther* **25**: 145–150.

Woollett, S. L. and Edelmann, R. J. (1988). Marital satisfaction in individuals with multiple sclerosis and their partners; its interactive effect with life satisfaction, social networks and disability. *Sex Marital Ther* **3**: 191–196.

Young, E. W. (1984). Patients' plea: tell us about our sexuality. *J Sex Educ Ther* **10**: 53–56.

Zilbergeld, B. (1978). *Men and Sex.* London: Fontana.

17

Rehabilitation of visual disorders after stroke

Stephanie Clarke and Claire Bindschaedler

Division de Neuropsychologie, Centre Hospitalier Universitaire Vaudois, Lausanne, Switzerland

Introduction

Postchiasmatic brain lesions are reported in association with a variety of visual disorders after stroke, including cortical blindness, visual field disorders, achromatopsia, akinetopsia, visual agnosia, prosopagnosia, visuospatial neglect and Balint's syndrome (for review see Grüsser and Landis, 1991). This chapter is devoted to the rehabilitation of these syndromes in the context of acquired brain lesions in adults who had normal vision and normal visuocognitive performance prior to the stroke.

As much as two-thirds of the hemispheres is devoted to visual analysis (Zilles and Clarke, 1997) and, therefore, it is not surprising that 20–40% of patients with stroke have visual disorders (Hier et al., 1983). Visual disorders often have very debilitating effects in everyday life and specific techniques for their rehabilitation have been developed (Zihl, 2000), often based on the understanding of visual processing derived from recent work in humans or in non-human primates.

Neurobiological basis of visual perception

Experimental work since the early 1970s has changed radically our understanding of visual processing. Three issues are of great importance to visual rehabilitation. First, although visual information is relayed to the cortex primarily via the retinogeniculo–primary visual cortex route, alternative, smaller routes have been identified via the pulvinar or the superior colliculus. This is highly relevant to the understanding of preserved capacities in those with brain lesions, such as blindsight (Stoerig and Cowey, 1997) or interhemispheric transfer of visual information following callosotomy (Clarke et al., 2000). Second, the visual association cortex contains a large number of specialized visual areas. This was shown to be the case in non-human primates, where over 30 visual areas were identified (Felleman and van Essen, 1991). Activation studies indicate that human extrastriate visual cortex also contains functionally defined visual areas, some of which are highly

Recovery after Stroke, ed. Michael P. Barnes, Bruce H. Dobkin and Julien Bogousslavsky. Published by Cambridge University Press. © Cambridge University Press 2005.

specialized. This is the case for area V4 , specialized for color perception (Zeki, 1990), and for area V5-MT, specialized for motion perception (Zeki, 1991). Selective deficits, such as achromatopsia or akinetopsia, are currently interpreted as the result of damage to these specialized areas. Third, the information flow within extrastriate visual cortex is directed along two streams: the ventral stream, subserving recognition and involving the inferior temporal cortex (the "What" stream), and the dorsal stream, subserving spatial aspects and involving the parietal cortex (the "Where" stream) (Mishkin *et al.,* 1983). This parallel processing forms the basis of compensatory strategies used by patients with apperceptive visual agnosia.

Cortical blindness

Cortical blindness is characterized by a sudden or gradual loss of vision within both hemifields, which may be affected at the same time or in succession. Most cases reported are associated with bilateral infarctions in the territory of the posterior cerebral artery and in particular the calcarine artery; other pathologies include traumatic injury, carbon monoxide poisoning, and intracranial hematoma. In some cases, but not all, denial of blindness and/or hallucinations are associated with the syndrome (Bergman, 1957; Symonds and Mackenzie, 1957; Aldrich *et al.,* 1987).

Spontaneous recovery of vision has been reported in patients who have sustained complete cerebral blindness. A meta-analysis (Zihl, 2000) of several studies (Bergman, 1957; Gloning *et al.,* 1962; Symonds and Mackenzie, 1957) revealed that approximately 70% of patients experience partial recovery and 6% complete recovery. Recovery occurs mostly within 8 to 12 weeks of injury, but improvement was also observed up to two years later. Recovery occurs progressively in an often-observed sequence (Poppelreuter, 1917; Teuber *et al.,* 1960; Gloning *et al.,* 1962): light perception, often without precise motion and color perception; approximate perception of contours; colors; motion; and then form recognition.

Blindsight

Blindsight is defined as residual vision in blind fields caused by cortical lesions involving the primary visual cortex (for review see Weiskrantz, 1986). The patients perform correctly in tests involving detection of targets placed in their blind field, but they are not aware of the presence and the nature of these targets. The successful discrimination that blindsight patients may perform includes color (Stoerig and Cowey, 1989) and motion (Weiskrantz *et al.,* 1995). In a series of patients with retrogeniculate damage, 20% were found to have blindsight (Blythe *et al.,* 1987).

The anatomical substrate of blindsight is under discussion. Initial observations and results in animal models suggest strongly the involvement of subcortical centers that receive direct retinal input, such as the superior colliculus (Weiskrantz, 1986; Stoerig and Cowey, 1997). An alternative explanation has stressed the role of spared islands within the primary visual area (Fendrich *et al.,* 1992; Wessinger *et al.,* 1997). Although the initial relay stages are under discussion, the involvement of extrastriate visual cortex is established. Functional imaging studies have demonstrated area V5 activity in tasks of motion discrimination (Barbur *et al.,* 1993; Sahraie *et al.,* 1997). In hemianopia, presentation of stimuli within the blind hemifield was shown to yield activation of extrastriate cortex ipsilateral to the striate lesion (Goebel *et al.,* 2001).

Blindsight does not improve functioning in everyday life, since the patients cannot make use of their unconscious visual capacities.

Visual field deficits

Injury to the visual pathway between the retina and the striate cortex is often associated with visual field deficits. Pre- and postchiasmatic lesions affect the visual field in a monocular or homonymous fashion, respectively.

Homonymous field loss can be uni- or bilateral and can affect different parts of the visual field to a varying extent. The quality of the disorder is an important issue for rehabilitation. The loss can be complete (anopia) or specific aspects may be affected, such as color and form perception (amblyopia).

Spontaneous recovery of visual field loss caused by postchiasmatic lesions does occur and has been reported to be between 12 and 30% within months following unilateral homonymous loss (Hier *et al.,* 1983; Zihl and von Cramon, 1985; Zihl, 1994). Control experiments showed that this field enlargement was not a result of eccentric fixation or other compensatory strategies, but rather reflected recovery of reversibly damaged parts of the primary visual cortex (Zihl and von Cramon, 1985).

In a series of patients with homonymous hemianopia that persisted several months after postgeniculate damage, 40% were found to have normal visual scanning behavior, while 60% scanned visual surroundings in a disorganized and sloweddown fashion (Zihl, 1995). The latter condition was often associated with additional damage to the ipsilateral posterior thalamus or the parieto-occipital cortex.

Successful functional recovery in everyday activities is based on gain in visual field (see above), on oculomotor compensation, and on rapid visual exploration and mental reconstruction of the perceived visual space (Zihl, 1994).

The rehabilitation of visual field disorders is based on three approaches that aim to enlarge the visual field, to enhance saccadic eye movements, and to improve visual exploration and integration of visual information.

Visual field enlargement

Several studies have demonstrated that visual training can enlarge a visual field. An early study showed that regular practice in visual tasks led to visual field enlargement (Pöppel *et al.*, 1978). More specific training involving systematic practice with stimuli presented in the border region of the visual field resulted in visual field enlargement in some, but not all, patients (Zihl and von Cramon, 1979). Training of visual saccades that consisted of stimuli presentation in the border zone and in the anopic field yielded significant visual field enlargement (Zihl, 1981; Zihl and von Cramon, 1982, 1985). Small, but significant enlargement of the visual field was found in a series of hemianopic patients who received specific reading training in the subacute or chronic stage following posterior hemispheric lesions (Kerkhoff *et al.*, 1992). The use of a computer-based training program for one hour a day and a total of 80 to 300 training hours has also been reported to increase the visual field; the degree of improvement correlated inversely with the age of the patient and the size of the lesion (Kasten and Sabel 1995; Poggel *et al.*, 2001).

Visual field enlargement probably relies on recovery of reversibly injured parts of the primary visual area (Zihl and von Cramon, 1985; Wessinger *et al.*, 1997; Sabel and Kasten, 2000). This is supported by functional imaging studies showing that recovery from hemianopia was accompanied by increased metabolism in the region of the primary visual area (Bosley *et al.*, 1987).

Enhancement of saccadic eye movements

Hypometria impairs visual exploration in patients with a visual field defect. Several techniques have been used to alleviate this problem.

A training program that significantly increased the visual search field (i.e. the visual field that is functionally explored) included three steps: training of large saccades to the blind field, improving visual search on projected slides, and transfer of both strategies to activities of daily living (Kerkhoff *et al.*, 1992). In this same study, only minor, though significant, increases in visual field size were observed in some patients. Visual search field enlargements were training-dependent and persisted at follow-up six months later. A later study using the same training program confirmed training-related increase in visual search field and visual field, the transfer of treatment gains to functional measures, the improvement of patients' subjective ratings, and the stability of improvement at follow-up at three months (Kerkhoff *et al.*, 1994).

Specific training involving the presentation of the fixation point and a target in different parts of the blind visual field has been shown to improve saccadic exploration (Pommerenke and Markowitsch, 1989; Zihl, 2000). In at least one study, this improvement of visual search strategies was not accompanied by training-related visual field enlargement (Pommerenke and Markowitsch, 1989).

Systematic visual scanning training in hemianopic patients whose functional recovery was compromised was shown to increase the visual search field. Successful rehabilitation with the saccadic eye movement technique may be, however, compromised if occipitoparietal structures and/or the posterior thalamus are included in the lesion (Zihl, 1995).

Even relatively short training of compensatory visual exploration strategies (four weeks) was shown to yield a lasting improvement of target detection and activities of daily living (Nelles *et al.*, 2001), although in this study no effect on the visual field was observed.

Visual exploration and integration of visual information

Parallel and serial visual search paradigms have been used to train visual exploration, starting with the easier parallel (pop-out) version, and yielded significant improvement both in search time and field of vision (Zihl, 2000).

Long-term effects of the combined approach to visual field rehabilitation have been documented, although some patients experience difficulties in confusing conditions, such as a crowded supermarket (Zihl, 2000).

Central amblyopia

Patients with posterior brain lesions and normal vision prior to it may complain of blurred vision. This may be related to reduced visual acuity (Symonds and MacKenzie, 1957; Pöppel *et al.*, 1978; Savino *et al.*, 1978), decreased spatial contrast sensitivity (Bodis-Wollner, 1972, 1976; Bodis-Wollner and Diamond, 1976; Bulens *et al.*, 1989; Hess *et al.*, 1990), and/or impaired light and dark adaptation (Zihl and Kerkhoff, 1990).

Specific training of contrast sensitivity has been shown to improve this capacity and decrease the visual handicap (Zihl, 2000).

Achromatopsia (lack of color vision)

Achromatopsia has been described within one or both hemifields following posterior lesions and is probably caused by damage to visual area V4 (Meadows, 1974; Albert *et al.*, 1975; Pearlman *et al.*, 1979; Damasio *et al.*, 1980; Henderson, 1982; Poulson *et al.*, 1994; Zeki, 1990). Patients showing no improvement over time had generally large posterior lesions (Pearlman *et al.*, 1979; Heywood *et al.*, 1987). Smaller lesions of V4 yielded initial achromatopsia with considerable improvement in the chronic stage; remaining deficits concerned color constancy and/or short-term memory for hues (Clarke *et al.*, 1998; Schoppig *et al.*, 1999; Bartels and Zeki, 2000).

Reports of specific rehabilitation of color-related functions are rare. Zihl (2000) reported two cases; in one of them hue discrimination was a professional necessity and in the second color discrimination was likely to improve visual recognition capacities. The rehabilitation approach was based on hue discrimination training with progressively increasing degree of difficulty and led in both cases to improvement.

Akinetopsia (inability to perceive motion)

Akinetopsia was reported for the first time following a bilateral posterior sinus thrombosis (Zihl et al., 1983). The patient failed to perceive naturally occurring motion, such as level of fluid rising in a cup or the flowing nature of water running from a tap. Psychophysical tests confirmed her inability to perceive motion. A follow-up study reported a residual perception of motion in specific situations (only one object moving, slow motion, motion limited to the horizontal or vertical direction; Zihl et al., 1991). This partial recovery of motion perception was not supported by visual area V5, which remained inactive, but by activity in another visual area (V3) and in superior parietal cortex. This residual motion vision was, however, not sufficient to bring improvement in everyday life, in which she relied rather on coping strategies that were based on a non-dependence to see objects or people in motion.

Unilateral damage to the lateral occipital cortex was associated with impaired motion perception in the contralateral visual field (Plant et al., 1993). Affected patients were not motion-blind as in the original case with bilateral occipital lesion described by Zihl et al. (1983) and, in particular, they were able to appreciate motion of objects within the affected hemifield. The residual, degraded motion perception within the affected hemifield had similar contrast and temporal properties to those subserving normal motion perception and was proposed to rely on the spared parts of the extrastriate cortex (Plant and Nakayama, 1993).

Visual agnosia

Visual agnosia denotes the inability or difficulty to recognize objects and is caused by different types of cognitive impairment (reviewed by Heilman and Valenstein, 1985; Grüsser and Landis, 1991).

Associative visual agnosia denotes the inability to attach meaning to a shape that is well perceived. A striking case was described by Rubens and Benson (1971); the patient perceived the visual shape extremely well and was even able to produce copies of drawings that enabled others to recognize the object. However, this perfect shape perception did not allow identification of the object. Associative visual agnosia is often associated with bilateral inferior occipitotemporal lesions (Grüsser and Landis, 1991).

The term apperceptive visual agnosia denotes conditions in which shape perception is affected. A severe form of apperceptive agnosia is characterized by the inability to perceive visual shapes at all; it is usually found in those with diffuse posterior damage, such as in anoxia (Benson and Greenberg, 1969; Alexander and Albert, 1983). Some of these patients stated that they could not even see the objects that they were asked to identify. However, they did not suffer from cortical blindness, since their visuomotor capacities and in particular their capacity to seize the object under visual control were preserved. This was well documented in a patient with a severe visual recognition deficit following a bilateral posterior brain injury caused by asphyxia; the patient did not discriminate even simple shapes but could perform visually guided activities both in test context and in everyday life (Milner *et al.,* 1991). The preserved visuomotor capacities lead in some cases to the identification of simple shapes by tracing the contours of a drawing either with a finger or with eye movements (Landis *et al.,* 1982).

A much milder form of apperceptive visual agnosia is characterized by deficient perceptual categorization. These patients are much less handicapped in everyday life than patients with the severe form, but they experience difficulties in situations in which a detailed shape analysis is required. This may be the case when object contours are superposed with other lines (Luria, 1959) or when objects are presented in unfamiliar views (Warrington and James, 1988). Deficient perceptual categorization is generally associated with parietal lesions involving the right side.

Diagnosis of the type of visual agnosia, based on the above described characteristics and anatomoclinical correlations, is essential for the planning of rehabilitation.

The degree of spontaneous recovery is reported to be poor in severe apperceptive visual agnosia following carbon monoxide poisoning, both after five years and after 40 years (Adler 1944, 1950; Sparr *et al.,* 1991).

Rehabilitation of visual agnosia relies on the use of spared capacities, such as analysis of details, as well as training of visual scanning (Zihl, 2000). Some patients with an apperceptive agnosia develop a tracing strategy for the recognition of line drawings by using their hand or their head; use of non-form information such as surface texture, brightness, stereo-depth, and motion parallax can help the identification of common objects. In associative visual agnosia, encouraging the patient to supply a verbal description of the object can lead to its recognition; the patients should be dissuaded from naming the object, as they subsequently base their recognition on their naming response. In both types of agnosia, multimodal cross-cueing helps the patient to identify objects.

As severe agnosia is relatively rare, there have been only a few individual attempts to analyze the particular stage of visual processing that is disturbed in an individual patient with regards to a cognitive model of visual recognition and allow the design and application of a training method specifically targeted at the damaged component. Even so, failure to observe any improvement on the trained task as well as in everyday life has been reported in a patient with apperceptive agnosia despite extensive practice on visual search tasks sensitive to grouping and segmentation (Humphreys and Riddoch, 1994).

Another approach undertaken with both aperceptive and associative agnosia has been to restore the visual recognition of specific items. It involves presenting a stimulus (an object or a pictured object), providing its right name, and asking the patient to write down its name in order to allow him or her to restore visual knowledge about the item. This approach can be combined with techniques known to enhance learning such as errorless learning (preventing the patient producing errors) and expanded rehearsal (increasing the intervals between practice trials). Patients with both types of agnosia have been shown to benefit from this procedure as they learn new visual–verbal associations. However, there is no generalization to untrained items and even no generalization to different pictures of the same object.

Prosopagnosia

Prosopagnosia is defined as failure to recognize previously known faces (Hecaen and Angelergues, 1962; de Renzi *et al.,* 1994). Prosopagnosia is described in isolation (i.e. for faces alone) but has been frequently reported in association with difficulties in identifying items from previously well-known categories, such as cows for farmers (Assal *et al.,* 1984), birds for birdwatchers (Bornstein *et al.,* 1969), mountains and landscapes for experienced mountaineers, or fish and plants for a professional in this domain (Clarke *et al.,* 1997). Other frequently associated disorders include achromatopsia (agnosia for colors), pure alexia, visuospatial or visuoconstructive disorders, memory deficits, and, in most patients, visual field deficits. Prosopagnosia without visual field deficit and without achromatopsia is relatively rare (for discussion see Clarke *et al.,* 1997).

In most reported cases, prosopagnosia was associated with bilateral or right unilateral inferior temporo-occipital lesions (Damasio *et al.,* 1982).

Prosopagnosia was reported without spontaneous recovery (Bruyer *et al.,* 1983). However, patients with prosopagnosia learn progressively to identify familiar faces by making use of additional information about hair style, head shape, height, dress, and gait (Benson, 1989). This same strategy, relying on the detailed and often verbal analysis of object characteristics, was also used for other affected categories (Clarke *et al.,* 1997).

Two individual attempts at retraining the structural analysis of faces with tasks involving analysis of physical features or same–different judgements on photographs or line drawings have met with no success (Ellis and Young, 1988; Polster and Rapcsak, 1996). Retraining face identification by asking the patient to learn the association between a face and a name has been demonstrated in prosopagnosic patients. Such learning can be facilitated by semantic processing of the faces: for instance, providing judgements of personality features on the basis of the face, or telling a story about the person (Polster and Rapcsak, 1996). However, as for visual agnosia, a major limitation of this approach is the absence of generalization to different views of the same face.

Visual localization

Patients with posterior brain lesions may present visual localization deficits and/or shifts in the vertical and horizontal axes (reviewed by Zihl, 2000). Visual localization tends to be impaired in the contralateral hemispace following unilateral lesions and in the whole space following bilateral lesions. Shifts in axes have been mainly described in patients with right occipitoparietal lesions (Kerkhoff, 1998). The majority of patients with right posterior hemispheric lesions were shown to have visuospatial deficits when tested with the rod orientation test, which required visuomotor coordination, at two weeks after the infarction (de Renzi *et al.*, 1971; Meerwaldt and van Harskamp, 1982). Spontaneous recovery was reported to occur mainly during the first six months and the speed of recovery was correlated with the size of lesion (Meerwaldt, 1983).

Early studies have demonstrated positive effects of specific visuospatial training in the trained task and in everyday activities (e.g. Weinberg *et al.*, 1979). Specific training using a computer-based program was shown to improve the adjustment of the visual vertical and horizontal axes, visual localization, discrimination of length of lines, line bisection, and line orientation (Kerkhoff, 1998).

Unilateral neglect

Hemineglect is characterized by lack or decrease of attention to stimuli and events on the left-hand side of the patient following a right hemispheric lesion. In extreme cases, patients do not react when they are spoken to from the left side, do not eat food on the left half of their plate, or read the left side of their newspaper. Hemineglect can affect, sometimes to a varying degree, visual, auditory, somatosensory, and motor modalities (Barbieri and de Renzi, 1989).

The neglect symptomatology has been interpreted in different ways. Kinsbourne (1993) proposed the existence of attentional gradients within hemispace and Mesulam (1981) proposed different roles for each hemisphere. Other models, based on studies in non-human primates, stressed the role of spontaneous eye movements in orienting attention (Gainotti, 1994).

The presence of hemineglect beyond the acute stage is associated with poor outcome in terms of independence (Denes *et al.*, 1982; Stone *et al.*, 1992) and considerable effort is, therefore, devoted to its rehabilitation.

Currently, several approaches are used in neglect rehabilitation (only group studies are quoted): (a) combined training of visual scanning, reading, copying, and figure description (e.g. Pizzamiglio *et al.*, 1992; Antonucci *et al.*, 1995; Vallar *et al.*, 1997); (b) visual scanning training alone (e.g. Weinberg *et al.*, 1977); (c) spatiomotor or visuospatiomotor cueing (e.g. Lin *et al.*, 1996; Kalra *et al.*, 1997; Frassinetti *et al.*, 2001); (d) visual cueing with kinetic stimuli (Butter *et al.*, 1990; Pizzamiglio *et al.*, 1990; Butter and Kirsch, 1995); (e) video feedback (Tham and Tegner, 1997); (f) training of sustained attention, increasing of alertness, or cueing of spatial attention (Hommel *et al.*, 1990; Ladavas *et al.*, 1994; Robertson *et al.*, 1995; Kerkhoff, 1998); (g) changes in trunk orientation (Wiart *et al.*, 1997); (h) use of prism goggles (Frassinetti *et al.*, 2002); (i) specific training of visual imagery (Niermeir, 1998); (j) forced use of left visual hemifield or left eye (Butter and Kirsch 1992; Walker *et al.*, 1996; Beis *et al.*, 1999); and (k) computer training (with mixed results) (Robertson *et al.*, 1990; Bergego *et al.*, 1997; Webster *et al.*, 2001).

In addition, transient effects on neglect, lasting only little longer than the therapeutic application, have been demonstrated for vestibular stimulation by cold water infusion into the left outer ear canal (Rode and Perenin, 1994; Rode *et al.*, 1998), galvanic vestibular stimulation (Rorsman *et al.*, 1999), or transcutaneous electrical stimulation of the left neck muscles (Vallar *et al.*, 1995; Guariglia *et al.*, 1998; Perennou *et al.*, 2001).

The effect of dopamine agonists on hemispatial neglect was investigated in studies involving small numbers of patients; four showed improvement (Fleet *et al.*, 1987; Geminiani *et al.*, 1998; Hurford *et al.*, 1998; Mukand *et al.*, 2001) and two worsening or mixed effects (Grujic *et al.*, 1998; Barrett *et al.*, 1999).

Balint's syndrome

Balint's syndrome is characterized by simultagnosia (inability to see more than one or two objects or object features at a time), psychic paralysis of gaze (difficulty in initiating gaze shifts), and ataxia (inability to point correctly to visual targets) (Balint, 1909). This syndrome was found in patients with bilateral parietal lesions and represents a very severe handicap in everyday life. It occurs relatively rarely, even in series of patients with posterior lesions (approximately 2%, Gloning *et al.*, 1962). Minor forms of this syndrome have been described in which the three elements are present but in a inconspicuous or transitory form (Hecaen and Ajuriaguerra, 1954).

Spontaneous recovery has been reported in patients with Balint's syndrome (Allison *et al.*, 1969; Montero *et al.*, 1982). Very little information is available, however, about the rehabilitation of Balint's syndrome. Zihl (2000) reported on three patients with a severe form of the syndrome. Treatment strategies aimed to improve oculomotor functions and included intensive practice in saccadic localization, as well as in touching and scanning visual displays. This training yielded improvement in fixation accuracy and in the enlargement of the field of oculomotor scanning. However, it did not result in better reading capacities, although in everyday life patients became better at finding their way in familiar surroundings. A recent case study reported significant improvement both in neuropsychological evaluation and in everyday activities as the result of a training program that started one year post-lesion and lasted for one year (Rosselli *et al.*, 2001). The training program included visuoperceptual retraining and rehabilitation in contexts that were meaningful to the patient.

Summary

Posterior hemispheric lesions, caused by stroke or other etiologies, are often associated with a variety of visual disorders, many of which significantly disturb activities of daily living. Group and single case studies have reported partial, or even complete, spontaneous recovery for most of these disorders. Specific rehabilitation programs have been developed for hemianopia and visuospatial neglect and their efficacy has been investigated in group studies. For other disorders, such as achromatopsia, akinetopsia, prosopagnosia, visual agnosia and Balint's syndrome, ad hoc rehabilitation has been developed, with variable success, for individual patients.

REFERENCES

Adler, A. (1944). Disintegration and restoration of optic recognition in visual agnosia: analysis of a case. *Arch Neurol Psychiat.*, **51**: 243–259.

(1950). Course and outcome of visual agnosia. *J Nerv Mental Dis* **111**: 41–51.

Albert, M. L., Reches, A., and Silverberg, R. (1975). Hemianopic color blindness. *J Neurol Neurosurg Psychiatry* **38**: 546–549.

Aldrich, M. S., Alessi, A. G., Beck, R. W., and Gilman, S. (1987). Cortical blindness: etiology, diagnosis, and prognosis. *Ann Neurol* **21**: 149–158.

Alexander, M. P. and Albert, M. L. (1983). The anatomical basis of visual agnosia. In *Localization in Neuropsychology*, ed. I. A. Kertesz. New York: Academic Press, pp. 393–415.

Allison, R. S., Hurwitz, L. J., White, G. J., and Wilmot, T. J. (1969). A follow-up study of a patient with Balint's syndrome. *Neuropsychologia* **7**: 319–333.

Antonucci, A., Guariglia, C., Judica, A., *et al.* (1995). Effectivness of neglect rehabilitation in a randomized group study. *J Clin Exp Neuropsychol* **17**: 383–389.

Assal, G., Favre, C., and Anderes, J. P. (1984). Non-reconnaissance d'animaux familiers chez un paysan. *Rev Neurol* (Paris) **140**: 580–584.

Balint, R. (1909). Seelenlähmung des "Schauens", optische Ataxie, räumliche Störung der Aufmerksamkeit. *Monatsschr Psychiat Neurol* **25**: 51–81.

Barbieri, C. and de Renzi, E. (1989). Patterns of neglect dissociation. *Behav Neurol* **2**: 13–24.

Barbur, J., Watson, J., Frackowiak, R., and Zeki, S. (1993). Conscious visual perception without V1. *Brain* **116**: 1293–1302.

Barrett, A. M., Crucian, G. P., Schwartz, R. L., and Heilman, K. M. (1999). Adverse effect of dopamine agonist therapy in a patient with motor-inattentional neglect. *Arch Phys Med Rehabil* **80**: 600–603.

Bartels, A. and Zeki, S. (2000). The architecture of the color center in the human visual brain: new results and a review. *Eur J Neurosci* **12**: 172–193.

Beis, J.-M., André, J.-M., Baumgarten, A., and Challier, B. (1999). Eye patching in unilateral spatial neglect: efficacy of two methods. *Arch Phys Med Rehabil* **80**: 71–76.

Benson, D. F. (1989). Disorders of visual gnosis. In *Neuropsychology of Visual Perception*, ed. J. W. Brown. Hillsdale, NY: Erlbaum, pp. 59–78.

Benson, D. F. and Greenberg, J. P. (1969). Visual form agnosia. *Arch Neurol* **20**: 82–89.

Bergego, C., Azouvi, P., Deloche, G., *et al.* (1997). Rehabilitation of unilateral neglect: a controlled multiple-baseline-across-subjects trial using computerised training procedures. *Neuropsychol Rehabil* **7**: 279–293.

Bergman, P. S. (1957). Cerebral blindness. *Arch Neurol Psychiatry* **78**: 568–584.

Blythe, I. M., Kennard, C., and Ruddock, K. H. (1987). Residual vision in patients with retrogeniculate lesions of the visual pathways. *Brain* **110**: 887–905.

Bodis-Wollner, I. (1972). Visual acuity and contrast sensitivity in patients with cerebral lesions. *Science* **178**: 769–771.

(1976). Vulnerability of spatial frequency channels in cerebral lesions. *Nature* **261**: 309–311

Bodis-Wollner, I. and Diamond, S. P. (1976). The measurement of spatial contrast sensitivity in cases of blurred vision associated with cerebral lesions. *Brain* **99**: 695–710.

Bornstein, B., Sroka, H., and Munitz, H. (1969). Prosopagnosia with animal face agnosia. *Cortex* **5**: 164–169.

Bosley, T. M., Dann, R., Silver, F. L., *et al.* (1987). Recovery of vision after ischemic lesions: positron emission tomography. *Ann Neurol* **21**: 444–450.

Bruyer, R., Laterre, C., Seron, F. X., *et al.* (1983). A case of prosopagnosia with some preserved covert remembrance of familiar faces. *Brain Cogn* **2**: 257–284.

Bulens, C., Meerwaldt, J. D., van der Wildt, G. J., and Keemink, C. J. (1989). Spatial contrast sensitivity in unilateral cerebral ischaemic lesions involving the posterior visual pathway. *Brain* **112**: 507–520.

Butter, C. M. and Kirsch, N. (1992). Combined and separate effects of eye patching and visual stimulation on unilateral neglect following a stroke. *Arch Phys Med Rehabil* **73**: 1133–1139.

(1995). Effect of lateralized kinetic visual cues on visual search in patients with unilateral spatial neglect. *J Clin Exp Neuropsychol* **17**: 856–867.

Butter, C. M., Kirsch, N. L., and Reeves, G. (1990). The effect of lateralized dynamic stimuli on unilateral spatial neglect following right hemisphere lesions. *Rest Neurol Neurosci* **2**: 39–46.

Clarke, S., Lindemann, A., Maeder, P., Borruat, F.-X., and Assal, G. (1997). Face recognition and postero-inferior hemispheric lesions. *Neuropsychologia* **35**: 1555–1563

Clarke, S., Walsh, V., Schoppig, A., Assal, G., and Cowey, A. (1998). Color constancy impairmentsin patients with lesions of the prestriate cortex. *Exp Brain Res* **123**: 154–158.

Clarke, S., Maeder, P., Meuli, R., *et al.* (2000). Interhemispheric transfer of visual motion information after a posterior callosal lesion: a neuropsychological and fMRI study. *Exp Brain Res* **132**: 127–133.

Damasio, A. R., Yamada, T., Damasio, H., Corbett, J., and McKee, J. (1980). Central achromatopsia: behavioral, anatomic and physiologic aspects. *Neurology* **30**: 1064–1071.

Damasio, A. R., Damasio, H., and Van Hoesen, G. W. (1982). Prosopagnosia: anatomic basis and behavioral mechanisms. *Neurology* **32**: 331–341.

Denes, G., Semenza, C., Stoppa, E., and Lis, A. (1982). Unilateral spatial neglect and recovery from hemiplegia. *Brain* **105**: 543–552.

de Renzi, E., Faglioni, P., and Scotti, G. (1971). Jugdement of spatial orientation in patients with focal brain damage. *J Neurol Neurosurg Psychiatry* **34**: 489–495.

de Renzi, E., Perani, D., Carlesimo, G. A., Silveri, M. C., and Fazio, F. (1994). Prosopagnosia can be associated with damage confined to the right hemisphere : an MRI and PET study and a review of the literature. *Neuropsychologia* **32**: 893–902

Ellis, H. D. and Young, A. W. (1988). Training in face-processing skills for a child with acquired prosopagnosia. *Dev Neuropsychol* **4**: 283–294.

Felleman, D. J. and van Essen, D. C. (1991). Distributed hierarchical processing in the primate cerebral cortex. *Cereb Cortex* **1**: 1–47.

Fendrich, R., Wessinger, C. M., and Gazzaniga, M. S. (1992). Residual vision in a scotoma: implications for blindsight. *Science* **258**: 1489–1491.

Fleet, W. S., Valenstein, E., Watson, R. T., and Heilman, K. M. (1987). Dopamine agonist therapy for neglect in humans. *Neurology* **37**: 1765–1770.

Frassinetti, F., Rossi, M., and Ladavas, E. (2001). Passive limb movements improve visual neglect. *Neuropsychologia* **39**: 725–733.

Frassinetti, F., Angeli, V., Meneghello, F., Avanzi, S., and Ladavas, E. (2002). Long-lasting amelioration of visuospatial neglect by prism adaptation. *Brain* **125**: 608–623.

Gainotti, G. (1994) The role of spontaneous eye movements in orienting attention and in unilateral neglect. In *Unilateral Neglect: Clinical and Experimental Studies*, ed. E. H. Robertson and J. C. Marshall. Hove, UK: Lawrence Erlbaum pp. 107–122.

Geminiani, G., Bottini, G., and Sterzi, R. (1998). Dopaminergic stimulation in unilateral neglect. *J Neurol Neurosurg Psychiatry* **65**: 344–347.

Gloning, L., Gloning, K., and Tschabitscher, H. (1962). Die occipitale Blindheit auf vaskulärer Basis. *Graefes Arch Ophthalmol* **165**: 138–177.

Goebel, R., Muckli, L., Zanella, F. E., Singer; W., and Stoerig, P. (2001). Sustained extrastriate cortical activation without visual awareness revealed by fMRI studies of hemianopic patients. *Vision Res* **41**: 1459–1474.

Grujic, Z., Mapstone, M., Gitelman, D. R., *et al.* (1998). Dopamine agonists reorient visual exploration away from the neglected hemispace. *Neurology* **51**: 1395–1398.

Grüsser, O. J. and Landis, T. (1991). Visual agnosias and other disturbances of visual perception and cognition. In *Vision and Visual Dysfunction*, vol. 12, ed. J. Cronly-Dillon. London: Macmillan Press.

Guariglia, C., Lippolis, G., and Pizzamiglio, L. (1998). Somatosensory stimulation improves imagery disorders in neglect. *Cortex* **34**: 233–241.

Hecaen, H. and de Angelergues, R. (1962). Agnosia for faces (prosopagnosia). *Arch Neurol* **7**: 92–100.

(1954). Balint's syndrome (psychic paralysis of fixation) and its minor forms. *Brain* **77**: 373–400.

Heilman, K. M. and Valenstein, E. (1985). *Clinical Neuropsychology*. Oxford: Oxford University Press.

Henderson, V. W. (1982). Impaired hue discrimination in homonymous visual fields. *Arch Neurol* **39**: 418–419.

Hess, R. F., Zihl, J., Pointer, S. J., and Schmid, C. (1990). The contrast sensitivity deficit in cases with cerebral lesions. *Clin Vision Sci* **5**: 203–215.

Heywood, C. A., Wilson, B., and Cowey, A. (1987). A case study of cortical color blindness with relatively intact achromatic discrimination. *J Neurol Neurosurg Psychiatry* **50**: 22–29.

Hier, D. B., Mondlock, J., and Caplan, L. R. (1983). Behavioral abnormalities after right hemisphere stroke. *Neurology* **33**: 337–344.

Hommel, M., Peres, B., Pollack, P., *et al.* (1990). Effects of passive tactile and auditory stimuli on left visual neglect. *Arch Neurol* **47**: 573–576.

Humphreys, G. W. and Riddoch, M. J. (1994). Visual object processing in normality and pathology: implications for rehabilitation. In *Cognitive Neuropsychology and Cognitive Rehabilitation*, ed. M. J. Riddoch and G. W. Humphreys. Hove, UK: Lawrence Erlbaum.

Hurford, P., Stringer, A. Y., and Jann, B. (1998). Neuropharmacological treatment of hemineglect: a case report comparing bromocriptine and methylphenidate. *Arch Phys Med Rehabil* **79**: 346–349.

Kalra, L., Perez, I., Gupta, S., and Wittink, M. (1997). The influence of visual neglect on stroke rehabilitation. *Stroke* **28**: 1386–1391.

Kasten, E., and Sabel, B. A. (1995). Visual field enlargement after computer training in braindamaged patients with homonymous deficits: an open pilot trial. *Rest Neurol Neurosci* **8**: 113–127.

Kerkhoff, G. (1998). Rehabilitation of visuospatial cognition and visual exploration in neglect: a cross-over study. *Rest Neurol Neurosci* **12**: 27–40.

Kerkhoff, G., Münssinger, U., Haaf, E., Eberle-Strauss, G., and Stögerer, E. (1992). Rehabilitation of homonymous scotomata in patients with postgeniculate damage of the visual system: saccadic compensation training. *Rest Neurol Neurosci* **4**: 245–254.

Kerkhoff, G., Münssinger, U., and Meier, E. (1994). Neurovisual rehabilitation in cerebral blindness. *Arch Neurol* **51**: 474–481.

Kinsbourne, M. (1993). Integrated cortical field model of consciousness. *Ciba Found Symp* **174**: 43–50.

Ladavas, E., Carletti, M., and Gori, G. (1994). Automatic and voluntary orienting of attention in patients with visual neglect: horizontal and vertical dimensions. *Neuropsychologia* **32**: 1195–1208.

Landis, T., Graves, R., Benson, F., and Hebben, N. (1982). Visual recognition through kinaesthetic mediation. *Psychol Med* **12**: 515–531.

Lin, K. -C., Cermark, S. A., Kinsbourne, M., and Trombly, C. A. (1996). Effects of left-sided movements on line bisection in unilateral neglect. *J Int Neuropsychol Soc* **2**: 404–411.

Luria, A. R. (1959). Disorders of "simultaneous perception" in a case of bilateral occipito-parietal brain injury. *Brain* **82**: 437–449.

Meadows, J. C. (1974). Disturbed perception of colors associated with localized cerebral lesion. *Brain* **97**: 615–632.

Meerwaldt, J. D. (1983). Spatial disorientation in right-hemisphere infarction: a study of the speed of recovery. *J Neurol Neurosurg Psychiatry* **46**: 426–429.

Meerwaldt, J. D. and van Harskamp, F. (1982). Spatial disorientation in right-hemisphere infarction. *J Neurol Neurosurg Psychiatry* **45**: 586–590.

Mesulam, M. M. (1981). A cortical network for directed attention and unilateral neglect. *Ann Neurol* **10**: 309–325.

Milner, A. D., Perrett, D. I., Johnston, R. S., *et al.* (1991). Perception and action in "visual form agnosia". *Brain* **114**: 405–428.

Mishkin, M., Ungerleider, L. G., and Macko, K. A. (1983). Object vision and spatial vision: two cortical pathways. *Trends Neurosci* **6**: 414–417.

Montero, J., Pena, J., Genis, D., *et al.* (1982). Balint's syndrome. *Acta Neurol Belg* **82**: 270–280.

Mukand, J. A., Guilmette, T. J., Allen, D. G., *et al.* (2001). Dopaminergic therapy with carbidopa L-dopa for left neglect after stroke: a case series. *Arch Phys Med Rehabil* **82**: 1279–1282.

Nelles, G., Esser, J., Eckstein, A., *et al.* (2001). Compensatory visual field training for patients with hemianopsia after stroke. *Neurosci Lett* **29**: 189–192.

Niermeir, J. P. (1998). The lighthouse strategy: use of a visual imagery technique to treat visual inattention in stroke patients. *Brain Injury* **12**: 399–406.

Pearlman, A. L., Birch, J., and Meadows, J. C. (1979). Cerebral color blindness: an acquired defect in hue discrimination. *Ann Neurol* **5**: 253–261.

Perennou, D. A., Leblond, C., Amblard, B., *et al.* (2001). Transcutaneous electric nerve stimulation reduces neglect-related postural instability after stroke. *Arch Phys Med Rehabil* **82**: 440–448.

Pizzamiglio, L., Frasca, R., Guariglia, C., Incoccia, C., and Antonucci, G. (1990). Effect of optokinetic stimulation in patients with visual neglect. *Cortex* **26**: 535–540.

Pizzamiglio, L., Antonucci, G., Judica, A., *et al.* (1992). Cognitive rehabilitation of the hemi-neglect disorder in chronic patients with unilateral right brain damage. *J Clin Exp Neuropsychol* **14**: 901–923.

Plant, G. T. and Nakayama, K. (1993). The characteristics of residual motion perception in the hemifield contralateral to lateral occipital lesions in humans. *Brain* **116**: 1337–1353.

Plant, G. T., Laxer, K. D., Barbaro, N. M., Schiffman, J. S., and Nakayama, K. (1993). Impaired visual motion perception in the contralateral hemifield following unilateral posterior cerebral lesions in humans. *Brain* **116**: 1303–1335.

Poggel, D. A., Kasten, E., Muller-Oehring, E. M., Sabel, B. A., and Brandt, S. A. (2001). Unusual spontaneous and training induced visual field recovery in a patient with a gunshot lesion. *J Neurol Neurosurg Psychiatry* **70**: 236–239.

Polster, M. R. and Rapcsak, S. Z. (1996). Representations in learning new faces: evidence from prosopagnosia. *J Int Neuropsychol Soc* **2**: 240–248.

Pommerenke, K. and Markowitsch, J. H. (1989). Rehabilitation training of homonymous visual field defects in patients with postgeniculate damage to the visual system. *Rest Neurol Neurosci* **1**: 47–63.

Pöppel, E., Brinkmann, R., von Cramon, D., and Singer, W. (1978). Association and dissociation of visual functions in a case of bilateral occipital lobe infarction. *Arch Psychiatr Nervenkrank* **225**: 1–21.

Poppelreuter, W. (1917). *Die psychischen Schädigungen durch Kopfschuss im Kriege 1914/16. Mit besonderer Berücksichtigung der pathopsychologischen, pädagogischen, gewerblichen und sozialen Beziehungen.* Vol. 1: *Die Störungen der nierderen und höheren Sehleistungen durch Verletzungen des Okzipitalhirns.* Leipzig: Voss.

Poulson, H. L., Galetta, S. L., Grossman, M., and Alavi, A. (1994). Hemiachromatopsia after occipitotemporal infarcts. *Am J Ophtalmol* **118**: 518–523.

Robertson, I. H., Gray, J., Pentland, B., and Waite, L. J. (1990). Microcomputer-based rehabilitation for unilateral left visual neglect: a randomized contolled trial. *Arch Phys Med Rehabil* **71**: 663–668.

Robertson, I. H., Tegnér, R., Tham, K., Lo, A., and Nimmo-Smith, I. (1995). Sustained attention training for unilateral neglect: theoretical and rehabilitation implications. *J Clin Exp Neuropsychol* **17**: 416–430.

Rode, G. and Perenin, M. T. (1994). Temporary remission of representational hemineglect through vestibular stimulation. *NeuroReport* **5**: 869–872.

Rode, G., Rossetti, Y., Li, L., and Boisson, D. (1998). Improvement of mental imagery after prism exposure in neglect: a case study. *Behav Neurol* **11**: 251–258.

Rorsman, I., Magnusson, M., and Johansson, B. B. (1999). Reduction of visuospatial neglect with vestibular galvanic stimulation. *Scand J Rehabil Med* **31**: 117–124.

Rosselli, M., Ardila, A., and Beltran, C. (2001). Rehabilitation of Balint's syndrome: a single case report. *Appl Neuropsychol* **8**: 242–247.

Rubens, A. B. and Benson, D. F. (1971). Associative visual agnosia. *Arch Neurol* **24**: 305–315.

Sabel, B. A. and Kasten, E. (2000). Restoration of vision by training of residual functions. *Curr Opin Ophthalmol* **11**: 430–436.

Sahraie, A., Weiskrantz, L., Barbur, J. L., *et al.* (1997). Pattern of neuronal activity associated with conscious and unconscious processing of visual signals. *Proc Natl Acad Sci USA* **94**: 9406–9411.

Savino, P. J., Paris, M., Schatz, N. J., and Corbett, J. J. (1978). Optic tract syndrome. *Arch Ophtalmol* **96**: 656–663.

Schoppig, A., Clarke, S., Walsh, V., *et al.* (1999). Short-term memory for color following posterior hemispheric lesions in man. *NeuroReport* **10**: 1379–1384.

Sparr, S. A., Jay, M., Drislane, F. W., and Venna, N. (1991). A historic case of visual agnosia revisited after 40 years. *Brain* **114**: 789–800.

Stoerig, P. and Cowey, A. (1989). Wavelength sensitivity in blindsight. *Nature* **342**: 916–918. (1997). Blindsight in man and monkey. *Brain* **120**: 535–559.

Stone, S. P., Patel, P., Greenwood, R. J., and Halligan, P. W. (1992). Measuring visual neglect in acute stroke and predicting its recovery: the visual neglect recovery index. *J Neurol Neurosurg Psychiatry* **55**: 431–436.

Symonds, C. and MacKenzie, I. (1957). Bilateral loss of vision from cerebral infarction. *Brain* **80**: 415–455.

Teuber, H. L., Battersby, W. S., and Bender, M. B. (1960). *Visual Field Defects after Penetrating Missile Wounds of the Brain.* Cambridge, MA: Harvard University Press.

Tham, K. and Tegnér, R. (1997). Video feedbeck in the rehabilitation of patients with unilateral neglect. *Arch Phys Med Rehabil* **78**: 410–413.

Vallar, G., Rusconi, M. L., Barozzi, S., *et al.* (1995). Improvement of left visuospatial hemineglect by left-sided transcutaneous electrical stimulation. *Neuropsychologia* **33**: 73–82.

Vallar, G., Guariglia, C., Magnotti, L., and Pizzamiglio, L. (1997). Dissociation between position sense and visual-spatial components of hemineglect through a specific rehabilitation treatment. *J Clin Exp Neuropsychol* **19**: 763–771.

Walker, R., Young, A. W., and Lincoln, N. B. (1996). Eye patching and he rehabilitation of visual neglect. *Neuropsychol Rehabil* **6**: 219–231.

Warrington, E. K. and James, M. (1988). Visual apperceptive agnosia: a clinico-anatomical study of three cases. *Cortex* **24**: 13–32.

Webster, J. S., McFarland, P. T., Rapport, L. J., *et al.* (2001). Computer-assisted training for improving wheelchair mobility in unilateral neglect patients. *Arch Phys Med Rehabil* **82**: 769–775.

Weinberg, J., Diller, L., Gordon, W. A., *et al.* (1977). Visual scanning training effect on reading-related tasks in acquired right brain damage. *Arch Phys Med Rehabil* **58**: 479–486.

Weinberg, J., Diller, L., Gordon, W. A., *et al.* (1979). Training sensory awareness and spatial organization in people with right brain damage. *Arch Phys Med Rehabil* **60**: 491–496.

Weiskrantz, L. (1986). *Blindsight. A Case Study and Implications.* Oxford: Clarendon Press.

Weiskrantz, L., Barbur, J. L., and Sahraie, A. (1995). Parameters affecting conscious versus unconscious visual discrimination with damage to the visual cortex (V1). *Proc Natl Acad Sci USA* **92**: 6122–6126.

Wessinger, C. M., Fendrich, R., and Gazzaniga, M. S. (1997). Islands of residual vision in hemianopic patients. *J Cogn Neurosci* **9**: 203–221.

Wiart, L., Bon Saint Côme, A., Debelleix, X., *et al.* (1997). Unilateral neglect syndrome rehabilitation by trunk rotation and scanning training. *Arch Phys Med Rehabil* **78**: 424–429.

Zeki, S. M. (1990). A century of cerebral achromatopsia. *Brain* **113**: 1721–1777. (1991). Cerebral akinetopsia (visual motion blindness). *Brain* **114**: 811–824.

Zihl, J. (1981). Recovery of visual functions in patients with cerebral blindness effect of specific practice with saccadic localization. *Exp Brain Res* **44**: 159–169. (1994) Rehabilitation of visual impairments in patients with brain damage. In *Low Vision,* ed. A. C. Koijman, P. L. Looijesijn, J. A. and Welling, G. J. van der Wildt. Amsterdam: IOS Press, pp. 287–295.

(1995). Visual scanning behavior in patients with homonymous hemianopia. *Neuropsychologia* **33**: 287–303.

(2000). *Rehabilitation of Visual Disorders after Brain Injury*. Hove, UK: Psychology Press.

Zihl, J. and Kerkhoff, G. (1990). Foveal photopic and scotopic adaptation in patients with brain damage. *Clin Vision Sci* **5**: 185–195.

Zihl, J. and von Cramon, D. (1979). Restitution of visual function in patients with cerebral blindness. *J Neurol Neurosurg Psychiatry* **42**: 312–322.

(1982). Restitution of visual field in patients with damage to the geniculostriate visual pathway. *Hum Neurobiol* **1**: 5–8.

(1985). Visual field recovery from scotoma in patients with postgeniculate damage. A review of 55 cases. *Brain* **108**: 335–365.

Zihl, J., von Cramon, D., and Mai, N. (1983). Selective disturbance of movement vision after bilateral brain damage. *Brain* **106**: 313–340.

Zihl, J., von Cramon, D., Mai, N., and Schmid, C. (1991). Disturbance of movement vision after bilateral posterior brain damage. Further evidence and follow up observations. *Brain* **114**: 2235–2252.

Zilles, K. and Clarke, S. (1997). Architecture, connectivity, and transmitter receptors of human extrastriate visual cortex. Comparison with nonhuman primates. *Cereb Cortex* **12**: 673–742.

18

Aphasia and dysarthria after stroke

Marjorie Nicholas

MGH Institute of Health Professions, Boston, MA, USA

Introduction

Disorders of communication following stroke are not uncommon. When the stroke affects the region of the left hemisphere known as the language zone, the chances of having a problem with language and/or speech are quite high in most right-handed individuals. Recovery from these disorders of language and speech is variable across individuals and dependent upon a number of factors, many of which are still unknown.

In this chapter, the common aphasia syndromes and stroke-caused dysarthria syndromes are reviewed with respect to lesion localization. This section is followed by a longer discussion of recovery that includes information on natural recovery patterns, recent trends in speech–language therapy and pharmacological treatments for aphasia, and mechanisms of recovery suggested by results of recent neuroimaging studies.

Aphasia after stroke

Aphasia is defined as a disorder of language caused by acquired brain damage. People with aphasia may have problems with a variety of activities that require linguistic knowledge or processing of language, such as understanding spoken language, formulating their own spoken messages, retrieving specific words, understanding written text, and writing. The incidence of aphasia after a stroke is estimated to be somewhere between 20 and 40%. Pedersen and colleagues (1995) found that the incidence of aphasia in a prospective study of over 800 acute stroke patients was 38%. After six months, approximately half of the surviving patients who initially had aphasia were still aphasic. Similar results were found by Laska and colleagues (2001), who suggested that aphasia in acute stroke was associated with higher mortality in a cohort of unselected stroke patients. The incidence of aphasia in left hemisphere stroke is, of course, much higher than in all cases of stroke, and estimated to be over 50%. For example, Scarpa *et al.* (1987) found that 55% of

Recovery after Stroke, ed. Michael P. Barnes, Bruce H. Dobkin and Julien Bogousslavsky. Published by Cambridge University Press. © Cambridge University Press 2005.

patients with left hemisphere stroke still had aphasia when examined between 15 and 30 days post-onset. Patients with stroke affecting the right hemisphere may have communication difficulties such as dysprosody, dysarthria, or higher-level disorders of communication pragmatics, but aphasias are rare from right hemisphere stroke. In fact, aphasia resulting from a right hemisphere stroke in a right-handed individual is such a rare syndrome that it has its own name: crossed aphasia.

The typical stroke patient with aphasia has suffered a stroke in the so-called language zone of the left hemisphere, a region supplied primarily by the middle cerebral artery, including portions of the frontal, parietal, and temporal lobes. The lesion causing the aphasia may be strictly cortical or strictly subcortical, although in many cases it affects both cortical and underlying subcortical regions. The important language-related regions of the left hemisphere have been recognized since the days of Paul Broca and Carl Wernicke and include Broca's area (Brodmann areas 44 and 45) in the frontal lobe, portions of the sensorimotor cortex in the frontal and parietal lobes, Heschl's gyrus and Wernicke's area (Brodmann area 22) in the temporal lobe, as well as association areas in all three lobes, including especially the supramarginal gyrus and the angular gyrus.

Aphasia syndromes

Although recent notions of brain–behavior relationships in the study of aphasic disorders stress the importance of widespread neural networks requiring the integrated functioning of several brain regions, older studies of lesion localization of the classic aphasia syndromes provided the foundation upon which these newer models are based. The classic "Boston" classification system of the aphasias was presented in Goodglass and Kaplan's 1972 test, the *Boston Diagnostic Aphasia Examination*, known as the *BDAE*. This test is now in its third revision and remains the worldwide standard for the assessment of aphasia (Goodglass *et al.*, 2001). The seven aphasia syndromes outlined on the BDAE are summarized in Table 18.1 with their most prominent language features and commonly associated lesion locations.

Many researchers seeking to clarify the neurolinguistic mechanisms underlying patterns of performance in individuals have criticized the use of aphasia syndromes (Caramazza, 1984). Nevertheless syndrome labels have continued to prove useful in clinical situations, because they are based on clinical descriptions of commonly observed clusters of symptoms. The syndrome labels used in BDAE represent a significant improvement over using the dichotomy of "expressive" versus "receptive" aphasia that was in vogue in the middle part of the last century, and unfortunately is still in use today in some medical settings. These terms are not useful and often prove to be quite misleading, as problems in both the expression and the reception of language are seen to differing degrees and in qualitatively different ways in every individual with aphasia. Many speech–language pathologists

Table 18.1 The Seven aphasia syndromes of the Boston Classification System

Aphasia syndrome	Language features	Common lesion location
Non-fluent aphasia syndromes		
Broca's aphasia	Non-fluent, sparse output, agrammatism, relatively preserved auditory comprehension, poor repetition	A large frontal lesion affecting Broca's area and surrounding cortical regions as well as white matter deep to Broca's area
Transcortical motor aphasia	Non-fluent output, relatively preserved auditory comprehension, strikingly preserved repetition	A frontal lobe lesion often anterior and/or superior to Broca's area, sometimes in the territory of the anterior cerebral artery
Global aphasia	Non-fluent severely restricted output, stereotypy or no speech, poor auditory comprehension, poor repetition	A large lesion affecting the frontal, parietal, and temporal lobes, or a smaller deep lesion affecting pathways from both anterior and posterior language regions
Fluent aphasia syndromes		
Wernicke's aphasia	Fluent, paraphasic, neologistic, empty output, poor auditory comprehension, poor repetition	A lesion affecting Wernicke's area in the temporal lobe, often with extension into other temporal regions and parietal lobe

Conduction aphasia	Fluent, paraphasic output, relatively good auditory comprehension, strikingly poor repetition	A lesion in supramarginal gyrus or arcuate fasciculus
Transcortical sensory aphasia	Fluent, paraphasic, neologistic output, poor auditory comprehension, strikingly preserved repetition	Borderzone regions of the territories of the middle cerebral and the posterior cerebral arteries, sparing Wernicke's area
Anomic aphasia	Fluent anomic output, relatively preserved auditory comprehension, preserved repetition	A variety of locations, often in posterior language regions, but some in frontal lobe

working with stroke patients have had the experience of receiving two identical referrals to evaluate two different patients described as having "expressive aphasia," only to find that one patient has sparse, non-fluent and agrammatic verbal output, while the other has an "expressive" problem characterized by fluent, neologistic verbal output as in classic Wernicke's aphasia. While the original use of the term "expressive" aphasia was not meant to cover cases like the second, in practice it sometimes is used erroneously to describe these cases.

Each of the seven syndromes in the Boston classification system is distinguished from the others by a specific pattern of performance in three areas: (a) fluency of spontaneous output, (b) degree of auditory comprehension impairment, and (c) status of repetition skills. Determination of preservation or impairment in each of these three areas theoretically allows the classification of the aphasia into one of the seven syndromes. Of course, the assessment of aphasia in an individual is not always straightforward, but Goodglass and colleagues (2001) stated that between 30 and 80% of people with aphasia will be classifiable with their system, depending on how rigorously the various criteria are applied.

Although commonalities have been found for lesion sites associated with the syndromes, there are also numerous exceptions. Furthermore, newer methods of neuroimaging are highlighting regions of hypoactivity (as measured by reduced blood flow) that may not show up as lesion on acute structural imaging scans. For example, Hillis and colleagues (2002) used perfusion-weighted magnetic resonance imaging (MRI) to study over 20 individuals with subcortical aphasia-producing lesions (seen on structural computed tomography or MRI) and found that, in every case, the images showed hypoperfusion in cortical regions. This type of imaging technique poses a challenge to some of our earlier notions of neuroanatomical correlations with the aphasia syndromes and will ultimately help to refine these correlations. However, for the most part, even the newer techniques provide results that are consistent with earlier clinicoanatomical patterns of correlations between aphasia syndromes and lesion location. Some of these earlier studies are briefly summarized in the next section, with the three non-fluent aphasia syndromes presented first (Broca's aphasia, transcortical motor aphasia, and global aphasia), followed by the four fluent aphasia syndromes (Wernicke's aphasia, conduction aphasia, transcortical sensory aphasia, and anomic aphasia.)

Lesion location and language characteristics of the aphasia syndromes

Broca's aphasia

Broca's aphasia is characterized by non-fluent, halting, frequently agrammatic spontaneous verbal output with relative preservation of auditory comprehension. In English-speaking aphasics, agrammatism refers to the omission of functor words and morphological endings in spontaneous verbal output, as well as problems in the production and comprehension of certain syntactic constructions. In an early land-mark study, Mohr and colleagues (1978) first suggested that the full-blown syndrome of Broca's aphasia was associated with a lesion that included Broca's area but was much more extensive, including nearby inferior frontal lobe regions, the insula, and white matter deep to these areas. A lesion restricted to Broca's area did not result in Broca's aphasia but rather a less-severe verbal output problem, variously described as aphemia or an articulatory motor programing disorder (a "dyspraxia of speaking aloud"). Lesion localization studies published in the years that followed generally confirmed these findings (Naeser and Hayward, 1978; Kertesz *et al.*, 1979; Mazzocchi and Vignolo, 1979; Dronkers, 1993.)

The motor speech disorder known as *apraxia of speech* is often found in patients who also have Broca's aphasia. This disorder has a somewhat controversial history because of its overlapping symptoms with the language disorder of Broca's aphasia as well as with some of the other aphasia syndromes. The difficulty of determining just what constitutes an apraxic speech error versus an aphasic language error lies at the heart of the controversy. McNeil and colleagues (2000) define apraxia of speech as a disorder of motor planning and programing that is distinct from the language disorder of Broca's aphasia but often coexists with it. Apraxia of speech very rarely occurs in isolation. There is no current consensus about the lesion location associated with apraxia of speech, perhaps because of the difficulty in determining just who has it and who does not. However, numerous left hemisphere regions have been associated with the disorder, including the insula (Dronkers, 1997), several different regions in the parietal and frontal lobes, as well as subcortical regions (Square-Storer *et al.*, 1997).

Transcortical motor aphasia

The transcortical aphasias, transcortical motor aphasia and transcortical sensory aphasia, are distinguished from other aphasic syndromes by their striking pre-servation of repetition skills. Transcortical motor aphasia is similar to Broca's aphasia in terms of non-fluency and comprehension but features preserved repetition abilities, even for lengthy sentences. Another symptom often associated with transcortical motor aphasia is lack of initiation, not only for language behaviors but also for other non-language behaviors. The lesions associated with transcortical motor aphasia are often subcortical in the white matter anterolateral to the left frontal horn and superior to Broca's area (Freedman *et al.*, 1984). The supplementary motor area of the frontal lobe is also often involved, and lesions in this region are believed to relate to the problem with initiation that is often seen. Many patients with transcortical motor aphasia had lesions in the anterior cerebral artery territory rather than the usual aphasia-producing lesion in the middle cerebral artery territory.

Global aphasia

In the common syndrome of global aphasia, there is severe disruption of all language skills. Spontaneous verbal output is severely restricted and may be limited to a verbal stereotypie (e.g. "ba ba ba" or "one two, one two") or there may be no verbal output at all. Auditory comprehension is also severely impaired, although usually some overlearned, personal, or highly emotional language is comprehended by individuals with global aphasia. The lesion associated with global aphasia is often large, affecting language areas in the frontal, parietal, and temporal lobes (Naeser and Hayward, 1978; Kertesz *et al.*, 1979; Mazzochi and Vignolo, 1979). Purely subcortical lesions can also result in global aphasia if the lesion disrupts enough important language pathways (Vignolo *et al.*, 1986).

While the typical patient with global aphasia also has an accompanying hemiparesis as a result of lesioning of the pyramidal tract at some point, a subset of patients with global aphasia is free of hemiparesis. This comparatively rare syndrome (global aphasia without hemiparesis) has been studied as well with respect to lesion location. Hanlon *et al.* (1999) identified three patterns of recovery within this subtype of global aphasia, each with a distinctive lesion profile: lesions in the superior temporal gyrus resulted in persistant global aphasia without persistent hemiparesis (lasting at least three months), lesions in the left inferior frontal gyrus and adjacent subcortical white matter led to evolving transcortical motor aphasia, and lesions in the left precentral and postcentral gyri led to evolving Wernicke's aphasia.

Wernicke's aphasia

Of the fluent types of aphasia, Wernicke's aphasia is perhaps the classic example of an aphasic disorder with a well-defined lesion location. Wernicke's aphasia is characterized by often excessively fluent output that contains numerous paraphasic errors and neologisms. Paraphasias are word substitution errors that may be related to the target word semantically (such as "chair" for stool) or phonemically (such as "spool" for stool). Neologisms are non-words that bear no relation to the target word or only a minimal relation (such as "beanstain" for stool). The verbal output of patients with Wernicke's aphasia is described as empty and anomic, but for the most part articulation and grammar are fairly normal. Auditory comprehension is moderately to severely impaired. People presenting with Wernicke's aphasia often have a lesion in Wernicke's area itself, with frequent extension into other association areas in the temporal and parietal lobes. Furthermore, the extent of lesion in Wernicke's area has been associated with the severity of the auditory comprehension impairment and also has been correlated with recovery of comprehension (Naeser *et al.*, 1987).

Conduction aphasia

Investigation of the lesion associated with conduction aphasia has been of interest to many researchers particularly after Geschwind (1965) suggested that the mechanism was a disconnection in the white matter tract known as the arcuate fasciculus, severing auditory input from motor speech pathways and leading to a severe disruption in repetition abilities as one of the primary clinical symptoms of the disorder. Conduction aphasia is classified as one of the fluent aphasia syndromes; however, many people with conduction aphasia are sometimes described as having halting "dysfluent" speech. Since auditory comprehension is relatively preserved in this syndrome, patients with conduction aphasia are able to monitor their own verbal output and, therefore, frequently attempt self-corrections of their paraphasic verbal errors. This results in a halting, starting and stopping pattern with frequent phonemic paraphasia.

Conduction aphasia is typically associated with lesions in the supramarginal gyrus, a cortical region overlying the arcuate fasciculus. While some studies of patients with conduction aphasia have found the expected lesion in the arcuate fasciculus itself (Naeser and Hayward, 1978; Damasio and Damasio, 1980), many other studies have not (Kertesz *et al.*, 1979; Mazzocchi and Vignolo, 1979). More recently, Selnes and colleagues (2001) reported on a patient with a documented lesion in the arcuate fasciculus using the newer method of MR diffusion-tensor imaging, which is particularly good at noting lesions in white matter tracts and their projections. The patient was severely aphasic yet had preserved repetition, leading to the conclusion that a lesion in the arcuate fasciculus was neither sufficient nor necessary to cause a disruption in repetition.

Transcortical sensory aphasia

Transcortical sensory aphasia has not been studied as extensively as some of the other syndromes, perhaps because of its relative rarity. It is characterized by fluent paraphasic output, not unlike that seen in Wernicke's aphasia, with concomitant impairment of auditory comprehension. Unlike Wernicke's aphasia, however, repetition is preserved. The lesions associated with this syndrome usually spare Wernicke's area itself, may be posterior and inferior to this region, and are sometimes exclusively subcortical (Kertesz *et al.*, 1979; Alexander *et al.*, 1989a; Damasio, 2001).

Anomic aphasia

Anomic aphasia is characterized by a significant impairment in word-finding ability in the presence of relative preservation of other spontaneous speech characteristics and auditory comprehension. As such, it is often described as the common end state for many recovered aphasics. In keeping with this characterization, a variety of lesion locations have been associated with anomic aphasia. Anomia as a symptom (i.e. the inability to produce the verbal "name" for a picture or a concept) has been studied extensively with respect to lesion location. Numerous patients have been described who present with category-specific naming deficits, for example difficulty with verbs and not nouns, or the reverse pattern, difficulty with nouns and not verbs. Other studies have investigated individuals with relative difficulty naming animate or living things versus inanimate items. Many reports point to various areas of the inferotemporal region of the left hemisphere as important to category-specific word retrieval skills (see Damasio, 2001.)

Subcortical aphasia syndromes

The seven aphasia syndromes described above are known as the "cortical" aphasia syndromes because of the common involvement of cortical language areas. Some clinicians and researchers have also found it useful to speak of subcortical aphasia syndromes. In contrast to the cortical aphasia syndromes, the subcortical aphasia syndromes are named for the location of the lesion. Common syndromes discussed in the literature include *thalamic aphasia* and *capsular–putaminal aphasia* (reviewed by Wallesch and Papagno, 1988; Nicholas, 1994). Thalamic aphasia, usually caused by a thalamic hemorrhage, shows features similar to the fluent aphasias, with relatively preserved repetition and an abundance of semantic paraphasias. Dysarthria, anomia, and memory deficits are also described in those with thalamic aphasia.

Several variations of capsular–putaminal aphasia have been recognized (Naeser *et al.*, 1982; Alexander *et al.*, 1987; Mega and Alexander, 1994), depending on the exact location of the lesion in the structures of the basal ganglia and the extent of involvement either in an anterior or posterior direction. One of these syndromes that stands out is posterior capsular–putaminal aphasia, which often has features similar to Wernicke's aphasia yet presents occasionally with a right hemiparesis owing to involvement of deep motor pathways. This constellation of symptoms would lead immediately to the supposition that the lesion was subcortical rather than cortical, because an accompanying hemiparesis is very rare in the "cortical" version of Wernicke's aphasia. Recent studies (e.g. Hillis *et al.*, 2002) have suggested that the symptoms seen in the subcortical aphasia syndromes, at least acutely, are caused not only by damage to the subcortical structures and white-matter pathways themselves but also by hypoperfusion of connected cortical regions.

Dysarthria after stroke

Dysarthria is a motor speech disorder resulting from impairments of any one or more of the speech subsystems of phonation, articulation, resonance, and prosody. It is distinct from the language disorder of aphasia although it often coexists with aphasia in patients who have suffered strokes that affect the functioning of the motor system at some level. Isolated dysarthria, or impairment of speech with fully intact language, is rare in stroke patients and is often described as one of the lacunar syndromes, implying a small lesion affecting a restricted area. Dysarthria as a neurological symptom, however, is fairly common and occurs in many with stroke, as well as in numerous degenerative disorders such as multiple sclerosis, amyotrophic lateral sclerosis, and Parkinson's disease, to name just a few.

In the classic differentiation of the dysarthrias by Darley *et al.* (1975), a number of dysarthria syndromes associated with stroke are described. These included flaccid dysarthria from lower motor neuron dysfunction (e.g. brainstem stroke), spastic dysarthria from bilateral upper motor neuron dysfunction (e.g. bilateral pyramidal tract lesions), and ataxic dysarthria from cerebellar dysfunction (e.g. cerebellar stroke). The other types of dysarthria in this classification system do not commonly occur with stroke but rather arise from degenerative brain diseases such as Parkinson's disease (hypokinetic dysarthria), Huntington's disease (hyper-kinetic dysarthria) or amyotrophic lateral sclerosis (mixed spastic-flaccid dysarthria). Each of these syndromes is associated with a cluster of speech symptoms that differentiates it from the other syndromes.

Darley *et al.* (1975) originally suggested that bilateral corticobulbar lesions were necessary to produce a permanent dysarthria after a stroke. A unilateral lesion in portions of the pyramidal tract important to motor control of the speech musculature might cause a dysarthria, but it was believed to be only transient. However, more recent investigations have questioned this belief and suggest that the syndrome of unilateral upper motor neuron (UUMN) dysarthria should be added to this list of syndromes (Duffy and Folger, 1996; Kent *et al.*, 2001). Occurrence of UUMN dysarthria may be masked by other disorders that affect communication in more drastic ways, such as aphasia and/or apraxia of speech. Duffy and Folger (1996) studied 56 patients with this form of dysarthria and found that over 60% had left hemisphere lesions, frequently involving the frontal lobe. The majority of lesions were in the internal capsule, pericapsular, or subcortical regions. The deviant speech characteristics were described as only mild or moderate, not severe, but in many cases they were persistent. The authors suggested that, in terms of symptomatology, UUMN dysarthrias overlapped with the categories of flaccid, spastic, and ataxic dysarthrias as originally described by Darley *et al.* (1975).

Kent and colleagues (2001) reviewed studies of dysarthria for which neuroimaging data were available. In this review, dysarthrias associated with stroke-caused lesions of the pyramidal system/upper motor neuron pathway included:

- UUMN: a mild-to-moderate dysarthria characterized by imprecise consonants, slow irregular alternating motion rates (repeating "puh-tuh-kuh"), slow rate, harsh vocal quality, and lingual weakness.

- the rare syndrome of isolated dysarthria associated with lesions in corona radiata, internal capsule, basal ganglia, or pons
- dysarthria clumsy-hand syndrome: associated typically with a pontine lesion, but other lesion locations also occurred.

Dysarthria was also seen from stroke-caused lesions of the cerebellar system, either in the cerebellar inflow or outflow pathways. This form of dysarthria, known as **ataxic dysarthria,** has some unique features that differentiate it from other stroke-caused dysarthria, such as irregular articulatory breakdown and vowel distortions.

Dysarthria in acute ischemic stroke was studied by Urban and colleagues (2001) with respect to lesion location and other factors. Patients who presented acutely with dysarthria and who had no aphasia or dementia were included in the study. They did not include patients with anarthria, a rare condition characterized by the total inability to produce speech that may be caused by a massive brainstem stroke as well as some other disorders. Approximately half of the patients with acute onset of dysarthria had lesions that were supratentorial and the others were infratentorial. Interestingly, most of the lesions were on the left side: 74% of supratentorial lesions and 91% of infratentorial lesions. About 60% of the lesions were small, qualifying as lacunar infarcts. All of the extracerebellar supratentorial lesions were located somewhere in the pyramidal tract. With respect to the dominance of left-sided lesions, the authors suggested that there might be a dominant speech pathway from the left hemisphere motor cortex region for mouth and tongue, analogous to the dominant left hemisphere language pathways. In an earlier study of dysarthria in lacunar stroke that used transcranial magnetic stimulation to investigate corticolingual responses, Urban *et al.* (1996) found that abnormalities of the corticolingual fibers were seen bilaterally in nearly every patient studied, even though the patients had unilateral lesions.

The syndrome of pure dysarthria (no other associated motor system impairments or language disorder) was studied by Okuda and colleagues (1999) using measures of blood flow as well as structural imaging. In 11 of the 12 patients studied, there were bilateral lacunar infarcts in the internal capsule or corona radiata. Cortical hypoperfusion was seen in the frontal lobe and in the anterior opercular and medial frontal regions, sparing sensorimotor, temporal, and parietal cortices. Given these findings, we may ask why these patients did not also show language deficits (associated with dysfunction of the frontal operculum/Broca's area region) or perhaps articulatory programming deficits in addition to the more elemental disorder of dysarthria. The dysarthria syndromes associated with stroke along with their most prominent speech features and commonly associated lesion locations are presented in Table 18.2.

Table 18.2 Dysarthria syndromes seen after stroke

Dysarthria syndrome	Speech features	Common lesion location
Spastic dysarthria	Imprecise consonants, monopitch, reduced stress, harsh vocal quality	Bilateral upper motor nueron pyramidal tract lesions
Unilateral upper motor neuron dysarthria	Imprecise consonants, slow alternating motor rates, phonatory abnormalities	Unilateral pyramidal tract lesions, more left than right
Flaccid dysarthria	Hypernasality, imprecise consonants, breathiness, monopitch	Lower motor neuron lesions, brainstem
Ataxic dysarthria	Imprecise consonants, excess and equal stess, irregular articulatory breakdown, distorted vowels	Cerebellum or cerebellar pathways
Pure or isolated dysarthria	Imprecise consonants	Lacunar infarcts in corona radiata or internal capsule

Speech features are from Darley *et al.* (1975) and Duffy and Folger (1996).

Recovery from aphasia

Recovery from the speech and language deficits caused by stroke is a broad topic that encompasses numerous subtopics. Before these can be addressed, the notion of recovery itself with respect to language and speech disorders needs to be further explained. When we speak of recovery from aphasia or dysarthria, there are two classes of behavioral change that we refer to: restoration of function and compensation for lost function. Restoration of function refers to the regaining or resumption of skills that were lost or damaged by the stroke, for example when a person with agrammatism as part of a Broca's aphasia syndrome recovers grammatical ability to pre-stroke levels. Compensation for lost function refers to the use of alternative functional systems to perform an activity, for example when a person with global aphasia uses drawing to communicate rather than spoken language. Many people who are using compensatory techniques effectively can be said to have good recovery of communication, yet they may have poor recovery of natural language. Therefore, when assessing recovery, it is important to specify what is being measured as an indicator of recovery. For perhaps the majority of patients with aphasia, the treatment plan attempts to influence both types of recovery by providing compensatory communication strategies while simultaneously facilitating the restoration of natural language functions.

Code (2001) highlighted the need for a theoretical model of recovery, which currently does not exist, and argued that a third concept, reorganization, underlies both restoration and compensation. He suggested that, in some cases, treatment directed towards compensation might actually inhibit restoration of function, a sentiment also echoed by Thompson (2000). Code further suggested that treatment which aims to restore functioning or compensate for impaired functioning would be more successful if it could "harness the natural recovery process." So, it must be asked what is meant by "natural recovery" in patients with aphasia and, most importantly, how exactly can it be harnessed. While the second question is probably unanswerable at the present time, in the next section we address the first.

Natural recovery from aphasia

Numerous researchers and clinicians have investigated recovery from aphasia in an attempt to isolate the set of factors that appears to be most important to recovery. Usually, recovery in this context refers to partial or full restoration of function rather than to compensation for a lost function. For example, it is often said that "spontaneous recovery" of language function will take place for up to six months post-stroke, but then improvement will plateau. Whatever deficits are seen at that point are presumed to be permanent or likely to show negligible improvements in the years to come. However, there are few studies that have followed stroke patients with aphasia for longer than one or two years post-onset at the most. The studies that have investigated outcomes for longer periods show that some language skills do continue to improve for many years after the stroke (Fitzpatrick, 1999.) Some recovery studies after stroke are also hampered by inadequate assessments for aphasia. For example, in one large-scale outcome study, aphasia was assessed using a gross 0–3 point scale that took into account only verbal expression and had no measure of auditory comprehension (Pedersen *et al.*, 1995.) Results pertaining to recovery from aphasia gained from an assessment such as this are likely to be quite different from studies that use more detailed analyses of language disorders. The lack of uniformity across studies in how aphasia is measured, as well as great variability in length of follow-up periods, has led to conflicting results with respect to what factors seem to be most important to recovery. Furthermore, it is clear that recovery from one type of aphasia may be quite different to recovery from a different type, and that those with severe aphasias may recover to a different extent and in different ways to those with mild aphasias.

Several reviews of the aphasia recovery literature have been published previously (e.g. Sarno, 1998; Cherney and Robey, 2001.) These have indicated that some personal factors such as age and gender appear to have little bearing on recovery from aphasia, while other variables such as lesion location and aphasia syndrome are relevant. It is not surprising that lesion location and aphasia syndrome should interact with aphasia recovery. If more of the language-related regions of the brain are damaged or rendered useless, then the aphasia is often more severe, and less full restoration of natural language function is to be expected over time. Generally, this is true; for example, people who have global aphasia persisting after a few weeks often remain severely aphasic for the rest of their lives. Auditory comprehension may show some improvements over time so that the syndrome label of "global aphasia" is no longer appropriate, yet verbal output usually remains severely non-fluent. Some clinical settings use the term "mixed non-fluent aphasia" for such cases.

Most people with persistent nonfluent aphasia remain nonfluent and most people with persistent fluent aphasia remain fluent over time. It is exceeding rare that a fluent syndrome ever evolves to a non-fluent syndrome and vice versa. Some of the more common syndrome progressions that are seen include Wernicke's aphasia evolving to conduction aphasia, with improvement of auditory comprehension, and global aphasia evolving to mixed non-fluent aphasia or severe Broca's aphasia, with improvement of auditory comprehension. In many cases, the aphasia syndrome evolves in terms of severity yet remains within the same syndrome classification (e.g. severe Broca's aphasia evolves to mild Broca's aphasia). For example, in a longitudinal study of patients with severe aphasia who were reassessed every six months after stroke onset, the majority of patients retained their original syndrome classifications even though significant improvements were noted in language assessments for up to 18 months post-onset (Nicholas et al., 1993).

Naeser and colleagues (Naeser et al., 1987, 1990; Gaddie et al., 1989) have investigated recovery of selected language skills with respect to lesion location. They found that extent of lesion in Wernicke's area was correlated with degree of recovery of auditory comprehension, and that patients with lesion in more than half of Wernicke's area showed much less recovery of auditory comprehension skills over time. Similarly, Hillis and colleagues (2001a) found that hypoperfusion of Wernicke's area in patients immediately after stroke *without infarct* in that region was related to severity of semantic language impairment. Furthermore, when this region was reperfused by raising blood pressure, language function was restored (Hillis et al., 2001b).

Naeser and colleagues (1989) also investigated recovery or non-recovery of speech fluency. Lesion in a combination of two white-matter pathways was identified as crucial to persistent non-fluency of verbal output in patients who had no speech or were only able to produce stereotypies for many years after their strokes.

The white-matter pathways they found that were critical were the subcallosal fasciculus in the medial portion of the frontal lobe and the middle one-third of the periventricular white matter. A review of 50 other cases in the literature revealed only one patient who had this lesion combination and yet had good recovery of spontaneous verbal output. In contrast to this finding, Dronkers and colleagues (1993) reported that verbal stereotypies were associated with lesion in the arcuate fasciculus, the region that had earlier been hypothesized as important for the repetition deficits of conduction aphasia.

Despite these correlations between lesion location and patterns of recovery, we see tremendous variability in recovery across individuals, even when they have the same lesion profiles. As Goodglass stated (1993, p. 220); "... one can predict a lesion from an observed syndrome much more successfully than one can predict a syndrome from a known lesion." One reason for this is that individuals may have "anomalous" brains, meaning that their personal pattern of dominance for various language functions may be idiosyncratic. Left-handers are more likely to show anomalous dominance than right-handers, but only about one-third of left-handers (or about 3% of the general population) are supposed to have anomalous dominance. The typical left-handed person with a left hemisphere stroke in the language areas will show the same behavioral deficits that a typical right-handed person would show. Nevertheless, when an unusual recovery pattern is observed in an individual, or the lesion does not seem to "match" the impairment, we sometimes try to explain this disparity by suggesting that perhaps the individual's brain is one of these anomalous ones. Alexander and colleagues (Alexander and Annett, 1996; Alexander et al., 1989b) have reported a wide variety of anomalous patterns of brain dominance for different language functions. For example, in one individual the left hemisphere may be dominant for comprehension of language, while the right may be dominant for phonological aspects of production; the reverse pattern may be seen in another individual.

Other factors that undoubtedly interact with recovery from aphasia to some extent but have received less scientific scrutiny include premorbid personality factors and psychosocial situation after the stroke. For example, patients with premorbid psychiatric disturbances (e.g. depression) probably will not respond as positively to various interventions for aphasia, particularly since depression is a common symptom post-stroke. Similarly, patients who premorbidly were socially withdrawn may have difficulty using compensatory communication strategies that require a lot of initiation and effort on their part, such as gesturing or drawing. Patients with aphasia also need to have *opportunities* for communication in order to demonstrate recovery from their aphasic disorder. If the patient is in a situation with few family members or conversational partners with whom he or she can interact, this lack of opportunity for communication may actually hamper the recovery process. Unfortunately, this is a reality for some patients with severe forms of aphasia, who may reside in less than optimal institutional settings.

Recent trends in speech–language treatment for aphasia

The role of treatment in recovery from aphasic disorders is a complex topic that can be summarized only briefly here. The efficacy of speech–language treatment for aphasia has received much attention in recent years. Despite overwhelming evidence that speech–language therapy is effective when appropriately provided to selected individuals (reviewed by Robey, 1998), the notion still persists in some circles that the effectiveness of speech–language therapy is as yet unproven (e.g. Pedersen *et al.*, 1995; Greener *et al.*, 2002a). It is true that many early studies were poorly designed and so did not allow conclusions as to the effectiveness of treatment. However, in recent years, clinical research has become increasingly sophisticated and numerous well-designed studies showing the effectiveness of specific treatment methods and approaches have been published. Many examples of these can be found in *Language Intervention Strategies in Aphasia and Related Neurogenic Communication Disorders*, a classic treatment text now in its fourth edition (Chapey, 2001.) This book describes a wide variety of treatment methods and approaches, some of which are designed to restore aspects of language functioning and some of which are designed to compensate for the communication impairments caused by aphasia.

One important trend in treatment for aphasia is the increasing use of single-subject designs in order to show the effectiveness of a given treatment method (Kearns, 2000). Some of the negative results seen in earlier efficacy studies that used group comparisons was likely the result of including groups of people with aphasia that were simply too heterogeneous. Intuitively, we would not expect a treatment that targets agrammatism, for example, to improve language in a patient with Wernicke's aphasia, nor would we expect a treatment targeting apraxia of speech to result in improved language output in someone who has global aphasia. Yet many of the early studies purporting to study treatment grouped together not only a variety of treatment methods but also a variety of patients with aphasia. It is not surprising then that the results of some of these studies are difficult to interpret with respect to treatment efficacy. Single-subject designs, by comparison, allow the researcher to tie changes in behavior in selected individuals directly to the application of a specific treatment. Some single-subject designs such as the multiple baseline design also provide a way to factor out the effect of spontaneous recovery and to isolate the effect of the specific treatment method being studied. Many earlier group treatment studies were plagued by this problem; that is, they included patients treated early post-onset so it was difficult to determine if behavioral changes were the result of "natural recovery" or the result of the treatment that was provided.

Another trend is the increasing use of neuropsychological models of cognition in the creation of treatment methods. Rather than developing a treatment method for "patients with Broca's aphasia," for example, treatment for a specific underlying neuropsychological deficit would be developed. Patients with this deficit, regardless of what type of aphasia they had, would receive treatment aimed either to restore or to repair the underlying deficit. An example of this type of approach is the treatment for agrammatic output developed by Thompson and colleagues (1993, 1996). In this treatment approach, people with agrammatism evident in their spontaneous verbal expression are trained to improve the production of question forms beginning with "wh" question words, such as "who" or "where." The treatment method is based on neurolinguistic theory and the hypothesis is that treatment aimed at the underlying deficit has a better chance of success than treatment aimed at more superficial aspects of language production. Numerous other treatment methods of this sort have been developed in recent years to address specific deficits in isolated language functions, such as various acquired alexia and agraphia deficits that are part of many aphasic disorders, (e.g. Beeson and Hillis, 2001).

Another important innovation in the treatment of aphasia is the recognition that many people with aphasia also have non-language deficits that are likely to affect response to treatment. Even though their aphasic disorder may be what is most obvious, many patients with left hemisphere damage show deficits in non-language functions as well. Furthermore, the extent of these non-language deficits seems to be independent of the severity of aphasia. For example, no correlation was found between performance on a set of non-verbal measures and overall aphasia severity (Helm-Estabrooks *et al.*, 1995; Helm-Estabrooks, 2002). Deficits in certain aspects of attention and other so-called executive functioning skills are currently being investigated (Hinckley and Carr, 2001; Helm-Estabrooks *et al.*, 2000; G. Ramsberger, personal communication 2002). Early results from some of these investigations indicate that selected non-language deficits may actually be more relevant to response to treatment than the specifics of the language deficit itself. For example, preliminary results from a study investigating response to an alternative communication treatment method on a computer (*C-Speak Aphasia*), indicate that subjects with poor performance on executive functioning tasks, such as symbol trails, design generation, and completing mazes, have more difficulty learning and using the *C-Speak Aphasia* system than subjects with good executive functioning skills, despite having identical aphasia profiles (Page *et al.*, 2003.)

This study is an example of another trend in the treatment for aphasia: the use of high-technology augmentative and alternative communication (AAC) approaches. These systems for people with aphasia do not aim to restore or repair language functioning but rather to compensate for the communication problems by providing an alternative means of expression. Electronic AAC systems for communication deficits are not new, but historically they have been used primarily for people with disturbances of motoric functioning, rather than language disturbances. Many of us are familiar with the AAC device ("Words Plus" software on a laptop computer) that the noted physicist Steven Hawking uses to assist his communication. This system relies on the fact that the user's language system is intact but compensates for impairment of motor control by providing an alternative means of accessing a keyboard, synthesized speech output, and abbreviated shortcuts for writing text. Patients with moderate-to-severe aphasia would not be able to use such a system because of their language disturbance, making it difficult for them to spell or read text, or even think of the words they might need to express themselves.

Any AAC system for aphasic patients must enable the user to create messages without placing heavy demands on the language system. Some approaches are low-technology, requiring no more than a pen and paper. Examples of these would be using drawing as a means of expression or pointing to pictures and text in an organized communication notebook. With advances in technology, high-technology electronic AAC devices have also been developed for use by people with severe aphasia, including computer-assisted visual communication (C-ViC: Steele *et al.*, 1989, 1992; Weinrich *et al.*, 1989a, b; Shelton *et al.*, 1996), Lingraphica (Tolfa Corp., Mountain View, CA, USA), and C-Speak Aphasia (Nicholas and Elliott, 1999). All of these are picture-based programs in which the user selects pictures to create a message. The C-Speak Aphasia program also has specialized screens to assist with communication in certain situation, such as speaking on the telephone or sending email messages. The user selects pictures to compose a message that can be spoken aloud by the computer's synthesized speech or sent as a text email message. (Fig. 18.1). Much of the basic efficacy research has not been conducted with these methods, so we do not yet have a clear sense of which patients will be able to use these to communicate effectively, nor do we know the optimal way to train patients to use these systems. One such study is currently underway in our laboratory investigating response to treatment with the *C-Speak Aphasia* system.

With these recent changes in the way speech–language therapy for aphasic disorders is being conceived, we can hope that treatment results published in the next few years will allow us to select more appropriate treatment methods and apply these methods to appropriate individuals with increasing accuracy.

Pharmacotherapy for aphasia

In addition to providing speech–language therapy, the approach to treatment of the patient with aphasia sometimes includes pharmacological interventions. Studies of pharmacotherapy for aphasia have focused on three medications: bromocriptine,

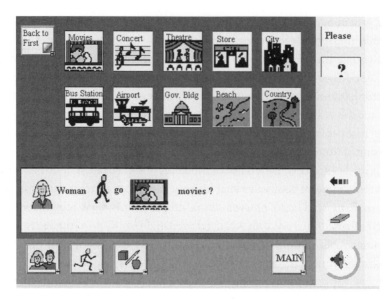

Fig. 18.1   Sample screen from *C-Speak Aphasia* showing a question in the message display area.

stimulants such as amphetamines, and piracetam. One problem with some of this research is that patients are often receiving two treatments simultaneously: both the drug under investigation and speech–language therapy. Therefore, isolating treatment effects to one or the other can be problematic. As will be seen, another major issue in pharmacotherapy for aphasia, as for any pharmacological intervention, is the undesirable side-effects of the medication.

Bromocriptine is a medication that works to increase the availability of the neurotransmitter dopamine in the brain. In patients with aphasia, bromocriptine has been used to help to improve speech initiation and verbal output. Generally, only modest improvements have been shown with bromocriptine (Albert *et al.*, 1988; Bragoni *et al.*, 2000; Gold *et al.*, 2000; Raymer *et al.*, 2001) or no differences between treated and untreated groups (Gupta *et al.*, 1995; Ozeren *et al.*, 1995; Sabe *et al.*, 1995). Furthermore, Altieri and colleagues (2002) discussed the high frequency of medical contraindication to bromocriptine administration, as well as an elevated occurrence of side-effects seen in their earlier study (Bragoni *et al.*, 2000).

Walker-Batson and colleagues (2001) reported on the first double-blind, placebo-controlled study of the use of dextroamphetamine on recovery from aphasia in stroke. Out of 850 stroke patients screened, only 21 were selected to receive either dextroamphetamine or placebo as well as speech–language therapy administered 30 minutes after the drug/placebo. Their findings indicated that the group receiving dextroamphetamine plus speech–language therapy had accelerated rates of recovery after 10 sessions with compared the group receiving placebo and speech–language therapy.

Perhaps the most promising of the pharmacological treatments for aphasia is the drug known as piracetam. Piracetam is a nootopic aminobutyric acid derivative that has been used clinically for the treatment of aphasia in Europe for several years. It is not yet approved as a treatment for aphasia in the USA. Numerous studies have reported positive effects of piracetam on language in patients with aphasia (Enderby *et al.*, 1994; de Deyn *et al.* 1997; Huber *et al.*, 1997; Orgogozo, 1999; Huber, 1999). In a recent review of 52 studies of various pharmacological treatments for aphasia, Greener *et al.* (2002b) concluded that only piracetam showed any effect on language functioning, but that the evidence for the positive effect of piracetam was only weak. Other drugs that were deemed even less effective in this review included bifemalane, piribedil, bromocriptine, idebenone, and Dextran 40. In general, the studies investigating response to drug treatments for aphasia have used a wide range of language measures to judge effectiveness of the treatment. We still do not know exactly which aspects of language are more likely to respond to treatment with specific medications, nor is there a good theoretical model guiding the selection of specific medications for certain types of deficit.

Kessler and colleagues (2000) have reported positive effects of piracetam given in conjunction with speech–language therapy in a group of patients with aphasia compared with a matched group given a placebo and speech–language therapy. The authors suggested that piracetam may benefit brain functioning by increasing release of acetylcholine and excitatory amino acids. The group receiving piracetam also showed increases in blood flow as measured by position emission tomography (PET) in language areas of the left hemisphere (Broca's area, Heschl's gyrus, and Wernicke's area). Neither group had increased flow in the right hemisphere but the piracetam group had a tendency to *suppress* blood flow in the right hemisphere homologous region to Broca's area. This finding led the authors to suggest that "...reactivation of temporal regions within the dominant hemisphere... might be more efficient for recovery from aphasia than facilitation of transcallosal transfer and restitution of functions within a bilateral network." This theory has been dominant in the neuroimaging studies investigating recovery from aphasia that we review in the next section.

Functional neuroimaging studies of recovery from aphasia

When recovery is seen in patients with aphasia, what is happening in the brain? This question has been of interest to aphasiologists since Broca's time. In fact, Broca himself suggested that perhaps the right hemisphere could "take over" some language functions if the left hemisphere were damaged. Many innovative treatment methods were also premised on this notion. For example, the aphasia treatment known as Melodic Intonation Therapy (Sparks *et al.*, 1974; Helm-Estabrooks *et al.*, 1989) uses singing and intonation, skills associated with the right hemisphere, to assist the production of propositional speech. Melodic Intonation Therapy is an example of a treatment method based on what the Russian aphasiologist A. R. Luria called "intersystemic reorganization." This term refers to the recruitment of an alternative functional system not ordinarily used in a behavior to assist a malfunctioning or inoperational functional system. In Melodic Intonation Therapy, the functional system used in production of melody is used to assist the malfunctioning system in the left hemisphere ordinarily used for overt language production. When melody is used to assist oral language production, does this really mean that the right hemisphere is being activated? Until recently, we could only speculate about what brain regions were involved when improvements were noted in language functioning during the course of recovery from aphasia. With the recent explosion of research using various functional imaging techniques, this is starting to change.

Some of the recovery hypotheses being investigated with functional imaging include: that language areas of the left hemisphere can resume functioning if they are not too severely damaged; that areas of the left hemisphere adjacent to the lesioned area are able to take over some language functions which they did not control premorbidly; and that language networks become extensively "reorganized," so that right hemisphere homologues to language areas of the left hemisphere are utilized for language activities. Some or all of these "reorganizations" may take place, depending on the time post-onset of the stroke and the extent of the damage to the left hemisphere. For example, the brain may first attempt to restore functioning within the left hemisphere, but if damage is extensive enough, control of some language functions might switch over time to the right hemisphere.

Observed activation in the right hemisphere has been subject to numerous and sometimes conflicting interpretations. In some studies, activation of the right hemisphere is seen as a positive indicator of how the brain reorganizes language to function more normally. In other studies, increased right brain activation is seen as pathological and associated with poorer recovery of language functions. Some researchers view the switchover of language control to the right hemisphere as a "last resort" effort. Both of these interpretations may be correct, depending upon the specific circumstances.

Stroke patients with very mild aphasias acutely may show full recovery when assessed after the initial acute period. Cappa and colleagues (1997) in a study using PET imaging found that early post-onset (two weeks) there was extensive bilateral depression of metabolism (diaschisis) in patients with mild aphasia. As the patients improved, activation increased in structurally unaffected regions, in particular in the right hemisphere, as seen in PET scans at six months post-onset. Functional MRI studies of patients with mild aphasias who subsequently showed full or nearly full recovery after six months have also indicated increased activity in the right hemisphere as well as in left hemispheric regions adjacent to the lesion (Heiss *et al.*, 1997, 1999; Cao *et al.*, 1999). However, these studies found better recovery of language if bilateral language networks could be reactivated rather than predominantly right hemisphere networks.

Heiss *et al.* (1997, 1999) suggested that the right hemisphere contributed to recovery but only if the left hemisphere language network was essentially destroyed. Furthermore, their results suggested that, because of the inferiority of the right hemisphere for language reorganization, language recovery would be complete only if left hemisphere language areas, particularly in the temporal lobe, were not destroyed and could be reactivated into the network. This idea received support in another longitudinal study using PET scanning performed at three to four weeks post-onset and then again after one year (Karbe *et al.*, 1998). In this study, the right hemisphere homologous region to Broca's area as well as the right supplementary motor area showed increased activation acutely. By one year post-onset, activation in the right hemisphere had diminished and left temporal activation had increased. Patients who showed persistent increased activation in the right supplementary motor area had persisting language problems and poorer recovery overall. Naeser and colleagues (2004) found similar results in a study using functional MRI in patients with nonfluent aphasia, claiming that "inadequate transcallosal inhibition and poor modulation of right SMA and right perisylvian language homologues may play a role in the hesitant, poorly articulated, agrammatic speech associated with nonfluent aphasia."

Interpreting increased right hemisphere activation as a maladaptive reaction may be analogous to viewing the glass as half empty, whereas it could also be viewed as the brain's attempt to do the best with what it has available: viewing the glass as half full. Consistent with this second interpretation, Mimura and colleagues (1998) found that recovery within the first year post-onset was clearly related to functional recovery of left hemisphere peri-lesional areas, but that subsequent recovery and long-term recovery (seven years post-onset) related to gradual compensation seen in increased activation in right frontal and thalamic regions. Patients who initially had moderate-to-severe Wernicke's aphasia were investigated with PET scanning by Weiller and colleagues (1995). At the time of scanning, the patients were five months to 12 years post-onset and all no longer scored as aphasic on language testing. Increased cerebral blood flow was noted in the right hemisphere homologous regions to Wernicke's area as well as in inferior premotor and lateral prefrontal cortex. Weiller *et al.*, (1995) suggested that patients with Wernicke's aphasia who recovered well were able to make use of a "pre-existing, extensive, and bilateral language network."

This brief review of some of the recent neuroimaging studies relevant to recovery from aphasia highlights how similar results can be interpreted in a variety of different ways. Our understanding of the recovery process will be enhanced as these studies become increasingly more sophisticated and we have a better understanding also of how the typical *non-damaged* brain processes language.

Recovery from dysarthria

Recovery from dysarthria in stroke patients has not been studied extensively. Partly this is because dysarthria is usually only one of many speech and language symptoms seen in stroke patients, and the other symptoms such as aphasia have taken center stage in studies of recovery. As stated above, dysarthria from UUMN damage is usually only mild or moderate, not severe, and so is not viewed as terribly important to the overall communication profile. Furthermore, when dysarthria is seen in isolation (pure dysarthria), it is also often mild, likely because the lesion producing it is small (lacunar) and so does not interrupt enough motor pathways to result in a more extensive speech deficit.

Likewise, there are few research studies pertaining to treatment of dysarthria from stroke that are rigorous enough to allow interpretation of treatment effects (see Sellars *et al.*, 2001.) Speech therapy for dysarthria includes a wide variety of techniques that have not been researched well in the stroke population. Common treatment methods include speech and articulation exercises such as using exaggerated speech or "over-articulation," improving intelligibility by reducing rate and speaking in a syllable-by-syllable manner, and improving loudness using a variety of techniques. Oral–motor exercises are also sometimes used (Robertson, 2001), although the efficacy of this approach is in doubt. In the rare cases where stroke-caused dysarthria significantly interferes with intelligibility of speech output, compensatory techniques such as the use of AAC devices may be tried. Some of the research on treatment techniques for patients with dysarthria arising as a result of other neurological disorders may also be relevant to stroke patients with dysarthria. See Duffy (1995) and Yorkston (1996) for further information on this topic.

Summary

Language and speech disorders are commonly seen as a result of stroke, particularly if the stroke damages the left hemisphere. Many different clinical syndromes of aphasia and dysarthria may occur, each with a unique pattern of language or speech deficits as well as commonly associated lesion locations. Nevertheless, it is well recognized that exceptions to these patterns are frequently seen in individuals. Recovery from aphasia depends upon many variables including extent and location of brain damage and what type of treatment is received. Recent trends in the treatment of aphasia include improvements in treatment research design, such as the increasing use of single-subject designs; the development of treatment methods for specific neurolinguistic deficits based on cognitive neuropsychological models; increasing consideration of non-language deficits in attention and executive functioning as factors that are potentially relevant to treatment response; improvements in electronic AAC devices for people with aphasia; and pharmacological interventions designed to ameliorate the language disorder. Advances in functional neuroimaging are helping us to investigate possible mechanisms underlying recovery from aphasia, including the notion that the right hemisphere or peri-lesional regions of the left hemisphere are able to reorganize language when a stroke damages the primary language areas of the brain.

REFERENCES

Albert, M. L., Bachman, D. L., Morgan, A., and Helm-Estabrooks, N. (1988). Pharmacotherapy for aphasia. *Neurology* **38**: 877–879.

Alexander, M. P. and Annett, M. (1996). Crossed aphasia and related anomalies of cerebral organization: case reports and a genetic hypothesis. *Brain Lang* **55**: 213–239.

Alexander, M. P., Naeser, M. A., and Palumbo, C. L. (1987). Correlations of subcortical CT lesion sites and aphasia profiles. *Brain* **110**: 961–991.

Alexander, M. P., Hiltbrunner, B., and Fischer, R. S. (1989a). Distributed anatomy of transcortical sensory aphasia. *Arch Neurol* **46**: 885–892.

Alexander, M. P., Fischette, M. R., and Fischer, R. S. (1989b). Crossed aphasia can be mirror image or anomalous. Case reports, review and hypothesis. *Brain* **112**: 953–973.

Altieri, M., Di Piero, V., and Luigi Lenzi, G. (2002). Drugs and recovery: a challenge for a few? *Stroke* **33**: 1170.

Beeson, P. M. and Hillis, A. E. (2001). Comprehension and production of written words. In *Language Intervention Strategies in Aphasia and Related Neurogenic Communication Disorders*, 4th edn., ed. R. Chapey. Philadelphia, PA: Lippincott Williams and Wilkins, PP. 572–604.

Bragoni, M., Altieri, M., DiPiero, V., *et al.* (2000). Bromocriptine and speech therapy in nonfluent chronic aphasia after stroke. *Neurol Scie* **21**: 19–22.

Cao, Y., Vikingstad, E. M., George, K. P., Johnson, A. F., and Welch, K. (1999). Cortical language activation in stroke patients recovering from aphasia with functional MRI. *Stroke* **30**: 2331–2340.

Cappa, S. F., Perani, D., Grassi, F., *et al.* (1997). A PET followup study of recovery after stroke in acute aphasics. *Brain Lang* **56**: 55–67.

Caramazza, A. (1984). The logic of neuropsychological research and the problem of patient classification in aphasia. *Brain Lang* **21**: 9–20.

Chapey, R. (ed.) (2001). *Language Intervention Strategies in Aphasia and Related Neurogenic Communication Disorders*, 4th edn. Philadelphia, PA: Lippincott Williams and Wilkins.

Cherny, L. R. and Robey, R. R (2001). Aphasia treatment: recovery, prognosis, and clinical effectiveness. In *Language Intervention Strategies in Aphasia and Related Neurogenic Communication Disorders*, 4th edn., ed. R. Chapey. Philadelphia, PA: Lippincott Williams and Wilkins, PP. 148–172.

Code, C. (2001). Multifactorial processes in recovery from aphasia: developing the foundations for a multileveled framework. *Brain Lang* 77: 25–44.

Damasio, H. (2001). Neural basis of language disorders. In *Language Intervention Strategies in Aphasia and Related Neurogenic Communication Disorders*, 4th edn., ed. R. Chapey. Philadelphia, PA: Lippincott Williams and Wilkins, PP. 18–36.

Damasio, H. and Damasio, A. R. (1980).The anatomical basis of conductive aphasia. *Brain* **103**: 337–350.

Darley, F. L., Aronson, A. E., and Brown, J. R. (1975). *Motor Speech Disorders*. Philadelphia, PA: W. B. Saunders Co.

de Deyn, P. P., de Reuck, J., Deberdt, W., Vlietinck, R., and Orgogozo, J.-M. (1997). Treatment of acute ischemic stroke with piracetam. *Stroke* **28**: 2347–2352.

Dronkers, N. (1993). *Cerebral Localization of Production Deficits in Aphasia*. [Tucson, AZ: Telerounds presentation.] National Center for Neurogenic Communication Disorders, University of Arizona.

Dronkers, N. (1997). A new brain region for coordinating speech coordination. *Nature* **384**: 159–161.

Duffy, J. R. (1995). *Motor Speech Disorders: Substrates, Differential Diagnosis, and Management*. St. Louis, MO: Mosby Year Book.

Duffy, J. R. and Folger, W. N. (1996). Dysarthria associated with unilateral central nervous system lesions: a retrospective study. *J Med Speech–Lang Pathol* **4**: 57–70.

Enderby, P., Broeckx, J., Hospers, W., Schildermans, F., and Deberdt, W. (1994). Effect of piracetam on recovery and rehabilitation after stroke: A double-blind, placebo-controlled study. *Clin Neuropharmacol* **17**: 320–331.

Fitzpatrick, P. (1999). Long-term recovery of naming and word-finding in narrative discourse in aphasia. PhD Thesis, Emerson College, Boston.

Freedman, M., Alexander, M. P., and Naeser, M. A. (1984). Anatomic basis of transcortical motor aphasia. *Neurology* **34**: 409–417.

Gaddie, A., Naeser, M. A., Palumbo, C., and Stiassny-Eder, D. (1989). Recovery of auditory comprehension after one year: a computed tomography scan study. In *Clinical Aphasiology*, vol. 18, ed. T. E. Prescott. Boston, MA: College-Hill, PP. 463–478.

Geschwind, N. (1965). Disconnexion syndromes in animals and man. *Brain* **88**: 237–294, 585–644.

Gold, M., van Dam, D., and Silliman, E. R. (2000). An open-label trial of bromocriptine in nonfluent aphasia: a qualitative analysis of word storage and retrieval. *Brain Lang* **74**: 141–156.

Goodglass, H. (1993). *Understanding Aphasia*. San Diego, CA: Academic Press.

Goodglass, H., Kaplan, E., and Barresi, B. (2001). *The Assessment of Aphasia and Related Disorders*, 3rd edn. Philadelphia, PA: Lippincott, Williams and Wilkins.

Greener, J., Enderby, P., and Whurr, R. (2002a). Speech and language therapy for aphasia following stroke. *Cochrane Database of Systematic Reviews*, Issue 3. Oxford: Update Software.

Greener, J., Enderby, P., and Whurr, R. (2002b). Pharmacological treatment for aphasia following stroke. *Cochrane Database of Systematic Reviews*. Issue 3. Oxford: Update software.

Gupta, S. R., Mlcoch, A. G., Scolaro, C., and Moritz, T. (1995). Bromocriptine treatment of nonfluent aphasia. *Neurology* **45**: 2170–3.

Hanlon, R. E., Lux, W. E., and Dromerick, A. W. (1999). Global aphasia without hemiparesis: language profiles and lesion distribution. *J Neurol Neurosurg Psychiatry* **66**: 365–369.

Heiss, W. D., Karbe, H., and Weber-Luxenberger, G., (1997). Speech-induced cerebral metabolic activation reflects recovery from aphasia. *J Neurol Sci* **145**: 213–217.

Heiss, W. D., Kessler, J., Thiel, A., Ghaemi, M., and Karbe, H. (1999). Differential capacity of left and right hemispheric areas for compensation of post-stroke aphasia. *Ann Neurol* **45**: 430–438.

Helm-Estabrooks, N. (2002). Cognition and aphasia: a discussion and a study. *J Commun Disord* **5215**: 1–16.

Helm-Estabrooks, N., Nicholas, M., and Morgan, A. R. (1989). *Melodic Intonation Therapy.* Austin, TX: Pro-ed.

Helm-Estabrooks, N., Bayles, K., Ramage, A., and Bryant, S. (1995). Relationship between cognitive performance and aphasia severity, age and education: females versus males. *Brain Lang* **51**: 139–141.

Helm-Estabrooks, N., Connor, L. T., and Albert, M. L. (2000). Treating attention to improve auditory comprehension in aphasia. *Annual Meeting of the Academy of Aphasia*, Montreal. [Poster Presentation.]

Hillis, A. E., Wityk, R. J., Tuffiash, E., *et al.* (2001a). Hypoperfusion of Wernicke's area predicts severity of semantic deficit in acute stroke. *Ann Neurol* **50**: 561–566.

Hillis, A. E., Kane, A., Tuffiash, E., *et al.* (2001b). Reperfusion of specific brain regions by raising blood pressure restores selective language functions in subacute stroke. *Brain Lang* **79**: 495–510.

Hillis, A. E., Wityk, R. J., Barker, P. B., *et al.* (2002). Subcortical aphasia and neglect in acute stroke: the role of cortical hyperperfusion. *Brain* **125**: 1094–1104.

Hinckley, J. J., and Carr, T. H. (2001). Differential contributions of cognitive abilities to success in skill-based versus context-based aphasia treatment. *Brain Lang* **79**: 3–6.

Huber, W. (1999). The role of piracetam in the treatment of acute and chronic aphasia. *Pharmacopsychiatry* **32**(Suppl. 1): 38–43.

Huber, W., Willmes, K., Poeck, K., van Vleymen, B., and Deberdt, W. (1997). Piracetam as an adjuvant to language therapy for aphasia: a randomized double-blind placebo-controlled pilot study. *Arch Phys Med Rehabil* **78**: 245–250.

Karbe, H., Thiel, A., Weber-Luxenberger, G., *et al.* (1998). Brain plasticity in post-stroke aphasia: what is the contribution of the right hemisphere? *Brain Lang* **64**: 215–230.

Kearns, K. (2000). Single-subject experimental designs in aphasia. In *Aphasia and Language: Theory to Practice*, ed. S. Nadeau, L. J. Gonzalez Rothi and B. Crosson New York: The Guilford Press PP. 421–441.

Kent, R. D., Duffy, J. R., Slama, A., Kent, J. F., and Clift, A. (2001). Clinicoanatomic studies of dysarthria: review, critique, and directions for research. *J Speech Lang Hear Res* **44**: 535–551.

Kertesz, A., Harlock, W., and Coates, R. (1979). Computer tomographic localization, lesion size, and prognosis in aphasia and nonverbal impairment. *Brain Lang* **8**: 34–50.

Kessler, J., Thiel, A., Karbe, H., and Heiss, W. D. (2000). Piracetam improves activated blood flow and facilitates rehabilitation of post-stroke aphasic patients. *Stroke* **31**: 2122–2116.

Laska, A. C., Hellblom, A., Murray, V., Kahan, T., and VonArbin, M. (2001). Aphasia in acute stroke and relation to outcome. *J Intern Med* **249**: 413–422.

Mazzocchi, F. and Vignolo, L. A. (1979). Localization of lesions in aphasia: clinical-CT scan correlations in stroke patients. *Cortex* **15**: 627–654.

McNeil, M. R., Doyle, P. J., and Wambaugh, J. (2000). Apraxia of speech: a treatable disorder of motor planning and programming. In *Aphasia and Language: Theory to Practice*, ed. S. Nadeau, L. J. Gonzalez Rothi and B. Crosson. New York: The Guilford Press PP. 221–266.

Mega, M. S. and Alexander, M. P. (1994). Subcortical aphasia: the core profile of capsulostriatal infarction. *Neurology* **44**: 1824–1829.

Mimura, M., Kato, M., Kato, M., *et al.* (1998). Prospective and retrospective studies of recovery in aphasia: changes in cerebral blood flow and language functions. *Brain* **121**: 2083–2094.

Mohr, J. P., Pessin, M. S., Finkelstein, S., *et al.* (1978). Broca aphasia: pathologic and clinical, *Neurology* **28**: 311–324.

Naeser, M. A. and Hayward, R. W. (1978). Lesion localization in aphasia with cranial computed tomography and the Boston Diagnostic Aphasia Examination. *Neurology* **28**: 545–551.

Naeser, M. A., Alexander, M. P., Helm-Estabrooks, N., *et al.* (1982). Aphasia with predominantly subcortical lesion sites: description of three capsular/putaminal syndromes. *Arch Neurol* **39**: 2–14.

Naeser, M. A., Helm-Estabrooks, N., Haas, G., Auerbach, S., and Srinivasan, M. (1987). Relationship between lesion extent in 'Wernicke's area' on computed tomographic scan and predicting recovery of comprehension in Wernicke's aphasia. *Arch Neurol* **44**: 73–82.

Naeser, M. A., Palumbo, C. L., Helm-Estabrooks, N., Stiassny-Eder, D., and Albert, M. L. (1989). Severe nonfluency in aphasia: role of the medial subcallosal fasciculus and other white matter pathways in recovery of spontaneous speech. *Brain* **112**: 1–38.

Naeser, M. A., Gaddie, A., Palumbo, C., and Stiassny-Eder, D. (1990). Late recovery of auditory comprehension in global aphasia: improved recovery observed with subcortical temporal isthmus lesion versus Wernicke's cortical area lesion. *Arch Neurol* **47**: 425–432.

Naeser, M. A., Hodge, S. M., Sczerzenie, S. E., *et al.* (2004). Overt, propositional speech in nonfluent aphasia studied with the dynamic susceptibility contrast fMRI method *Neuroimage* **22**: 29–41.

Nicholas, M. (1994). CT scan studies of localization and recovery of function in aphasia. *Crit Rev Phys Rehabil Med* **6**: 391–408.

Nicholas, M. and Elliot, S. (1999). *C-Speak Aphasia. A Communication System for Adults with Aphasia.* Solana Beach, CA: Mayer-Johnson Co.

Nicholas, M. L., Helm-Estabrooks, N., Ward-Lonergan, J., and Morgan, A. R. (1993). Evolution of severe aphasia in the first two years post onset. *Arch Phys Med Rehabil* **74**: 830–836.

Okuda, B., Kawabata, K., Tachibana, H., and Sugita, M., (1999). Cerebral blood flow in pure dysarthria: role of frontal cortical hypoperfusion. *Stroke* **30**: 109–113.

Orgogozo, J. M. (1999). Piracetam in the treatment of acute stroke. *Pharmacopsychiatry* **32** Suppl. 1: 25–32.

Ozeren, A., Sarica, Y., and Demirkiran, M. (1995). Bromocriptine is ineffective in the treatment of chronic nonfluent aphasia. *Acta Neurol Belg* **95**: 235–238.

Page, M., Nicholas, M, and Helm-Estabrooks, N. (2003). Cognitive skills predict response to alternative communication aphasia treatment. International Neuropsychological Meeting, Honolulu. [Poster Presentation.]

Pedersen, P. M., Jorgensen, H. S., Nakayama, H., Raaschou, H. O., and Olsen, T. S. (1995). Aphasia in acute stroke: incidence, determinants and recovery. *Ann Neurol*, **38**: 659–666.

Raymer, A. M., Bandy, D., Adair, J. C., *et al.* (2001). Effects of bromocriptine in a patient with crossed nonfluent aphasia: a case report. *Arch Phys Med Rehabil* **82**: 139–144.

Robertson, S. (2001). The efficacy of oro-facial and articulation exercises in dysarthria following stroke. *Int J Lang Commun Disord* **36**: (Suppl.) 292–297.

Robey, R. (1998). A meta-analysis of clinical outcomes in the treatment of aphasia. *J Speech Lang Hear Res* **41** 172–87.

Sabe, L., Salvarezza, F., Garcia Cuerva, A., Leiguarda, R., and Starkstein, S. (1995). A randomized, double-blind, placebo-controlled study of bromocriptine in nonfluent aphasia. *Neurology* **45**: 2272–2274.

Sarno, M. T. (1998). Recovery and rehabilitation in aphasia. In *Acquired Aphasia*, 3rd edn., ed. M. T. Sarno., San Diego CA: Academic Press, pp. 595–631.

Scarpa, M., Colombo, P., Sorgato, P., and DeRenzi, E. (1987). The incidence of aphasia and global aphasia in left brain-damaged patients. *Cortex* **23**: 331–336.

Sellars, C., Hughes, T., and Langhorne, P. (2001).Speech and language therapy for dysarthria due to non-progressive brain damage. *Cochrane Database of Systematic Reviews*. Oxford: Update Software.

Selnes, O. A., Mori, S., Barker, P. B., Hillis, A. E., and van Zijl, P. C. M. (2001). Preserved repetition in a patient with MR diffusion tensor imaging documented arcuate fasciculus lesion. *Brain Lang* **79**: 95–98.

Shelton, J. R., Weinrich, M., McCall, D., and Cox, D. M. (1996). Differentiating globally aphasic patients: data from in-depth language assessments and production training using C-ViC. *Aphasiology* **10**: 319–342.

Sparks, R. W., Helm, N., and Albert, M. L. (1974). Aphasia rehabilitation resulting from Melodic Intonation Therapy, *Cortex* **10**: 303–316.

Square-Storer, P. A., Roy, E. A., and Martin, R. E. (1997). Apraxia of speech: another form of praxis disruption. In *Apraxia: The Neuropsychology of Action,* ed. L. J. G. Gonzalez Rothi and K. M. Heilman. Hove, England: Psychology Press, pp. 173–206.

Steele, R. D., Weinrich, M., Wertz, R. T., Kleczewska, M. K., and Carlson, G. S. (1989). Computer-based visual communication in aphasia. *Neuropsychologia* **27**: 409–426.

Steele, R. D., Kleczewska, M. K., Carlson, G. S., and Weinrich, M. (1992). Computers in the rehabilitation of chronic, severe aphasia: C-ViC 2.0 cross-modal studies. *Aphasiology* **6**: 185–194.

Thompson, C. K. (2000). The neurobiology of language recovery in aphasia. *Brain Lang* **71**: 245–248.

Thompson, C. K., Shapiro, L. P., and Roberts, M. M. (1993). Treatment of sentence production deficits in aphasia: a linguistic-specific approach to wh-interrogative training and generalization. *Aphasiology* **7**: 111–133.

Thompson, C. K., Shapiro, L. P., Tait, M. E., Jacobs, B. J., and Schneider, S. L. (1996). Training wh-question production in agrammatic aphasia: analysis of argument and adjunct movement. *Brain Lang* **52**: 175–228.

Urban, P., Hopf, H., Zorowka, P., Fleischer, S., and Jorg, A. (1996). Dysarthria and lacunar stroke: pathophysiologic aspects. *Neurology* **47**: 1135–1141.

Urban, P. P., Wicht, S., Vukurevic, G., *et al.* (2001). Dysarthria in acute ischemic stroke: lesion topography, clinicoradiologic correlation, and etiology. *Neurology* **24**: 1021–1027.

Vignolo, L. A., Boccardi, E., and Caverni, L. (1986). Unexpected CT-scan findings in global aphasia. *Cortex* **22**: 55–69.

Walker-Batson, D., Curtis, S., Natarajan, R., *et al.* (2001). A double-blind, placebo-controlled study of the use of amphetamine in the treatment of aphasia. *Stroke* **32**: 2093–2098.

Wallesch, C. W. and Papagno, C. (1988). Subcortical aphasia. In *Aphasia*, ed. F. C. Rose, R. Whurr, and M. A. Wyke. London: Whurr. pp. 256–287.

Weiller, C., Isensee, C., Rijntjes, M., *et al.* (1995). Recovery from Wernicke's aphasia: a positron emission tomographic study. *Ann Neurol* **37**: 723–732.

Weinrich, M., Steele, R. D., Kleczewska, M. K., *et al.* (1989a). Representation of "verbs" in a Computerized Visual Communication System. *Aphasiology* **3**: 501–512.

Weinrich, M., Steele, R. D., Carlson, G. S., *et al.* (1989b). Processing of visual syntax in a globally aphasic patient. *Brain Lang* **36**: 391–405.

Yorkston, K. M. (1996). Treatment efficacy: dysarthria. *J Speech Hear Res* **39**: S46–S57.

19

Cognitive recovery after stroke

Antonio Carota, Radek Ptak and Armin Schnider.

University Hospital Geneva, Switzerland.

Introduction

Cognitive manifestations of stroke depend primarily on the lesion location. The area of brain destruction partly depends on individual variations in vascular organization, but also on the type of stroke: ischemic stroke tends to produce lesions with relatively stable patterns, defined by the affected vascular territory. Hemorrhages produce damage beyond vascular territories with, nonetheless, preferential lesion distribution: spontaneous intracerebral hemorrhage preferentially occurs in deep structures (basal ganglia, thalamus) or in hemispheric lobes. By contrast, hemorrhage from aneurysm rupture occurs with the arteries at the base of the skull, thus producing specific syndromes, although definitive lesion extension may widely vary with vascular spasms.

The brain's division into vascular territories is only partially congruent with its subdivision in functional neural networks and circuitries. The consequence is that cognitive syndromes caused by ischemic lesions (Table 19.1) are rarely pure and, frequently, several functional systems can be involved (McNeil *et al.*, 1991; Posner, 1995; Robertson, 2001).

It would be beyond the scope of this chapter to discuss in depth the cognitive syndromes occurring after stroke. We will discuss the typical cognitive failures associated with stroke in different cerebral areas as shown in Fig. 19.1 (Schnider, 1997) and then we will focus on some aspects of recovery of the main cognitive disorders occurring after stroke.

Localization of cognitive failures

Prefrontal lesions

Whereas damage of the posterior part of the frontal lobes (motor strip) gives rise to motor syndromes, damage of the area in front of and below the motor strip often produces cognitive and intellectual problems. The prefrontal cortex

Recovery after Stroke, ed. Michael P. Barnes, Bruce H. Dobkin and Julien Bogousslavsky. Published by Cambridge University Press. © Cambridge University Press 2005.

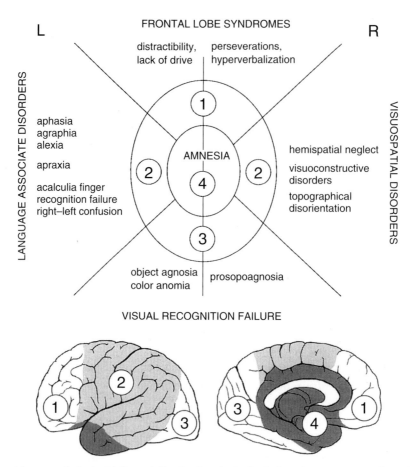

Fig. 19.1   Neuropsychological failures following hemispheric dysfunction. Area 1, prefrontal cortex; area 2, left or right hemisphere, area 3, posterior hemisphere, area 4, midline structures (limbic and paralimbic areas).

(Fig. 19.1, area 1) can be defined as the part of the frontal lobes receiving afferents from the dorsomedial thalamic nucleus (Fuster, 1997). It is eminently important for the ability to plan, initiate, and monitor actions; to concentrate on an action; and, at the same time, remain flexible to integrate new incoming information relevant for Behaviors (Fuster, 1997; Miller and Cohen, 2001). The precise cognitive failures emanating from prefrontal damage depend on the lesion location. At least three distinct syndromes can be distinguished (Stuss and Benson, 1986; Cummings, 1993). The first is seen in patients with lesions of the dorsolateral frontal region, following lobar hemorrhage or watershed infarct. They may manifest decreased drive, failure to recognize concepts, and lack of flexibility, together with perseveration and stereotyped motor behavior (e.g. grasping). Manifestations

Table 19.1 Cognitive syndromes reported with ischemic stroke in circumscribed vascular territories

		Cognitive syndromes	
Cerebral arteries	Right Side	Left Side	Bilateral lesions
Middle cerebral artery (MCA)			
Complete MCA superficial territory	Left neglect; anosodiaphoria; constructive and dressing apraxia; acute confusional state; sensory aprosodia	Global or Broca's aphasia; ideomotor apraxia	
MCA superior or anterior division	Left neglect; dysprosodia; anosognosia of hemiplegia; acute confusional state	Mutism evolving over few days in aphemia or in Broca's aphasia, bucco-linguo-facial apraxia; Wernicke's aphasia is very rare	
MCA inferior or posterior division	Left neglect; constructional apraxia; delirium or confusional states; sensory aprosodia	Wernicke's aphasia; conduction aphasia; global aphasia	
Orbitofrontal artery (usually associated with prefrontal and central artery territory infarction)	Disinhibition; spontaneous confabulations	Disinhibition; spontaneous confabulations	
Prefrontal artery	Delusions	Transcortical motor aphasia	Loss of planning abilities, utilization and imitation behaviors, grasp reflex, perseverations, poor abstraction and categorization, reduced mental flexibility, apathy and abulia

Table 19.1 (cont.)

Cerebral arteries	Cognitive syndromes		
	Right Side	Left Side	Bilateral lesions
Precentral (prerolandic or precentral sulcus) artery	"Frontal" neglect	Transcortical motor aphasia and limb kinetic apraxia; global aphasia without hemiparesis (if there is a second lesion in the posterior language areas); aphemia or pure apraxia of speech pure anarthria; transcortical sensory aphasia; agraphia with or without acalculia	
Central sulcus artery	–	Mild Broca's aphasia	
Anterior parietal (or postcentral sulcus) artery	Left neglect; "acute hemiconcern"	Acute conduction aphasia associated or not with ideomotor apraxia, anomia, acalculia or agraphia	
Posterior parietal artery (usually in association with angular artery territory infarction)	Hemiextinction; visuospatial and visuoconstructive dysfunction	Wernicke's aphasia; Gerstmann's syndrome; ideomotor apraxia; anomic aphasia; phonologic agraphia	
Angular artery	Spatial neglect; hemiextinction; asomatognosia; visuoconstructive and visuospatial disturbancies	Gerstmann's syndrome; trasncortical sensory aphasia; anomic aphasia; Wernicke's aphasia	Balint's syndrome, sometimes associated with anterograde and partially retrograde amnesia
Temporal arteries	Left visual neglect; left-side extinction; constructional apraxia; agitated confusional state; manic symptoms expressive instrumental amusia	Wernicke's aphasia; difficulties in identification of melodies or rhythm perception	Cortical deafness that can be associated with delusions about time; pure word deafness

Lenticulostriate arteries			
Internal capsule, anterior limb	Infarcts affecting the anterior thalamic peduncle induce frontal lobe signs and motor neglect;	Infarcts affecting the anterior thalamic peduncle induce frontal lobe signs and motor neglect;	Akinetic mutism
Upper part of the internal capsule and corona radiata adjacent to the lateral ventricle	Neglect or constructional apraxia	Aphasia	
External capsule – subinsular – infarcts		Aphasia	
Lentiform nucleus	Micrographia	Aphasia and agraphia	
The head of the caudate nucleus	Aphasia; abulia, akinesia, frontal lobe signs (disinhibition, inappropriateness); defective recall; psychotic mood changes	Neglect; abulia, akinesia, frontal lobe signs (disinhibition, inappropriateness); defective recall; psychotic mood changes	Dementia
Striatocapsular infarcts	Motor and visuospatial neglect; visual memory dysfunction; neglect (good prognosis)	Transcortical motor aphasia; anomia; verbal memory deficits; aphasia (good prognosis)	
Anterior cerebral artery			
Cortical infarcts	Abulia or akinetic mutism	Abulia or akinetic mutism; transcortical motor aphasia	Abulia or akinetic mutism tend to be persistent in case of bilateral infarctions; infarction in the mesial frontal lobe can cause emotional liability, euphoria, stuttering, mirror writing, grasp phenomenon

Table 19.1 (*cont.*)

Cerebral arteries	Cognitive syndromes		
	Right Side	Left Side	Bilateral lesions
Corpus callosum			Signs of callosal dysconnection (left unilateral ideomotor apraxia, left-hand agraphia, unilateral tactile anomia, unilateral constructional apraxia of the right hand, bilateral crossed pseudoneglect, alien-hand sign, diagonistic dyspraxia)
Caudate infarcts (Heubner's artery): see the head of the caudate nucleus above			
Anterior choroidal artery (deep branch of internal carotid artery)	In most cases without cognitive deficits; visual neglect, constructional apraxia, anosognosia and motor impersistence	In most cases without cognitive deficits; thalamic aphasia; slight language processing difficulties and short-term verbal memory deficit	
Posterior cerebral artery (PCA)			
Superficial PCA territory	Neglect; constructional apraxia; topoagnosia	Alexia without agraphia and anomia for colors or color agnosia or achromatopsia; elements of Gerstmann's syndrome; elements of conduction aphasia; anomic aphasia; transcortical sensory aphasia; visual agnosia; persistent amnesia	Inferior bank infarcts: amnesia; prosopagnosia; "ventral" agnosia Superiorbank infarcts: Balint's syndrome; difficulty in revisualizing directions; "dorsal" agnosia

Arterial territory	Clinical findings	
Proximal PCA disease with thalamic infarction	The clinical findings are those of the lateral thalamic infarction as a result of the occlusion of the thalamogeniculate or posterior choroidal arteries combined with temporal and occipital deficits including anomia, transcortical sensory aphasia or visual neglect	The clinical findings are those of the lateral thalamic infarction as a result of the occlusion of the thalamogeniculate or posterior choroidal arteries combined with temporal and occipital deficits including anomia, transcortical sensory aphasia or visual neglect
Thalamic infarcts		
Thalamogeniculate arteries	Cognition and behaviors are generally preserved	
Infarcts in the territory of the polar artery	Abulia; apathy; akinetic mutism; loss of self-psychic-activation; acute amnesia; verbal recall impairment is more common	Abulia; apathy; akinetic mutism; loss of self-psychic-activation; acute amnesia; visual-memory deficits predominate
Paramedian thalamic–subthalamic arteries	Hypersomnolence, lethargy, amnesia, confabulations	Hypersomnolence, lethargy, amnesia, confabulations; Abulia and amnestic disturbancies are severe and persistent; Cognitive impairment is more severe and long-lasting, utilization behavior, palypsychism
Posterior choroidal artery	Aphasia, amnesia, abulia and visual hallucinosis	

Adapted From Bogousslavsky and Caplan (2001).

may vary according to the laterality of the lesion, with left-sided lesions interfering with language production and verbal fluency, right-sided lesions interfering with production of visuospatial ideas (non-verbal fluency). The second is seen in patients with frontomedial lesions, particularly in the area of the anterior cingulate cortex. These lesions tend markedly to impair the ability to initiate behavior. The lesions may result from the occlusion of the anterior cerebral artery or from spasms after rupture of an anterior communicating artery aneurysm. In the initial stage, patients may be entirely unable to initiate motor acts and communicate (akinetic mutism; Bogousslavsky and Regli, 1990). The third syndrome is the orbitofrontal syndrome, which has often been associated with disinhibition (Cummings, 1993; DeLuca and Diamond, 1995). In our experience, clinically evident disinhibition is not more common in these patients than in patients with dorsolateral prefrontal lesions.

Acute damage of the posterior medial orbitofrontal cortex, generally associated with basal forebrain damage, typically emanating from rupture of an aneurysm of the anterior communicating artery, produces a distinct syndrome: "spontaneous confabulations." Here thought is guided by memories, which may have justly guided a subject's behavior in the past but, do not pertain to ongoing reality (Schnider, 2001). Anterior orbitofrontal lesions involving the frontal pole may produce social failure, often through altered decision-making faculty and personality modifications (Eslinger and Damasio, 1985; Schnider, 1997; Bechara *et al.*, 2000). To our knowledge, frank sociopathy (e.g. stealing, aggressive behavior) has not been described after vascular lesions.

Lateral left hemisphere lesions

Lesions in the middle part of the left hemisphere (Fig. 19.1, area 2), essentially in the distribution of the middle cerebral artery, preferentially produce failures of language-associated capacities. This area involves the motor association areas in the posterior frontal lobes, inferior parietal lobe, and lateral temporal lobe. Damage here may result from occlusion of a branch of the middle cerebral artery or from an intracerebral hemorrhage following the rupture of an aneurysm of the middle cerebral or posterior communicating artery. The best-known cognitive failure resulting in such a lesion is aphasia. The aphasia profile depends on the precise lesion location (Alexander and Benson, 1991; Benson and Ardila, 1996; Kreisler *et al.*, 2000). Anterior lesions, involving the frontal operculum and the surrounding frontal tissue provoke Broca's aphasia (Mohr *et al.*, 1978), characterized by word-finding difficulties, frequently interrupted and effortful speech, phonemic and phonetic paraphasias, syntax failures, and relatively spared comprehension. The verbal output of these patients is non-fluent and repetition is also impaired.

In contrast, lesions of the temporal lobe tend to interfere particularly with language comprehension; the patients produce a fluent, seemingly effortless speech, which may be unintelligible because of the semantic paraphasias and neologisms (jargon aphasia; Wernicke's aphasia). The patients seem to ignore the incomprehensibility of their verbal output.

Global aphasia is the more severe form with failure of all linguistic abilities. Oral production is limited to few stereotyped sounds or syllables pronounced with effort. Communication relies on facial expressions and intonation, for which the right hemisphere is dominant.

Other forms of aphasia are characterized by repetition abilities (preserved in transcortical and subcortical aphasias, impaired in conduction aphasia). Aphasic individuals often present with language disorders that cannot be definitely classified or that modify during recovery.

Aphasia frequently includes an inability to produce written language (agraphia) and to understand written text (alexia), although these failures may occur in isolation.

Aphasic disorders have been described after subcortical lesions involving the basal ganglia, the thalamus, or deep white matter and are often accompanied by a dysarthric speech (Mega and Alexander, 1994).

Another syndrome pointing to left hemisphere dysfunction is ideomotor apraxia: the inability to produce skilled movements to verbal commands, in particular pantomimes of tool use (Alexander et al., 1992; Heilman and Gonzalez Rothi, 1993; Schnider et al., 1997). It is often associated with aphasia, but dissociation in individual patients shows that the two disorders have independent mechanisms.

The combination of agraphia, the inability to recognize one's own fingers (finger agnosia or localization failure), the inability to make calculations (acalculia) and right–left confusion is known as Gerstmann's syndrome and indicates a dysfunction at the temporal–parietal junction (angular gyrus). It may occur without an accompanying aphasic disorder and is probably based on a core defect in spatial processing (Mayer et al., 1999).

Lateral right hemisphere lesions

Damage of the middle part of the right hemisphere (Fig. 19.1, area 2) results in impairment of spatial processing. The most specific failure, resulting from inferior parietal or superior temporal damage, is hemispatial neglect: the unawareness of stimuli presented to the contralesional space (Heilman et al., 2000). Neglect may depend on the position of the trunk (Karnath et al., 1991), the head, or the eyes and whether an object is within or outside reachable space (Vuilleumier et al., 1998).

Neglect is often associated with visuospatial failures: the patient may fail to copy or to respect the spatial proportions of complex drawings or to make three-dimensional constructions (visuoconstructive disorder; de Renzi, 1997). These failures may also occur after left hemisphere damage but are usually more severe after right hemispheric lesions. Neglect, even in a discrete form, is a major impediment to an independent life (Denes *et al.*, 1982), as patients putting themselves risk in danger when crossing the streets or utilizing the cooker.

Posterior hemispheric lesions

Damage to posterior hemispheric areas (Fig. 19.1, area 3) produce failures of visual recognition. These areas are within the vascular territory of the posterior cerebral arteries and include the occipital lobes and the inferior temporal lobes. Particularly, right-sided, lateral lesions of the occipital lobes impair visual recognition; patients may fail to recognize fractionated or overlapping visual information or even simple drawings (apperceptive agnosia; de Renzi and Spinnler, 1966).

Damage to left temporal–parietal association areas may compromise the attribution of a meaning to visual information that has been correctly perceived or to an object correctly copied (associative agnosia) (Rubens and Benson, 1971; Schnider *et al.*, 1994a). A lesion in this area can affect word reading but not copying (pure alexia; Damasio and Damasio, 1983; Binder and Mohr, 1992). Stroke in the right inferior temporal cortex (superficial territory of the posterior cerebral artery) may disturb the recognition of previously familial visual information, in particular individual faces (prosopagnosia; Damasio *et al.*, 1982; de Renzi *et al.*, 1991) or famous places (associative topographagnosia; Landis *et al.*, 1986; Takahashi *et al.*, 1995).

Limbic and paralimbic lesions

Lesions of midline structures (limbic and paralimbic areas; Fig. 19.1 central area 4) often produce memory failures and affective changes. Ischemic strokes in the distribution of the posterior cerebral artery may involve, apart from visual and deep limbic areas, the hippocampus and the surrounding cortex (von Cramon *et al.*, 1988). These lesions produce a failure to learn and retain new information (anterograde amnesia). The amnesia is particular severe if the lesion is bilateral and extends beyond the hippocampus itself (Schnider *et al.*, 1994b; Zola-Morgan *et al.*, 1986). Depending on the extension of the lesions toward inferior and lateral temporal areas, patients may lose information acquired before the brain damage (retrograde amnesia; Schnider *et al.*, 1994b). Patients with medial temporal lesions typically have a severe failure of encoding new information.

Severe anterograde amnesia accompanied by impaired vigilance and oculomotor disorders may result from bilateral medial (paramedian) thalamic infarction;

the involvement of the mamillothalamic tract seems to be particularly important for inducing a true amnesic syndrome those with thalamic stroke (von Cramon *et al.*, 1985; Graff-Radford *et al.*, 1990).

A different disorder results from anterior limbic damage, particularly after the rupture of an anterior communicating artery aneurysm damaging the basal forebrain and the posterior orbitofrontal cortex. Even though the patients fail in common memory tests (Alexander and Freedman, 1984; DeLuca and Diamond, 1995), they often remain unaware of the brain damage, act according to previous habits rather than currently relevant memories, and are disoriented. We have recently shown that these patients fail to suppress (deactivate) activated memories that do not pertain to ongoing reality, a syndrome called spontaneous confabulation (Schnider, 2001).

Principles of recovery

Early prediction of functional outcome is important in stroke management to fix optimal rehabilitation programs with realistic objectives. These objectives should be periodically checked and readapted with the salient clinical aspects of the patient recovery.

Outcome is generally better for deep cerebral hemorrhage than for subarachnoid hemorrhage and ischemic stroke. The influence of the lesion size and side is controversial, but the best predictor remains the severity of the deficits at the onset (Chang *et al.*, 2002; Sumer *et al.*, 2003). Most sensorimotor and cognitive recovery occurs in the first three months (Skilbeck *et al.*, 1983; Bach-y-Rita, 1990; Nakayama *et al.*, 1994) and continues at a slower pace throughout the first year (Kotila *et al.*, 1984), although some recovery can be found up to several years (Katz *et al.*, 1966). Low-level functions (sensorimotor deficits processed by primary cerebral areas) often improve before than more complex functions (attention, memory, language, and the other faculties processed by integrative or associative areas) (Skilbeck *et al.*, 1983).

Age, sitting balance, severity of paresis, disability on admission, urinary incontinence, comorbidities, psychotropic drugs, previous stroke, interval before the onset of the rehabilitation treatment, and the adequacy of social support emerged as factors directly and indirectly influencing functional recovery (Denes *et al.*, 1982; Ween *et al.*, 1996; Paolucci *et al.*, 1998, 2000; Giaquinto *et al.*, 1999; Katz *et al.*, 1999; Pettersen *et al.*, 2002; Troisi *et al.*, 2002).

Cognitive deficits (particularly aphasia, neglect, and executive dysfunction; Paolucci *et al.*, 1998; Pohjasvaara *et al.*, 2002a), low Mini-Mental State Examination scores (Pohjasvaara *et al.*, 2002b), and mood disturbances (depression and anxiety; Singh *et al.*, 2000; Gainotti *et al.*, 2001) have a strong negative impact on the degree of autonomy after stroke.

In the earliest phases, recovery depends on resolution of edema and reperfusion of the ischemic penumbra. During the following weeks, months and years, recovery is enhanced by the plasticity of the brain.

Mechanisms of brain plasticity are both structural (sprouting of fibers from the surviving neurons with formation of new synapses) and functional (extension of the cortical map, the emergency of alternative pattern of activation within the neural network including the damaged area, unmasking of previously existing but functionally inactive pathways, the use of alternative strategies and brain circuitries to resolve the same task).

All these mechanisms of recovery have been demonstrated in humans and animals and are modulated by experience and training (Nudo *et al.*, 1996; Buonomano and Merzenich, 1998; Kempermann *et al.*, 1998; Nakatomi *et al.*, 2002).

Functional neuroimaging studies have provided considerable evidence that the reorganization of the injured brain can be modulated by activity, behavior, and skill acquisition, even after a long delay after injury (Carey *et al.*, 2002; Jang *et al.*, 2003). These studies suggest that combining therapies, greater intensities of therapy, and increasing overall afferent inputs may improve stroke outcome.

While there is evidence that recovery of cognitive functions is supported by mechanisms of brain plasticity, the actual challenge is to identify which of the processes identified are important and how they can be enhanced by specific behavioral or pharmacological interventions.

Cognitive therapies for the individual patient should be supported by high-quality evidence-based practice. Randomized controlled trials and rigorous meta-analysis studies are widely accepted as the more robust methodology for research into clinical treatments. Nevertheless, cognitive rehabilitation is a particularly hostile field for application for this methodology because the great interindividual variability may be often, unfortunately, responsible for significant sampling errors.

Recovery from aphasia

Aphasia is the most frequent cognitive deficit in the early (20–38%) and late (12–28%) phases of stroke (Wade *et al.*, 1986a; Dobkin, 1995; Pedersen *et al.*, 1995).

Most patients undergo at least some degree of spontaneous recovery of language over time (Basso, 1992). The greatest improvement occurs in the first two weeks and most final recovery takes place during the first one to three months (Basso, 1992). After the third month, the recovery is slower until the sixth month and in some cases until one year; after this, very little if any spontaneous recovery is to be expected. Nevertheless, interindividual variability is high and improvement may be significant even after six months.

The role of gender (females recover better than males in oral production and auditory comprehension; Basso *et al.*, 1982; Pizzamiglio *et al.*, 1985), higher IQ, and higher education (better recovery; Connor *et al.*, 2001) on prognosis has been advanced in some studies but not found by others (David and Skilbeck, 1984; Ferro *et al.*, 1999). A better and faster recovery is frequently observed on clinical ground for left-handers and ambidextrous people (Subirana, 1969; Gloning *et al.*, 1976). However, these factors have little impact in rehabilitation programs.

Older patients have the poorest prognosis. Different distributions of infarcts with age (Ferro and Madureira, 1997; Godefroy *et al.*, 2002), decreased brain plasticity, and limited capacity for learning are additional plausible explanations for this difference.

Post-stroke mood disorders have a negative influence on aphasia outcome (Kauhanen *et al.*, 2000). The link is often bidirectional: depression can worsen aphasia but is also often its consequence.

Severity of aphasia at the stroke onset and the lesion size are significantly correlated with the residual deficit (especially spontaneous fluency decrement) (Pedersen *et al.*, 1995; Code, 2001). Aphasia outcome is better with subcortical lesions and is generally a result of reversal of cortical hypometabolism (Hillis *et al.*, 2000, 2002).

Some aspects of recovery reflect, to a certain extent, some general principles of the organization and functioning of the language system in the brain and are valid for every aphasic syndrome independent from the lesion localization: comprehension and repetition usually shows faster recovery; naming and verbal output recovery is slower and often incomplete; and oral language improves better than written language (Kertesz and McCabe, 1977).

Global aphasia and Wernicke's aphasia, characterized by a severe impairment of comprehension, have the poorest prognosis, while transcortical aphasias, anomic aphasia, and conduction aphasia generally have a more favorable outcome (Valles *et al.*, 1997). Restricted lesions of Broca's area induce a mild and transient language deficit (Mohr *et al.*, 1978), while recovery is less favorable (especially for spontaneous fluency) with damage to adjacent cortical and subcortical areas (Knopman *et al.*, 1983).

Patients with Wernicke aphasia and particularly severe and persisting lexical–semantic deficits (referring to the relationships between words and their underlying meanings) generally have large temporal lobe lesions (Selnes *et al.*, 1984). However, even for these patients, some single-word comprehension is often achieved. Lexical–semantic deficits are indeed transient for patients with smaller temporal lesions, and, within the first year of recovery, they resolve into less-severe forms of aphasia (anomic or conduction aphasia) (Benson *et al.*, 1973).

The contributions of the right and the left hemisphere to the recovery of language have been investigated with functional neuroimaging (regional cerebral blood flow analysis, single photon emission and position emission tomography, functional magnetic resonance imaging, and transcranial Doppler sonography) in resting or activating linguistic conditions. These studies have associated aphasia recovery with the activation of the right hemisphere (Silvestrini *et al.*, 1998; Musso *et al.*, 1999; Thulborn *et al.*, 1999), reactivation of language areas in the left hemisphere (Cao *et al.*, 1999; Warburton *et al.*, 1999), or activation of both hemispheres (Cappa *et al.*, 1997; Mimura *et al.*, 1998). The role of the right hemisphere in aphasia recovery is probably more relevant for comprehension and semantic tasks than for expression, especially in the earliest phases of stroke (Weiller *et al.*, 1995; Musso *et al.*, 1999). Its contribution probably varies with individual differences for the hemispheric dominance for language and appears to be greater when the degree of impairment of the left areas is particular severe (Gainotti, 1993; Heiss *et al.*, 1999). Undamaged or peri-lesional areas in the left hemisphere are probably more relevant for the final outcome and, specifically, for speech output, syntax, and lexical tasks (Heiss *et al.*, 1997, 1999; Warburton *et al.*, 1999).

The cognitive–neuropsychological approach to aphasia therapy involves the use of cognitive models of linguistic functions in assessing the language disorder and choosing or designing a therapy program for individual patients. This approach provides the therapist with a theoretical basis for suggesting that a particular therapy might result in improvement in a person's language performance and also a framework that has the potential to explain why a given treatment works for one patient and not another. This approach is founded on evidence that patients with aphasia have unique deficits and that multiple factors may determine the same clinical picture (Saffran *et al.*, 1980; Kay and Ellis, 1987; Marshall *et al.*, 1990; Basso *et al.*, 2001).

This approach has specially been used for anomia, agrammatism, alexia, and agraphia, and there are well-documented single case studies showing its effectiveness (Hillis, 1991, 1998; Robson *et al.*, 1998). Cognitive therapy for aphasia has also proved its effectiveness with computer-assisted programs (Crerar *et al.*, 1996; Fink *et al.*, 2002; Laganaro *et al.*, 2003).

The cognitive approach often requires detailed baseline measures and time-consuming evaluation during treatment, and the treatment of any particular language function according to a linguistic model may not necessarily be adapted to all the affected patients in group studies. The approach emphasizes restitution of function of damaged cognitive components, rather than merely encouraging strategies that compensate for those impairments; it is best suited for moderately impaired individuals with relatively circumscribed deficits, for whom cognitive problems can be isolated and decomposed.

Melodic Intonation Therapy (Sparks *et al.*, 1974), the enhanced gestural performance (Hanlon *et al.*, 1990), lexical–semantic therapy (Mazzoni and Vista,

1997), the mapping technique for the treatment of agrammatism (Marshall, 1995), and the writing therapy for jargon aphasia (Robson *et al.*, 2001) are specific techniques used in aphasia therapy that particularly focus on the linguistic channels of inputs and outputs and even, within specific guidelines, are applicable to larger groups of patients.

Other techniques such as promoting aphasic communicative effectiveness (PACE) are founded on the pragmatic aspects of communication (Davis and Wilcox, 1985). Here quality and quantity of information in conversational speech is increased by the need to transmit new information to the listener. This is in contrast with the traditional therapies where the therapist aims to reduce the chances that an aphasic will fail to get the message by asking only for known information.

Several procedures of non-verbal communications are used for the treatment of global aphasia, such as visual analogue and iconic communication (Johannsen-Horbach *et al.*, 1985), the visual action therapy (Helm-Estabrooks *et al.*, 1982), drawing therapies (Sacchett *et al.*, 1999), and the acquisition and use of the American Indian Gestural Code (Amerind) or the American Sign Language (Guilford *et al.*, 1982). Nevertheless, even if these therapies are attractive, patients with global aphasia do not often have sufficient residual semantic capacities for their effective learning and use.

Computerized visual communication is indeed a sort of verbal prosthesis, specifically designed for patients with severe aphasia who manipulate pictures or icons loaded into a computer for the purpose of communication (Baker *et al.*, 1976; Gardner *et al.*, 1976; Steele *et al.*, 1989). Despite encouraging results, teaching patients with severe aphasia to master the mechanisms of the system may be very difficult. A very practical attitude to train communicative aspects of language, or alternative strategies, is adopted in group treatments (Holland, 1991; Elman, 1998). It has been shown that some social context (meaningful to the patient) significantly increases motivation and promotes active participation (Lyon *et al.*, 1997).

Computer-aided therapies used in community-based programs can be adapted to the patients' progress and can satisfy the desires of caregivers to participate in rehabilitation therapies at home, even for patients with chronic aphasia (Aftonomos *et al.*, 1997).

Aphasic individuals often present with an impairment of other cognitive functions, such as attention or memory. The treatment of these non-linguistic deficits can improve communication. For example, speech therapy focused on verbal perseverations ameliorated symptoms in patients with Broca's aphasia (Helm-Estabrooks *et al.*, 1987). Within the same holistic perspective, several studies have indicated the beneficial effect of antidepressant drugs or relaxation therapy, both combined with aphasia therapy (Marshall and Watts, 1976; Murray and Heather Ray, 2001).

Lesion size and location influence not only the spontaneous recovery of aphasia but also the capacity to profit from language therapy (Goldenberg and Spatt, 1994; Naeser *et al.*, 1998). Non-fluent aphasics with bilateral lesions or a lesion including Wernicke's area or the temporal isthmus have poor response to Melodic Intonation Therapy (Naeser and Helm-Estabrooks, 1985). Patients with bilateral lesions and with lesions in critical areas (temporal lobe, supraventricular frontal lobe, and subcortical medial subcallosal fasciculus) are inappropriate candidates for learning on an icon-based computer-assisted visual communication system (Naeser *et al.*, 1998).

Efficacy of professional speech therapy has been shown in both the early and the late phases of stroke (Basso *et al.*, 1979; Wertz *et al.*, 1981; Shewan and Kertesz, 1984; Mazzoni *et al.*, 1995; and may extend beyond the sixth month post-onset (Wertz *et al.*, 1986). However, there also negative reports (reviewed by Ferro *et al.*, 1999). The difference between studies with positive and negative effects is probably explained by the different intensity and times of therapy. Early and more-intensive (daily) therapies are more efficacious and individuals with aphasia benefit from treatments that are specific to their own situation (Carlomagno *et al.*, 2001). Although the effect of aphasia therapy on recovery appears to be limited in meta-analysis or randomized studies (Greener *et al.*, 2000), it is questionable whether these types of study are really suited for evaluation and treatment of the individual stroke patient with aphasia. The reasons are the great interindividual variability of patients with aphasia, even within the same aphasic syndrome, and the fact that aphasia is a very highly dynamic (time-related) phenomenon after stroke.

A further perspective to consider is that therapeutic changes during the course of therapies should be included within theoretical frameworks that cover all the possible (neural, linguistic, cognitive, and behavioral) variables involved in language recovery (Code, 2001).

The role of pharmacological interventions (nootropic drugs; psycho-stimulants; drugs acting on noradrenergic, dopaminergic, or cholinergic systems) also need further validation (Greener *et al.*, 2001; Walker-Batson *et al.*, 2001), while new therapies such as the "constraint-induced therapy for aphasia" (Pulvermuller *et al.*, 2001) or transcranial magnetic stimulation (Sakai *et al.*, 2002) are promising.

The use of biotechnology in the field of neural regeneration will probably influence the future of aphasia therapy; however, patients with transplanted or pharmacologically modified neural networks will continue to require active language training.

Recovery from visuospatial neglect

Visuospatial neglect (VSN) is formally diagnosed with tasks evaluating spatial processing, such as cancellation tasks, line-bisection, writing, reading, or drawing. It is particularly sensitive to ipsilesional distracters; the more distracting information present on the ipsilesional side, the less will such patients explore the controlateral hemispace. The sensitivity of a neglect test does, therefore, often depend on the number and complexity of ipsilesional distracters.

Visuospatial neglect may operate in different spatial coordinates. Patients may ignore stimuli presented on the body (somatic space) or near the body (peripersonal space) as well as outside of reaching distance (extrapersonal space) (Bisiach *et al.*, 1986; Halligan and Marshall, 1991; Vuilleumier *et al.*, 1998).

Within these spatial frames, VSN may depend on egocentric coordinates (retinal axes, the sagittal midplane of head or trunk, the axis of a limb moving) or allocentric coordinates (i.e. object-based frames) (Marshall and Halligan, 1994; Driver, 1995). However, often, the different contributions of egocentric and allocentric reference frames may only be detected with extended testing.

Occasionally, neglect may only be found in mental representation (Bisiach *et al.*, 1979; Guariglia *et al.*, 1993; Ortigue *et al.*, 2001) or may only be evident when a motor response is produced (Adair *et al.*, 1998).

Patients with VSN often show spatial extinction on double simultaneous stimulation (in auditory, visual, and tactile modalities), other visuospatial disorders (constructional apraxia or agnosia), and sometimes alloesthesia (the mislocalization of contralesional stimuli to symmetrical or asymmetrical points of the ipsilesional somatic or extrasomatic space).

In conclusion, VSN is not a unitary disorder and requires detailed assessment. The existence of multiple dissociations among neglect patients, and the different evaluation methods used, probably explains the variable findings of the degree of VSN recovery after stroke, from 0 to 100% (Bowen *et al.*, 1999; Ferro *et al.*, 1999), among the different follow-up studies.

Spontaneous recovery of acute neglect occurs in the first 10 days and continues thereafter to reach a plateau at three months post-stroke (Stone *et al.*, 1992).

According to Hier and collaborators (1983a), different VSN signs recover in the following order: drawing, visual and auditory orienting, anosognosia, and sensory extinction. However, the extent of the lesion appears to be a crucial variable.

Neuroimaging and clinical studies indicate that spatial attention is processed predominantly in the right hemisphere in a widely distributed network, including the posterior parietal and dorsolateral frontal cortex, the cingulate cortex, the basal ganglia, and the reticulothalamic system (Leibovitch *et al.*, 1998; Kirk, 2001; Karnath *et al.*, 2002). Persistent neglect has, therefore, to be expected after large cortical strokes involving frontal and parietal areas (Hier *et al.*, 1983a). In contrast, VSN is in general less severe and more transient after subcortical lesions and VSN recovery is associated with resolution of ipsilesional diaschisis on cingulate, frontal, and parietal cortical areas (Hillis *et al.*, 2000, 2002). According to functional imaging studies, the controlateral hemisphere may be dominant for early VSN recovery and the ispilateral for late recovery (Pizzamiglio *et al.*, 1998).

Persistent deficits of visuospatial attention predict a negative functional outcome (Jehkonen *et al.*, 2000a; Cherney *et al.*, 2001; Paolucci *et al.*, 2001), an increased probability of accidents, fewer transfers with physiotherapeutic training, and dressing problems. Therefore, the need for VSN rehabilitation has been recognized and several approaches have been proposed.

The efficacy of neuropharmacological treatment of VSN with bromocriptine (Fleet *et al.*, 1987) and apomorphine (Corwin *et al.*, 1996; Geminiani *et al.*, 1998) is limited to case reports or uncontrolled case series with conflicting results.

Systematic training of visual scanning by presenting facilitating contralesional cues (e.g. a colored bar that the patient has to fixate before reading a line of the text) and gradually modulating the task difficulty has been used in early rehabilitation studies to improve spatial exploration.

Cueing techniques have been applied in reading (Weinberg *et al.*, 1977), figure description (Pizzamiglio *et al.*, 1992), sensory awareness (by proprioceptive cueing), and spatial organization training (Weinberg *et al.*, 1979). Proprioceptive cueing with touch or movement of the contralesional limb also ameliorates VSN (Ladavas *et al.*, 1997). These cueing techniques may show some benefits for the task trained but often show a lack of generalization to other tasks.

Several authors have, therefore, attempted to increase awareness of the deficit in neglect patients by verbal (Robertson and North, 1992) or visual (Tham and Tegner, 1997) feedback of their exploration behaviors.

Visual–motor treatments try to improve spatial deficits by requiring actions towards a particular object or a position in space such as assembling pieces to complete a figure, drawing, or pointing to a location (Weinberg *et al.*, 1982). Another strategy is to stimulate ipsilesional limb movements into the neglected hemispace. This can be achieved with a Neglect Alert Device placed on the contralesional limbs, which emits a loud buzzing noise if its switch is not pressed at regular intervals (Robertson *et al.*, 1992), or with glasses with a reminder beep if the patient fails to move the eyes to the left (Fanthome *et al.*, 1995).

All these methods increase awareness of the deficits and stimulate the patient to maintain attention to the contralesional side of space. A different approach consists in recalibrating the biased egocentric reference frame in a more implicit manner. An example is the blinding of the right eye coupled with a dynamic visual stimulation on the left side (Butter and Kirsch, 1992; Arai *et al.*, 1997; Zeloni *et al.*, 2002). However, since patients with VSN often have left visual field deficits, right-eye blinding limits even more the already restricted visual and perceptual abilities needed for daily activities.

Several studies have found that the ipsilesional bias of neglect patients may be recalibrated by different kinds of sensory stimulation. Vestibular and optokinetic stimulation (Rubens, 1985; Pizzamiglio *et al.*, 1990; Rorsman *et al.*, 1999), transcutaneous mechanical vibration (Karnath *et al.*, 1993), electrical vibration (Vallar *et al.*, 1995), and prism adaptation (Rossetti *et al.*, 1998; Frassinetti *et al.*, 2002), have all been reported to influence positively SVN. The influence of prism adaptation is particularly interesting because it also improves mental spatial representations (Rossetti *et al.*, 1998) and because its effect can be sustained over time (Frassinetti *et al.*, 2002). The findings of studies using prism adaptation to rehabilitate VSN are promising but suffer from a lack of satisfactory explanations for the observed effects.

Future studies of VSN recovery and therapy need to answers questions concerning the specificity of the intervention on different neglect subtypes, the durability of effects, and their functional relevance in natural settings, especially for daily life activities (Bowen *et al.*, 2002; Pierce and Buxbaum, 2002).

Recovery from visual disturbances

Ischemic lesions in the part of the visual system responsible for low-level perceptual analysis and in the oculomotor system may induce impairments of functions that are easily measurable (visual acuity, contrast sensitivity, photopic and scotopic foveal adaptation, stereopsis, convergent fusion, and scotoma). Their recovery can be relatively easily evaluated, quantified, and correlated with therapeutic interventions. When the lesion involves the associative visual areas such as the peristriate cortex, the occipitotemporal and parietal association cortex, the resulting visual disorders are more complex and often inadequately investigated; their recovery is more difficult to measure.

Neurophysiological and neuropsychological studies suggest the existence of at least two visual functional pathways: a ventral stream (occipitotemporal) involved in form, color, and pattern analysis (the "what" stream) and a dorsal stream (occipitoparietal) processing spatial information (the "where" stream) (Mishkin *et al.*, 1982; Perenin and Vighetto, 1988; Jeannerod *et al.*, 1994; Milner, 1998). Both systems act in parallel to coordinate motor responses to visual stimuli. Schematically, lesions in the ventral stream manifest with visual agnosia; lesions in the dorsal stream manifest with reaching or grasping errors of seen objects (optic ataxia) or in defective localization of stimuli.

Visual agnosia corresponds to a failure of object recognition that is not explained by elementary visual deficits and that is modality (visual) specific. In most cases, the differentiation of visual agnosia from basic perceptual deficits requires extensive testing (Riddoch and Humphreys, 1993). Probably for this reason, and since patients with relatively pure agnosia are rare, there are few data on prevalence and recovery of visual agnosia after stroke.

Recovery from visual agnosia is generally considered favorable (Hier *et al.*, 1983b) but this notion could be biased by exercise effects on the same paradigm tests and by the fact that functional consequences of visual agnosia on daily life activities may be mild. Recovery is probably limited in those with bilateral or diffuse disseminated lesions.

Rehabilitation studies with patients with visual agnosia are rare, and specific programs must be elaborated on an individual basis. In patients with chronic problems, the aim is to encourage compensation of the visual deficits by using unimpaired channels. Functional programs should be designed to train compensation in natural contexts that are meaningful to the patient.

In contrast to ventral lesions, damage to the dorsal stream may lead to a profound deficit of spatial processing and localization: Balint's syndrome. This comprises impaired fixation of gaze (gaze apraxia); defective visually guided reaching (optic ataxia and apraxia), especially in the controlateral hemispace; impaired simultaneous perception of more than one or a few objects (simultanagnosia); reading inability; defective depth perception; and severe visuospatial disorders (Rizzo and Vecera, 2002).

Balint's syndrome is a rare disorder in stroke because it occurs with bilateral lesions of the superior regions of the posterior parietal lobule, and it is likely that mild forms of the disorder are often overlooked or misdiagnosed (Rizzo and Vecera, 2002).

Reports on rehabilitation techniques are rare (Perez *et al.*, 1996; Rosselli *et al.*, 2001) and mostly based on systematic training of visual exploration and fixation. Eye blinking may eliminate confusing visual images or seeing the same object at multiple locations.

Finally, effective treatment strategies are poorly developed and evaluated. Rehabilitation of "higher" visual functions is a newly developing field needing to combine findings from neuropsychology, neurolasticity, neurophthalmology, and neurophysiology .

Recovery from memory failures

The failure to store and retrieve new information is relatively common after stroke (Wade *et al.*, 1986b). By contrast, pure amnesia, with no other cognitive failures, is comparatively rare. Extremely severe, persistent amnesia has been reported after bilateral medial temporal damage involving the hippocampus and adjacent cortex in the parahippocampal gyrus (Schnider *et al.*, 1994b). Unilateral lesions tend to be less severe and modality specific (e.g. for names, rather than faces of people) (von Cramon *et al.*, 1988). However, such reports of individual cases constitute a negative selection and do not necessarily reflect the full spectrum of outcomes after medial temporal lesions. The same is valid for thalamic lesions: whereas modality-specific memory failures after unilateral lesions are well known (Speedie and Heilman, 1983), severe amnesia appears to require a lesion involving, apart from the dorsomedial nucleus, the mamillothalamic tract (von Cramon *et al.*, 1985; Graff-Radford *et al.*, 1990; Hodges and McCarthy, 1993). As with medial temporal lesions, patients with severe and persistent amnesia have been reported after bilateral lesions, but rates of absence of, or recovery from, amnesia after thalamic lesions are unknown.

The course of spontaneous confabulation after anterior limbic lesions has been described in some detail. Patients with anterior medial orbitofrontal lesions (frontal pole) tend to have relatively fast recovery of their ability to adapt behavior to ongoing reality; some patients even have full neuropsychological recovery (Schnider *et al.*, 2000). By contrast, patients with posterior orbitofrontal and basal forebrain damage tend to remain in a state of spontaneous confabulation with confusion of ongoing reality for more than three months and up to one year (Schnider *et al.*, 2000). Although they may later regain their ability to adapt behaviors to ongoing reality, and thus lead a life of relative independence, they often remain severely amnesic (D'Esposito *et al.*, 1996).

Unfortunately, rehabilitative techniques do not seem to improve directly memory capacity in patients with stable deficits. Therefore, therapy focuses on strategies that are also efficacious when healthy subjects try to improve encoding of information: patients are trained to visualize information and repetitively encode it without guessing or giving it meaning (deep encoding) (Richardson, 1992; Thoene and Glisky, 1995). Such strategies do not induce recovery of memory but help to exploit fully residual memory or encoding capacities. When amnesia is severe, compensatory aides such as a memory booklet or a pager system can help patients to attain a certain degree of independence (Wilson *et al.*, 2001).

Recovery from emotional changes

Emotional factors influence recovery from stroke in two major ways that have important consequences for recovery. One view is that emotional changes derive from a strong psychological reaction to the disabilities caused by stroke. In this context, any form of stroke affecting motor, cognitive, and sensory abilities can be accompanied by mood changes. This postulate is supported by a similar prevalence of mood disorders in stroke as in other chronic non-neurological debilitating diseases (Aben *et al.*, 2003).

An alternative view is that damage to neural networks mediating emotional processes leads to a pattern of psychological changes specific to the locality of the stroke.

In reality, these two factors, the "psychological" and the "organic," are often intermingled in stroke patients. Extensive analysis of both factors is required to predict functional recovery and plan adequate treatments. For example, patients with lacunar strokes and leukoaraiosis respond less well to antidepressant drugs (Fujikawa *et al.*, 1993, 1996; Greenwald *et al.*, 1998).

Post-stroke mood disorders are treated elsewhere in this volume and we will focus only on emotional changes where the link with regional brain dysfunction is more direct.

Among patients with right hemisphere stroke, anosognosia for hemiplegia is a disorder involving surprisingly insufficient emotional activation or arousal. Multiple mechanisms have been postulated (Gold *et al.*, 1994; Jehkonen *et al.*, 2000b; Meador *et al.*, 2000) as the origin of the anosognosia, such as inattention to the left hemibody; reduced sensory feedback; impairment of general attention resources; a defect in body schemata, self awareness, internal representation or mental flexibility; mental deterioration; or loss of expectancy of movement owing to the failure of updating an internal comparator about impending movements.

Anosognosia may dramatically improve in a few hours or days after the stroke onset, more rapidly and completely than spatial neglect (Bisiach *et al.*, 1986). Anosognosia for hemiplegia significantly recovers in the first three months after stroke (Hier *et al.*, 1983b; Jehkonen *et al.*, 2001), but its association with neglect at the initial presentation is an indication for poorer functional outcomes, increased dependence, disability, and longer medical as well as institutional care (Hartman-Maeir *et al.*, 2001; Jehkonen *et al.*, 2001). Nevertheless, as for neglect, the role of anosognosia as an independent factor of negative outcome has been questioned in several studies (Jehkonen *et al.*, 2001). Anosognosia for neglect (which has been the object of fewer investigations) may be more lasting and results in a poorer outcome (Jehkonen *et al.*, 2001).

There is no standardized treatment for anosognosia.

Arousal or activation of neural networks subserving emotional processing is often reduced after right hemisphere stroke. Patients with right stroke have less emotional expressivity in the voice, face, and gestures, as well as less-accurate perception of facial and vocal emotional communication. Affective dysprosodia is frequent in the acute phase of stroke but, as for aphasia, rapid improvement usually occurs.

In contrast to the reduced emotional arousal observed with right hemisphere damage, two other syndromes, the catastrophic reaction and emotionalism, are indeed characterized by a strong emotional content.

The catastrophic reaction, a syndrome of the left hemisphere, refers to an outburst of frustration, depression, and anger suddenly building up to an overwhelming degree when the patient is confronted with an unsolvable task. It is observed in aphasic patients during the days or weeks after stroke onset (Carota *et al.*, 2001). Opercular lesions have been associated with this syndrome, for which an insular–amygdala limbic disconnection has been hypothesized as the causative process (Carota *et al.*, 2001). Patients with catastrophic reactions are at risk of developing emotionalism and post-stroke depression in the following months.

Emotionalism is an increase in the frequency of crying or laughing starting with little or no warning (House *et al.*, 1989). This syndrome is frequent in the acute phase of stroke (40% in personal data) and at one month follow-up (21%), but the prevalence declines over the first six months (Calvert *et al.*, 1998). A specific correlation with localization of stroke has not yet been demonstrated. The biochemical substrate may be serotoninergic because patients respond well to selective serotonin reuptake inhibitors (Brown *et al.*, 1998).

Frontal lobe damage with stroke leads to impairment in the regulation and expression of emotion (e.g. akinesia, apathy, hypomania) as well as in the role of emotion in motivation, decision making, and social interactions (e.g. affective empathy, drive). Dysfunction of dopaminergic frontosubcortical loops may be specifically involved in amotivational syndromes, and psychostimulants or direct (bromocriptine, pergolide) or indirect (apomorphine) dopamine agonists may prove helpful (Marin *et al.*, 1995).

Empathy refers to cognitive processes such as identifying a behavioral perspective or inferring the intentions and mental states of others. This faculty is fundamental for human relationships and social integration and is based on very highly dynamic and active cognitive and emotional processes. Its correct functioning allows continuous behavioral adjustments in order to enhance interpersonal relations and achievement of personal goals. Its impairment results in the absence of tact and inhibition, a childish behavior, acting on simple motivations, impulsiveness, self-centeredness, and immorality. These failures often have important consequences on social integration, partnership, and return to work. These disturbances are poorly understood and should be also researched in the early phases of stroke.

Damage of the dorsolateral prefrontal cortex has been associated with diminition of both empathy and cognitive flexibility (Grattan *et al.*, 1994). The orbital frontal cortex appears to underlie some social functions, such as empathy, through its involvement in the generation of somatic states anticipating important decisions. Deep white matter lesions of the frontal lobe disconnecting frontal–limbic pathways have also been associated with impaired empathy and negative social adaptation. Patients with right posterior stroke may be impaired in understanding sarcasm (Shamay *et al.*, 2002) a task that requires "theory of mind" capabilities.

Emotion-related processing disorders are still minimally understood; their course of recovery is uncertain, and remediation techniques are just beginning to receive attention.

Summary

Issues surrounding cognitive recovery after stroke are an increasing concern in neurology, neuropsychology, neurorehabilitation, neuropsychiatry, descriptive psychopathology, geriatrics, neuroradiology, neurophysiology, and neuropharmacology.

Stroke, within the fixed limits of the brain vascular architecture, is a privileged field of research for brain–mind correlations and for mechanisms of brain plasticity.

Future studies may investigate aspects of cognitive recovery after stroke in individual patients and will relate them to the aspects of brain plasticity. Where are synapses sprouting? Are cortical maps enlarging? Are homologous or non-homologous areas activated? On which hemisphere? The results of such analyses integrated into cognitive and behavioral models of recovery should clarify if restoration or compensation of function are occurring and should allow planning and monitoring of high-quality rehabilitation treatments.

REFERENCES

Aben, I., Verhey, F., Strik, J., *et al.* (2003). A comparative study into the one year cumulative incidence of depression after stroke and myocardial infarction. *J Neurol Neurosurg Psychiatry* **74**: 581–585.

Adair, J. C., Na, D. L., Schwartz, R. L., and Heilman, K. M. (1998). Analysis of primary and secondary influences on spatial neglect. *Brain Cogn* **37**: 351–367.

Aftonomos, L. B., Steele, R. D., and Wertz, R. T. (1997). Promoting recovery in chronic aphasia with an interactive technology. *Arch Phys Med Rehabil* **78**: 841–846.

Alexander M. P. and Benson D. F. (1991). The aphasias and related disturbances. In *Clinical Neurology*, vol.1, revised edn, ed. R. J. Joynt. Philadelphia, PA: J. B. Lippincott, pp. 1–58.

Alexander, M. P. and Freedman, M. (1984). Amnesia after anterior communicating artery aneurysm rupture. *Neurology* **34**: 452–757.

Alexander, M. P, Baker, E., Naeser, M. A., Kaplan, E., and Palumbo, C. (1992). Neuropsychological and neuroanatomical dimensions of ideomotor apraxia. *Brain* **115**: 87–107.

Arai, T., Ohi, H., Sasaki, H., Nobuto, H., and Tanaka, K (1997). Hemispatial sunglasses: effect on unilateral spatial neglect. *Arch Phys Med Rehabil* **78**: 230–232.

Bach-y-Rita, P. (1990). Brain plasticity as a basis for recovery of function in humans. *Neuropsychologia* **28**: 547–554.

Baker, E. H., Berry, T., Gardner, H., *et al.* (1976). Can linguistic competence be dissociated from natural language formations. *Nature* **254**: 609–619.

Basso, A. (1992). Prognostic factors in aphasia. *Aphasiology* **6**: 337–342.

Basso, A., Capitani, E., and Vignolo, L. A. (1979). Influence of rehabilitation on language skills in aphasic patients. A controlled study. *Arch Neurol* **36**: 190–196.

Basso, A., Capitani, E., and Moraschini, S. (1982). Sex differences in recovery from aphasia. *Cortex* **18**: 469–475.

Basso, A., Marangolo, P., Piras, F., and Galluzzi, C. (2001). Acquisition of new "words" in normal subjects: a suggestion for the treatment of anomia. *Brain Lang* **77**: 45–59.

Bechara, A., Damasio, H., and Damasio, A. R. (2000). Emotion, decision making and the orbitofrontal cortex. *Cereb Cortex* **10**: 295–307.

Benson, D. F. and Ardila, A. (1996) *Aphasia. A Clinical Perspective.* New York: Oxford University Press.

Benson, D. F., Sheremata, W. A., Bouchard, R., *et al.* (1973). Conduction aphasia. A clinico-pathological study. *Arch Neurol* **28**: 339–346.

Binder, J. R. and Mohr, J. P. (1992). The topography of callosal reading pathways. A case–control analysis. *Brain* **115**: 1807–1826.

Bisiach, E., Luzzatti, C., and Perani, D. (1979). Unilateral neglect, representational schema and consciousness. *Brain* **102**: 609–618.

Bisiach, E., Perani, D., Vallar, G., and Berti, A. (1986). Unilateral neglect: personal and extra-personal. *Neuropsychologia* **24**: 759–767.

Bogousslasvky, J. and Caplan L.R. (2001) *Stroke Syndromes*, 2nd edn. Cambridge: Cambridge University Press.

Bogousslavsky, J. and Regli, F. (1990). Anterior cerebral artery territory infarction in the Lausanne stroke registry. Clinical and etiologic patterns. *Arch Neurol* **47**: 144–150.

Bowen, A., McKenna, K., and Tallis, R. C. (1999). Reasons for variability in the reported rate of occurrence of unilateral spatial neglect after stroke. *Stroke* **30**: 1196–1202.

Bowen, A., Lincoln N. B., and Dewey, M. (2002) Cognitive rehabilitation for spatial neglect following stroke. *Cochrane Database of Systematic Reviews.* Oxford: Update software, CD003586.

Brown, K. W., Sloan, R. L., and Pentland, B. (1998). Fluoxetine as a treatment for post-stroke emotionalism. *Acta Psychiatr Scand* **98**: 455–458.

Buonomano, D. V. and Merzenich, M. M. (1998). Cortical plasticity: from synapses to maps. *Annu Rev Neurosci* **21**: 149–186.

Butter, C. M. and Kirsch, N. (1992). Combined and separate effects of eye patching and visual stimulation on unilateral neglect following stroke. *Arch Phys Med Rehabil* **73**: 1133–1139.

Calvert, T., Knapp, P., and House, A. (1998). Psychological associations with emotionalism after stroke. *J Neurol Neurosurg Psychiatry* **65**: 928–929.

Cao, Y., Vikingstad, E. M., George, K. P., Johnson, A. F., and Welch, K. M. (1999). Cortical language activation in stroke patients recovering from aphasia with functional MRI. *Stroke* **30**: 2331–2340.

Cappa, S. F., Perani, D., Grassi, F., *et al.* (1997). A PET follow-up study of recovery after stroke in acute aphasics. *Brain Lang* **56**: 55–67.

Carey, J. R., Kimberley, T. J., Lewis, S. M., *et al.* (2002). Analysis of fMRI and finger tracking training in subjects with chronic stroke. *Brain* **125**: 773–788.

Carlomagno, S., Pandolfi, M., Labruna, L., Colombo, A., and Razzano, C. (2001). Recovery from moderate aphasia in the first year post-stroke: effect of type of therapy. *Arch Phys Med Rehabil* **82**: 1073–1080.

Carota, A., Rossetti, A. O., Karapanayiotides, T., and Bogousslavsky, J. (2001). Catastrophic reaction in acute stroke: a reflex behavior in aphasic patients. *Neurology* **57**: 1902–1905.

Chang, K. C., Tseng, M. C., Weng, H. H., *et al.* (2002). Prediction of length of stay of first-ever ischemic stroke. *Stroke* **33**: 2670–2674.

Cherney, L. R., Halper, A. S., Kwasnica, C. M., Harvey, R. L., and Zhang, M. (2001). Recovery of functional status after right hemisphere stroke: relationship with unilateral neglect. *Arch Phys Med Rehabil* **82**: 322–328.

Code, C. (2001). Multifactorial processes in recovery from aphasia: developing the foundations for a multileveled framework. *Brain Lang* **77**: 25–44.

Connor, L. T., Obler, L. K., Tocco, M., Fitzpatrick, P. M., and Albert, M. L. (2001). Effect of socioeconomic status on aphasia severity and recovery. *Brain Lang* **78**: 254–257.

Corwin, J. V., Burcham, K. J., and Hix, G. I. (1996). Apomorphine produces an acute dose-dependent therapeutic effect on neglect produced by unilateral destruction of the posterior parietal cortex in rats. *Behav Brain Res* **79**: 41–49.

Crerar, M. A., Ellis, A. W., and Dean, E. C. (1996). Remediation of sentence processing deficits in aphasia using a computer-based microworld. *Brain Lang* **52**: 229–275.

Cummings, J. L. (1993). Frontal-subcortical circuits and human behavior. *Arch Neurol* **50**: 873–880.

D'Esposito, M., Alexander, M. P., Fischer, R., McGlinchey-Berroth, R., and O'Connor, M. (1996). Recovery of memory and executive function following anterior communicating artery aneurysm rupture. *J Int Neuropsychol Soc* **2**: 565–570.

Damasio, A. R. and Damasio, H. (1983). Anatomical basis of pure alexia. *Neurology* **33**: 1573–1583.

Damasio, A. R., Damasio, H., and van Hoesen, G. W. (1982). Prosopagnosia: anatomic basis and behavioral mechanisms. *Neurology* **32**: 331–341.

David, R. M. and Skilbeck, C. E. (1984). Raven IQ and language recovery following stroke. *J Clin Neuropsychol* **6**: 302–308.

Davis, G. A. and Wilcox, M. J. (1985) *Adult Aphasia Rehabilitation: Applied Pragmatics.* San Diego, CA: College Hill Press.

DeLuca, J. and Diamond, B. J. (1995). Aneurysm of the anterior communicating artery: a review of neuroanatomical and neuropsychological sequelae. *J Clin Exp Neuropsych* **17**: 100–121.

Denes, G., Semenza, C., Stoppa, E., and Lis, A. (1982). Unilateral spatial neglect and recovery from hemiplegia: a follow-up study. *Brain* **105**: 543–552.

de Renzi E (1997) Visuospatial and constructional disorders. In *Behavioral Neurology and Neuropsychology*, ed. M. J. Farah. New York: McGraw-Hill, pp. 297–307.

de Renzi, E. and Spinnler, H. (1966). Visual recognition in patients with unilateral cerebral disease. *J Nerv Ment Dis* **142**: 515–525.

de Renzi, E., Faglioni, P., Grossi, D., and Nichelli, P. (1991). Apperceptive and associative forms of prosopagnosia. *Cortex* **27**: 213–221.

Dobkin, B. (1995). The economic impact of stroke. *Neurology* **45**: S6–S9.

Driver, J. (1995). Object segmentation and visual neglect. *Behav Brain Res* **71**: 135–146.

Elman, R. J. (1998). *Group Treatment for Aphasia*. Newton, MA: Butterworth-Heinemann.

Eslinger, P. J. and Damasio, A. R. (1985). Severe disturbances of higher cognition after bilateral frontal lobe ablation: patient EVR. *Neurology* **35**: 1731–1741.

Fanthome, Y., Lincoln, N. B., Drummond, A., and Walker, M. F. (1995). The treatment of visual neglect using feedback of eye movements: a pilot study. *Disabil Rehabil* **17**: 413–417.

Ferro, J. M. and Madureira, S. (1997). Aphasia type, age and cerebral infarct localisation. *J Neurol* **244**: 505–509.

Ferro, J. M., Mariano, G., and Madureira, S. (1999). Recovery from aphasia and neglect. *Cerebrovasc Dis* **5**: 6–22.

Fink, R. B., Brecher, A., Schwartz, M. F., and Robey, R. R. (2002). A computer-implemented protocol for treatment of naming disorders: evaluation of clinicial-guided and partially self-guided instructions. *Aphasiology* **16**: 1061–1086.

Fleet, W. S., Valenstein, E., Watson, R. T., and Heilman, K. M. (1987). Dopamine agonist therapy for neglect in humans. *Neurology* **37**: 1765–1770.

Frassinetti, F., Angeli, V., Meneghello, F., Avanzi, S., and Ladavas, E. (2002). Long-lasting amelioration of visuospatial neglect by prism adaptation. *Brain* **125**: 608–623.

Fujikawa, T., Yamawaki, S., and Touhouda, Y. (1993). Incidence of silent cerebral infarction in patients with major depression. *Stroke* **24**: 1631–1634.

Fujikawa, T., Yokota, N., Muraoka, M., and Yamawaki, S. (1996). Responses of patients with major depression and silent cerebral infarction to antidepressant drug therapy, with emphasis on central nervous system advers reactions. *Stroke* **27**: 2040–2042.

Fuster J.M. (1997) *The Prefrontal Cortex. Anatomy, Physiology, and Neuropsychology of the Frontal Lobes*, 3rd edn. New York: Raven Press.

Gainotti, G. (1993). The riddle of the right hemisphere's contribution to the recovery of language. *Eur J Disord Commun* **28**: 227–246.

Gainotti, G., Antonucci, G., Marra, C., and Paolucci, S. (2001). Relation between depression after stroke, antidepressant therapy, and functional recovery. *J Neurol Neurosurg Psychiatry* **71**: 258–261.

Gardner, H., Zurif, E. B., Berry, T., and Baker, E. (1976). Visual communication in aphasia. *Neuropsychologia* **14**: 275–292.

Geminiani, G., Bottini, G., and Sterzi, R. (1998). Dopaminergic stimulation in unilateral neglect. *J Neurol Neurosurg Psychiatry* **65**: 344–347.

Giaquinto, S., Buzzelli, S., Di Francesco, L., *et al.* (1999). On the prognosis of outcome after stroke. *Acta Neurol Scand* **100**: 202–208.

Gloning, K., Trappi, R., Heiss, W., and Quatember, R. (1976). Prognosis and speech therapy in aphasia. In *Recovery in Aphasics*, ed. Y. Lebrun and R. Hoops. Amsterdam: Swets and Zettlinger, pp. 57–64.

Godefroy, O., Dubois, C., Debachy, B., Leclerc, M., and Kreisler, A. (2002). Vascular aphasias: main characteristics of patients hospitalized in acute stroke units. *Stroke* **33**: 702–705.

Gold, M., Adair, J. C., Jakobs, D. H., and Heilman, K. M. (1994). Anosognosia for hemiplegia: an electrophysiologic investigation of the feed-forward hypothesis. *Neurology* **44**: 1804–1808.

Goldenberg, G. and Spatt, J. (1994). Influence of size and site of cerebral lesions on spontaneous recovery of aphasia and on success of language therapy. *Brain Lang* **47**: 684–698.

Graff-Radford, N. R., Tranel, D., Van, H. G. W., and Brandt, J. P. (1990). Diencephalic amnesia. *Brain* **113**: 1–25.

Grattan, L. M., Bloomer, R. H., Archambault, F. X., and Eslinger, P. J. (1994). Cognitive flexibility and empathy after frontal lobe lesion. *Neuropsychiatry Neuropsychol Behav Neurol* **7**: 251–259.

Greener, J., Enderby, P., and Whurr, R. (2000) Speech and language therapy for aphasia following stroke. *Cochrane Database of Systematic Reviews*. Oxford: Update Software, CD000425.

Greener, J., Enderby, P., and Whurr, R. (2001) Pharmacological treatment for aphasia following stroke. *Cochrane Database of Systematic Reviews*. Oxford: Update Software, CD000424.

Greenwald, B., Kramer-Ginsberg, E., Krishnank, R., *et al.* (1998). Neuroanatomic localization of magnetic resonance imaging signal hyperintensities in geriatric depression. *Stroke* **29**: 613–617.

Guariglia, C., Padovani, A., Pantano, P., and Pizzamiglio, L. (1993). Unilateral neglect restricted to visual imagery. *Nature* **364**: 235–237.

Guilford, A. M., Scheuerle, J., and Shirek, P. G. (1982). Manual communication skills in aphasia. *Arch Phys Med Rehabil* **63**: 601–604.

Halligan, P. W. and Marshall, J. C. (1991). Left neglect for near but not far space in man. *Nature* **350**: 498–500.

Hanlon, R. E., Brown, J. W., and Gerstman, L. J. (1990). Enhancement of naming in nonfluent aphasia through gesture. *Brain Lang* **38**: 298–314.

Hartman-Maeir, A., Soroker, N., and Katz, N. (2001). Anosognosia for hemiplegia in stroke rehabilitation. *Neurorehabil Neural Repair* **15**: 213–222.

Heilman, K. M. and Gonzalez Rothi, L. J. (1993) Apraxia. In *Clinical Neuropsychology*, 3rd edn., ed. E. Valenstein. New York: Oxford University Press, pp. 141–163.

Heilman, K. M., Valenstein, E., and Watson, R. T. (2000). Neglect and related disorders. *Semin Neurol* **20**: 463–470.

Heiss, W. D., Karbe, H., Weber-Luxenburger, G., *et al.* (1997). Speech-induced cerebral metabolic activation reflects recovery from aphasia. *J Neurol Sci* **145**: 213–217.

Heiss, W. D., Kessler, J., Thiel, A., Ghaemi, M., and Karbe, H. (1999). Differential capacity of left and right hemispheric areas for compensation of post-stroke aphasia. *Ann Neurol* **45**: 430–438.

Helm-Estabrooks, N., Fitzpatrick, P. M., and Barresi, B. (1982). Visual action therapy for global aphasia. *J Speech Hear Disord* **47**: 385–389.

Helm-Estabrooks, N., Emery, P., and Albert, M. L. (1987). Treatment of aphasic perseveration (TAP) program. A new approach to aphasia therapy. *Arch Neurol* **44**: 1253–1255.

Hier, D. B., Mondlock, J., and Caplan, L. R. (1983a). Behavioral abnormalities after right hemisphere stroke. *Neurology* **33**: 337–344.

Hier, D. B., Mondlock, J., and Caplan, L. R. (1983b). Recovery of behavioral abnormalities after right hemisphere stroke. *Neurology* **33**: 345–350.

Hillis, A. E. (1991) The effects of separate treatments for distinct impairments within the naming process. In *Clinical Aphasiology*, ed. T. Prescott. Austin, TX: Pro-Ed.

Hillis, A. E. (1998). Effects of separate treatments for distinct impairment within the naming process. *J Int Neuropsychol Soc* **4**: 648–660.

Hillis, A. E., Barker, P. B., Beauchamp, N. J., Gordon, B., and Wityk, R. J. (2000). MR perfusion imaging reveals regions of hypoperfusion associated with aphasia and neglect. *Neurology* **55**: 782–788.

Hillis, A. E., Wityk, R. J., Barker, P. B., *et al.* (2002). Subcortical aphasia and neglect in acute stroke: the role of cortical hypoperfusion. *Brain* **125**: 1094–1104.

Hodges, J. R. and McCarthy, R. A. (1993). Autobiographical amnesia resulting from bilateral paramedian thalamic infarction. *A study in cognitive neurobiology. Brain* **116**: 921–940.

Holland, A. (1991). Pragmatic aspects of intervention in aphasia. *J Neurolinguist* **6**: 197–211.

House, A., Dennis, M., Molyneux, A., Warlow, C., and Hawton, K. (1989). Emotionalism after stroke. *BMJ* **298**: 991–994.

Jang, S. H., Kim, Y. H., Cho, S. H., *et al.* (2003). Cortical reorganization induced by task-oriented training in chronic hemiplegic stroke patients. *NeuroReport* **14**: 137–141.

Jeannerod, M., Decety, J., and Michel, F. (1994). Impairment of grasping movements following a bilateral posterior parietal lesion. *Neuropsychologia* **32**: 369–380.

Jehkonen, M., Ahonen, J. P., Dastidar, P., *et al.* (2000a). Visual neglect as a predictor of functional outcome one year after stroke. *Acta Neurol Scand* **101**: 195–201.

Jehkonen, M., Ahonen, J. P., Dastidar, P., Laippala, P., and Vilkki, J. (2000b). Unawareness of deficits after right hemisphere stroke: double-dissociations of anosognosias. *Acta Neurol Scand* **102**: 378–384.

Jehkonen, M., Ahonen, J. P., Dastidar, P., *et al.* (2001). Predictors of discharge to home during the first year after right hemisphere stroke. *Acta Neurol Scand* **104**: 136–141.

Johannsen-Horbach, H., Cegla, B., Mager, U., Schempp, B., and Wallesch, C. W. (1985). Treatment of chronic global aphasia with a nonverbal communication system. *Brain Lang* **24**: 74–82.

Karnath, H. O., Schenkel, P., and Fischer, B. (1991). Trunk orientation as the determining factor of the 'contralateral' deficit in the neglect syndrome and as the physical anchor of the internal representation of body orientation in space. *Brain* **114**: 1997–2014.

Karnath, H. O., Christ, K., and Hartje, W. (1993). Decrease of contralateral neglect by neck muscle vibration and spatial orientation of trunk midline. *Brain* **116**: 383–396.

Karnath, H. O., Himmelbach, M., and Rorden, C. (2002). The subcortical anatomy of human spatial neglect: putamen, caudate nucleus and pulvinar. *Brain* **125**: 350–360.

Katz, N., Hartman-Maeir, A., Ring, H., and Soroker, N. (1999). Functional disability and rehabilitation outcome in right hemisphere damaged patients with and without unilateral spatial neglect. *Arch Phys Med Rehabil* **80**: 379–384.

Katz, S., Ford, A., Chinn, A., and Newill, V. (1966). Prognosis after strokes. Part II. Long term course of 159 patients. *Medicine (Baltimore)* **45**: 236–246.

Kauhanen, M. L., Korpelainen, J. T., Hiltunen, P., *et al.* (2000). Aphasia, depression, and non-verbal cognitive impairment in ischaemic stroke. *Cerebrovasc Dis* **10**: 455–461.

Kay, J. and Ellis, A. (1987). A cognitive neuropsychological case study of anomia. Implications for psychological models of word retrieval. *Brain* **110**: 613–629.

Kempermann, G., Brandon, E. P., and Gage, F. H. (1998). Environmental stimulation of 129/SvJ mice causes increased cell proliferation and neurogenesis in the adult dentate gyrus. *Curr Biol* **8**: 939–942.

Kertesz, A. and McCabe, P. (1977). Recovery patterns and prognosis in aphasia. *Brain* **1**: 1–18.

Kirk, A. (2001). Spatial neglect. *Curr Neurol Neurosci Rep* **1**: 541–546.

Knopman, D. S., Selnes, O. A., Niccum, N., *et al.* (1983). A longitudinal study of speech fluency in aphasia: CT correlates of recovery and persistent nonfluency. *Neurology* **33**: 1170–1178.

Kotila, M., Waltimo, O., Niemi, M. L., Laaksonen, R., and Lempinen, M. (1984). The profile of recovery from stroke and factors influencing outcome. *Stroke* **15**: 1039–1044.

Kreisler, A., Godefroy, O., Delmaire, C., *et al.* (2000). The anatomy of aphasia revisited. *Neurology* **54**: 1117–1123.

Ladavas, E., Berti, A., Ruozzi, E., and Barboni, F. (1997). Neglect as a deficit determined by an imbalance between multiple spatial representations. *Exp Brain Res* **116**: 493–500.

Laganaro, M., Di Pietro, M., and Schnider, A. (2003). Computerised treatment of anomia in chronic and acute phasia: an exploratory study. *Aphasiology* **17**: 709–721.

Landis, T., Cummings, J. L., Benson, D. F., and Palmer, E. P. (1986). Loss of topographic familiarity: an environmental agnosia. *Arch Neurol* **43**: 132–136.

Leibovitch, F. S., Black, S. E., Caldwell, C. B., *et al.* (1998). Brain–behavior correlations in hemispatial neglect using CT and SPECT: the Sunnybrook Stroke Study. *Neurology* **50**: 901–908.

Lyon, J., Carisky, D., Keisler, L., *et al.* (1997). Communication partner: enhancing participation in life and communication for adults with aphasia in natural settings. *Aphasiology* **11**: 693–708.

Marin, R. S., Fogel, B. S., Hawkins, J., Duffy, J., and Krupp, B. (1995). Apathy: a treatable syndrome. *J Neuropsychiatry Clin Neurosci* **7**: 23–30.

Marshall, J. (1995). The mapping hypothesis and aphasia therapy. *Aphasiology* **9**: 517–539.

Marshall, J., Pound, C., White-Thomson, M., and Pring, T. (1990). The use of picture/word matching tasks to assist word retrieval in aphasic patients. *Aphasiology* **4**: 167–184.

Marshall, J. C. and Halligan, P. W. (1994). The Yin and the Yang of visuospatial neglect: a case study. *Neuropsychologia* **32**: 1037–1057.

Marshall, R. C. and Watts, M. T. (1976). Relaxation training: effects on the communicative ability of aphasic adults. *Arch Phys Med Rehabil* **57**: 464–467.

Mayer, E., Martory, M. D., Pegna, A. J., *et al.* (1999). A pure case of Gerstmann syndrome with a subangular lesion. *Brain* **122**: 1107–1120.

Mazzoni, M. and Vista, M. (1997). Lexical semantic therapy. *Aphasiology* **11**: 1096–1100.

Mazzoni, M., Vista, M., Geri, E., *et al.* (1995). Comparison of language recovery in rehabilitated and matched, non-rehabilitated aphasic patients. *Aphasiology* **9**: 553–563.

McNeil, M., Odell, K., and Tseng, C. (1991). Toward the integration of resource allocation into a general theroy of aphasia. *Clin Aphasiol* **20**: 21–39.

Meador, K. J., Loring, D. W., Feinberg, T. E., Lee, G. P., and Nichols, M. E. (2000). Anosognosia and asomatognosia during intracarotid amobarbital inactivation. *Neurology* **55**: 816–820.

Mega, M. S. and Alexander, M. P. (1994). Subcortical aphasia: the core profile of striatocapsular infarction. *Neurology* **44**: 1824–1829.

Miller, E. K. and Cohen, J. D. (2001). An integrative theory of prefrontal cortex function. *Annu Rev Neurosci* **24**: 167–202.

Milner, A. D. (1998). Neuropsychological studies of perception and visuomotor control. *Philos Trans R Soc Lond B Biol Sci* **353**: 1375–1384.

Mimura, M., Kato, M., Sano, Y., *et al.* (1998). Prospective and retrospective studies of recovery in aphasia. Changes in cerebral blood flow and language functions. *Brain* **121**: 2083–2094.

Mishkin, M., Lewis, M. E., and Ungerleider, L. G. (1982). Equivalence of parieto-preoccipital subareas for visuospatial ability in monkeys. *Behav Brain Res* **6**: 41–55.

Mohr, J. P., Pessin, M. S., Finkelstein, S., *et al.* (1978). Broca aphasia: pathologic and clinical. *Neurology* **28**: 311–324.

Murray, L. L., and Heather Ray, A. (2001). A comparison of relaxation training and syntax stimulation for chronic nonfluent aphasia. *J Commun Disord* **34**: 87–113.

Musso, M., Weiller, C., Kiebel, S., *et al.* (1999). Training-induced brain plasticity in aphasia. *Brain* **122**: 1781–1790.

Naeser, M. A. and Helm-Estabrooks, N. (1985). CT scan lesion localization and response to melodic intonation therapy with nonfluent aphasia cases. *Cortex* **21**: 203–223.

Naeser, M. A., Baker, E. H., Palumbo, C. L., *et al.* (1998). Lesion site patterns in severe, nonverbal aphasia to predict outcome with a computer-assisted treatment program. *Arch Neurol* **55**: 1438–1448.

Nakatomi, H., Kuriu, T., Okabe, S., *et al.* (2002). Regeneration of hippocampal pyramidal neurons after ischemic brain injury by recruitment of endogenous neural progenitors. *Cell* **110**: 429–441.

Nakayama, H., Jorgensen, H. S., Raaschou, H. O., and Olsen, T. S. (1994). Recovery of upper extremity function in stroke patients: the Copenhagen Stroke Study. *Arch Phys Med Rehabil* **75**: 394–398.

Nudo, R. J., Wise, B. M., SiFuentes, F., and Milliken, G. W. (1996). Neural substrates for the effects of rehabilitative training on motor recovery after ischemic infarct. *Science* **272**: 1791–1794.

Ortigue, S., Viaud-Delmon, I., Annoni, J. M., *et al.* (2001). Pure representational neglect after right thalamic lesion. *Ann Neurol* **50**: 401–404.

Paolucci, S., Antonucci, G., Pratesi, L., *et al.* (1998). Functional outcome in stroke inpatient rehabilitation: predicting no, low and high response patients. *Cerebrovasc Dis* **8**: 228–234.

Paolucci, S., Grasso, M. G., Antonucci, G., *et al.* (2000). One-year follow-up in stroke patients discharged from rehabilitation hospital. *Cerebrovasc Dis* **10**: 25–32.

Paolucci, S., Antonucci, G., Grasso, M. G., and Pizzamiglio, L. (2001). The role of unilateral spatial neglect in rehabilitation of right brain-damaged ischemic stroke patients: a matched comparison. *Arch Phys Med Rehabil* **82**: 743–749.

Pedersen, P. M., Jorgensen, H. S., Nakayama, H., Raaschou, H. O., and Olsen, T. S. (1995). Aphasia in acute stroke: incidence, determinants, and recovery. *Ann Neurol* **38**: 659–666.

Perenin, M. T., and Vighetto, A. (1988). Optic ataxia: a specific disruption in visuomotor mechanisms. I. Different aspects of the deficit in reaching for objects. *Brain* **111**: 643–674.

Perez, F. M., Tunkel, R. S., Lachmann, E. A., and Nagler, W. (1996). Balint's syndrome arising from bilateral posterior cortical atrophy or infarction: rehabilitation strategies and their limitation. *Disabil Rehabil* **18**: 300–304.

Pettersen, R., Dahl, T., and Wyller, T. B. (2002). Prediction of long-term functional outcome after stroke rehabilitation. *Clin Rehabil* **16**: 149–159.

Pierce, S. R., and Buxbaum, L. J. (2002). Treatments of unilateral neglect: a review. *Arch Phys Med Rehabil* **83**: 256–268.

Pizzamiglio, L., Mammucari, A., and Razzano, C. (1985). Evidence for sex differences in brain organization in recovery in aphasia. *Brain Lang* **25**: 213–223.

Pizzamiglio, L., Frasca, R., Guariglia, C., Incoccia, C., and Antonucci, G. (1990). Effect of optokinetic stimulation in patients with visual neglect. *Cortex* **26**: 535–540.

Pizzamiglio, L., Antonucci, G., Judica, A., *et al.* (1992). Cognitive rehabilitation of the hemineglect disorder in chronic patients with unilateral right brain damage. *J Clin Exp Neuropsychol* **14**: 901–923.

Pizzamiglio, L., Perani, D., Cappa, S. F., *et al.* (1998). Recovery of neglect after right hemispheric damage: H^2 (15)O positron emission tomographic activation study. *Arch Neurol* **55**: 561–568.

Pohjasvaara, T., Leskela, M., Vataja, R., *et al.* (2002a). Post-stroke depression, executive dysfunction and functional outcome. *Eur J Neurol* **9**: 269–275.

Pohjasvaara, T., Vataja, R., Leppavuori, A., Kaste, M., and Erkinjuntti, T. (2002b). Cognitive functions and depression as predictors of poor outcome 15 months after stroke. *Cerebrovasc Dis* **14**: 228–233.

Posner, M. (1995) Attention in cognitive neurosciences: an overview. In *The Cognitive Neurosciences*, ed. M. Gazzaniga. Cambridge, MA: MIT Press.

Pulvermuller, F., Neininger, B., Elbert, T., *et al.*(2001). Constraint-induced therapy of chronic aphasia after stroke. *Stroke* **32**: 1621–1626.

Richardson, J. T. E. (1992). Imagery mnemonics and memory remediation. *Neurology* **42**: 283–286.

Riddoch, M. and Humphreys, G. (1993) *BORB. Birmingham Object Recognition Battery.* Hove, UK: Lawrence Erlbaum.

Rizzo, M., and Vecera, S. P. (2002). Psychoanatomical substrates of Balint's syndrome. *J Neurol Neurosurg Psychiatry* **72**: 162–178.

Robertson, I. H. (2001). Do we need the "lateral" in unilateral neglect? Spatially nonselective attention deficits in unilateral neglect and their implications for rehabilitation. *Neuroimage* **14**: S85–90.

Robertson, I. H. and North, N. (1992). Spatio-motor cueing in unilateral left neglect: the role of hemispace, hand and motor activation. *Neuropsychologia* **30**: 553–563.

Robertson, I. H., North, N. T., and Geggie, C. (1992). Spatiomotor cueing in unilateral left neglect: three case studies of its therapeutic effects. *J Neurol Neurosurg Psychiatry* **55**: 799–805.

Robson, J., Marshall, J., Pring, T., and Chiat, S. (1998). Phonological naming therapy in jargon aphasia: positive but paradoxical effects. *J Int Neuropsychol Soc* **4**: 675–686.

Robson, J., Marshall, J., Chiat, S., and Pring, T. (2001). Enhancing communication in jargon aphasia: a small group study of writing therapy. *Int J Lang Commun Disord* **36**: 471–488.

Rorsman, I., Magnusson, M., and Johansson, B. B. (1999). Reduction of visuospatial neglect with vestibular galvanic stimulation. *Scand J Rehabil Med* **31**: 117–124.

Rosselli, M., Ardila, A., and Beltran, C. (2001). Rehabilitation of Balint's syndrome: a single case report. *Appl Neuropsychol* **8**: 242–247.

Rossetti, Y., Rode, G., Pisella, L., *et al.* (1998). Prism adaptation to a rightward optical deviation rehabilitates left hemispatial neglect. *Nature* **395**: 166–169.

Rubens, A. B. (1985). Caloric stimulation and unilateral visual neglect. *Neurology* **35**: 1019–1024.

Rubens, A. B. and Benson, D. F. (1971). Associative visual agnosia. *Arch Neurol* **24**: 305–316.

Sacchett, C., Byng, S., Marshall, J., and Pound, C. (1999). Drawing together: evaluation of a therapy program for severe aphasia. *Int J Lang Commun Disord* **34**: 265–289.

Saffran, E. M., Schwartz, M. F., and Marin, O. S. (1980). The word order problem in agrammatism. II. Production. *Brain Lang* **10**: 263–280.

Sakai, K. L., Noguchi, Y., Takeuchi, T., and Watanabe, E. (2002). Selective priming of syntactic processing by event-related transcranial magnetic stimulation of Broca's area. *Neuron* **35**: 1177–1182.

Schnider, A. (1997). *Verhaltensneurologie. Die neurologische Seite der Neuropsychologie.* Stuttgart: Thieme.

(2001). Spontaneous confabulation, reality monitoring, and the limbic system: a review. *Brain Res Rev* **36**: 150–160.

Schnider, A., Benson, D. F., and Scharre, D. W. (1994a). Visual agnosia and optic aphasia: are they anatomically distinct? *Cortex* **30**: 445–457.

Schnider, A., Regard, M., and Landis, T. (1994b). Anterograde and retrograde amnesia following bitemporal infarction. *Behav Neurol* **7**: 87–92.

Schnider, A., Hanlon, R. E., Alexander, D. N., and Benson, D. F. (1997). Ideomotor apraxia. Behavioral and neuroanatomical dimensions. *Brain Lang* **58**: 125–136.

Schnider, A., Ptak, R., von Däniken, C., and Remonda, L. (2000). Recovery from spontaneous confabulations parallels recovery of temporal confusion in memory. *Neurology* **55**: 74–83.

Selnes, O. A., Niccum, N., Knopman, D. S., and Rubens, A. B. (1984). Recovery of single word comprehension: CT-scan correlates. *Brain Lang* **21**: 72–84.

Shamay, S. G., Tomer, R., and Aharon-Peretz, J. (2002). Deficit in understanding sarcasm in patients with prefronal lesion is related to impaired empathic ability. *Brain Cogn* **48**: 558–563.

Shewan, C. M. and Kertesz, A. (1984). Effects of speech and language treatment on recovery from aphasia. *Brain Lang* **23**: 272–299.

Silvestrini, M., Troisi, E., Matteis, M., Razzano, C., and Caltagirone, C. (1998). Correlations of flow velocity changes during mental activity and recovery from aphasia in ischemic stroke. *Neurology* **50**: 191–195.

Singh, A., Black, S. E., Herrmann, N., *et al.* (2000). Functional and neuroanatomic correlations in post-stroke depression: the Sunnybrook Stroke Study. *Stroke* **31**: 637–644.

Skilbeck, C. E., Wade, D. T., Hewer, R. L., and Wood, V. A. (1983). Recovery after stroke. *J Neurol Neurosurg Psychiatry* **46**: 5–8.

Sparks, R., Helm, N., and Albert, M. (1974). Aphasia rehabilitation resulting from melodic intonation therapy. *Cortex* **10**: 303–316.

Speedie, L. J. and Heilman, K. M. (1983). Anterograde memory deficits for visuospatial material after infarction of the right thalamus. *Arch Neurol* **40**: 183–186.

Steele, R. D., Weinrich, M., Wertz, R. T., Kleczewska, M. K., and Carlson, G. S. (1989). Computer-based visual communication in aphasia. *Neuropsychologia* **27**: 409–426.

Stone, S. P., Patel, P., Greenwood, R. J., and Halligan, P. W. (1992). Measuring visual neglect in acute stroke and predicting its recovery: the visual neglect recovery index. *J Neurol Neurosurg Psychiatry* **55**: 431–436.

Stuss, D. T. and Benson, D. F. (1986). *The Frontal Lobes.* New York: Raven Press.

Subirana, A. (1969) Handedness and cerebral dominance. In *Handbook of Clinical Neurology*, ed. B. Vinken and G. Bruyn. Amsterdam: North-Holland pp 248–272.

Sumer, M. M., Ozdemir, I., and Tascilar, N. (2003). Predictors of outcome after acute ischemic stroke. *Acta Neurol Scand* **107**: 276–280.

Takahashi, N., Kawamura, M., Hirayama, K., Shiota, J., and Isono, O. (1995). Prosopagnosia: a clinical and anatomical study of four patients. *Cortex* **31**: 317–329.

Tham, K. and Tegner, R. (1997). Video feedback in the rehabilitation of patients with unilateral neglect. *Arch Phys Med Rehabil* **78**: 410–413.

Thoene, A. I. and Glisky, E. L. (1995). Learning of name-face associations in memory impaired patients: a comparison of different training procedures. *J Int Neuropsychol Soc* **1**: 29–38.

Thulborn, K. R., Carpenter, P. A., and Just, M. A. (1999). Plasticity of language-related brain function during recovery from stroke. *Stroke* **30**: 749–754.

Troisi, E., Paolucci, S., and Silvestrini, M., (2002). Prognostic factors in stroke rehabilitation: the possible role of pharmacological treatment. *Acta Neurol Scand* **105**: 100–106.

Vallar, G., Rusconi, M. L., Barozzi, S., *et al.* (1995). Improvement of left visuospatial hemineglect by left-sided transcutaneous electrical stimulation. *Neuropsychologia* **33**: 73–82.

Valles, E., Roig, J., and Navarra, J. (1997). The development of verbal communication in aphasic patients treated by neuropsychological therapy. *Rev Neurol* **25**: 1387–1393.

von Cramon, D. Y., Hebel, N., and Schuri, U. (1985). A contribution to the anatomical basis of thalamic amnesia. *Brain* **108**: 993–1008.

(1988). Verbal memory and learning in unilateral posterior cerebral infarction. A report on 30 cases. *Brain* **111**: 1061–1077.

Vuilleumier, P., Valenza, N., Mayer, E., Reverdin, A., and Landis, T. (1998). Near and far visual space in unilateral neglect. *Ann Neurol* **43**: 406–410.

Wade, D. T., Hewer, R. L., David, R. M., and Enderby, P. M. (1986a). Aphasia after stroke: natural history and associated deficits. *J Neurol Neurosurg Psychiatry* **49**: 11–16.

Wade, D. T., Parker, V., and Langton Hewer, R. (1986b). Memory disturbance after stroke: frequency and associated losses. *Int Rehabil Med* **8**: 60–64.

Walker-Batson, D., Curtis, S., Natarajan, R., *et al.* (2001). A double-blind, placebo-controlled study of the use of amphetamine in the treatment of aphasia. *Stroke* **32**: 2093–2098.

Warburton, E., Price, C. J., Swinburn, K., and Wise, R. J. (1999). Mechanisms of recovery from aphasia: evidence from positron emission tomography studies. *J Neurol Neurosurg Psychiatry* **66**: 155–161.

Ween, J. E., Alexander, M. P., D'Esposito, M., and Roberts, M. (1996). Factors predictive of stroke outcome in a rehabilitation setting. *Neurology* **47**: 388–392.

Weiller, C., Isensee, C., Rijntjes, M., *et al.* (1995). Recovery from Wernicke's aphasia: a positron emission tomographic study. *Ann Neurol* **37**: 723–732.

Weinberg, J., Diller, L., Gordon, W. A., *et al.* (1977). Visual scanning training effect on reading-related tasks in acquired right brain damage. *Arch Phys Med Rehabil* **58**: 479–486.

Weinberg, J., Diller, L., Gordon, W. A., *et al.* (1979). Training sensory awareness and spatial organization in people with right brain damage. *Arch Phys Med Rehabil* **60**: 491–496.

Weinberg, J., Piasetsky, E., Diller, L., and Gordon, W. (1982). Treating perceptual organization deficits in nonneglecting RBD stroke patients. *J Clin Neuropsychol* **4**: 59–75.

Wertz, R. T., Collins, M. J., Weiss, D., *et al.* (1981). Veterans Administration Cooperative Study on Aphasia: a comparison of individual and group treatment. *J Speech Hear Res* **24**: 580–594.

Wertz, R. T., Weiss, D. G., Aten, J. L., *et al.* (1986). Comparison of clinic, home, and deferred language treatment for aphasia. A Veterans Administration Cooperative Study. *Arch Neurol* **43**: 653–658.

Wilson, B. A., Emslie, H. C., Quirk, K., and Evans, J. J. (2001). Reducing everyday memory and planning problems by means of a paging system: a randomised control crossover study. *J Neurol Neurosurg Psychiatry* **70**: 477–482.

Zeloni, G., Farne, A., and Baccini, M. (2002). Viewing less to see better. *J Neurol Neurosurg Psychiatry* **73**: 195–198.

Zola-Morgan, S., Squire, L. R., and Amaral, D. G. (1986). Human amnesia and the medial temporal region: enduring memory impairment following a bilateral lesion limited to field CA1 of the hippocampus. *J Neurosci* **6**: 2950–2967.

20

Stroke-related dementia

José G. Merino

University of Florida, Jacksonville, FL, USA

Vladimir Hachinski

University of Western Ontario, London, ON, Canada

Introduction

Stroke can lead to significant cognitive decline (Kase *et al.*, 1998). Population-based epidemiological studies in Italy (Prencipe *et al.*, 1997), Rotterdam (van Kooten *et al.*, 1998), and Stockholm (Zhu *et al.*, 1998) have shown that the prevalence of dementia is higher in individuals with a history of stroke than in stroke-free individuals (Table 20.1). While population studies show that a history of cerebrovascular disease increases the risk of dementia, they do not prove causality, since a temporal association between stroke and the development of dementia cannot be established with certainty. In order to test hypotheses regarding the etiology of dementia after stroke, the characteristics of the subjects and the stroke need to be studied carefully, and the patients must be assessed serially with detailed neuropsychological evaluations. In 1990, Tatemichi proposed that the prospective study of stroke cohorts could lead to the verification of testable hypotheses regarding the risk factors for, and the etiology and course of, post-stroke dementia. Multiple groups have taken up the challenge, and, despite the use of different diagnostic criteria and methods for evaluating cognitive impairment, have found that one-quarter to one-third of patients have dementia after stroke (Table 20.2).

Incidence and prevalence of dementia after stroke

In a pooled analysis of two cohorts totaling 453 patients, researchers at Columbia University (Tatemichi *et al.*, 1992a; Desmond *et al.*, 2000) found that 26.3% (95% confidence interval [CI], 22.2–30.3) had dementia as defined in the *Diagnostic and Statistical Manual* (DSM)-III-R (American Psychiatric Association, 1987) three

Recovery after Stroke, ed. Michael P. Barnes, Bruce H. Dobkin and Julien Bogousslavsky. Published by Cambridge University Press. © Cambridge University Press 2005.

Table 20.1 Prevalence of dementia associated with stroke in population studies

Series	Subjects	Age (years)	Prevalence of dementia among subjects with stroke (%)	Prevalence of dementia among stroke-free subjects (%)	Odds ratio for dementia among subjects with stroke (95% confidence interval)
van Kooten et al., 1998	7983	≥55	24.3	5.1[a]	N/A
Prencipe et al., 1997	1032	≥65	30.0	5.7	5.8 (3.1–10.8)
Zhu et al., 1998	1810	≥75	32.0	10.6	3.6 (2.3–5.5)

[a] Prevalence of dementia in the entire sample.

Table 20.2 Prevalence of dementia in stroke cohorts, series listed in chronological order 1996–2001

Series	Number[a]	Mean age (years)	Time to follow-up (months)	Diagnostic criteria[b]	Pre-existing cognitive impairment (%)	Percentage with dementia
Censori et al., 1996	110[c]	65	3–4	NINDS-AIREN	N/A	13.6
Pohjasvaara et al., 1997	451[d]	70.2	3	DSM-III-R	N/A	20.0
Inzitari et al., 1998	339[e]	71	12	ICD-10[f]	7.5	16.8[g]
van Kooten et al., 1998[h]	300[e]	72.9	3	DSM-III-R	N/A	23.7
Desmond et al., 2000[i]	453[d]	72	3	DSM-III-R[f]	10.2	26.3
Barba et al., 2000	251[e]	69	3	DSM-III-R	10	30
Madureira et al., 2000	237[e]	59	3	NINDS-AIREN	N/A	6

[a] Used to calculate post-stroke dementia (doers not include those with pre-stroke decline in some series).
[b] See Table 20.3 for sources of diagnostic criteria.
[c] First ischemic stroke.
[d] Ischemic stroke.
[e] Ischemic and hemorrhagic stroke.
[f] Proxy interview
[g] After excluding those with pre-stroke cognitive decline.
[h] Includes only patients in the Rotterdam Stroke Data Bank.
[i] Includes 251 patients from Tatemichi (1992a).
[j] Modified criteria.

months after the stroke. After adjusting for age, education, and race, the odds ratio for dementia was 9.4 (95% CI, 4.2–21.2). The risk increased with age, doubling every 10 years. Groups from Milan (Censori et al., 1996), Helsinki (Pohjasvaara et al., 1997) Florence (Inzitari et al., 1998), Rotterdam (van Kooten et al., 1998),

Table 20.3 Prevalence of dementia three months after stroke according to different diagnostic criteria

Diagnostic criteria	Prevalence (%)
DSM-III (American Psychiatric Association, 1980)	25.5
DSM-III-R (American Psychiatric Association, 1987)	20.0
DSM-IV (American Psychiatric Association, 1994)	18.4
ICD-10 (WHO, 1989)	6.0
NINDS-AIREN (Roman *et al.*, 1993)	21.1

Data from Pohjasvaara *et al.* (1997).

Madrid (Barba *et al.*, 2000), and Lisbon (Madureira *et al.*, 2000) have published similar results (see Table 20.2). Since dementia is differentially associated with early patient attrition, the frequency of dementia may be even higher when allowance is made for patients with stroke whose death or severity of neurological impairment precludes neuropsychological testing (Desmond *et al.*, 1998a). The prevalence of dementia depends on the cognitive domains that are tested and the diagnostic criteria that are used. The number of patients that are classified as demented differs by a factor of 10 according to the criteria that are used (Erkinjuntti *et al.*, 1997; Chui *et al.*, 2000); DSM-III was the most sensitive and the World Health Organization (WHO) *International Classification of Diseases* (ICD)-10 criteria (WHO, 1989) the most specific for dementia in a stroke cohort (Table 20.3) (Pohjasvaara *et al.*, 1997).

The risk of incident dementia in patients with stroke is high (Tatemichi *et al.*, 1994a). The group at Columbia University found that the crude incidence rate of new dementia (using criteria modified from DSM-III-R) was 8.49 cases per 100 person-years in the stroke group and 1.37 cases per 100 person-years in the control group (Desmond *et al.*, 2002a). Patients with stroke had an almost six-fold higher risk of dementia during long-term follow-up (relative risk [RR], 6.12; 95% CI, 3.57–10.50). After adjusting for demographic variables and baseline Mini Mental State Examination (MMSE) score, the RR was 3.83 (95% CI, 2.14–6.84) (Desmond *et al.*, 2002a). Hénon and colleagues (2001) followed for three years a consecutive group of 169 stroke patients who did not have cognitive impairment before the stroke. After 294 person-years of follow-up, 36 patients developed dementia (diagnosed using ICD-10 criteria). The incidence rate was 12.3 cases per 100 person-years. Loeb (1992) found that 23.2% of patients with lacunar stroke developed incident dementia after four years of follow-up, and among the 81 patients followed by Samuelsson (1996), 4.9% and 9.9% had incident dementia after 1 and 3 years of follow-up, respectively.

Stroke leads to impairment in several cognitive domains, even in the absence of frank dementia (Tatemichi *et al.*, 1994b; Pohjasvaara *et al.*, 1998a; Madureira *et al.*, 2000). Single supratentorial lacunar infarcts produce subtle cognitive abnormalities in language, concept shifting, abstraction, incidental memory, and verbal fluency (van Zandvoort *et al.*, 2000, 2001). Tatemichi and his group (1994b) used a comprehensive neuropsychological battery to evaluate 227 patients with stroke but without pre-existing cognitive impairment, and 249 stroke-free controls. Three months after a stroke 35.2% of patients but only 3.8% of controls were cognitively impaired. The most significant areas of impairment were visuospatial ability, memory, orientation, language, attention, and executive function. Pohjasvaara and coworkers (1998a) found cognitive decline in one, two, and three or more domains in 61.7%, 34.8%, and 26.8%, respectively, of their patients three months after a stroke. The domains most frequently impaired were visuospatial and memory, but 25% of patients had executive function deficit. In a separate study of 286 stroke patients, they found executive dysfunction in 40.5%, a similar proportion of patients were impaired in the study of (Madureira *et al.*, 2000). Patients with stroke and memory impairment at three months always had deficits in one or more additional cognitive domains, and most patients had deficits in two or more (Desmond *et al.*, 1998b).

Determinants of dementia after stroke

Multiple factors (host characteristics, risk factor profile, and clinical and radiological characteristics of the stroke) contribute to the risk of cognitive decline after a cerebrovascular insult (Tatemichi *et al.*, 1993). Independent predictors of prevalent dementia after a stroke have been identified. Not all groups have identified the same predictors; this may be because of differences in the population studied, how clinical and radiological features are defined, and time elapsed between the stroke and the evaluation. Age is a significant factor in most series (Inzitari *et al.*, 1998; Barba *et al.*, 2000; Desmond *et al.*, 2000). It may be a surrogate for concomitant Alzheimer disease (as will be discussed below) since the odds ratio for dementia among stroke subjects ≥ 80 years of age (versus those 60–69) declined from 12.73 (95% CI, 6.12–26.47) to 7.83 (95% CI, 3.17–19.31) when only subjects with vascular dementia and not those with probable Alzheimer disease were entered into the model (Desmond *et al.*, 2000). Low educational level is an independent predictor of dementia in several prevalence studies (Pohjasvaara *et al.*, 1998a; Desmond *et al.*, 2000) but not in incidence (Desmond *et al.*, 2002a), as is a history of diabetes (Censori *et al.*, 1996; Desmond *et al.*, 2000). Interestingly, although prior stroke is a predictor in some series (Inzitari *et al.*, 1998; Pohjasvaara *et al.*, 1998a; Desmond *et al.*, 2000), other traditional vascular risk factors are not. The fact that prior stroke increases the risk of developing dementia suggests that the effect of multiple infarcts may be cumulative (Hachinski *et al.*, 1974). Severe hemispheral syndromes (Censori *et al.*, 1996; Pohjasvaara *et al.*, 1998a; Desmond *et al.*, 2000), particularly in the dominant side (Pohjasvaara *et al.*, 1998a), are relevant. However, since non-verbal memory was not always considered when making the diagnosis of dementia, aphasia was sometimes (Censori *et al.*, 1996; Inzitari *et al.*, 1998; Pohjasvaara *et al.*, 1998a) but not always related to intellectual decline (Desmond *et al.*, 2000). The left hemisphere has been implicated in patients with post-stroke dementia (Ladurner *et al.*, 1982; Liu *et al.*, 1992; Gorelick *et al.*, 1993) and was an independent predictor in the series from New York (Desmond *et al.*, 2000) and Helsinki (Pohjasvaara *et al.*, 1998a). Tatemichi *et al.* (1994a) and Desmond *et al.* (2000) found that strokes in the pooled territories of the anterior and posterior cerebral arteries (including medial frontal and medial temporal lobes; all important for memory) were more likely to lead to dementia than strokes in other territories. This may reflect the use of diagnostic criteria that feature memory loss as a prominent characteristic of the dementia syndrome. Other authors, however, found that middle cerebral artery infarcts were stronger predictors of cognitive loss (Censori *et al.*, 1996; Pohjasvaara *et al.*, 2000a). Lacunar strokes were predictors in the original cohort of Tatemichi *et al.* (1993), but not in the analysis of a larger cohort (Desmond *et al.*, 2000).

The predictors of incident dementia beyond three months after the stroke are similar. Hénon *et al.* (2001) found as that the predictors of incident post-stroke dementia were aging, pre-existing cognitive decline, severity of deficit at admission, diabetes mellitus, silent infarcts, and, when pre-stroke cognitive decline is not taken into account, leukoaraiosis. In addition to older age and recurrent stroke, Desmond and colleagues (2002a) found that intercurrent medical illnesses that could lead to cerebral hypoxia or ischemia (such as myocardial infarction, congestive heart failure, arrhythmias, syncope, pneumonia, seizures, and sepsis) were predictors of incident dementia. This association between hypoxic–ischemic illnesses and incident dementia has been reported previously (Sulkava and Erkinjuntti, 1987; Cooper and Mungas, 1993; Skoog *et al.*, 1993; Brun, 1994; Longstreth *et al.*, 1996; Moroney *et al.*, 1997a; Hénon *et al.*, 2001). Significantly, the location of the index stroke, the presence of vascular risk factors, educational level, and other demographic variables were unrelated to incident dementia.

Prognosis in patients with dementia after a stroke

The risk of incident dementia is greatest in the first few months after stroke. In a retrospective study in Rochester, Kokmen and coworkers (1996) found that the number of patients with stroke who became demented was nine times higher than expected in the first year after the stroke, but only four times higher three years

Table 20.4 Dependency after stroke

Series	Cognitive status	Odds ratio of dependency (95% confidence interval)
		Dependency after stroke
Tatemichi *et al.*, 1994b	Cognitive impairment	2.4 (1.30–4.40)
Barba *et al.*, 2000	Cognitive impairment	4.5 (1.97–11.20)
	Dementia	3.9 (1.52–10.67)

later. In a large population study of elderly subjects, history of stroke was a risk factor for incident dementia, but a "fresh" stroke (in previous three years) doubled the risk of dementia (RR, 2.4; 95% CI, 1.4–4.2), while older strokes did not (RR, 1.1; 95% CI 0.6–2.3) (Zhu *et al.*, 1998). Although in the series of Tatemichi *et al.* (1994a), 30% of patients who were not demented at three months had new-onset dementia within three years, only 7% of French patients not demented at six months developed dementia within that period of time (Hénon *et al.*, 2001).

Some patients with cognitive impairment after a stroke can improve (Kotila *et al.*, 1984; Wade *et al.*, 1986). In New York, almost 15% of 151 patients assessed three months after a stroke had cognitive improvement by the time of the one-year examination (Desmond *et al.*, 1996). When only those who met prespecified criteria for cognitive impairment were considered, 36% had improvement. Correlates of improvement were a left hemispheric infarct, independent of aphasia status, and a major hemispheral stroke syndrome. Patients with diabetes mellitus tended to do less well.

Cognitive impairment and dementia after stroke are associated with higher risk of stroke recurrence (Moroney *et al.*, 1997b), poor functional recovery (Tatemichi *et al.*, 1994b; Pohjasvaara *et al.*, 1998b), and mortality (Tatemichi *et al.*, 1994c; Barba *et al.*, 2002; Desmond *et al.*, 2002b). In a series of 242 patients who were alive three months after a stroke and were subsequently followed-up for a mean of 34.5 months, the cumulative stroke recurrence rate was 24%. The incidence of recurrent stroke was doubled among patients with dementia three months after the index stroke (RR, 2.71; 95% CI 1.36–5.42) (Moroney *et al.*, 1997b). Independent of stroke recurrence, patients with dementia or cognitive impairment after stroke have a two- to four-fold higher risk of being dependent (requiring daily assistance, home attendant help, or admission to a nursing home) three months after a stroke (Tatemichi *et al.*, 1994b; Pohjasvaara *et al.*, 1998b) (Table 20.4). Independent correlates of dependent living three months after the stroke were the presence of a major hemispheral syndrome, and a combination of handicap, cognition, and performance of activities of daily living. Handicap, as measured on the Rankin

Table 20.5 Mortality after stroke in patients with and without dementia

Series	Mean follow-up (months)	Survivors with dementia (%)	Survivors without dementia (%)	Relative risk of confidence interval[a] death (95%)
With no pre-stroke dementia				
Tatemichi et al., 1994c	58.6	38.9	74.5	3.1 (1.8–5.4)
Barba et al., 2002	22.1	58.3[b]	95.4	6.3 (2.3–17.3)
	20.9	51.4[c]	95.5	8.5 (3.4–20.9)
With pre-stroke dementia				
Hénon et al., 1997	6	N/A	N/A	4.2 (2.0–9.2)
Barba et al., 2002	16.1	20.4	72.6	2.1 (1.2–3.6)

[a] Adjusted for other coexistent predictors of mortality (demographic variables, medical illnesses, recurrent stroke and stroke syndrome, location, and severity).
[b] Stroke-related dementia: previously non-demented patients that had dementia after the stroke.
[c] Post-stroke dementia: all those with dementia three months after the stroke, irrespective of the time of onset.

Scale, explained 51.%, performance of activities of daily living (measured with the Functional Activities Questionnaire) 5.9%, and the presence of dementia or cognitive decline 3.4% of the total variance between dependent and independent patients after stroke (Pohjasvaara et al., 1998b).

Compared with non-demented patients, patients with dementia have an increased risk of death (Molsa et al., 1986; Katzman et al., 1994; Rockwood et al., 2000). The mortality rate in the original cohort of Tatemichi et al. (1994c) was 19.8 and 6.1 deaths per 100 person-years among stroke patients that did and did not, respectively, develop dementia. The proportion of survivors after follow-up and the RR of death among patients with dementia in several series (Tatemichi et al., 1994c; Henon et al., 1997; Barba et al., 2002; Desmond et al., 2002b) are given in Table 20.5. Several mechanisms have been postulated to explain the association between dementia and poor outcomes (Barba et al., 2002; Desmond et al., 2002b); dementia after stroke may be a surrogate for greater cerebrovascular disease burden (Tatemichi et al., 1994c; Desmond et al., 2002b), patients with dementia may be treated less aggressively for stroke prophylaxis and other conditions (Gurwitz et al., 1997; Moroney et al., 1999), and patients with cognitive impairment may be less compliant with treatment (Moroney et al., 1999; Richards et al., 2000).

Given the high risk of adverse outcomes, it is important to identify patients with dementia after a stroke to reduce complications. The use of a comprehensive neuropsychological evaluation and operationalized paradigms for the diagnosis of dementia has superior predictive validity compared with conventional methods (such as the use of the MMSE and clinical judgement) in the diagnosis of dementia after stroke (Desmond *et al.*, 1996). Research of possible interventions in a carefully selected population is sorely needed.

Mechanisms of dementia after stroke

Dementia after stroke can result from the stroke itself, from pre-existing neurodegenerative processes, or from a combination of both. It is likely that multiple factors interact to produce dementia in patients with stroke (Scheinberg, 1988; Pohjasvaara *et al.*, 2000a). Since the stroke may be a causal or a confounding factor, the use of broad terms, such as dementia after or associated with stroke, instead of vascular dementia, may be prudent until the precise contribution of the stroke can be determined (Hachinski, 1994; Gorelick *et al.*, 1996). The National Institute of Neurological Disorders and Stroke-Association Internationale pour la Recherche et l'Enseignement en Neurosciences (NINDS-AIREN) (Roman *et al.*, 1993) criteria specify the vascular lesions that may be responsible for dementia: multiple large vessel (Hachinski *et al.*, 1974) and single strategically placed (Tatemichi *et al.*, 1995) infarcts, multiple basal ganglia and white matter lacunes, and extensive periventricular white matter lesions (Pasquier *et al.*, 2000), or combinations thereof. In addition, hemorrhages and regional or global hypoperfusion have also been implicated in the genesis of dementia.

Tomlinson *et al.* (1970) postulated that there is "an upper limit or threshold of cerebral degeneration beyond which some degree of intellectual deterioration usually occurs" and concluded that in "cerebral softening this is apparently around 100 ml." Subsequently, several groups have shown that stroke patients that develop dementia have larger infarcts but have not identified a threshold above which dementia invariably develops (Del Ser *et al.*, 1990; Pohjasvaara *et al.*, 2000a). Furthermore, there are data to suggest that the level of functional tissue loss owing to cortical deafferentation, rather than the total volume, is critical for the development of dementia (Mielke *et al.*, 1992; Kwan *et al.*, 1999). Location is at least as important as size. In the series of Pohjasvaara *et al.* (2000a), patients with and without dementia could be differentiated by the volume of lesions in the superior middle cerebral artery territory of either hemisphere and in the left thalamocortical projection (genu and anterior internal capsule, anterior corona radiata, and anterior centrum semiovale). In the series of Tatemichi *et al.* (1993), infarcts in the pooled anterior and posterior cerebral arteries were more likely to lead to dementia than lesions in other territories.

Strategically placed lesions can lead to intellectual decline when they damage strategic cortical or subcortical areas, thereby interrupting frontal–subcortical pathways that are critical for cognition (Tatemichi *et al.*, 1995). Structures that have been implicated include left angular gyrus (Benson and Cummings, 1982), inferomesial temporal lobe (Caplan and Hedley-Whyte, 1974; Ott and Saver, 1993), mesial frontal lobe (Alexander and Freedman, 1984; Damasio *et al.*, 1985), anterior limb and genu of the internal capsule (Tatemichi *et al.*, 1992b, 1995), thalamus (Castaigne *et al.*, 1981; Michel *et al.*, 1982; Choi *et al.*, 1983; Guberman and Stuss, 1983; Tatemichi *et al.*, 1992b), caudate nucleus (Mendez *et al.*, 1989; Caplan *et al.*, 1990), and mesencephalon (Trimble and Cummings, 1981; Katz *et al.*, 1987). However, the interpretation of these reports is problematic since many are based on computed tomographic imaging, which may miss some cortical lesions. In addition, the contribution of Alzheimer-type pathology cannot be excluded (Leys *et al.*, 1999). Further research on the location of lesions that lead to dementia, using modern neuroimaging techniques and prolonged follow-up, is warranted.

Lacunar strokes are independent predictors of dementia (Tatemichi *et al.*, 1993), and microvascular damage, but not macroscopic infarcts, may distinguished those with vascular dementia from those with stroke without dementia (Esiri, 2000). Small-vessel disease leads to lacunar infarctions and subcortical ischemic white matter changes (Roman *et al.*, 2002) and, when widespread, can produce a distinct syndrome characterized by cognitive impairment, personality changes, gait disturbance, motor deficits, and urinary incontinence (Inzitari *et al.*, 1999; Erkinjuntti *et al.*, 2000a; Roman *et al.*, 2002). Lipohyalinosis of the penetrating vessels (caused by hypertension) is the most common cause of lacunes with leukoencephalopathy, but other conditions, such as infiltration of cerebral microvessel walls by hyaline eosinophilic material (amyloid; Vinters, 1987) and mutations in the gene *NOTCH-3* on chromosome 19 (Tournier-Lasserve *et al.*, 1993), have also been implicated.

Cerebrovascular and Alzheimer-type pathology are common in the elderly and frequently occur together. In a large multicenter, community-based study, vascular and Alzheimer-type pathology were seen in a majority of patients, and most patients had features of both (MRC CFAS, 2001). Some patients with dementia after stroke have Alzheimer's disease; in this group, the Alzheimer's disease may have been subclinical prior to the cerebrovascular event. Stroke and Alzheimer disease have similar vascular risk factors (de la Torre, 2002), and both pathological processes, when present in the same brain, are synergistic (Snowdon *et al.*, 1997). It is not known at present if risk factors act by leading to stroke or whether they have a direct effect on the brain (Desmond *et al.*, 1993). Lacunes in the basal ganglia increase the risk of the clinical expression of dementia in patients with Alzheimer disease (Snowdon *et al.*, 1997), and infarcts lead to a greater severity of dementia (Snowdon *et al.*, 1997; Heyman *et al.*, 1998). In the Framingham Study, half the people who developed cognitive impairment after stroke had pre-existing difficulties (Kase *et al.*, 1998). In stroke cohorts evaluated with a standardized questionnaire that assessed cognitive function in the preceding 10 years, cognitive decline preceded the stroke in up to 20% of patients (Hénon *et al.*, 1997; Barba *et al.*, 2000), and two-thirds of patients had a course suggestive of Alzheimer's disease (Hénon *et al.*, 1997). Confusional syndromes are more common in patients with pre-existing impairment (Hénon *et al.*, 1999). In the cohorts from New York, functional and cognitive deficits preceded the index stroke in 40% of patients who had dementia after stroke (Tatemichi *et al.*, 1992a; Desmond *et al.*, 2000). Medial temporal lobe atrophy is strongly associated with Alzheimer disease (Jobst *et al.*, 1992) and is more common in stroke patients with pre-stroke dementia than in those without (Hénon *et al.*, 1998). It is a predictor of dementia after stroke (Pohjasvaara *et al.*, 2000b), and hippocampal and cerebral atrophy may be critical factors in determining dementia after stroke (Fein *et al.*, 2000). Patients with subcortical ischemic vascular dementia have smaller volumes of the entorhinal cortex and hippocampus than normal controls; however, for similar degrees of dementia, the volumes are smaller in patients with Alzheimer's disease than in those with vascular dementia (Du *et al.*, 2002). After excluding patients with pre-stroke dementia, 30% of patients with post-stroke dementia meet criteria for Alzheimer disease (Hénon *et al.*, 2001), and in population series, the incidence of Alzheimer disease among patients with stroke is 50% higher than expected (Kokmen *et al.*, 1996).

Prevention and treatment

It is important to identify and treat subjects at risk for stroke and cognitive impairment before dementia develops (Hachinski, 1994). As discussed above, dementia after stroke may result from the effect of the vascular lesions or a coexisting stroke and Alzheimer's disease. Both conditions have risk factors in common, many of which are modifiable (Gorelick *et al.*, 1999; Breteler, 2000). Well-designed clinical trials have proved the value of several interventions to prevent new and recurrent stroke (Straus *et al.*, 2002). Some studies have focused on the management of vascular risk factors, particularly hypertension (Amenta *et al.*, 2002), and the incidence of dementia. In a large trial of elderly people with isolated systolic hypertension, antihypertensive treatment was associated with a lower incidence of dementia (Forette *et al.*, 1998); this may have been a result of a neuroprotective effect of calcium channel blockers in patients with Alzheimer's disease or it may result from a reduction in the number of infarcts in these subjects (Leys and Pasquier, 1999). The use of statin agents has been linked to a lower incidence of dementia (Jick *et al.*, 2000). The recognition that dementia is common in patients with cerebrovascular and cardiovascular disease has been acknowledged in recent clinical trials that now include dementia as a primary or secondary outcome measure (Yusuf, 2002); this will result in concrete evidence to help us to improve targeting of these interventions.

Several studies of pharmacological agents for the treatment of vascular dementia have been published. Many have been underpowered to detect both cognitive and global change (Schneider, 2002) and have included heterogeneous groups of patients; this may explain some of the equivocal results (Inzitari *et al.*, 1999; Erkinjuntti *et al.*, 2000b; Roman *et al.*, 2002). Some agents may be efficacious in patients with subcortical ischemic disease but not in those with cortical or strategic strokes (Pantoni *et al.*, 2000a, 2000b; Wilcock *et al.*, 2002). Long-term benefits have been inconsistent, and none of the studies has been carried out in cohorts of stroke patients. Cognitive evaluations that address the cognitive, behavioral, and physical limitations of patients with stroke-related dementia have not been published (Ball *et al.*, 2002).

Neuroprotective agents have shown mild benefit when used in patients with vascular dementia. In two recent clinical trials, memantidine (an antagonist at *N*-methyl-D-aspartate [NMDA] receptors) improved cognition consistently across different cognitive scales in patients with mild-to-moderate dementia, but it did not have an effect in global functioning and behavior (Orgogozo *et al.*, 2002; Wilcock *et al.*, 2002). Pooled analysis showed that the cognitive improvement was most pronounced in patients with small vessel disease (Mobius and Stoffler, 2002). Several trials have examined the effect of the calcium channel blocker nimodipine in patients with vascular and mixed dementias, and a meta-analysis showed that its use led to improvements on global function and cognition but did not affect activities of daily living. The authors did not recommend widespread use because there are no data on the long-term effects of its use (Lopez-Arrieta and Birks, 2002). It may be more effective in patients with subcortical disease (Pantoni *et al.*, 2000a). Propentofylline (a glial cell modulator that interferes with neuroinflammatory processes implicated in the genesis of dementia) has shown a consistent improvement over placebo in efficacy assessments for patients with Alzheimer's disease and vascular dementia, and drug-withdrawal studies suggest that it can slow progression of the disease itself (Marcusson *et al.*, 1997; Rother *et al.*, 1998).

Some patients with vascular dementia have cholinergic deficits (Carlsson, 1987; Markstein, 1989; Wallin *et al.*, 1989; Gottfries *et al.*, 1994; Tohgi *et al.*, 1996) and, in addition, a significant proportion of patients with dementia after stroke have Alzheimer's disease, as discussed above. The use of acetylcholinesterase inhibitors is, therefore, a promising strategy in these patients. A small, open-label trial of rivastigmine versus aspirin showed improvement in executive function stabilization of behavioral symptoms (Moretti *et al.*, 2002). A randomized, double-blinded, placebo-controlled trial of rivastigmine in patients with Alzheimer's disease showed that it led to better cognitive outcomes, particularly in patients with vascular risk factors (Kumar *et al.*, 2000). Galantamine showed a positive effect on cognitive and non-cognitive abilities in patients with Alzheimer's disease and stroke and in patients with vascular dementia (Erkinjuntti *et al.*, 2002). The trial was inadequately powered to allow subgroup analyses but there is a suggestion that among the former group galantamine stabilized cognitive function while among the latter it led to cognitive improvement (Schneider, 2002). Partial published data from two large trials in patients with probable or possible vascular dementia suggest that cognitive and global scales improved significantly among patients treated with donepezil when compared with placebo (Pratt, 2002). Further clinical trials that are sufficiently powered and that enroll homogeneous groups of patients, preferably from well-defined stroke cohorts, will extend these observations and will potentially provide us with data to prevent, when possible, and to treat dementia after stroke.

REFERENCES

Alexander, M. P. and Freedman, M. (1984). Amnesia after anterior communicating artery aneurysm rupture. *Neurology* **34**: 752–757.

Amenta, F., Mignini, F., Rabbia, F., Tomassoni, D., and Veglio, F. (2002). Protective effect of anti-hypertensive treatment on cognitive function in essential hypertension. Analysis of published clinical data. *J Neurol Sci* **203–204**: 147–151.

American Psychiatric Association (1980). *Diagnostic and Statistical Manual of Mental Disorders,* 3rd edn. Washington, DC: American Psychiatric Press.

 (1987). *Diagnostic and Statistical Manual of Mental Disorders,* 3rd edn. revised Washington, DC: American Psychiatric Press.

American Psychiatric Association (1994). *Diagnostic and Statistical Manual of Mental Disorders,* 4th edn. Washington, DC: American Psychiatric Press.

Ball, K., Berch, D. B., Helmers, K. F., *et al.* (2002). Effects of cognitive training interventions with older adults: a randomized controlled trial. *JAMA* **288**: 2271–2281.

Barba, R., Martinez-Espinosa, S., Rodriguez-Garcia, E., *et al.* (2000). Post-stroke dementia: clinical features and risk factors. *Stroke* **31**: 1494–1501.

Barba, R., Morin, M. D., Cemillan, C., *et al.* (2002). Previous and incident dementia as risk factors for mortality in stroke patients. *Stroke* **33**: 1993–1998.

Benson, D. F. and Cummings, J. L. (1982). Angular gyrus syndrome simulating Alzheimer's disease. *Arch Neurol* **39**: 616–620.

Breteler, M. M. (2000). Vascular risk factors for Alzheimer's disease: an epidemiologic perspective. *Neurobiol Aging* **21**: 153–160.

Brun, A. (1994). Pathology and pathophysiology of cerebrovascular dementia: pure subgroups of obstructive and hypoperfusive etiology. *Dementia* **5**: 145–147.

Caplan, L. R. and Hedley-Whyte, T. (1974). Cuing and memory dysfunction in alexia without agraphia. A case report. *Brain* **97**: 251–262.

Caplan, L. R., Schmahmann, J. D., Kase, C. S., *et al.* (1990). Caudate infarcts. *Arch Neurol* **47**: 133–143.

Carlsson, A. (1987). Brain neurotransmitters in aging and dementia: similar changes across diagnostic dementia groups. *Gerontology* **33**: 159–167.

Castaigne, P., Lhermitte, F., Buge, A., *et al.* (1981). Paramedian thalamic and midbrain infarct: clinical and neuropathological study. *Ann Neurol* **10**: 127–148.

Censori, B., Manara, O., Agostinis, C., *et al.* (1996). Dementia after first stroke. *Stroke* **27**: 1205–1210.

Choi, D., Sudarsky, L., Schachter, S., Biber, M., and Burke, P. (1983). Medial thalamic hemorrhage with amnesia. *Arch Neurol* **40**: 611–613.

Chui, H. C., Mack, W., Jackson, J. E., *et al.* (2000). Clinical criteria for the diagnosis of vascular dementia: a multicenter study of comparability and interrater reliability. *Arch Neurol* **57**: 191–196.

Cooper, J. K. and Mungas, D. (1993). Risk factor and behavioral differences between vascular and Alzheimer's dementias: the pathway to end-stage disease. *J Geriatr Psychiatry Neurol* **6**: 29–33.

Damasio, A. R., Graff-Radford, N. R., Eslinger, P. J., Damasio, H., and Kassell, N. (1985). Amnesia following basal forebrain lesions. *Arch Neurol* **42**: 263–271.

de la Torre, J. C. (2002). Alzheimer disease as a vascular disorder: nosological evidence. *Stroke* **33**: 1152–1162.

Del Ser, T., Bermejo, F., Portera, A., *et al.* (1990). Vascular dementia. A clinicopathological study. *J Neurol Sci* **96**: 1–17.

Desmond, D. W., Tatemichi, T. K., Paik, M., and Stern, Y. (1993). Risk factors for cerebrovascular disease as correlates of cognitive function in a stroke-free cohort. *Arch Neurol* **50**: 162–166.

Desmond, D. W., Moroney, J. T., Sano, M., and Stern, Y. (1996). Recovery of cognitive function after stroke. *Stroke* **27**: 1798–1803.

Desmond, D. W., Bagiella, E., Moroney, J. T., and Stern, Y. (1998a). The effect of patient attrition on estimates of the frequency of dementia following stroke. *Arch Neurol* **55**: 390–394.

Desmond, D. W., Moroney, J. T., Bagiella, E., Sano, M., and Stern, Y. (1998b). Dementia as a predictor of adverse outcomes following stroke: an evaluation of diagnostic methods. *Stroke* **29**: 69–74.

Desmond, D. W., Moroney, J. T., Paik, M. C., *et al.* (2000). Frequency and clinical determinants of dementia after ischemic stroke. *Neurology* **54**: 1124–1131.

Desmond, D. W., Moroney, J. T., Sano, M., and Stern, Y. (2002a). Incidence of dementia after ischemic stroke: results of a longitudinal study. *Stroke* **33**: 2254–2262.

(2002b). Mortality in patients with dementia after ischemic stroke. *Neurology* **59**: 537–543.

Du, A. T., Schuff, N., Laakso, M. P., *et al.* (2002). Effects of subcortical ischemic vascular dementia and AD on entorhinal cortex and hippocampus. *Neurology* **58**: 1635–1641.

Erkinjuntti, T., Ostbye, T., Steenhuis, R., and Hachinski, V. (1997). The effect of different diagnostic criteria on the prevalence of dementia. *N Engl J Med* **337**: 1667–1674.

Erkinjuntti, T., Inzitari, D., Pantoni, L., *et al.* (2000). Research criteria for subcortical vascular dementia in clinical trials. *J Neural Transm Suppl* **59**: 23–30.

Erkinjuntti, T., Kurz, A., Gauthier, S., *et al.* (2002). Efficacy of galantamine in probable vascular dementia and Alzheimer's disease combined with cerebrovascular disease: a randomised trial. *Lancet* **359**: 1283–1290.

Esiri, M. M. (2000). Which vascular lesions are of importance in vascular dementia?. *Ann N Y Acad Sci* **903**: 239–243.

Fein, G., Di, S., V, Tanabe, J., *et al.* (2000). Hippocampal and cortical atrophy predict dementia in subcortical ischemic vascular disease. *Neurology* **55**: 1626–1635.

Forette, F., Seux, M. L., Staessen, J. A., *et al.* (1998). Prevention of dementia in randomised double-blind placebo-controlled Systolic Hypertension in Europe (Syst-Eur) trial. *Lancet* **352**: 1347–1351.

Gorelick, P. B., Brody, J., Cohen, D., *et al.* (1993). Risk factors for dementia associated with multiple cerebral infarcts. A case–control analysis in predominantly African-American hospital-based patients. *Arch Neurol* **50**: 714–720.

Gorelick, P. B., Nyenhuis, D. L., Garron, D. C., and Cochran, E. (1996). Is vascular dementia really Alzheimer's disease or mixed dementia? *Neuroepidemiology* **15**: 286–290.

Gorelick, P. B., Erkinjuntti, T., Hofman, A., *et al.* (1999). Prevention of vascular dementia. *Alzheimer Dis Assoc Disord* **13**(Suppl. 3): S131–S139.

Gottfries, C. G., Blennow, K., Karlsson, I., and Wallin, A. (1994). The neurochemistry of vascular dementia. *Dementia* **5**: 163–167.

Guberman, A. and Stuss, D. (1983). The syndrome of bilateral paramedian thalamic infarction. *Neurology* **33**: 540–546.

Gurwitz, J. H., Monette, J., Rochon, P. A., Eckler, M. A., and Avorn, J. (1997). Atrial fibrillation and stroke prevention with warfarin in the long-term care setting. *Arch Intern Med* **157**: 978–984.

Hachinski, V. (1994). Vascular dementia: a radical redefinition. *Dementia* **5**: 130–132.

Hachinski, V. C., Lassen, N. A., and Marshall, J. (1974). Multi-infarct dementia. A cause of mental deterioration in the elderly. *Lancet* **2**: 207–210.

Hénon, H., Pasquier, F., Durieu, I., *et al.* (1997). Pre-existing dementia in stroke patients. Baseline frequency, associated factors, and outcome. *Stroke* **28**: 2429–2436.

Hénon, H., Pasquier, F., Durieu, I., Pruvo, J. P., and Leys, D. (1998). Medial temporal lobe atrophy in stroke patients: relation to pre-existing dementia. *J Neurol Neurosurg Psychiatry* **65**: 641–647.

Hénon, H., Lebert, F., Durieu, I., *et al.* (1999). Confusional state in stroke: relation to pre-existing dementia, patient characteristics, and outcome. *Stroke* **30**: 773–779.

Hénon, H., Durieu, I., Guerouaou, D., *et al.* (2001). Post-stroke dementia: incidence and relationship to prestroke cognitive decline. *Neurology* **57**: 1216–1222.

Heyman, A., Fillenbaum, G. G., Welsh-Bohmer, K. A., *et al.* (1998). Cerebral infarcts in patients with autopsy-proven Alzheimer's disease: CERAD, part XVIII. Consortium to Establish a Registry for Alzheimer's Disease. *Neurology* **51**: 159–162.

Inzitari, D., Di Carlo, A., Pracucci, G., *et al.* (1998). Incidence and determinants of post-stroke dementia as defined by an informant interview method in a hospital-based stroke registry. *Stroke* **29**: 2087–2093.

Inzitari, D., Erkinjuntti, T., Wallin, A., Del Ser, T., and Pantoni, L. (1999). Is subcortical vascular dementia a clinical entity for clinical drug trials? *Alzheimer Dis Assoc Disord* **13**:(Suppl. 3): S66–S68.

Jick, H., Zornberg, G. L., Jick, S. S., Seshadri, S., and Drachman, D. A. (2000). Statins and the risk of dementia. *Lancet* **356**: 1627–1631.

Jobst, K. A., Smith, A. D., Szatmari, M., *et al.* (1992). Detection in life of confirmed Alzheimer's disease using a simple measurement of medial temporal lobe atrophy by computed tomography. *Lancet* **340**: 1179–1183.

Kase, C. S., Wolf, P. A., Kelly-Hayes, M., *et al.* (1998). Intellectual decline after stroke: the Framingham Study. *Stroke* **29**: 805–812.

Katz, D. I., Alexander, M. P., and Mandell, A. M. (1987). Dementia following strokes in the mesencephalon and diencephalon. *Arch Neurol* **44**: 1127–1133.

Katzman, R., Hill, L. R., Yu, E. S., *et al.* (1994). The malignancy of dementia. Predictors of mortality in clinically diagnosed dementia in a population survey of Shanghai, China. *Arch Neurol* **51**: 1220–1225.

Kokmen, E., Whisnant, J. P., O'Fallon, W. M., Chu, C. P., and Beard, C. M. (1996). Dementia after ischemic stroke: a population-based study in Rochester, Minnesota (1960–1984). *Neurology* **46**: 154–159.

Kotila, M., Waltimo, O., Niemi, M. L., Laaksonen, R., and Lempinen, M. (1984). The profile of recovery from stroke and factors influencing outcome. *Stroke* **15**: 1039–1044.

Kumar, V., Anand, R., Messina, J., Hartman, R., and Veach, J. (2000). An efficacy and safety analysis of Exelon in Alzheimer's disease patients with concurrent vascular risk factors. *Eur J Neurol* **7**: 159–169.

Kwan, L. T., Reed, B. R., Eberling, J. L., *et al.* (1999). Effects of subcortical cerebral infarction on cortical glucose metabolism and cognitive function. *Arch Neurol* **56**: 809–814.

Ladurner, G., Iliff, L. D., and Lechner, H. (1982). Clinical factors associated with dementia in ischaemic stroke. *J Neurol Neurosurg Psychiatry* **45**: 97–101.

Leys, D. and Pasquier, F. (1999). Prevention of dementia: Syst-Eur trial. *Lancet* **353**: 236–237.

Leys, D., Erkinjuntti, T., Desmond, D. W., *et al.* (1999). Vascular dementia: the role of cerebral infarcts. *Alzheimer Dis Assoc Disord* **13**(Suppl. 3): S38–S48.

Liu, C. K., Miller, B. L., Cummings, J. L., *et al.* (1992). A quantitative MRI study of vascular dementia. *Neurology* **42**: 138–143.

Loeb, C., Gandolfo, C., Croce, R., and Conti, M. (1992). Dementia associated with lacunar infarction. *Stroke* **23**: 1225–1229.

Longstreth, W. T., Jr., Manolio, T. A., Arnold, A., *et al.* (1996). Clinical correlates of white matter findings on cranial magnetic resonance imaging of 3301 elderly people. The Cardiovascular Health Study. *Stroke* **27**: 1274–1282.

Lopez-Arrieta, J. M. and Birks, J. (2002), Nimodipine for primary degenerative, mixed and vascular dementia *Cochrane Database of Systematic Reviews*, Issue 3. Oxford: Update Software, CD000147.

Madureira, S., Canhao, P., Guerreiro, M., and Ferro, J. M. (2000). Cognitive and emotional consequences of perimesencephalic subarachnoid hemorrhage. *J Neurol* **247**: 862–867.

Marcusson, J., Rother, M., Kittner, B., *et al.* (1997). A 12-month, randomized, placebo-controlled trial of propentofylline (HWA 285) in patients with dementia according to DSM III-R. The European Propentofylline Study Group. *Dement Geriatr Cogn Disord* **8**: 320–328.

Markstein, R. (1989). Pharmacological approaches in the treatment of senile dementia. *Eur Neurol* **29**(Suppl. 3): 33–41.

Mendez, M. F., Adams, N. L., and Lewandowski, K. S. (1989). Neurobehavioral changes associated with caudate lesions. *Neurology* **39**: 349–354.

Michel, D., Laurent, B., Foyatier, N., Blanc, A., and Portafaix, M. (1982). Left paramedian thalamic infarct. Memory and language study. *Rev Neurol (Paris)* **138**: 533–550.

Mielke, R., Herholz, K., Grond, M., Kessler, J., and Heiss, W. D. (1992). Severity of vascular dementia is related to volume of metabolically impaired tissue. *Arch Neurol* **49**: 909–913.

Mobius, H. J. and Stoffler, A. (2002). New approaches to clinical trials in vascular dementia: memantine in small vessel disease. *Cerebrovasc Dis* **13**(Suppl. 2): 61–66.

Molsa, P. K., Marttila, R. J., and Rinne, U. K. (1986). Survival and cause of death in Alzheimer's disease and multi-infarct dementia. *Acta Neurol Scand* **74**: 103–107.

Moretti, R., Torre, P., Antonello, R. M., Cazzato, G., and Bava, A. (2002). Rivastigmine in subcortical vascular dementia. An open 22-month study. *J Neurol Sci* **203–204**: 141–146.

Moroney, J. T., Bagiella, E., Desmond, D. W., *et al.* (1997a). Cerebral hypoxia and ischemia in the pathogenesis of dementia after stroke. *Ann N Y Acad Sci* **826**: 433–436.

Moroney, J. T., Bagiella, E., Tatemichi, T. K., *et al.* (1997b). Dementia after stroke increases the risk of long-term stroke recurrence. *Neurology* **48**: 1317–1325.

Moroney, J. T., Tseng, C. L., Paik, M. C., Mohr, J. P., and Desmond, D. W. (1999). Treatment for the secondary prevention of stroke in older patients: the influence of dementia status. *J Am Geriatr Soc* **47**: 824–829.

MRC CFAS (2001), Pathological correlates of late-onset dementia in a multicentre, community-based population in England and Wales. Neuropathology Group of the Medical Research Council Cognitive Function and Aging Study (MRC CFAS). *Lancet* **357**: 169–175.

Orgogozo, J. M., Rigaud, A. S., Stoffler, A., Mobius, H. J., and Forette, F. (2002). Efficacy and safety of memantine in patients with mild to moderate vascular dementia: a randomized, placebo-controlled trial (MMM 300). *Stroke* **33**: 1834–1839.

Ott, B. R., and Saver, J. L. (1993). Unilateral amnesic stroke. Six new cases and a review of the literature. *Stroke* **24**: 1033–1042.

Pantoni, L., Bianchi, C., Beneke, M., *et al.* (2000a). The Scandinavian Multi-Infarct Dementia Trial: a double-blind, placebo-controlled trial on nimodipine in multi-infarct dementia. *J Neurol Sci* **175**: 116–123.

Pantoni, L., Rossi, R., Inzitari, D., *et al.* (2000b). Efficacy and safety of nimodipine in subcortical vascular dementia: a subgroup analysis of the Scandinavian Multi-Infarct Dementia Trial. *J Neurol Sci* **175**: 124–134.

Pasquier, F., Henon, H., and Leys, D. (2000). Relevance of white matter changes to pre- and post-stroke dementia. *Ann N Y Acad Sci* **903**: 466–469.

Pohjasvaara, T., Erkinjuntti, T., Vataja, R., and Kaste, M. (1997). Dementia three months after stroke. Baseline frequency and effect of different definitions of dementia in the Helsinki Stroke Aging Memory Study (SAM) cohort. *Stroke* **28**: 785–792.

Pohjasvaara, T., Erkinjuntti, T., Ylikoski, R., *et al.* (1998a). Clinical determinants of post-stroke dementia. *Stroke* **29**: 75–81.

Pohjasvaara, T., Erkinjuntti, T., Vataja, R., and Kaste, M. (1998b). Correlates of dependent living 3 months after ischemic stroke. *Cerebrovasc Dis* **8**: 259–266.

Pohjasvaara, T., Mantyla, R., Salonen, O., *et al.* (2000a). How complex interactions of ischemic brain infarcts, white matter lesions, and atrophy relate to post-stroke dementia. *Arch Neurol* **57**: 1295–1300.

Pohjasvaara, T., Mantyla, R., Salonen, O., *et al.* (2000b). MRI correlates of dementia after first clinical ischemic stroke. *J Neurol Sci* **181**: 111–117.

Pratt, R. D. (2002). Patient populations in clinical trials of the efficacy and tolerability of donepezil in patients with vascular dementia. *J Neurol Sci* **203–204**: 57–65.

Prencipe, M., Ferretti, C., Casini, A. R.., *et al.* (1997). Stroke, disability, and dementia: results of a population survey. *Stroke* **28**: 531–536.

Richards, S. S., Emsley, C. L., Roberts, J., *et al.* (2000). The association between vascular risk factor-mediating medications and cognition and dementia diagnosis in a community-based sample of African-Americans. *J Am Geriatr Soc* **48**: 1035–1041.

Rockwood, K., Wentzel, C., and Hachinski, V. (2000). Prevalence and outcomes of vascular cognitive impairment. Vascular Cognitive Impairment Investigators of the Canadian Study of Health and Aging. *Neurology* **54**: 447–451.

Roman, G. C., Tatemichi, T. K., Erkinjuntti, T., *et al.* (1993). Vascular dementia: diagnostic criteria for research studies. Report of the NINDS-AIREN International Workshop. *Neurology* **43**: 250–260.

Roman, G. C., Erkinjuntti, T., Wallin, A., Pantoni, L., and Chui, H. C. (2002). Subcortical ischaemic vascular dementia. *Lancet Neurol* **1**: 426–436.

Rother, M., Erkinjuntti, T., and Roessner, M. (1998). Propentofylline in the treatment of Alzheimer's disease and vascular dementia: a review of phase III trials. *Dement Geriatr Cogn Disord.* **9**(Suppl. 1): 36–43.

Samuelsson, M., Soderfeldt, B., and Olsson, G. B. (1996). Functional outcome in patients with lacunar infarction. *Stroke* **27**: 842–846.

Scheinberg, P. (1988). Dementia due to vascular disease: a multifactorial disorder *Stroke* **19**: 1291–1299.

Schneider, L. S. (2002). Galantamine for vascular dementia: some answers, some questions. *Lancet* **359**: 1265–1266.

Skoog, I., Nilsson, L., Palmertz, B., Andreasson, L. A., and Svanborg, A. (1993). A population-based study of dementia in 85-year-olds. *N Engl J Med* **328**: 153–158.

Snowdon, D. A., Greiner, L. H., Mortimer, J. A., *et al.* (1997). Brain infarction and the clinical expression of Alzheimer disease. The Nun Study. *JAMA* **277**: 813–817.

Straus, S. E., Majumdar, S. R., and McAlister, F. A. (2002). New evidence for stroke prevention: scientific review. *JAMA* **288**: 1388–1395.

Sulkava, R. and Erkinjuntti, T. (1987). Vascular dementia due to cardiac arrhythmias and systemic hypotension. *Acta Neurol Scand* **76**: 123–128.

Tatemichi, T. K. (1990). How acute brain failure becomes chronic: a view of the mechanisms of dementia related to stroke. *Neurology* **40**: 1652–1659.

Tatemichi, T. K., Desmond, D. W., Mayeux, R., *et al.* (1992a). Dementia after stroke: baseline frequency, risks, and clinical features in a hospitalized cohort. *Neurology* **42**: 1185–1193.

Tatemichi, T. K., Desmond, D. W., Prohovnik, I., and Stern, Y. (1992b). Confusion and memory loss from capsular genu infarction: a thalamocortical disconnection syndrome? *Neurology* **42**: 1966–1979.

Tatemichi, T. K., Desmond, D. W., and Paik, M. (1993). Clinical determinants of dementia related to stroke. *Ann Neurol* **33**: 568–575.

Tatemichi, T. K., Paik, M., and Bagiella, E. (1994a). Risk of dementia after stroke in a hospitalized cohort: results of a longitudinal study. *Neurology* **44**: 1885–1891.

Tatemichi, T. K., Desmond, D. W., Stern, Y. *et al.* (1994b). Cognitive impairment after stroke: frequency, patterns, and relationship to functional abilities. *J Neurol Neurosurg Psychiatry* **57**: 202–207.

Tatemichi, T. K., Paik, M., Bagiella, E., *et al.* (1994c). Dementia after stroke is a predictor of long-term survival. *Stroke* **25**: 1915–1919.

Tatemichi, T. K., Desmond, D. W., and Prohovnik, I. (1995). Strategic infarcts in vascular dementia. A clinical and brain imaging experience. *Arzneimittelforschung* **45**: 371–385.

Tohgi, H., Abe, T., Kimura, M., Saheki, M., and Takahashi, S. (1996). Cerebrospinal fluid acetylcholine and choline in vascular dementia of Binswanger and multiple small infarct types as compared with Alzheimer-type dementia. *J Neural Transm* **103**: 1211–1220.

Tomlinson, B. E., Blessed, G., and Roth, M. (1970). Observations on the brains of demented old people. *J Neurol Sci* **11**: 205–242.

Tournier-Lasserve, E., Joutel, A., Melki, J., *et al.* (1993). Cerebral autosomal dominant arteriopathy with subcortical infarcts and leukoencephalopathy maps to chromosome 19q12. *Nat Genet* **3**: 256–259.

Trimble, M. R., and Cummings, J. L. (1981). Neuropsychiatric disturbances following brainstem lesions. *Br J Psychiatry* **138**: 56–59.

van Kooten, F., Bots, M. L., Breteler, M. M., *et al.* (1998). The Dutch Vascular Factors in Dementia Study: rationale and design. *J Neurol* **245**: 32–39.

van Zandvoort, M. J., Aleman, A., Kappelle, L. J., and de Haan, E. H. (2000). Cognitive functioning before and after a lacunar infarct. *Cerebrovasc Dis* **10**: 478–479.

van Zandvoort, M. J., de Haan, E. H., and Kappelle, L. J. (2001). Chronic cognitive disturbances after a single supratentorial lacunar infarct. *Neuropsychiatry Neuropsychol Behav Neurol* **14**: 98–102.

Vinters, H. V. (1987). Cerebral amyloid angiopathy. A critical review. *Stroke* **18**: 311–324.

Wade, D. T., Parker, V., and Langton, H. R. (1986). Memory disturbance after stroke: frequency and associated losses. *Int Rehabil Med* **8**: 60–64.

Wallin, A., Alafuzoff, I., Carlsson, A., *et al.* (1989). Neurotransmitter deficits in a non-multi-infarct category of vascular dementia. *Acta Neurol Scand* **79**: 397–406.

Wilcock, G., Mobius, H. J., and Stoffler, A. (2002). A double-blind, placebo-controlled multicentre study of memantine in mild to moderate vascular dementia (MMM500). *Int Clin Psychopharmacol* **17**: 297–305.

WHO (1989), *The International Classification of Diseases*, 10th edn. Geneva: World Health Organization.

Yusuf, S. (2002). From the HOPE to the ONTARGET and the TRANSCEND studies: challenges in improving prognosis. *Am J Cardiol* **89**: 18A–25A.

Zhu, L., Fratiglioni, L., Guo, Z., *et al.* (1998). Association of stroke with dementia, cognitive impairment, and functional disability in the very old: a population-based study. *Stroke* **29**: 2094–2099.

21

Depression and fatigue after stroke

Fabienne Staub

University of Lausanne, Lausanne, Switzerland

Antonio Carota

University Hospital Geneva, Switzerland

Introduction

Post-stroke depression (PSD) is a significant factor affecting functional and social disability, even long after neurological and neuropsychological recovery. Fatigue is a commonly reported complaint in clinical practice. Fatigue after stroke (PSF), often disabling, is frequently reported and can in some cases be the only significant sequelae. It is often neglected or is considered as one aspect of PSD.

Post-stroke depression

The occurrence of PSD has been extensively investigated, with over 200 scientific papers published between 1985 and 1995 (Gordon and Hibbard, 1997). However, major methodological differences between the studies prevent straightforward conclusions being drawn and the following paragraphs are more descriptive than synthetic. For example, PSD has been reported in both less than 25% and in more than 75% of patients. The role of the side and site of stroke also remains controversial.

Diagnosis

The diagnostic accuracy of the standardized psychiatric assessment for patients with neurological impairment is questionable. Psychiatric criteria of mood disorders rely heavily on patients' reports of their own symptoms. This requires patients to be aware of their situation and to be capable of providing an accurate report of it, a task that can be difficult or impossible in patients with aphasia and other cognitive impairment caused by stroke. The presence of neurobehavioral sequelae such as aphasia, psychomotor slowing, anosognosia, and denial often compromises the validity of patients' answers. The presence of conditions

Recovery after Stroke, ed. Michael P. Barnes, Bruce H. Dobkin and Julien Bogousslavsky. Published by Cambridge University Press. © Cambridge University Press 2005.

Table 21.1 Diagnostic confounders of depressive syndromes after stroke

Type	Confounders
Indirect and common to many severely ill hospitalized patients	Controlled appetite (e.g. no oral feeding, tube feeding); frequently awakened; confined to bed; delirium (acute confusional states)
Indirect of special concern in stroke patients	Immobility (potential confusion with apathy); dysphagia (interferes with eating habits); slurred speech (and resultant miscommunication)
Direct	Aphasia; amnesia and cognitive impairment; anosognosia and denial of depressive signs; aprosody; neurological apathy syndromes; isolated abulia/apathia; loss of psychic auto-activation; frontal lobe syndrome; Klüver–Bucy syndrome; Korsakoff's syndrome; Post-stroke fatigue; special behavioral syndromes (emotional lability or emotionalism, catastrophic reaction); dementia; pseudobulbar syndrome

interfering with the appreciation of the symptoms of depression should be carefully considered. (Table 21.1).

The diagnosis of mood disorders caused by medical conditions, including stroke, is actually based on the DSM-IV criteria (American Psychiatric Association, 1994). According to these criteria, the diagnosis of PSD requires the presence of persistent symptoms and cannot be made in the very acute phase of stroke. It is also uncertain if the DSM-IV diagnosis of PSD is valid for all depressive episodes occurring at any time after stroke. It is still a subject of controversy whether behavioral changes and subjective symptoms of PSD, and endogenous depression are equivalent (Robertson, 1998) or at least partially different (Lipsey *et al.*, 1986), and whether the two conditions share the dysfunction of the same cerebral areas and neurotransmitters. The "non-reactive" or "unmotivated" aspects (e.g. feelings of worthlessness, guilt, and suicidal ideation) and morning aggravation prevail in endogenous depression, while anxiety, diurnal mood fluctuation, and the "motivated" or "reactive" aspects (e.g. low mood, reduced appetite, and anergia) are prevalent for PSD (Gainotti *et al.*, 2001).

Differentiating between "major" and "minor" forms of depression is another aspect of great clinical relevance. The symptoms of major depression include low mood, insomnia or hypersomnia, reduced appetite, weight loss, anergia, psychomotor retardation, difficulty in concentrating, forgetfulness, anhedonia, loss of interest in sex, feelings of worthlessness, pathological guilt, and recurrent thoughts of death or suicide. The DSM-IV diagnosis of a "major depressive-like episode" is based on the existence of five or more of these depressive symptoms, two of which must be a depressed mood and a loss of interest and pleasure in almost all activities. Minor depression is defined as a less-severe form of depression with the presence of two, but fewer than five, of the symptoms of major depression, including either a depressed mood or loss of interest. The DSM-IV distinction between major and minor depression seems reasonable and clinically adequate in both stroke patients (Paradiso and Robinson, 1999) and endogenous depression but it is uncertain if the two forms of depression correspond to different etiologies and outcomes.

The DSM-IV definition of depression is based on the assumption that a unique postulate exists for all the depressive syndromes. For the DSM-IV, the depressive dimension is a function where all the clinical forms of depression, ranging from dysthimia to melancholia, are represented in a continuum with several degrees of severity. Within this unidimensional perspective, an artificial threshold is empirically adopted to separate the major from the minor depression. In DSM-IV, the qualitative dimensions of depression (depressive temperament or traits, neuroticism, emotionalism, anedonia), such as they are observed in the clinical practice, are mostly neglected.

The role of personal events, as main determinants of mood changes, corresponds to a clinical reality for stroke patients. Victims of stroke experience the destruction of the body integrity with loss of autonomy and self-esteem. The presence of cognitive, motor, and perceptive impairment strongly modifies the whole life project of the individual patient. Spouse and social conflicts, isolation, the loss of a professional activity, application to rehabilitative programs, environmental changes, and financial problems are source of anxiety and emotional changes. These "reactive" aspects of depression, which very often impregnate the conversations between doctors and patients, could have a different origin than changes caused by the brain lesion.

The reactive phenomena of depression could correspond to two models: the first considers the depressive syndrome as autonomous from the trigger event; while for the second the trigger event reactions are interactive phenomena. In the first model, the occurrence of a depressive syndrome is indicative of the trauma of the precipitating event. In this model, the depression is a pathological disease of more general importance and the trigger event is part of a process of causality that allows an analysis of the depression in terms of precipitating events, pre-existing vulnerability, sensitivity, and reactivation of latent or unconscious conflicts. In the second model, the trigger is considered a trauma but the reaction, consisting of some of a defined variety of responses, gives a specific configuration to the occurrence of depression. The interactivity model locates the depression in the dimension of the adaptive disorders next to the cognitive models of stress.

Finally, the possibility of different forms of PSD should be considered for each individual patient and for purposes related to clinical studies.

Incidence, prevalence, and demographic data

In the vast literature, PSD prevalence varies between 20 and 40% in the first two weeks, is 31–53% at three to four months, 19–55% at one year, 19% at two years, and 9–41% at three years (Feibel and Springer, 1982; House *et al.*, 1990a,b; Astrom *et al.*, 1993; Burvill *et al.*, 1995; Angeleri *et al.*, 1997; Kauhanen *et al.*, 1999; Kotila *et al.*, 1999). Similar prevalences are reported in community-based (27–62%; Wade *et al.*, 1987; Burvill *et al.*, 1997; Kotila *et al.*, 1998), outpatient (40%; Burvill *et al.*, 1995; Pohjasvaara *et al.*, 1998), and rehabilitation unit (27.4–55%; Ebrahim *et al.*, 1987; Schwartz *et al.*, 1993; Hermann *et al.*, 1998; Pohjasvaara *et al.*, 1998; Paolucci *et al.*, 1999) studies.

Major depression accounts for a minority of cases, with a prevalence of 10–20% in stroke patients (Eastwood *et al.*, 1989; Palomaki *et al.*, 1999), the prevalence of minor depression varying between 5 and 40% (Eastwood *et al.*, 1989; Burvill *et al.*, 1995). These large variations result from the use of different structured interviews, differing study sizes and selection criteria, and different times of investigation.

The incidence of PSD varies slightly with age (Neau *et al.*, 1998) and gender. In women, major depression correlates with a high level of education, cognitive impairment, and previous psychiatric antecedents, while, in men, it is more dependent on physical impairment (Paradiso and Robinson, 1998).

There are no neuroanatomical, functional, and genetic models that can explain either sexual differences or a different hemispheral risk profile for the ischemic lesion.

In conclusion, PSD incidence and prevalence are very high; risk factors are not yet clearly understood, and stroke patients should be investigated for PSD even when several years have elapsed after the acute event.

Role of lesion localization

In endogenous depression, computed tomographic and magnetic resonance imaging studies are not diagnostic but show a trend towards a reduction in volume of the basal ganglia (Rabins *et al.*, 1991; Parashos *et al.*, 1998), hippocampus (Bremner *et al.*, 2000; Mervaala *et al.*, 2000), and amygdala (Mervaala *et al.*, 2000); cortical and subcortical atrophy (Rabins *et al.*, 1991); white matter hyperintensities (Kramer and Garralda, 1998); and ventricular enlargement (Pantel *et al.*, 1998).

Positron emission (Merriam *et al.*, 1999; Lai *et al.*, 2000) and single photon emission (Willeit *et al.*, 2000) computed tomography show reduced metabolism with normalization after therapy in the left frontosubcortical and paralimbic circuits, left anterior cingulate, superior temporal and parietal cortex, and caudate.

A major role for the anterior cingulate cortex is apparent from a wealth of neuropsychological, neuroanatomical, and functional imaging data (Auer *et al.*, 2000), consistent with increasingly sophisticated models that place it at the interface of emotion, cognition, drive, and motor control (Devinsky *et al.*, 1995; Carter *et al.*, 1999; Paus, 2001). Orbital and dorsolateral regions of the prefrontal cortex have also been implicated in mood disorder on structural and clinical grounds (Goodwin, 1997; Merriam *et al.*, 1999; Lai *et al.*, 2000; Ongur and Price, 2000).

Most clinical studies on PSD have tried to identify dysfunction of specific cerebral regions with the underlying hypothesis that these regions are also determinant for endogenous depression. Such regions should be part of, or connected to, the limbic and temporal lobes, which are involved in emotional processing, but also include basal ganglia and premotor areas to enhance or inhibit oriented-goal behaviors.

Several studies (Bokura and Robinson, 1997; Lauterbach *et al.*, 1997), but not all (Sato *et al.*, 1999; Berg *et al.*, 2003), have suggested the role of the limbic connected areas and basal ganglia in the development of PSD.

Beblo *et al.* (1999) studied, with detailed neuropsychological examination, 20 selected patients with PSD but without severe physical impairment, psychiatric antecedents, concomitant morbidity, or aphasia. They found an implication of basal ganglia structures in the majority and a positive association between depression and impairment in executive functions. Kim and Choi-Kwon (2000) found a similar distribution of lesions in patients with PSD and emotional lability.

In patients with acute traumatic brain injury, the presence of left dorsolateral frontal or basal ganglia lesions is associated with an increased risk of developing major depression (Greenwald *et al.*, 1998).

The role of subcortical lesions and frontal–subcortical dysfunction is suggested by retrospective magnetic resonance imaging studies (Greenwald *et al.*, 1998; Yanai *et al.*, 1998; Ballard *et al.*, 2000; Moresco *et al.*, 2000; Tupler *et al.*, 2002), which have shown a relationship between major unipolar depression and silent cerebral infarctions among elderly people. For these patients, the severity of depression is greater and the response to pharmacological treatment is less prompt. These studies suggest that approximately half of those with presenile-onset major depression and probably the majority of those with senile-onset major depression might have the diagnosis of post-stroke or "secondary" depression. Health strategies aimed at preventing cerebrovascular disease may, therefore, lessen depressive vulnerability in the elderly.

Robinson and colleagues (Robinson and Stitt, 1981) indicated that the location of the lesion in the left hemisphere and the proximity of its anterior border to the frontal pole are the determinant factors for developing PSD. According to Robinson *et al.* (Pearlson and Robinson, 1981; Robinson and Stitt, 1981), the neuroanatomy of the biogenic amine-containing pathways in the cerebral cortex, which have a more anterior distribution, might explain the linear correlation between anterior lesion location and severity of depression. These conclusions have been the subject of great criticism because patients with severe aphasia or cognitive impairment were generally excluded, diffuse lesions in the territory of the medial cerebral artery are frequently proximal to both poles, PSD symptoms may be the result of metabolic dysfunction of distant cerebral areas connected with the lesions, and because many other clinical studies failed to find any lateralization or any anteroposterior gradient for PSD (Ebrahim *et al.*, 1987; Dam *et al.*, 1989; Eastwood *et al.*, 1989; House *et al.*, 1990b; Malec *et al.*, 1990; Morris *et al.*, 1990; Schwartz *et al.*, 1993), while others found that right, rather than left, hemispheral lesions were significantly associated with PSD (Dam *et al.*, 1989; Finset *et al.*, 1989; Machale *et al.*, 1998).

Finally lesion location may contribute only to a small extent to the risk of developing PSD (Carson *et al.*, 2000) but the association of PSD with a specific cognitive syndrome (psychomotor slowing, executive and verbal learning dysfunction, amotivational states), and the presence of equivalent mood changes in other neurological diseases with a documented regional pattern of lesion (CADASIL, vascular dementia, multiple sclerosis, Hungtington's disease, Parkinson's disease, human immunodeficiency virus encephalopathy) are further arguments for the role of the prefrontal regions, the frontal–subcortical networks (including striatum, caudate nucleus, and the thalamus), and the limbic and paralymbic regions (temporal lobe and amygdala).

Association with cognitive impairment

A significant association between PSD and cognitive deficits has been reported in several studies (Bolla-Wilson *et al.*, 1989; Eastwood *et al.*, 1989; Kase *et al.*, 1998), even though stroke itself may be followed by a significant decline in cognitive performance when pre and post-stroke measurements are compared (Pohjasvaara *et al.*, 1999).

The main question is whether it is depression that negatively influences the outcome of cognitive impairment or whether cognitive impairment leads to depression. Data from numerous studies (Kauhanen *et al.*, 1999; Sato *et al.*, 1999) fail to provide an insight into the problem, because of differences of methods and of the time considered elapsed since the stroke.

The majority of these studies adopted the Mini Mental State Examination (MMSE), a test with obvious limitations including its dependence on verbal skills, the different degrees of sensitivity of its various items (which overestimate deficits in patients with left lesions), and its inability to assess frontal or executive functions accurately (Bolla-Wilson *et al.*, 1989).

Although non-comparable, some of these studies provide evidence that depression is the main factor leading to, or aggravating, cognitive impairment post-stroke. This hypothesis is summarized by the term "dementia of depression" (Bolla-Wilson *et al.*, 1989; Kimura *et al.*, 2000). We will briefly describe the data in favor of this hypothesis. Fronto-amnesic deficits caused by disruption of cortical projections to the caudate nucleus have been suggested to explain the progressive deterioration of patients with PSD and lesions of the caudate nucleus (Bokura and Robinson, 1997). In a group of 53 patients with unique ischemic lesion, Bolla-Wilson *et al.* (1989) found that patients with left hemispheral lesions and major depression were more impaired in terms of orientation, language (naming), verbal learning, visuoperceptual and visuoconstructional tasks, executive functions (attention, concentration, non-verbal problem solving, and psychomotor speed) than those with left lesion without depression, data confirmed by other studies (Veiel Ho, 1997; Kauhanen *et al.*, 1999). The presence of dysphasia seems particularly correlated to a higher risk of major depression (Kauhanen *et al.*, 1999). Furthermore, greater severity and longer duration of cognitive impairment has been observed in patients with PSD and left lesions (Bolla-Wilson *et al.*, 1989; Andersen *et al.*, 1996).

However, other studies have favored the opposite hypothesis: in patients with stroke, depressive symptoms are part of, or determined by, a dementia syndrome. This condition corresponds to the "depression of dementia" (Andersen *et al.*, 1996).

In other community studies, using MMSE (House *et al.*, 1990a; Malec *et al.*, 1990; Morris *et al.*, 1990) or other measurements (Morris *et al.*, 1992), no evidence was found to support a correlation between cognitive impairment and major depression one year after first-ever stroke (House *et al.*, 1990a).

In conclusion, despite inconclusive findings indicating depression to be a factor leading to dementia in patients with cerebrovascular lesions, the link between PSD and cognitive impairment is probably bidirectional and prompt treatment of PSD is warranted to enhance recovery of cognitive functions.

Neurological deficits and outcome

PSD may be the consequence of the individual adaptive reaction to the neurological deficits caused by stroke. In this sense, PSD could correspond to a "reactive depression" and originate from psychodynamic processes more than from organic factors. In some studies, the development and intensity of depressive symptoms correlate strongly with the grade of functional impairment (Burvill *et al.*, 1997; Neau *et al.*, 1998; Kauhanen *et al.*, 1999) during the acute phase and the first six months (Robinson *et al.*, 1983), but others studies failed to reproduce these results (Feibel and Springer, 1982; Finklestein *et al.*, 1982).

No definite conclusion can be drawn from the literature, although the association of PSD with stroke severity and functional outcome seems likely.

In the study of Neau *et al.* (1998) of young adult patients with stroke, multivariate analysis showed a low score on the US National Institute of Health (NIHSS) scale on admission to be a significant predictor for return to work, absence of PSD, and a good quality of life. The hypothesis that functional impairment could be one of the major causal factors for depression is also based on studies that showed a similar incidence or prevalence of depression in patients with stroke and patients with similar functional disability caused by other medical illness (Lieberman *et al.*, 1999). In the study of Singh *et al.* (2000), disability correlated temporally with the progress of PSD and was a better longitudinal predictor of depressive symptoms than lesion location.

The other issue is whether it is the functional impairment that leads to depression or whether the depression itself can compromise the motor and cognitive outcome of deficits caused by the stroke. Many studies (Angeleri *et al.*, 1997; Kotila *et al.*, 1998; Gainotti *et al.*, 2001; Paolucci *et al.*, 2001), but not all, have reported that depressive feelings themselves negatively influence the prognosis and functional outcome of patients with stroke, at short- and long-term follow-up. A comparison of groups of stroke patients with or without mood disorders, but with the same functional disability, showed that physical functioning, bodily pain, somatic symptoms, and social functioning were worse in patients with affective disorders (Carson *et al.*, 2000). Depressive patients with stroke may not have the energy or motivation to participate in rehabilitation therapy. They might also feel helpless or hopeless about the future and, therefore, fail to put any effort into rehabilitation treatments.

Surprisingly, patients with great disability and depressive mood frequently express little enthusiasm about receiving psychiatric treatment. The reason is probably the negative correlation between physical impairment, reduced functional autonomy, and self-esteem. Self-esteem is significantly correlated to functional independence at short- and long-term follow-up (Chang and Mackenzie, 1998).

Depressive feelings at the time of initial inpatient evaluation result in a greater than three-fold increase in the risk of subsequent mortality over the following 10 years for patients with PSD compared with patients with stroke but no depression (Morris *et al.*, 1993). This risk is independent of other cardiovascular risk factors, age, sex, social class, type of stroke, lesion location, and level of social functioning; however, it may also be associated with social isolation (Morris *et al.*, 1993). Patients who are depressed may return to detrimental habits, such as smoking or consuming excessive alcohol, and might not comply with treatment recommendations.

The effect of negative mood states in increasing mortality is probably also mediated by modifications of the cardiovascular system (Everson *et al.*, 1998). Patients with endogenous depression experience a higher grade of arterial hypertension (Jonas *et al.*, 1997) (especially elevation of the systolic pressure) and myocardial infarction (Hippisley-Cox *et al.*, 1998) and exhibit enhanced platelet aggregation (Kusumi *et al.*, 1991).

The few studies that have examined depression as a risk factor of mortality over the period from 15 months to two years in patients with stroke found a significant association of mortality with either depression prior to stroke or depression during the first weeks after stroke (Morris *et al.*, 1993; Everson *et al.*, 1998).

Psychiatric antecedents and psychosocial factors

It is important to have an understanding of the patient baseline characteristics, particularly with regard to a previous history of depression, in order to ensure that evidence of a current disorder represents a meaningful change from a premorbid level of function. The process of adjustment to serious physical illness can be understood in terms of personal vulnerability, low self-esteem, conflict within close relationships, and negative experiences in the developmental history. Acting on this vulnerability are stressful life events (e.g. illness or stroke). In this perspective, it is understandable that physical illness could dramatically precipitate a preexisting psychiatric condition (Morris and Raphael, 1987) or allow a genetic trait for mood disorders to emerge. Particular personality traits and especially neuroticism are also possible factor risks for PSD (Aben *et al.*, 2002).

An increased incidence of personal or familial history of psychiatric disorders in patients with PSD suggests the role of a genetic predisposition (Morris *et al.*, 1990).

The quality of social functioning and depression are strongly associated with physical and cognitive recovery after stroke (Morris *et al.*, 1992). An impaired relationship with the patient's spouse or closest other relative prior to the stroke and limited social activities are both associated with depression immediately after stroke and depression at long-term follow-up (Baker, 1993; Robinson *et al.*, 1999).

Other factors to consider are job loss or reduction in job satisfaction, social isolation, financial security, and adequacy of living arrangements. For some authors, the available evidence supports PSD as being consistent with the biopsychosocial models of mental illness (Whyte and Mulsant, 2002).

Treatment of PSD

Several pharmacological treatments have been proposed for patients with PSD (Table 21.2).

Table 21.2 Drugs used in post-stroke depression

Drug	References
Selective serotonin reuptake inhibitors	
Sertraline	Burns *et al.*, 1999
Fluoxetine	Dam *et al.*, 1996; Stamenkovic *et al.*, 1996; Robinson *et al.*, 2000
Citalopram	Anderson *et al.*, 1995
Paroxetine	Derex *et al.*, 1997
Psychostimulants	
Methylphenidate	Masand *et al.*, 1991; Johnson *et al.*, 1992
Dextroamphetamine	Masand *et al.*, 1991
Tricyclic antidepressants	
Imipramine	Lauritzen *et al.*, 1994
Amitriptyline	
Desipramine	Lauritzen *et al.*, 1994
Amoxapine	
Nortriptyline	Lipsey *et al.*, 1984; Robinson *et al.*, 2000
Monoamine oxidase inhibitors	
Moclobemide	
Other drugs	
Trazodone	
Maprotiline (tetracyclic)	Dam *et al.*, 1996
Mianserin fa	Lauritzen *et al.*, 1994; Palomaki *et al.*, 1999

Tricyclic antidepressants are no longer the first choice (Gustafson *et al.*, 1995), because of the severity and high frequency of adverse effects (orthostatic hypotension, atrioventricular block, delirium or confusion, drowsiness, agitation, life-threatening cardiac arrhythmias, heart block, urinary outlet obstruction, and narrow-angle glaucoma).

The preference is currently given to the selective serotonin reuptake inhibitors (SSRIs), which have been shown to be more effective than placebo and tricyclic drugs and to have fewer side-effects. The side-effects of SSRIs are similar in frequency and expression in patients with PSD and endogenous depression. They are rare and consist of gastrointestinal effects (particularly nausea), headache, agitation, anxiety, and insomnia. Fluoxetine-induced mania has been described in patients with stroke (Berthier and Kulisevsky, 1993).

Fluoxetine, nortriptiline, and sertraline are among the more commonly employed SSRI. Fluoxetine may not be the first choice if a rapid onset is required, as steady-state concentrations are not reached until after four or five weeks. By comparison, sertraline requires less than one week (Edwards and Anderson, 1999). The advantages of Fluoxetine could be the long half-life, which may allow less-frequent administration in non-compliant patients and result in less-severe discontinuation effects. Sertraline seems to be more efficacious in the treatment of emotionalism and is better tolerated than Fluoxetine, with minor probability of agitation, weight loss, and dermatological adverse effects, and fewer interactions with drugs influencing P450 enzymes.

A recent study comparing combinations of drugs with either noradrenergic effects (desipramine plus mianserin) or noradrenergic and serotonergic effects (imipramine plus mianserin) indicated that drugs with the dual effect may be more effective (Lauritzen et al., 1994).

Some studies have demonstrated that improvement of mood disorders by SSRIs can also enhance recovery of neurological function and that this effect can be quite large (30% recovery; van der Weg et al., 1999). Nevertheless, a close relationship between appropriate early treatment and recovery has not emerged in all studies (Palomaki et al., 1999; Robinson et al., 2000).

Prophylactic treatment for depression in all patients with first-ever stroke may not affect the outcome (Palomaki et al., 1999).

Finally, a placebo effect may also account for therapeutic response in trials of antidepressants (Enserink, 1999). Spontaneous remissions might be frequent in the immediate period following stroke in minor depression and after a longer interval (one or two years) in major depression (Parikh et al., 1987). At present the natural course of PSD and the effect of pharmacological therapy remain partly undetermined.

The use of psychostimulant drugs seems an interesting alternative to SSRIs; their beneficial effects are probably a result of their capacity to overcome the fatigue and apathy components of depression. Unfortunately, adverse reactions necessitating the interruption of drugs of this class are not rare, including adrenergic-like symptoms (tachycardia and hypertension).

Cognitive–behavior therapy may be an appropriate and alternative treatment for PSD (Baker, 1993; Nichol et al., 2002).

Conclusion

PSD is an ever-present and often unrecognized problem after stroke, with multiple dimensions including both psychodynamic and organic causes and with a great impact on stroke outcome. The estimation of the PSD rates must be considered carefully because of the different methods used for diagnosis and the possibility of several subtypes.

There is no definite consensus on the link between PSD and regional brain dysfunction. Lesion location in other neurological diseases with a depressive syndrome similar to PSD, low incidence of PSD with vertebrobasilar stroke, and the specific neuropsychological PSD profile (executive functions and recall deficits) suggest a role for frontosubcortical, temporolimbic and basal ganglia areas.

Finally, although depression is an frequent consequence of stroke, it is diagnosed and treated in only a minority of patients. The SSRI drugs seem to be both safe and effective in the treatment of PSD.

Post-stroke fatigue

The first issue related to fatigue as a symptom or a disease is its definition. Although there is a popular consensus about the meaning of this term and phenomenon, the vagueness that surrounds the concept makes difficult any operational definition.

The first and most obvious distinction is between the objective and subjective dimensions of fatigue. Objective fatigue corresponds to the observable and measurable decrement in performance occurring with the repetition of a physical or mental task, while subjective fatigue is the feeling of early exhaustion, weariness, and aversion to effort.

It can also be useful to distinguish between the fatigue that develops in connection with activities requiring a sustained effort (fatigability) and the fatigue that occurs as a primary state, which is closer to a lack of initiative owing to an imbalance between motivation (preserved) and effectiveness (decreased).

It is also possible to divide the concept of fatigue into various subtypes: "physical" fatigue occurring after muscular exertion, "somatic" fatigue related to the occurrence of a medical illness, "mental" fatigue appearing with cognitively demanding tasks or with the presence of neuropsychological disorders, and "psychological" fatigue associated with lack of interest, poor motivation, or depressive ruminations and themes.

These subtypes of fatigue, which are not mutually exclusive, can be revealed at a behavioral level (corresponding to the objective fatigue) or at a psychological level (corresponding to the subjective fatigue).

Fatigue is a very common complaint in clinical practice, the feeling of fatigue being the usual symptom reported, often dissociated of an objective component.

There are only a few studies on PSF (Leegaard, 1983; van Zandvoort et al., 1998; Ingles et al., 1999; van der Werf et al., 2001; Glader et al., 2002) By comparison, among other brain disorders, the cooccurrence of fatigue with multiple sclerosis has been the object of a great number of investigations. Some studies have also evaluated the association of fatigue with Parkinson's disease, post-polio syndrome, immune-mediated polyneuropathies, systemic lupus erythematosus, Lyme disease, and amyotrophic lateral sclerosis.

In clinical practice, many neurologists have observed that stroke patients frequently complain of a disabling fatigue, which is, in some cases, the only significant sequela from the stroke. Nevertheless, this complaint is often neglected (probably because fatigue is an evil of our modern society) or included in the problematic of PSD.

In our experience, it is patients with good recovery who appear to be the most disabled by the presence of fatigue. The explanation is probably that individuals with severe cognitive and neurological impairment experience fatigue as a "minor" symptom compared with others. Furthermore, patients with major disability are generally partially or completely dependent and so are not being confronted with the demands of an active social and professional life.

Fatigue assessment

The causes leading to a fatigue syndrome after stroke could be varied. Neuropsychological deficits could generate mental fatigue, not only because of the increase in cognitive demands but also because they force the subject to produce additional mental effort to match prior performances. Even with apparent total recovery in standardized psychometric assessment, performing at the former level may be possible only at higher psychophysiological costs. Furthermore, the necessity to accept neurological and cognitive deficits as well as the attempt to mask or overcome deficits can lead to psychological stress, anxiety, and sadness, with subsequent "psychological" fatigue. Stroke patients also experience physical fatigue owing to the presence of motor disability and vegetative symptoms. In addition, post-stroke sleep disturbances have to be considered, since they may cause somnolence and fatigue (Mohsenin and Valor, 1995; Blanco et al., 1999).

For the clinician neurologist, neuropsychologist, psychiatrist, and geriatrician, the main consideration is to access the size of the subjective component of fatigue. The development of an evaluative instrument is not an easy matter; first, the feeling of fatigue is a complex disorder with multimodal components (motor perceptive, emotional, and cognitive); second, fatigue is poorly correlated with objective measures and assessments mostly rely on the psychological attributes of the experience. A variety of self-reported instruments have been developed to measure fatigue as a feeling state. Some have been created for specific disorders (Schwartz et al., 1993; Fisk et al., 1994); others have more general applications and are included in a less-specific health inquiry. Some questionnaires assess a general condition of fatigue (Lee et al., 1991); others assess more selectively the mental (Bentall et al., 1993) or physical dimensions of fatigue, while still others are more comprehensive (Schwartz et al.,1993; Fisk et al., 1994). At present, there are no validated scales for a specific evaluation of PSF.

The distinction between fatigue and depression, and other related phenomena

The feeling of fatigue is often described using related terms, such as asthenia, apathy, weariness, lassitude, abulia, exhaustion, boredom, or lack of energy. This diversity illustrates well the variety of phenomena commonly included, sometimes inappropriately, under the heading of fatigue. It is therefore essential to clarify the field of the subjective fatigue and to distinguish it from distinct, although closely related, phenomena such as depression and abulia. The overlap between fatigue and depression is undeniable, and the presence of fatigue constitutes one of the main diagnostic criteria for depression in most standardized scales for assessment of depression. Nevertheless, fatigue can also occur in the absence of depression, a dissociation that has been already highlighted for patients with Parkinson's disease (Friedman and Friedman, 1993) and multiple sclerosis (Vercoulen et al., 1996; van der Werf et al., 1998). This dissociation is similarly valid for stroke patients (Ingles et al., 1999; van der Werf et al., 2001). Van der Werf et al. (2001) found that only 38% of patients with severe fatigue after stroke were depressed. Clinicians must be aware of this dissociation: fatigue syndrome can develop independently of depression, even in the absence of obvious neurological or cognitive impairment, and the distinction between fatigue, depression, and abulia should be considered. Apathy, anhedonia (severe reduction of initiative), and emotional flatness are the hallmarks of the abulic states but they can be differentiated from PSF or PSD.

As previously reported, sleep disturbances could also contribute to the development of PSF. Insomnia, hypersomnia, and obstructive apnea have been frequently reported after stroke and they manifest, on clinical grounds, with diurnal fatigue (Mohsenin and Valor, 1995; Blanco et al., 1999). Fatigue induced by concomitant sleep disorders is usually characterized by diurnal somnolence rather than loss of drive, but this distinction may be particularly difficult on clinical grounds.

Current data about post-stroke fatigue

Ingles et al. (1999) studied PSF in 88 subjects with a first acute stroke. Fatigue, defined as a feeling of physical tiredness and lack of energy, was assessed through a self-report, specifically assessing the PSF impact on daily cognitive, physical, and psychosocial functioning. Depression was similarly evaluated with a self-report. The authors found that fatigue was significantly more common in patients (68%) than in healthy elderly controls (36%). Stroke-related features, such as infarct type, severity of neurological, and functional impairment, and lesion location, did not seem to be independent predictors of fatigue. This study demonstrated that fatigue affected functional abilities, especially in physical and psychosocial domains, often independently from depression. As many as 40% of patients considered that fatigue was the worst, or one of the worst sequelae of stroke.

Leegaard (1983) examined 44 survivors of cerebral infarction below the age of 70 years, fully active, and in good health at the time of stroke. All patients were autonomous for walking and able to manage activities at home, and only 17 had neurological deficits. Between 6 and 26 months after stroke, patients were questioned about 13 general symptoms, including fatigue, emotional lability, forgetfulness, and concentration difficulties. These complaints, which were taken into account only if they had started after the vascular episode, were present in 93% of patients (mainly fatigue, impaired concentration, emotional instability, irritability, and depression). More than the half of them reported at least 5 of the 13 symptoms, fatigue being particularly frequent. No association was found with the site or size of lesion, and symptoms were not significantly related to cognitive impairment or neurological deficits. Since some of these complaints could sometimes be found in survivors of myocardial infarction, the author suggested that fatigue was a psychological stress response syndrome resulting from inadequate "coping" with the consequences of a medical disorder.

Van Zandvoort et al. (1998) studied fatigue, defined as a decreased capacity for mental effort, with detailed psychometric assessment but also considering the patients' performances in everyday life activities. The study population comprised 16 patients examined at 6 to 45 months after a single supratentorial lacunar or small infarction and 16 healthy controls matched for age and gender. The authors selected this population because lacunar or small subcortical strokes do not usually lead to cognitive dysfunction. The quality of life of these patients was often less favorable than expected. They commonly complained of fatigue and of "being different from before stroke," despite good functional recovery. Although globally "normal," the patients' performances in testing were inferior to controls in 6 of 17 neuropsychological tests, the ones with more attentional demands, independently from the specific cognitive domain of the test. Subtle attentional deficits seemed to be the main determinants of fatigue, reflecting a problem of performance rather than competence, because stroke patients appeared to be required to provide additional mental efforts to that needed by control subjects.

Van der Werf et al. (2001) examined the possible associations of experienced fatigue with both depression and physical impairment using questionnaires mailed to 138 outpatients with clinical diagnosis of stroke at least one year earlier. A group of 90 patients and 50 controls completed the Checklist Individual Strength for physical fatigue assessment and the Beck Depression Inventory for Primary Care. General disability was measured with the Sickness Impact Scale, the different subscales providing a measure of functional impairments in home management, mobility, alertness, sleep/rest, ambulation, social interactions, and recreation/pastimes. The authors found that persistent and severe fatigue was experienced by a significantly larger proportion of the respondents with stroke

(51%) than by controls (16%). Depressive symptoms did not correlate with levels in experienced fatigue in the stroke group whereas they explained most of the variance in fatigue in the control group. Impairment of locomotion was the better predictor of fatigue severity for stroke patients.

Finally, Glader *et al.* (2002) tried to estimate the prevalence of PSF among long-term survivors after stroke and to determine its impact on survival and daily living. Mailed questionnaires, including items on the patient's self-perceived fatigue, depression, and anxiety, were sent to more than 5000 patients, two years after stroke. After excluding patients who responded that they always felt depressed, the authors found that nearly 40% of the remaining patients complained of fatigue (10% reporting they always felt tired and 29.2% they often felt tired). Fatigue was an independent predictor for institutionalization and for a reduced autonomy in daily-living activities. Furthermore, fatigue had a negative impact on survival.

The principal message from these studies is that fatigue is a frequent and potentially invaliding post-stroke sequelae. Just like depression, it can have a negative influence on functional outcomes, daily living, and survival. Although fatigue is often associated with depression, it is important to emphasize that it can also occur independently. Finally, PSF is a complex phenomenon with predictors that are difficult to evaluate. In the studies published so far, no clear risk factors emerge as determinant for developing PSF, apart from depression. It is interesting that stroke characteristics, and particularly the side and site of infarct, do not seem to have relevant influence.

Fatigue and stroke location

Contrary to the results of the studies described in the previous paragraphs, our group found some interesting data concerning potential links between PSF and stroke location (Staub *et al.*, 2000, 2002). We are currently conducting a three-year longitudinal prospective study (The Lausanne Post-stroke Fatigue Study) on a study population with a first-ever acute "non-disabling" stroke (that means a NIH stroke scale smaller or equal to 6 at discharge and/or smaller or equal to 3 at six months). At the six-month follow-up, each patient underwent a neurological and psychiatric assessment together with an evaluation of fatigue. Patients with a standard diagnosis of depression were excluded in order to focus on subjects with "pure" fatigue. We found that patients with lesions involving the cortex had higher fatigue severity scores, fatigue being often associated with specific cognitive disorders. The term "task-specific" fatigue was chosen to refer to this kind of fatigue, the typical example being a subject with residual aphasia who develops mental fatigue when speaking for a certain time. The group of patients with brainstem strokes had similar fatigue severity scores whereas subjects with subcortical or cerebelar lesions had lower scores. Patients with brainstem strokes appear interesting because they *a priori* do not have relevant cognitive dysfunction. We think that they may be particularly at risk to develop the condition we called "primary" PSF. We hypothesize that primary PSF is the result of subtle attentional deficits in association with specific damage to the reticular formation and other cortex-activating systems.

Future developments

Until now, the study of PSF has been almost completely neglected in clinical follow-up series, and there are many questions that have not been answered, or even asked (Staub and Bogousslavsky, 2001). Further longitudinal prospective studies are needed to understand the pre-, per-, and post-stroke characteristics that are associated with the development of PSF, as well as its relationships with depression, post-stroke neurological and neuropsychological sequelae, psychological and social factors, and sleep disorders. It appears obvious to us that there are different types of PSF. The challenge is to identify, delineate, and distinguish from changes related to mood disorders, which frequently coexist. We emphasize the concept of primary PSF, which may develop in the absence of depression or significant cognitive impairment, and which may be linked to specific damage to the reticular activating system participating in the functioning of the neural attentional network. If primary PSF exists, another challenge is establishing a pathophysiological model, such as the brain fatigue model developed by Bruno *et al.* (1998). These authors recently postulated that viral damage (in chronic fatigue syndromes after polio and other viral infections) to reticular formation, lenticular, hypothalamic, and thalamic nuclei, cortical motor areas, and, particularly, dopaminergic neurons in the substantia nigra was responsible for the development of a feeling of fatigue, exhaustion, and aversion to effort, mediated by a decrement in cortical activation, with attentional impairment, slowing of information-processing, and motor activity inhibition.

Summary

PSF has been misleadingly regarded as a mere component of PSD. It is now established that these two phenomena could develop independently even if they are often strongly correlated. As well as PSD, PSF may be a frequent and disabling sequela of stroke. Its study is complex, first, because of difficulties in producing an operational definition; second, because of the lack of objective tools to measure it; third, because of the diversity of its manifestations; and, finally, because of our ignorance of the underlying neurobiological mechanisms. In patients with excellent neurological and neuropsychological recovery, PSF may be the only persisting sequela, which may severely limit return to previous activities. For these reasons, recognition of PSF may be critical during recovery and rehabilitation after stroke.

Further studies are needed to understand the clinical and biological pathophysiology of PSF. This could lead to the treatment of PSF, which is, to date, only experimental and anecdotal.

REFERENCES

Aben, I., Denollet, J., Lousberg, R., *et al.* (2002). Personality and vunerability to depression in stroke patients: a 1-year prospective follow-up study. *Stroke* **33**: 2391–2395.

American Psychiatric Association (1994). *DSM-IV: Diagnostic and Statistical Manual of Mental Disorders,* 4th edn, revised. Washington, DC: American Psychiatric Press.

Andersen, G., Vestergaard, K., and Lauritzen, L. U. (1995). Effective treatment of depression following apoplexy with citalopram. *Ugeskr Laeg* **157**: 2000–2003.

Andersen, G., Vestergaard, K., Riis, J. O., and Ingeman-Nielsen, M. (1996). Dementia of depression or depression of dementia in stroke? *Acta Psychiatr Scand* **94**: 272–278.

Angeleri, F., Angeleri, V. A, Foschi, N., *et al.* (1997). Depression after stroke: an investigation through catamnesis. *J Clin Psychiatry* **58**: 261–265.

Astrom, M., Adolfsson, R., and Asplund, K. (1993). Major depression in stroke patients. A 3-year longitudinal study. *Stroke* **24**: 976–982.

Auer, D. P., Putz, B., Kraft, E., *et al.* (2000). Reduced glutamate in the anterior cingulate cortex in depression: an *in vivo* proton magnetic resonance spectroscopy study. *Biol Psychiatry* **47**: 305–313.

Baker, A. C. (1993). The spouse's positive effect on the stroke patient's recovery. *Rehabil Nurs* **18**: 30–33.

Ballard, C., Mckeith, I., O'Brien, J., *et al.* (2000). Neuropathological substrates of dementia and depression in vascular dementia, with a particular focus on cases with small infarct volumes. *Dement Geriatr Cogn Disord* **11**: 59–65.

Beblo, T., Wallesch, C. W., and Herrmann, M. (1999). The crucial role of frontostriatal circuits for depressive disorders in the post-acute stage after stroke. *Neuropsychiatry Neuropsychol Behav Neurol* **12**: 236–246.

Bentall, R. P., Wood, G. C., Marrinan, T., Deans, C., and Edwards, R. H. (1993). A brief mental fatigue questionnaire. *Br J Clin Psychol* **32**: 375–379.

Berg, A., Palomaki, H., Lehtihalmes, M., Lonnqvist, J., and Kaste, M. (2003). Post-stroke depression: an 18-month follow-up. *Stroke* **34**: 138–143.

Berthier, M. L. and Kulisevsky, J. (1993). Fluoxetine-induced mania in a patient with post-stroke depression. *Br J Psychiatry* **163**: 698–699.

Blanco, M., Espinosa, M., Arpa, J., Barreiro, P., and Rodriguez-Albarino, A. (1999). Hypersomnia and thalamic and brain stem stroke: a study of seven patients. *Neurologia* **14**: 307–314.

Bokura, H. and Robinson, R. G. (1997). Long-term cognitive impairment associated with caudate stroke. *Stroke* **28**: 970–975.

Bolla-Wilson, K., Robinson, R. G., Starkstein, S. E., Boston, J., and Price, T. R. (1989). Lateralization of dementia of depression in stroke patients. *Am J Psychiatry* **146**: 627–634.

Bremner, J. D., Narayan, M., Anderson, E. R., *et al.* (2000). Hippocampal volume reduction in major depression. *Am J Psychiatry* **157**: 115–118.

Bruno, R. L., Creange, S. J., and Frick, N. M. (1998). Parallels between post-polio fatigue and chronic fatigue syndrome: a common pathophysiology? *Am J Med* **105**(Suppl.1): 66–73.

Burns, A., Russell, E., Stratton-Powell, H., *et al.* (1999). Sertraline in stroke-associated lability of mood. *Int J Geriatr Psychiatry* **14**: 681–685.

Burvill, P. W., Johnson, G. A., Jamrozik, K. D., *et al.* (1995). Prevalence of depression after stroke: the Perth Community Stroke Study. *Br J Psychiatry* **166**: 320–327.

Burvill, P., Johnson, G., Jamrozik, K., Anderson, C., and Stewart-Wynne, E. (1997). Risk factors for post-stroke depression. *Int J Geriatr Psychiatry* **12**: 219–226.

Carson, A. J., Machale, S., Allen, K., *et al.* (2000). Depression after stroke and lesion location: a systematic review. *Lancet* **356**: 122–126.

Carter, C. S., Botvinick, N. M., and Cohen, J. D. (1999). The contribution of the anterior cingulate cortex to executive processes in cognition. *Rev Neurosci* **10**: 49–57.

Chang, A. M. and Mackenzie, A. E. (1998). State self-esteem following stroke. *Stroke* **29**: 2325–2328.

Dam, H., Pedersen, H. E., and Ahlgren, P. (1989). Depression among patients with stroke. *Acta Psychiatr Scand* **80**: 118–124.

Dam, M., Tonin, P., Deboni, A., *et al.* (1996). Effects of fluoxetine and maprotiline on functional recovery in post-stroke hemiplegic patients undergoing rehabilitation therapy. *Stroke* **27**: 1211–1214.

Derex, L., Ostrowsky, K., Nighoghossian, N., and Trouillas, P. (1997). Severe pathological crying after left anterior choroidal artery infarct. Reversibility with paroxetine treatment. *Stroke* **28**: 1464–1466.

Devinsky, O., Morrell, M. J., and Vogt, B. A. (1995). Contributions of anterior cingulate cortex to behavior. *Brain* **118**: 279–306.

Eastwood, M. R., Rifat, S. L., Nobbs, H., and Ruderman, J. (1989). Mood disorder following cerebrovascular accident. *Br J Psychiatry* **154**: 195–200.

Ebrahim, S., Barer, D., and Nouri, F. (1987). Affective illness after stroke. *Br J Psychiatry* **151**: 52–56.

Edwards, J. G. and Anderson, I. (1999). Systematic review and guide to selection of selective serotonin reuptake inhibitors. *Drugs* **57**: 507–533. [Published erratum in *Drugs* (1999). **58**: 1207–1209.]

Enserink, M. (1999). Can the placebo be the cure? *Science* **284**: 238–240.

Everson, S. A., Roberts, R. E., Goldberg, D. E., and Kaplan, G. A. (1998). Depressive symptoms and increased risk of stroke mortality over a 29-year period. *Arch Intern Med* **158**: 1133–1138.

Feibel, J. H. and Springer, C. J. (1982). Depression and failure to resume social activities after stroke. *Arch Phys Med Rehabil* **63**: 276–277.

Finklestein, S., Benowitz, L. I., Baldessarini, R. J., *et al.* (1982). Mood, vegetative disturbance, and dexamethasone suppression test after stroke. *Ann Neurol* **12**: 463–468.

Finset, A., Goffeng, L., Landro, N. I., and Haakonsen, M. (1989). Depressed mood and intra-hemispheric location of lesion in right hemisphere stroke patients. *Scand J Rehabil Med* **21**: 1–6.

Fisk, J. D., Ritvo, P. G., Ross, L., *et al.* (1994). Measuring the functional impact of fatigue: initial validation of the fatigue impact scale. *Clin Infect Dis* **21**: 9–14.

Friedman, J. and Friedman, H. (1993). Fatigue in Parkinson's disease. *Neurology* **43**: 2016–2019.

Gainotti, G., Antonucci, G., Marra, C., and Paolucci, S. (2001). Relation between depression after stroke, antidepressant therapy, and functional recovery. *J Neurol Neurosurg Psychiatry* **71**: 258–261.

Glader, E. L., Stegmayr, B., and Asplund, K. (2002). Post-stroke fatigue: a 2-year follow-up study of stroke patients in Sweden. *Stroke* **33**: 1327–1333.

Goodwin, G. M. (1997). Neuropsychological and neuroimaging evidence for the involvement of the frontal lobes in depression. *J Psychopharmacol* **11**: 115–122.

Gordon, W. A. and Hibbard, M. R. (1997). PSD: an examination of the literature. *Arch Phys Med Rehabil* **78**: 658–663.

Greenwald, B. S., Kramer-Ginsberg, E., Krishnan, K. R., *et al.* (1998). Neuroanatomic localization of magnetic resonance imaging signal hyperintensities in geriatric depression. *Stroke* **29**: 613–617.

Gustafson, Y., Nilsson, I., Mattsson, M., Astrom, M., and Bucht, G. (1995). Epidemiology and treatment of post-stroke depression. *Drugs Aging* **7**: 298–309.

Hermann, N., Black, S. E., Lawrence, J., Szekely, C., and Szalai, J. P. (1998). The Sunnybrook stroke study: a prospective study of depressive symptoms and functional outcome. *Stroke* **29**: 618–624.

Hippisley-Cox, J., Fielding, K., and Pringle, M. (1998). Depression as a risk factor for ischaemic heart disease in men: population based case–control study. *BMJ* **316**: 1714–1719 [Published erratum in *BMJ* 1998 Jul 18; **317**(7152): 185] [see (1998). **317**: 185.]

House, A., Dennis, M., Warlow, C., Hawton, K., and Molyneux, A. (1990a). The relationship between intellectual impairment and mood disorder in the first year after stroke. *Psychol Med* **20**: 805–814.

(1990b). Mood disorders after stroke and their relation to lesion location. A CT scan study. *Brain* **113**: 1113–1129.

Ingles, J. L., Eskes, G. A., and Phillips, S. J. (1999). Fatigue after stroke. *Arch Phys Med Rehabil* **80**: 173–178.

Johnson, M. L., Roberts, M. D., Ross, A. R., and Witten, C. M. (1992). Methylphenidate in stroke patients with depression. *Am J Phys Med Rehabil* **71**: 239–241.

Jonas, B. S., Franks, P., and Ingram, D. D. (1997). Are symptoms of anxiety and depression risk factors for hypertension? Longitudinal evidence from the National Health and Nutrition Examination Survey I Epidemiologic Follow-up Study. *Arch Fam Med* **6**: 43–49.

Kase, C. S., Wolf, P. A., Kelly-Hayes, M., *et al.* (1998). Intellectual decline after stroke: the Framlingham Study. *Stroke* **29**: 805–812.

Kauhanen, M., Korpelainen, J. T., Hiltunen, P., *et al.* (1999). Post-stroke depression correlates with cognitive impairment and neurological deficits. *Stroke* **30**: 1875–1880.

Kim, J. S. and Choi-Kwon, S. (2000). Post-stroke depression and emotional incontinence: correlation with lesion location. *Neurology* **54**: 1805–1810.

Kimura, M., Robinson, R. G., and Kosier, J. T. (2000). Treatment of cognitive impairment after post-stroke depression: a double-bind treatment trial. *Stroke* **31**: 1482–1486.

Kotila, M., Numminen, H., Waltimo, O., and Kaste, M. (1998). Depression after stroke: results of the Finn Stroke Study. *Stroke* **29**: 368–372.

(1999). Post-stroke depression and functional recovery in a population-based stroke register. The Finn Stroke Study. *Eur J Neurol* **6**: 309–312.

Kramer, T. and Garralda, M. E. (1998). Psychiatric disorders in adolescents in primary care. *Br J Psychiatry* **173**: 508–513.

Kusumi, I., Koyama, T., and Yamashita, I. (1991). Serotonin-stimulated Ca^{2+} response is increased in the blood platelets of depressed patients. *Biol Psychiatry* **30**: 310–312.

Lai, T., Payne, M. E., Byrum, C. E., Steffens, D. C., and Krishnan, K. R. (2000). Reduction of orbital frontal cortex volume in geriatric depression. *Biol Psychiatry* **48**: 971–975.

Lauritzen, L., Bendsen, B. B., Vilmar, T., *et al.* (1994). Post-stroke depression: combined treatment with imipramine or desipramine and mianserin. A controlled clinical study. *Psychopharmacology (Berl)* **114**: 119–122.

Lauterbach, E. C., Jackson, J. G., Wilson, A. N., Dever, G. E., and Kirsh, A. D. (1997). Major depression after left posterior globus pallidus lesions. *Neuropsychiatry Neuropsychol Behav Neurol* **10**: 9–16.

Lee, K. A., Hicks, G., and Nino-Murcia, G. (1991). Validity and reliability of a scale to assess fatigue. *Psychiatry Res* **36**: 291–298.

Leegaard, O. F. (1983). Diffuse cerebral symptoms in convalescents from cerebral infarction and myocardial infarction. *Acta Neurol Scand* **67**: 348–355.

Lieberman, D., Friger, M., Fried, V., *et al.* (1999). Characterization of elderly patients in rehabilitation: stroke versus hip fracture. *Disabil Rehabil* **21**: 542–547.

Lipsey, J. R., Robinson, R. G., Pearlson, G. D., Rao, K., and Price, T. R. (1984). Nortriptyline treatment of post-stroke depression: a double-blind study. *Lancet* **i**: 297–300.

Lipsey, J. R., Spencer, W. C., Rabins, P. V., and Robinson, R. G. (1986). Phenomenological comparison of post-stroke depression and functional depression. *Am J Psychiatry* **143**: 527–529.

Machale, S. M., O'Rourke, S. J., Wardlaw, J. M., and Dennis, M. S. (1998). Depression and its relation to lesion location after stroke. *J Neurol Neurosurg Psychiatry* **64**: 371–374.

Malec, J. F., Richardson, J. W., Sinaki, M., and O'Brien, M. W. (1990). Types of affective response to stroke. *Arch Phys Med Rehabil* **71**: 279–284.

Masand, P., Murray, G. B., and Pickett, P. (1991). Psychostimulants in post-stroke depression. *J Neuropsychiatry Clin Neurosci* **3**: 23–27.

Merriam, E. P., Thase, M. E., Haas, G. L., Keshavan, M. S., and Sweeney, J. A. (1999). Prefrontal cortical dysfunction in depression determined by Wisconsin Card Sorting Test performance. *Am J Psychiatry* **156**: 780–782.

Mervaala, E., Fohr, J., Kononen, M., *et al.* (2000). Quantitative MRI of the hippocampus and amygdala in severe depression. *Psychol Med* **30**: 117–125.

Mohsenin, V. and Valor, R. (1995). Sleep apnea in patients with hemispheric stroke. *Arch Phys Med Rehabil* **76**: 71–76.

Moresco, R. M., Colombo, C., Fazio, F., *et al.* (2000). Effects of fluvoxamine treatment on the in vivo binding of [F-18] FESP in drug naive depressed patients: a PET study. *Neuroimagery* **12**: 452–465.

Morris, P. L. and Raphael, B. (1987). Depressive disorder associated with physical illness. The impact of stroke. *Gen Hosp Psychiatry* **9**: 324–330.

Morris, P. L., Robinson, R. G, and Raphael, B. (1990). Prevalence and course of depressive disorders in hospitalized stroke patients. *Int J Psychiatry Med* **20**: 349–364.

Morris, P. L., Robinson, R. G., Raphael, B., Samuels, J., and Molloy, P. (1992). The relationship between risk factors for affective disorder and post-stroke depression in hospitalised stroke patients. *Aust N Z J Psychiatry* **26**: 208–217.

Morris, P. L., Robinson, R. G., Andrzejewski, P., Samuels, J., and Price, T. R. (1993). Association of depression with 10-year post-stroke mortality. *Am J Psychiatry* **150**: 124–129.

Neau, J. P, Ingrand, P, Mouille-Brachet, C., *et al.* (1998). Functional recovery and social outcome after cerebral infarction in young adults. *Cerebrovasc Dis* **8**: 296–302.

Nicholl, C. R., Lincoln, N. B., Muncaster, K., and Thomas, S. (2002). Cognitions and post-stroke depression. *Br J Clin Psychol* **41**: 221–231.

Ongur, D., and Price, J. L. (2000). The organization of networks within the orbital and medial prefrontal cortex of rats, monkeys and humans. *Cereb Cortex* **10**: 206–219.

Palomaki, H., Kaste, M., Berg, A., *et al.* (1999). Prevention of post-stroke depression: 1 year randomised placebo controlled double blind trial of mianserin with 6 month follow up after therapy. *J Neurol Neurosurg Psychiatry* **66**: 490–494.

Pantel, J., Schroder, J., Essig, M., *et al.* (1998). Volumetric brain findings in late depression. A study with quantified magnetic resonance tomography. *Nervenarzt* **69**: 968–974.

Paolucci, S., Antonucci, G., Pratesi, L., *et al.* (1999). Post-stroke depression and its role in rehabilitation of inpatients. *Arch Phys Med Rehabil* **80**: 985–990.

Paolucci, S., Antonucci, G., Grasso, M. G., *et al.* (2001). Post-stroke depression, antidepressant treatment and rehabilitation results. A case–control study. *Cerebrovasc Dis* **12**: 264–271.

Paradiso, S. and Robinson, R. G. (1998). Gender differences in post-stroke depression. *J Neuropsychiatry Clin Neurosci* **10**: 41–47.

(1999). Minor depression after stroke: an initial validation of the DSM-IV construct. *Ame J Geriatr Psychiatry* **7**: 244–251.

Parashos, I. A., Tupler, L. A., Blitchington, T., and Krishnan, K. R. (1998). Magnetic-resonance morphometry in patients with major depression. *Psychiatry Res* **84**: 7–15.

Parikh, R. M., Lipsey, J. R., Robinson, R. G., and Price, T. R. (1987). Two-year longitudinal study of post-stroke mood disorders: dynamic changes in correlates of depression at one and two years. *Stroke* **18**: 579–584.

Paus, T. (2001). Primae anterior cingulate cortex: where motor control, drive and cognition interface. *Nat Rev Neurosci* **2**: 417–424.

Pearlson, G. D. and Robinson, R. G. (1981). Suction lesions of the frontal cerebral cortex in the rat induce asymmetrical behavioral and catecholaminergic responses. *Brain Res* **218**: 233–242.

Pohjasvaara, T., Leppavuori, A., Siira, I., *et al.* (1998). Frequency and clinical determinants of post-stroke depression. *Stroke* **29**: 2311–2317.

Pohjasvaara, T., Mantyla, R., Aronen, H. J., *et al.* (1999). Clinical and radiological determinants of prestroke cognitive decline in a stroke cohort. *J Neurol Neurosurg Psychiatry* **67**: 742–748.

Rabins, P. V., Pearlson, G. D., Aylward, E., Kumar, A. J., and Dowell, K. (1991). Cortical magnetic resonance imaging changes in elderly inpatients with major depression. *Am J Psychiatry* **148**: 617–620.

Reding, M. J., Orto, L. A., Winter, S. W., *et al.* (1986). Antidepressant therapy after stroke. A double-blind trial. *Archives of Neurology* **43**: 763–765.

Robertson J. T. (1998). *The Clinical Neuropsychiatry of Stroke.* New York: Cambridge University Press.

Robinson, R. G. and Stitt, T. G. (1981). Intracortical 6-hydroxydopamine induced an asymmetrical behavioral response in the rat. *Brain Res* **213**: 387–395.

Robinson, R. G., Starr, L. B., Kubos, K. L., and Price, T. R. (1983). A two-year longitudinal study of post-stroke mood disorders: findings during the initial evaluation. *Stroke* **14**: 736–741.

Robinson, R. G., Murata, Y., and Shimoda, K. (1999). Dimensions of social impairment and their effect on depression and recovery following stroke. *Int Psychogeriatr* **11**: 375–384.

Robinson, R. G., Schultz, S. K., Castillo, C., *et al.* (2000). Nortriptyline versus fluoxetine in the treatment of depression and in short-term recovery after stroke: a placebo-controlled, double-blind study. *Am J Psychiatry* **157**: 351–359.

Sato, R., Bryan, R. N., and Fried, L. P. (1999). Neuroanatomic and functional correlates of depressed mood: the Cardiovascular Health Study. *Am J Epidemiol* **150**: 919–929.

Schwartz, J. A., Speed, N. M., Brunberg, J. A., *et al.* (1993). Depression in stroke rehabilitation. *Biol Psychiatry* **33**: 694–699.

Singh, A., Black, S. E., Herrmann, N., *et al.* (2000). Functional and neuroanatomic correlations in post-stroke depression: the Sunnybrook Stroke Study. *Stroke* **31**: 637–644.

Stamenkovic, M., Schindler, S., and Kasper, S. (1996). Post-stroke depression and fluoxetine. *Am J Psychiatry* **153**: 446–447.

Staub, F. and Bogousslavsky, J. (2001). Fatigue after stroke: a major but neglected issue. *Cerebrovasc Dis* **12**: 75–81.

Staub, F., Annoni, J. M., and Bogousslavsky, J. (2000). Fatigue after stroke: a pilot study. *Cerebrovasc Dis* **10**: 62.

Staub, F., Annoni, J. M., and Bogousslavsky, J. (2002). Post-stroke fatigue: a major problem in "non-disabling" stroke. *Cerebrovasc Dis* **13**: 96.

Tupler, L. A., Krishnan, K. R., McDonald, W. M., *et al.* (2002). Anatomic location and laterality of MRI signal hyperintensities in late-life depression. *Psychosom Res* **53**: 665–676.

van der Werf, S. P., Jongen, P. J., Lycklama, A., *et al.* (1998). Fatigue in multiple sclerosis: interrelations between fatigue complaints, cerebral MRI abnormalities and neurological disability. *J Neuro Sci* **160**: 164–170.

van der Weg, F. B., Kuik, D. J., and Lankhorst, G. J. (1999). Post-stroke depression and functional outcome: a cohort study investigating the influence of depression on functional recovery from stroke. *Clin Rehabil* **13**: 268–272.

van der Werf, S. P., van den broek, H. L. P., Anten, H. W. M., and Bleijenberg, G. (2001). Experience of severe fatigue long after stroke and its relation to depressive symptoms and disease characteristics. *Eur Neurol* **45**: 28–33.

van Zandvoort, M. J. E., Kappelle, L. J., Algra, A., and de Haan, E. H. F. (1998). Decreased capacity for mental effort after single supratentorial lacunar infarct may affect performance in everyday life. *J Neurol Neurosurg Psychiatry* **65**: 697–702.

Veiel, H. O. (1997). A preliminary profile of neuropsychological deficits associated with major depression. *J Clin Exp Neuropsychol* **19**: 587–603.

Vercoulen, J., Hommes, O. R., Swanink, C., *et al.* (1996). The measurement of fatigue in patients with multiple sclerosis: a multidimensional comparison with patients with chronic fatigue syndrome and healthy subjects. *Arch Neurol* **53**: 642–649.

Wade, D. T., Legh-Smith, J., and Hewer, R. A. (1987). Depressed mood after stroke. A community study of its frequency. *Br J Psychiatry* **151**: 200–205.

Whyte, E. M. and Mulsant, B. H. (2002). Post stroke depression: epidemiology, pathophysiology, and biological treatment. *Bio Psychiatry* **52**: 253–264.

Willeit, M., Praschak-Rieder, N., *et al.* (2000). [123 I]-beta-CIT SPECT imaging shows reduced brain serotanin transporter availability in dmg-free depressed patients with seasonal affective disorder. *Biol Psychiatry* **47**: 482–489.

Yanai, I., Fujikawa, T., Horiguchi, J., Yamawaki, S., and Touhouda, Y. (1998). The 3-year course and outcome of patients with major depression and silent cerebral infarction. *J Affec Disord* **47**: 25–30.

22

Sleep disorders after stroke

Dirk M. Hermann
University Hospital, Zürich, Switzerland

Claudio L. Bassetti
University Hospital, Zürich, Switzerland

Introduction

Sleep disorders are commonly found in the general population. In stroke patients, their frequency is even higher, because brain damage can affect sleep–wake mechanisms and because cerebrovascular and sleep disorders can arise from similar predisposing factors. Sleep disorders often influence negatively general well-being, physical and mental performance, and, as a consequence, rehabilitation and final outcome. In addition, sleep-disordered breathing (SDB) – one of the most common forms of post-stroke sleep disorders – may increase the risk of stroke recurrence. For these reasons, sleep disturbances should be adequately diagnosed and treated after stroke.

Historical remarks

Changes in sleep and breathing were reported in stroke patients as early as in the beginning of the nineteenth century. Cheyne (1818) first described periodic breathing in a patient with cardiac disease and "apoplexy." Jackson later recognized that this breathing pattern frequently accompanies bilateral hemispheric stroke (quoted by Brown and Plum, 1961). Symptoms of obstructive sleep apnea (OSA) were first reported in a patient with intracerebral hemorrhage by Broadbent (1877). In the nineteenth century, it was also already known that stroke may cause profound changes of sleep patterns. Post-stroke hypersomnia was recognized by MacNish as early as 1830 (see Lavie, 1991), but it was only in the beginning of the twentieth century that its preferential association with thalamic and mesencephalic strokes was recognized (Freund, 1913). Neurogenic insomnia (agrypnia) related to thalamomesecephalic stroke was first described by Lhermitte (1922) and van Bogaert (1926). Lhermitte (1922) coined the term peduncular hallucinosis to describe vivid, colorful, and dream-like hallucinations following midbrain

Recovery after Stroke, ed. Michael P. Barnes, Bruce H. Dobkin and Julien Bogousslavsky. Published by Cambridge University Press. © Cambridge University Press 2005.

stroke. Asymmetries of the electroencephalogram (EEG) during sleep, with a reduction of spindle activity over the affected hemisphere, were first reported by Cress and Gibbs (1948). During subsequent decades, other authors described abnormalities in rapid eye movement (REM) and non-REM sleep in patients with supra- and infratentorial strokes. More recently, the link between SDB and vascular disease has been suggested.

Circadian rhythms and stroke

Cerebrovascular events, such as myocardial infarction and sudden death, appear most frequently in the morning hours – between 6 a.m. and noon – and particularly within the first hour after awakening. A meta-analysis of 31 publications with 11 816 patients found a 49% increase in all types of stroke (ischemic, hemorrhagic, transient ischemic attack) during that time of the day compared with other times (Elliott, 1998). Interestingly, one study found a higher frequency of strokes on awakening when strokes were of thrombotic (29%) and lacunar (28%) origin than with those of embolic (19%) origin (Lago et al., 1998). There was no difference in circadian rhythm between first and recurrent stroke. In general, stroke onset appears to be correlated with physical activity, as suggested by a recent study on hypertensive patients (Stergiou et al., 2002). In this study, both blood pressure and heart rate were closely associated with the physical activity level, and all three physiological variables paralleled the incidence pattern of stoke onset, the peaks and minima of these variables being located at about the same times of day.

While intracerebral and subarachnoid hemorrhages rarely occur during the night hours, 20–40% of all ischemic strokes present at night, that is, during sleep (Elliott, 1998; Bassetti and Aldrich, 1999a). This suggests indeed that sleep might represent a vulnerable phase at least for a subset of stroke patients. A recent study assessed patients with stroke onset during sleep and found an association with SDB but not with other factors (Iranzo et al., 2002). This indicates that SDB may trigger stroke in some patients.

Sleep-disordered breathing after stroke

Prevalence

As first shown in the mid 1990s (Bassetti et al.,1996a; Good et al.,1996; Bassetti and Aldrich, 1999a,b) and also confirmed in more recent papers (Parra et al., 2000; Wessendorf et al., 2000a; Iranzo et al., 2002; Harbison et al., 2002; Hui et al., 2002; Turkington et al., 2002), approximately 50–70% of all stroke patients exhibit SDB, as defined by an apnea–hypopnea index (AHI; measuring the number of apneic and hypopneic events per hour) $\geq 10/h$. As many as 40% of patients have an AHI $\geq 25/h$. Although AHI may partially improve from the acute to the subacute phase of cerebrovascular infarction, up to 60% of patients still exhibit an AHI $\geq 10/h$ three months after their stroke event (Parra *et al.*, 2000; Harbison *et al.*, 2002; Hui *et al.*, 2002). Since SDB is associated with transient hypoxemic episodes and rapid blood pressure changes, SDB is suspected to influence stroke outcome and promote the recurrence of further stroke events.

The most common form of SDB in stroke patients is OSA; some patients have Cheyne–Stokes breathing (CSB) or a combination of both OSA and CSB (Bassetti *et al.*, 1997; Bassetti and Aldrich, 1999a). Central hypoventilation and failure of automatic breathing (Ondine's curse) are uncommon.

Sleep disordered breathing can present with a variety of symptoms and signs that are sometimes misinterpreted and attributed to the underlying neurological disorder. Night-time symptoms of SDB include difficulties falling asleep, respiratory noises (snoring, stridor), irregular or periodic respiration, apneas, agitated sleep with increased motor activity and frequent awakenings, sudden awakenings with choking sensations, shortness of breath, palpitations, "panic attacks," orthopnea, and increased sweating. In patients with severe hypoventilation, arousal responses can be suppressed by increasing sleep debt and lead to death during sleep. Daytime symptoms of SDB can be headaches, excessive daytime sleepiness, altered mentation with concentration and memory difficulties, irritability, and depression. Some patients may exhibit also breathing abnormalities during wakefulness including dyspnea, apneas, inspiratory breath holding, irregular breathing, rapid-shallow breathing, CSB, hiccup, and many more. Disturbances of sleep–wake, bulbar (phonation, deglutition, coughing) and cardiovascular functions can also be observed.

In patients with stroke, SDB is often of multifactorial origin. In addition to brain damage per se (see below), pre-existing cardiorespiratory conditions (e.g. OSA and heart failure) and indirect complications of brain damage (e.g. aspiration, lung edema, immobility, respiratory infection) may favor the appearance of SDB.

Brain damage and sleep-disordered breathing

Considering the complexity in anatomy and physiology of breathing control, brain damage would be expected to impair breathing during wakefulness and/or sleep in different ways according to the type, extension, and topography of the lesion (Bassetti and Gugger, 2002). Because of the convergence/overlap in the brainstem of mechanisms controlling respiration and other somatic and vegetative functions, disorders of breathing in stroke patients are often associated with a variety of sleep–wake and autonomic deficits. The mechanisms involved in stroke patients with disordered breathing can be differentiated based on the topography of the lesion.

1. Lesions involving afferent inputs to the medullary respiratory neurons (e.g. posterior spinal cord stroke) may lead to reduction or cessation of airflow of obstructive or non-obstructive type (central and obstructive hypopneas and apneas).
2. Direct dysfunction of medullary respiratory neurons (e.g. in medullary stroke) can manifest with central apneas, irregular breathing (Biot's or ataxic breathing) and failure of automatic breathing (Ondine's curse) during both wakefulness and sleep.
3. Lesions involving the efferent respiratory control at the level of respiratory neurons (e.g. anterior medullary or spinal stroke) may be accompanied by central or obstructive hypopneas and apneas.
4. Lesions causing dysfunction of supramedullary breathing control mechanisms can present with a variety of forms of disordered breathing. Cortical, corticobulbar, and corticospinal lesions may affect volitional breathing partially (respiratory apraxia) or completely (failure of voluntary breathing) (Munschauer et al., 1991). The lesion may be as high as in the frontal cortex and as low as at the cervicomedullary junction (Newsom-Davis, 1974). These patients cannot hold their breath or voluntary change their respiratory rate. Bilateral lesions in the ventrotegmental pons were reported to cause inspiratory breath holding (apneustic breathing) or metronomically regular and rapid breathing (central neurogenic hyperventilation). In patients with pontomedullary lesions, complex abnormalities of voluntary and automatic breathing can be observed. Patients may exhibit irregular breathing (cluster breathing), central apneas, hiccup, inspiratory breath holding, and stridor during wakefulness and sleep (Plum and Swanson, 1959; Plum and Alvord, 1964).

The contribution of brain damage to the pathophysiology of the two most common forms of SDB in stroke victims – OSA (Fig. 22.1) and CSB (Fig. 22.2) – remains poorly understood. The cycling fluctuation in breathing amplitude, with periods of central apneas/hypopneas alternating with periods of hyperpnea, called CSB, may be related to carbon dioxide hypersensitivity induced by bilateral supratentorial lesions (Brown and Plum, 1961). This abnormality is also reflected by the presence in these patients of a post-hyperventilation apnea during wakefulness. The presence of bilateral supratentorial or pontine lesions may be crucial for the appearance of CSB during wakefulness (Brown and Plum, 1961; Lee et al., 1974, 1976). In these patients, a decreased level of consciousness and especially heart failure are additional predisposing factors. Conversely, CSB present only during sleep can be seen also in patients with unilateral lesions of variable topography and without disturbed level of consciousness or heart failure (Nachtmann et al., 1995; Bassetti et al., 1997). A disturbed coordination of upper airway, intercostal, and diaphragmatic muscles caused by brainstem or hemispheric lesions may favor the appearance of OSA. Finally, CSB and OSA may potentiate each other (Bassetti and Aldrich, 1999a).

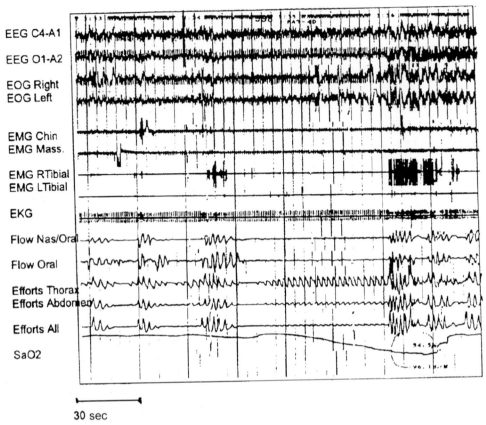

| EEG C4-A1 |
| EEG O1-A2 |
| EOG Right |
| EOG Left |
| EMG Chin |
| EMG Mass. |
| EMG RTibial |
| EMG LTibial |
| EKG |
| Flow Nas/Oral |
| Flow Oral |
| Efforts Thorax |
| Efforts Abdomen |
| Efforts All |
| SaO2 |

30 sec

Fig. 22.1   Obstructive sleep apnea in acute ischemic stroke in a 50-year-old patient with mild, unilateral middle cerebral artery infarction (National Institute of Health Stroke Score of 8). Sleep study was carried out three days after the stroke event. Note the severe, mainly obstructive sleep apnea syndrome (apnea–hypopnea index, 47/h). In the figure, a prolonged obstructive respiratory event during non-REM sleep with oxygen desaturation to 54% is shown (standard polysomnography). (Reproduced with permission from Bassetti and Gugger *Swiss Medical Weekly* (2002) 132, 109–115.)

Snoring and sleep-disordered breathing as vascular risk factors

Following a few mainly Finnish works in the 1980s and early 1990s, several more recent studies support the hypothesis that SDB may represent an independent risk factor for cerebrovascular disease (Shamsuzzaman *et al.*, 2003). A large analysis including 71 779 female nurses aged 40–65 years without previously diagnosed cardiovascular disease or cancer found that self-reported snoring increased the risk for hypertension, coronary heart disease, and stroke within eight years from study inclusion (Hu *et al.*, 1999, 2000). The association between snoring and coronary heart disease, but not with stroke, was still significant after statistical adjustment

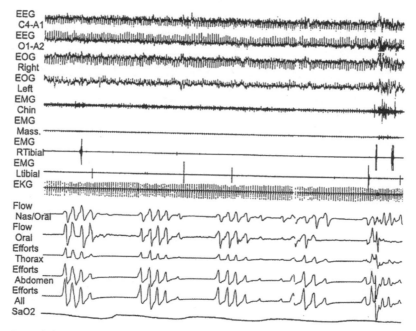

Fig. 22.2   Central sleep apnea in acute ischemic stroke in a 68-year-old patient with moderately severe, unilateral thalamomesencephalic infarction (National Institutes of Health Stroke Score, 12). Sleep studies were carried out two days after stroke. Note again the severe, now mainly central sleep apnea syndrome (apnea–hypopnea index, 45/h). In the figure, periodic central apneas are shown (standard polysomnography). (Reproduced with permission from Bassetti and Gugger *Swiss Medical Weekly* (2002) 132, 109–115.)

for age, smoking, body mass index and other covariates (Hu *et al.*, 2000). The lack of an association between snoring and stroke may be because strokes had a lower incidence (398) than coronary heart disease (644).

The association between SDB and vascular disease was further corroborated by a cross-sectional study performed by the Sleep Heart Health Study Group, who examined the prevalence of self-reported cardiovascular disease in 6424 free-living individuals who underwent overnight polysomnography at home (Shahar *et al.*, 2001). A total of 1023 participants reported at least one manifestation of vascular disease in their personal history (myocardial infarction, angina, coronary revascularization procedure, heart failure, or stroke). Occurrence of SDB was associated more strongly with self-reported heart failure and stroke than with self-reported coronary heart disease, the relative odds ratio (upper versus lower AHI quartile) being 2.38, 1.58, and 1.27, respectively.

In patients with ischemic heart disease, a pathogenic role of OSA in the development of cardiac ischemia was suggested in a study combining Holter electrocardiograms with whole-night polysomnographies (Peled *et al.*, 1999). In that study, cardiac ischemias were noticed in about 20% of patients. Interestingly, ischemic events were found predominantly during the rebreathing phase of obstructive apneas (Peled *et al.*, 1999). The events were characterized by an increased heart rate and nocturnal double product. Six out of ten patients with nocturnal ST depression had subjective symptoms (angina pectoris) on awakening. These observations provide a possible link between vascular events on awakening and SDB.

Mechanisms involved in the increased cardiovascular risk with sleep-disordered breathing

The immediate consequences of respiratory apneic events include hypoxemia, hypercapnia, arousal from sleep, intrathoracic pressure changes, and sympathetic activation (Shamsuzzaman *et al.*, 2003). A series of hemodynamic, neural, metabolic, and inflammatory changes result and may be involved in the increased vascular risk secondary to SDB.

1. High levels of sympathetic activity (during night and daytime) occur, with elevated pulse rate, sharp swings of arterial blood pressure (and consequently of cerebral blood flow) (Balfors and Franklin, 1994) and blunted nocturnal arterial blood pressure dips (Phillips *et al.*, 2000).
2. Disturbances can be detected in endothelial function, particularly of nitric oxide synthetase (Ip *et al.*, 2000) and endothelin (Phillips *et al.*, 1999) pathways.
3. Prothrombotic shift occurs in the coagulation balance, with increased factor VII clotting activity (Chin *et al.*, 1996, 1998); this factor is a marker of the extrinsic coagulation pathway, increased platelet activation and aggregation, which have been previously demonstrated by flow cytometry both *in vitro* and *in vivo* (Bokinsky *et al.*, 1995; Eisensehr *et al.*, 1998; Sanner *et al.*, 2000; Geiser *et al.*, 2002; Reinhart *et al.*, 2002).
4. Metabolic dysregulation results in increased leptin levels and impaired glucose tolerance (Shamsuzzaman *et al.*, 2003).
5. Inflammatory processes increase, with elevated levels of fibrinogen (Wessendorf *et al.*, 2000b), C-reactive protein (Shamsuzzaman *et al.*, 2002), inflammatory cytokines, and adhesion molecules (Shamsuzzaman et al., 2003).
6. There is increased oxidative stress related to intermittent hypoxia and normoxia (Shamsuzzaman *et al.*, 2003).

Cerebrovascular disease and sleep-disordered breathing

The exact nature of the link between SDB and stroke remains speculative, and chronic as well as acute mechanisms may be involved.

Chronically, patients with SDB, and in particular OSA, are found (partly as a consequence of the factors listed above) to have an increased frequency of cardiovascular diseases, including hypertension, congestive heart failure, cardiac arrhythmias, and cardiac ischemia (Shamsuzzaman *et al.*, 2003); these all increase the risk for stroke. The observation of an almost 50% increase in the intima–media thickness of the common carotid artery documented by ultrasound techniques in patients with OSA compared with controls matched for age and vascular risk factors (diabetes, hypertension, hyperlipidemia, and smoking) (Silvestrini *et al.*, 2002) gives further support for an increased (chronic) atherogenesis in SDB.

Acutely, paradoxical embolization resulting from right-to-left shunting in patients with patent foramen ovale during long apneas (Beelke *et al.*, 2002) and decreased cerebral blood flow in patients with pre- or intracranial stenoses may trigger or decompensate cerebrovascular events in patients with SDB.

Whether SDB represents an independent risk factor for stroke remains controversial. It is indeed possible that the increased vascular risk associated with SDB may be a consequence of the frequent presence, possibly genetically codetermined, in these patients of associated vascular risk factors/diseases. Davies *et al.* (2001) conducted a magnetic resonance imaging (MRI) study in asymptomatic subjects with and without OSA who were matched for age, body mass index, alcohol and cigarette consumption, treated hypertension, and ischemic heart disease. The percentage of patients with high-intensity signals in brain MRI did not differ between those with OSA and normal control (33 versus 35%), despite higher mean daytime as well as night-time blood pressure values in patients with SDB (Davies *et al.*, 2001). The authors concluded that the frequency of subclinical cerebrovascular disease was similar in patients with and without OSA, and they questioned the hypothesis of OSA as an independent risk factor for stroke.

The presence of SDB in patients with cerebrovascular disorders may, however, be detrimental even in the absence of a direct causative link between SDB and stroke. In a recent study, SDB detected the first night after brain infarction was found to be associated with early neurological worsening (Iranzo *et al.*, 2002). Interestingly, patients with and without stroke progression did not differ with respect to other risk factors, such as body mass index, arterial hypertension, smoking, diabetes, or hyperlipidemia. It remains unclear, however, why SDB worsened early clinical evolution in this study without influencing functional long-term outcome, which was unaffected.

Continuous positive airway pressure treatment

Effect on arterial hypertension and vascular disease
A pathogenic role of SDB in vascular disease has been suggested also from continuous positive airway pressure (CPAP) treatment studies comparing effects of therapeutical and subtherapeutical pressures (sham CPAP). Most (Engleman *et al.*, 1996; Faccenda *et al.*, 2001; Pepperell *et al.*, 2002) but not all (Barbé *et al.*, 2001) studies have shown favorable effects of CPAP on mean arterial blood

pressure. Faccenda *et al.* (2001) found a small but statistically significant decrease in diastolic blood pressure (77.8 versus 79.2 mmHg) in CPAP-treated patients compared with sham-treated patients. Desaturation frequency appeared to be the best predictor of the diastolic pressure fall (Faccenda *et al.*, 2001). Pepperell *et al.* (2002) reported that therapeutic CPAP reduced mean arterial blood pressure by 2.5 mmHg, whereas subtherapeutic CPAP levels increased blood pressure by 0.8 mmHg. In this study, a benefit was seen both for systolic and diastolic blood pressure during sleep as well as during wakefulness (Pepperell *et al.*, 2002). The reduction in blood pressure values was independent from pre-existing values. Effects were, however, more pronounced in patients with severe OSA. Becker *et al.* (2003) conducted a further trial in patients with severe OSA syndrome (mean AHI before treatment was 62.5/h and 65.0/h, respectively, in the therapeutic and control group). A more pronounced therapeutic effect was seen in that study than in any other previous report, with reductions in mean arterial blood pressure by 9.9 mmHg with effective CPAP treatment (6–12 cmH$_2$O) and no significant pressure changes with subtherapeutic pressure values (3–4 cmH$_2$O). Notably, mean diastolic and systolic pressure values were similarly decreased by approximately 10 mmHg, and pressure reductions were seen both during the night and in the day. The authors extrapolated that a fall in mean arterial blood pressure of 10 mmHg should reduce the risk for coronary heart disease by 37% and that for stroke by 56%. The authors claimed that the striking effect on blood pressure in their study may, at least to some extent, be related to the fact that treatment was performed over as long as nine weeks, which is longer than in earlier studies (Becker *et al.*, 2003). In fact, the duration of CPAP treatment may be an important factor influencing the blood pressure decline.

More direct evidence that CPAP ameliorates vascular disease was obtained in patients with OSA and ischemic heart disease (Peled *et al.*, 1999). In this study, which assessed nocturnal ST depression time as well as the maximum double product values, CPAP treatment significantly ameliorated the ST depression time (from 78 to 33 minutes) and the maximum double product values (from 14.1 to 12.1) (Peled *et al.*, 1999). The reduction in cardiac ischemia events was associated with a reduction of heart rate by CPAP in patients with OSA. Since AHI reduction leads to a decrease of both intrathoracic pressure and myocardial wall stress, the authors concluded that amelioration of myocardial ischemia by CPAP may be related not only to an improved oxygen supply but also to a reduction in tissue oxygen demands (Peled *et al.*, 1999).

Treatment with CPAP may also favorably influence surrogate markers of vascular disease. Chin *et al.* (1998) were able to demonstrate in their study that CPAP treatment led to a progressive decrease in factor VII clotting activity, which steadily improved over as long as 18 months after onset of treatment. The decrease in exogenous clotting activity was associated with a decrease in systolic as well as diastolic blood pressure (Chin *et al.*, 1998). Bokinsky *et al.* (1995) reported that CPAP improved platelet activation/aggregation immediately: already in the first night after treatment was started.

Effect on cerebrovascular diseases

Recently, a few outcome studies have also appeared in patients with stroke and SDB treated with CPAP. Wessendorf *et al.* (2001) reported an improvement of subjective well-being and night-time blood pressure values in a group of 41 and 16 patients, respectively, with stroke and SDB who were treated with CPAP over 10 days. Noteworthy is that the same authors described a compliance of about 70% in their patients' group to continue CPAP treatment in the subacute stage of their stroke, that is after admission to the rehabilitation unit (Wessendorf *et al.*, 2001). The improvement of subjective well-being in stroke patients with SDB may partially be related to changes of mood: Sandberg *et al.* (2001a) reported that treatment of SDB was associated with improved ratings for depression in post-stroke patients, as revealed by the Montgomery Asberg Depression Rating Scale (MADRS). No improvement was found on neurological recovery, as assessed by the Barthel Activities of Daily Living Scale (Sandberg *et al.*, 2001b).

Practical guidelines for the management of sleep-disordered breathing in stroke patients

In the acute stroke setting, SDB is best diagnosed by respiratory polygraphy, in which nasal airflow and thoracic and abdominal respiratory movements are monitored in addition to oxymetry (capillary oxygen saturation) (see also Hermann and Bassetti, 2003a,b). Conventional polysomnography offers additional informations (e.g. on sleep architecture, motor activity, etc.) but is much more expensive and less-commonly available in acute settings; it should, therefore, be reserved for unclear/more complex situations. Based on nasal airflow, respiratory movements and oxygen desaturation recordings, various forms of SDB can be defined, including OSA, central sleep apnea or CSB. The number of apneic and hypopneic events per hour of sleep (AHI) and the number/severity of desaturations are indicators of the severity of breathing disturbances.

Treatment of SDB in stroke patients represents a major clinical, technical, and logistic challenge (Hermann and Bassetti, 2003b). Treatment strategies should always include prevention and early treatment of secondary complications (e.g. aspiration, respiratory infections, pain) and a cautious use/avoidance of alcohol and sedative–hypnotic drugs, which may all negatively affect breathing control during sleep. CPAP ventilation is the treatment of choice for OSA. This treatment prevents the collapse of the upper airway, acting as a pneumatic guide rail. Two types of CPAP device are available: classical and automatic CPAP (also called the "intelligent" or auto-CPAP). Auto-CPAP systems can be used for simultaneous detection of upper airway obstructions and treatment, which is made possible by automatic titration of CPAP pressure. As mentioned above, CPAP can be highly beneficial in stroke patients with OSA, with compliance rates of up to 70% in some (Wessendorf et al., 2001) but not all (Hui et al., 2002) series. Compliance to CPAP is reduced in stroke patients with dementia, delirium, aphasia, anosognosia or pseudobulbar/bulbar palsy.

Besides CPAP, surgical interventions (e.g. uvulopalatopharyngoplasty) and oral appliances, including mandibular repositioners and tongue-retaining devices, may be considered for use at least in some patients with anatomical abnormalities.

Most drugs, such as theophylline, have been shown, in general, to have little or no effect on SDB (reviewed by Robinson and Zwillich, 2000). In patients with central apneas, however, improvements of breathing disturbances may be achieved with oxygen.

In addition, a novel method of ventilatory support called "adaptive servoventilation" may be considered in patients with central apneas. One study has shown that adaptive servoventilation prevented central apneas in stroke patients with heart failure more efficiently than CPAP or oxygen (Teschler et al., 2001).

Tracheostomy and mechanical ventilation may become necessary in patients with central hypoventilation.

Sleep–wake disorders

Sleep–wake functions depend on the integrity of the brain. Therefore, it is not astonishing that stroke may lead to profound sleep–wake changes and their neurophysiological correlates. In healthy subjects, sleep exhibits cyclic patterns of non-REM (stages 1–4) and REM sleep, which typically last about 90 minutes each and are followed by subsequent sleep cycles. During the night, three to up to five sleep cycles follow each other, depending on the duration of the patient's resting period. Sufficient amounts of NREM sleep stage 3–4 (deep sleep) and sleep continuity are considered essential for the recovery value of sleep. In stroke patients, alterations of sleep architecture are frequently found.

Prevalence of sleep–wake disorders in stroke patients

In stroke, sleep–wake disorders (SWD) are found in at least 20–40% of patients, and most commonly present with increased sleep needs (hypersomnia), excessive daytime sleepiness, or insomnia (Leppävuori et al., 2002; Vock et al., 2002). In some patients, episodes of hypersomnia, mutism, and akinesia alternate with episodes of insomnia, psychomotor agitation or confusion state (Façon et al., 1958; Fisher, 1983; Rondot et al., 1986; Bogousslavsky et al., 1988; Caplan et al.,

1990). Sometimes, the transition from wakefulness to sleep and vice versa is impaired and patients may present a dream–reality confusion (oneiric state). Fortunately, SWD are often mild or only transient.

In patients with stroke, SWD are often of multifactorial origin. In addition to brain damage per se, environmental factors, including noise, light, and intensive medical monitoring, may contribute to the development of SWD. Furthermore, cardiorespiratory disorders, seizures, infections, fever, and drugs may aggravate sleep fragmentation and result in sleep disturbances. The importance of these factors is well illustrated by the high occurrence rate of SWD even among patients in intensive care units who do not have brain damage (Krachmann *et al.*, 1995).

Hypersomnia/excessive daytime sleepiness

Hypersomnia is defined by an increased sleep propensity with excessive daytime sleepiness and/or abnormal sleep (or sleep behavior). Sleep behavior may either mimic physiological sleep or be accompanied by abnormal features, such as altered posturing and breathing, particularly in patients with large hemispheric or brain-stem lesions. Patients with deep hemispheric and thalamic stroke may also exhibit so-called pre-sleep behavior, during which they yawn, stretch, close their eyes, curl up, and assume a normal sleeping posture while complaining of a constant sleep urge (Catsman-Berrevoets *et al.*, 1988). When stimulated or given explicit tasks, however, these patients are able to suppress their behavior patterns. For this peculiar dissociation between lack of autoactivation in the presence of preserved heteroactivation, Laplane *et al.* (1984) suggested the term athymormia or "pure psychic akinesia." These cases illustrate the overlap between disorders of motor and mental arousal. In some patients, hypersomnia evolves to extreme apathy, with lack of spontaneity and initiative, slowness, poverty of movement, and catalepsy, a condition for which the term akinetic mutism has been coined (Cairns *et al.*, 1941). Akinetic mutism and its less severe form, usually referred to as abulia, may persist despite normalization of vigilance or even after appearance of insomnia.

The majority of post-stroke hypersomnias are caused by decreased arousal because of lesions involving the ascending reticular activating system. This "passive" hypersomnia may be reflected by focal, multifocal, or diffuse cortical hypometa-bolism, as examined by positron emission tomography (Levasseur *et al.*, 1992). The most severe and persisting forms of de-arousal are seen in patients with bilateral lesions of the thalamus, subthalamic area, tegmental midbrain, and upper pons, where fibers of the ascending reticular activating system are bundled and can be severely injured even by a single small lesion (Fig. 22.3). Mental arousal seems to be affected more severely by medial lesions, while motor arousal is impaired more strongly by lateral lesions of the ascending reticular activating system (Castaigne and Escourolle, 1967; Passouant *et al.*, 1967). In deep

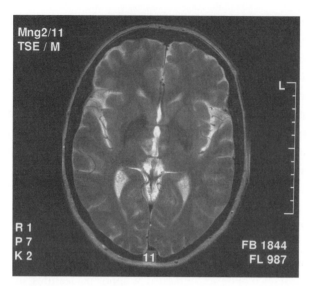

Fig. 22.3   Hypersomnia after bilateral paramedian thalamic stroke in a 54-year-old patient. After an
initial sopor, the patient presented with vertical gaze palsy, severe amnesia, childish behavior,
dysphonia, moderate increase in sleep needs (12 hours/day compared with seven before
stroke), mild excessive daytime sleepiness, loss of dream recall, and weight gain. Levels of
hypocretin/orexin in the cerebrospinal fluid were normal. Improvement of hypersomnia
was achieved with levodopa 250 mg daily (modafinil was stopped because of headaches).
At 14 months after stroke, the patient reported a decrease in sleep needs (10 hours/day)
and the return of dreaming experiences but still had the persistence of memory deficits
and of a disturbed time perception ("Zeitgefühl").

hemispheric lesions sparing the thalamus, de-arousal is usually mild and transient,
probably because of the widespread distribution of activating system projections at
this level. In large hemispheric strokes, de-arousal results from disruption of the
ascending reticular activating system in the upper brainstem secondary to vertical
(transtentorial) or horizontal displacement of the brain caused by brain edema
(Ropper, 1989). The occurrence of SWD following cortical or striatal strokes
without mass effect supports the assumption that the role of these structures in
maintenance of arousal and more generally in sleep–wake regulation may have
been underestimated in the past (Villablanca *et al.*, 1976).

Hypersomnia with increased sleep per 24 hours ("active" hypersomnia) has
occasionally been documented by polysomnography in patients with thalamic,
hypothalamic, mesencephalic, and pontine strokes (Rivera *et al.*, 1986; Arpa *et al.*,
1995; Scammell *et al.*, 2001). In a 51-year-old man, anarcolepsy-like symptom
(excessive daytime sleepiness, hypnagogic hallucinations, sleep paralysis, and cata-
plexy) appeared following cerebral hypoxia caused by cardiac arrest (Rivera *et al.*,
1986). Another case of secondary narcolepsy has been reported after bilateral

diencephalic stroke in a 23-year-old man following surgical removal of a cranio-pharyngeoma. In this patient, cerebrospinal fluid orexin levels were low, suggesting that orexinergic neurons in the posterior hypothalamus were destroyed (Scammell et al., 2001).

Hypersomnia with increased REM sleep can be induced in the cat by a small, bilateral lesion of the ventrolateral periaqueductal gray at the level of the trochlear nucleus (Petitjean et al., 1975; Sastre et al., 1996). Pharmacological studies revealed that this alteration is mediated by gamma-amminobutyric acid type A receptors and that stimulation of these receptors by muscimol leads to a pronounced increase in REM sleep to >50% and up to 100% of the recording time (Sastre et al., 1996). In humans, patients with similarly high proportions of REM sleep have not been described.

Hypersomnia with hyperphagia (Kleine–Levin-like syndrome) has been reported after multiple cerebral strokes (Drake, 1987).

Insomnia

Mild-to-moderate insomnia is a frequent, usually non-specific and multifactorial complication of acute strokes. Recurrent arousals, sleep discontinuity, and sleep deprivation may result from pre-existing disorders (e.g. heart failure, pulmonary disease), SDB, medications, infections and fever, inactivity, environmental disturbances (e.g. being in the intensive care unit), stress, and depression. In a recent study, the use of psychotropic agents, anxiety, dementia, pre-existing insomnia, and stroke severity (as estimated by the Barthel index) were found to be risk factors for post-stroke insomnia (Leppävuori et al., 2002).

Insomnia may also be related to brain damage, a situation for which the term agrypnia has been suggested (Autret et al., 2001). Insomnia may be accompanied by an inversion of the sleep–wake cycle particularly in patients with thalamic, thalamomesencephalic and large tegmental pontine stroke. Van Bogaert (1926) reported a patient with thalamohypothalamic stroke who experienced almost complete insomnia during more than two months. One patient with locked-in syndrome as a result of a bilateral basal pontine stroke with extension to the pontine tegmentum furthermore experienced nearly complete, polysomnographically proven insomnia over as long as six months (Girard et al., 1962).

Parasomnias

Parasomnias are less common forms of SWD following stroke. Strokes in the pontine tegmentum, for example, may result in REM sleep-behavior disorder, in which patients act out their dreams because of a loss of physiological REM atonia (Culebras and Moore, 1989).

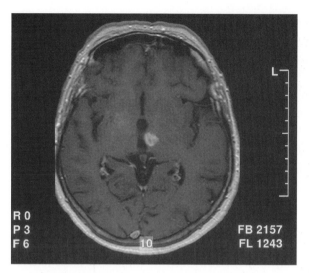

Fig. 22.4   Dream-like hallucinations after unilateral (left) paramedian thalamic stroke in a
62-year-old patient. After an initial confusional state, the patient had abulia, anomia and
moderate–severe amnesia, in the absence of major sleep–wake disturbances. In the first few
days after hospital admission, recurrent episodes of visual and acoustic hallucinations in the
form of human figures (mostly relatives), seen on the right side of the visual field, developed,
which the patient experienced as dreaming. At seven months after stroke, the patient had
persistent memory problems and reported almost daily episodes of psychic hallucinations
("sensed presence') and a disturbed time perception ("Zeitgefühl').

Patients with dorsal pontine/mesencephalic or paramedian thalamic strokes
may experience Lhermitte's peducular hallucinosis, characterized by complex,
often colorful, dream-like visual hallucinations, particular in the evenings and at
sleep onset. Uni- and multimodal dream-like hallucinations can be reported by
patients with hemispheric, thalamic, and brainstem strokes.

Seizures and "release" phenomena after thalamic, temporal, parietal, and occipital
strokes can lead to increased dreaming, recurrent nightmares, or to a syndrome of
dream–reality confusion (Fig.22.4) (Grünstein, 1924; Boller et al., 1975).

A persistent decrease or cessation of dreaming/dream recall (Charcot–Wildbrand
syndrome) can occur in patients with occipital, deep frontal, or parietal lesions
(Fig. 22.5) (Grünstein, 1924; Solms, 1997).

Sleep architecture changes

Abnormalities of sleep architecture are common after acute strokes but result only in
part from acute brain damage (see also above). The importance of non-specific
influences on sleep is well illustrated by the occurrence of SWD among hospitalized
patients without brain damage (Krachmann et al., 1995). Some changes of sleep
architecture, however, are more specifically related to brain damage.

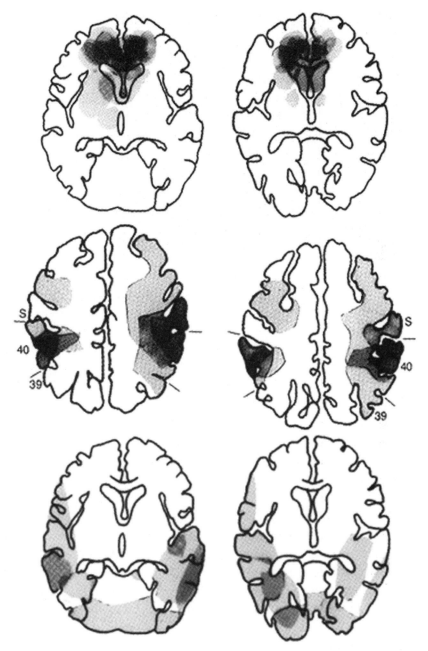

Fig. 22.5   Loss of dreaming in patients with frontal, parietal, and occipital lesions. (Modified figure reproduced with permission from M. Solms, *Neuropsychology of Dreams*, 1997.)

Supratentorial strokes

Reductions in NREM sleep, total sleep time, and sleep efficiency can follow acute supratentorial stroke. In some cases, decreased spindles, K complexes, and slow-wave sleep may predict poor outcome when found after large hemispheric strokes (Cress and Gibbs, 1948; Hachinski *et al.*, 1978; Bassetti and Aldrich, 2001). Reduction of spindling can be ipsilateral (Greenberg, 1966) or bilateral (Hachinski *et al.*, 1978, 1990; Bassetti and Aldrich 2001; Gottselig *et al.*, 2002; Vock *et al.*, 2002) after unilateral stroke. Changes in sleep spindling and slow-wave sleep usually, but not always, coincide (Bassetti and Aldrich, 2001; Gottselig *et al.*, 2002; Müller *et al.*, 2002). Transient reductions in REM sleep can occur in the first few days after supratentorial stroke (Hachinski *et al.*, 1978, 1990; Bassetti and Aldrich, 2001) and may persist after large hemispheric strokes, with poor outcome (Giubiliei *et al.*, 1992). Sawtooth waves can be decreased bilaterally after large hemispheric lesions (Hachinski *et al.*, 1990; Bassetti and Aldrich, 2001).

Changes of sleep architecture after hemispheric stroke do not have a specific localizing value. Cortical blindness has been associated with a reduction in rapid eye movements (Appenzeller *et al.*, 1968). Spindling and, to a lesser extent, slow-wave activity and K complexes appear to be particularly reduced in paramedian thalamic strokes (Guilleminault *et al.*, 1993; Bassetti *et al.*, 1996b). In severe hypersomnia following paramedian thalamic strokes, prolonged polysomnographic recordings can demonstrate an almost continuous state of light NREM stage 1 sleep, perhaps reflecting inability to make the transition from wakefulness to sleep or to produce full wakefulness (Guilleminault *et al.*, 1993; Bassetti *et al.*, 1996b).

Like EEG of wakefulness, the sleep EEG probably undergoes a reorganization after acute brain damage, but data on this subject are scarce. In patients with paramedian thalamic stroke, recovery from hypersomnia may occur despite the persistence of significant NREM sleep changes (Guilleminault *et al.*, 1993; Bassetti *et al.*, 1996b).

Infratentorial strokes

Bilateral paramedian infarcts of the pontine tegmentum or large bilateral infarcts in the ventrotegmental pons can lead to a reduction in non-REM and, especially, REM sleep (Cummings and Greenberg, 1977; Tamura *et al.*, 1983; Autret *et al.*, 1988; Arpa *et al.*, 1995). Physiological EEG sleep features such as sleep spindles, K complexes and vertex waves may be completely lost (Markand and Dyken, 1976; Autret *et al.*, 1988). Patients usually present clinically with crossed or bilateral sensorimotor deficits, oculomotor disturbances, and, at least initially, disturbances of consciousness. In rare instances, the only focal finding in a patient with severe sleep EEG changes may be horizontal gaze palsy (Valldeoriola *et al.*, 1993. Isolated

REM sleep loss can persist for years without cognitive or behavioral consequences (Obrador et al., 1975).

Practical guidelines for the management of sleep–wake disorders in stroke patients

In stroke patients, the correlation of SWD and sleep EEG is often poor (Vock et al., 2002). For example, patients with the clinical picture of hypersomnia, may reveal in sleep EEG either a reduction or, less commonly, an increase of non-REM and/or REM sleep. For this reason, multiple sleep latency tests may be inadequate for assessment of post-stroke SWD (Bassetti et al., 1996b). Actigraphy, conversely, may be helpful to estimate changes in sleep–wake rhythms and sleep needs following stroke.

There are almost no systematic studies on treatment of SWD in stroke patients. Nonetheless, practical guidelines for the treatment of patients have recently been presented (Hermann et al., 2003b). Unfortunately, treatment of post-stroke hypersomnia is often ineffective. In single patients, some improvement was seen in thalamic and mesencephalic stroke with amphetamines, modafinil, methylphenidate, and dopaminergic agents. Catsman-Berrevoets and Harskamp (1988) reported, for example, improvement of apathy and pre-sleep behavior in patients with paramedian thalamic stroke with 20–40 mg bromocriptine. Autret et al. (2001) described a dramatic improvement of alertness with 200 mg modafinil in a patient with bilateral mesodiencephalic paramedian infarct. Treatment of an associated depression with stimulating antidepressants may also improve post-stroke hypersomnia. It is noteworthy that a favorable influence on early post-stroke rehabilitation was reported both for methylphenidate (5–30 mg daily in a three week trial) and levodopa (100 mg daily in a three week trial), an effect that may at least in parts be related to improved alertness in these patients (Grade et al., 1998; Scheidtmann et al., 2001).

Treatment of insomnia occurring acutely after stroke should include placement of patients in private rooms at night, protection from nocturnal noise and light, increased mobilization with exposure to light during the day, and, when unavoidable, temporary use of hypnotics that are relatively free of cognitive side-effects, such as zolpidem and benzodiazepines. It should be kept in mind that benzodiazepines may not only enhance sedation and neuropsychological deficits in stroke patients but also lead to the reemergence of other neurological symptoms (Lazar et al., 2002). Treatment of an associated depression with sedative antidepressants may also improve post-stroke insomnia. In a recent study of 51 stroke patients 60 mg mianserin daily led to a better improvement of insomnia complaints than placebo, even in patients without associated depression (Palomäki et al., 2003). Antidepressants may be preferable for long-term management of post-stroke insomnia.

REFERENCES

Appenzeller, O. and Fisher, A. P. (1968). Disturbances of rapid eye movements during sleep in patients with lesions of the nervous system. *Electroencephalograph Clin Neurophysiol* **25**: 29–35.

Arpa, J., Rodriguez-Albarino, R., Izal, E., *et al.* (1995). Hypersomnia after tegmental pontine hematoma: case report. *Neurology* (Spain) **10**: 140–144.

Autret, A., Laffont, F., de Toffol, B., and Cathala, H. P. (1988). A syndrome of REM and non-REM sleep reduction and lateral gaze paresis after medial tegmental pontine stroke. *Arch Neurol* **45**: 1236–1242.

Autret, A., Lucas, B., Mondon, K., *et al.* (2001). Sleep and brain lesions: a critical review of the literature and additional new cases. *Neurophysiol Clin* **31**: 356–375.

Balfors, E. M. and Franklin, K. A. (1994). Impairment of cerebral perfusion during obstructive sleep apneas. *Am J Resp Crit Care Med* **150**: 1587–1591.

Barbé, F., Mayoralas, L. R., Duran, J., *et al.* (2001). Treatment with continuous positive airway pressure is not effective in patients with sleep apnea but no daytime sleepiness. A randomized, controlled trial. *Ann Intern Med* **134**: 1015–1023.

Bassetti, C., and Aldrich, M. S. (1999a). Sleep apnea in acute cerebrovascular diseases: final report on 128 patients. *Sleep* **22**: 217–223.

(1999b). Nighttime versus daytime transient ischemic attack and ischemic stroke: a prospective study of 110 patients. *J Neurol Neurosurg Psychiatry* **67**: 463–469.

(2001). Sleep electroencephalogram changes in acute hemispheric stroke. *Sleep Med* **2**: 185–194.

Bassetti, C., and Gugger, M. (2002). Sleep disordered breathing in neurological diseases. *Swiss Med Wkly* **132**: 109–115.

Bassetti, C., Aldrich, M. S., Chervin, R., and Quint, D. (1996a). Sleep apnea in the acute phase of TIA and stroke. *Neurology* **47**: 1167–1173.

Bassetti, C., Mathis, J., Gugger, M., Lovblad, K. O., and Hess, C. W. (1996b). Hypersomnia following thalamic stroke. *Ann Neurol* **39**: 471–480.

Bassetti, C., Aldrich, M. S., and Quint, D. (1997). Sleep-disordered breathing in patients with acute supra- and infratentorial stroke. *Stroke* **28**: 1765–1772.

Becker, H. F., Jerrentrup, A., Ploch, T., *et al.* (2003). Effect of nasal continuous positive airway pressure treatment on blood pressure in patients with obstructive sleep apnea. *Circulation* **107**: 68–73.

Beelke, M., Angeli, S., Del Sette, M., *et al.* (2002). Obstructive sleep apnea can be provocative for right-to-left shunting through a patent foramen ovale. *Sleep* **25**: 856–862.

Bogousslavsky, J., Ferrazzini, M., Regli, F., *et al.* (1988). Manic delirium and frontal-lobe syndrome with paramedian infarction of the right thalamus. *J Neurol Neurosurg Psychiatr* **51**: 116–117.

Bokinsky, G., Miller, M., Ault, K., Husband, P., and Mitchell, J. (1995). Spontaneous platelet activation and aggregation during obstructive sleep apnea and its response to therapy with nasal continuous positive airway pressure. A preliminary investigation. *Chest* **108**: 625–630.

Boller, F., Wright, D., Cavallieri, R., *et al.* (1975). Paroxysmal "nightmares." *Neurology* **25**: 1026–1030.

Broadbent, W. H. (1877). On Cheyne–Stokes respiration in cerebral hemorrhage. *Lancet* **i**: 307–309.

Brown, H. W. and Plum, F. (1961). The neurological basis of Cheyne–Stokes respiration. *Am J Med* **30**: 849–869.

Cairns, H., Oldfield, R. C., Pennybacker, J. B., and Whitteridge, D. (1941). Akinetic mutism with an epidermoid cyst of the 3rd ventricle. *Brain* **64**: 273–290.

Caplan, L. R., Schmahmann, J. D., Kase, C. S., *et al.* (1990). Caudate infarcts. *Arch Neurol* **47**: 133–143.

Castaigne, P. and Escourolle, R. (1967). Etude topographique des lésions anatomiques dans les hypersomnies. *Rev Neurol* **116**: 547–584.

Catsman-Berrevoets, C. E. and Harskamp, F. (1988). Compulsive pre-sleep behavior and apathy due to bilateral thalamic stroke. *Neurology* **38**: 647–649.

Cheyne, A. (1818). A case of apoplexy in which the fleshy part of the heart was converted into fat. *Dublin Hosp Rep* **2**: 216–218.

Chin, K., Ohi, M., Kita, H., *et al.* (1996). Effects of NCPAP therapy on fibrinogen levels in obstructive sleep apnea syndrome. *Am J Respir Crit Care Med* **153**: 1972–1976.

Chin, K., Kita, H., Noguchi, T., *et al.* (1998). Improvement of factor VII clotting activity following long-term NCPAP treatment in obstructive sleep apnoea syndrome. *Q J Med* **91**: 627–633.

Cress, C. H. and Gibbs, E. L. (1948). Electroencephalographic asymmetry during sleep. *Dis Nerv Syst* **9**: 327–329.

Culebras, A. and Moore, J.T (1989). Magnetic resonance imaging in REM sleep behavior disorder. *Neurology* **39**: 1519–1523.

Cummings, J. L. and Greenberg, R. (1977). Sleep patterns in the "locked-in" syndrome. *Electroencephalograph Clin Neurophysiol* **43**: 270–271.

Davies, C. W., Crosby, J. H., Mullins, R. L., *et al.* (2001). Case control study of cerebrovascular damage defined by magnetic resonance imaging in patients with OSA and normal matched control subjects. *Sleep* **24**: 715–720.

Drake, M. E. (1987). Kleine-Levine-syndrome after multiple cerebral infarctions. *Psychosomatics* **28**: 329–330.

Eisensehr, I., Ehrenberg, B. L., Noachtar, S., *et al.* (1998). Platelet activation, epinephrine, and blood pressure in obstructive sleep apnea syndrome. *Neurology* **51**: 188–195.

Elliott, W. J. (1998). Circadian variation in the timing of stroke onset: a meta-analysis. *Stroke* **29**: 992–996.

Engleman, H. M., Gough, K., Martin, S. E., *et al.* (1996). Ambulatory blood pressure on and off continuous positive airway pressure therapy for the sleep apnea/hypopnea syndrome: effects in "non-dippers." *Sleep* **19**: 378–381.

Faccenda, J. F., Mackay, T. W., Boon, N. A., and Douglas, N. J. (2001). Randomized placebo-controlled trial of continuous positive airway pressure on blood pressure in the sleep apnea-hypopnea syndrome. *Am J Respir Crit Care Med* **163**: 344–348.

Façon, E., Steriade, M., and Wertheim, N. (1958). Hypersomnie prolongée engendrée par des lésions bilatérale du système activateur médial. Le syndrome thrombotique de la bifurcation du tronc basilaire. *Rev Neurol* **98**: 117–133.

Fisher, C. M. (1983). Abulia minor versus agitated behavior. *Clin Neurosurg* **31**: 9–31.

Freund, S. C. (1913). Zur Klinik und Anatomie der vertikalen Blicklähmung. *Neurol Zentralbl* **32**: 1215–1229.

Geiser, T., Buck, F., Meyer, B. J., *et al.* (2002). In vivo platelet activation is increased during sleep in patients with obstructive sleep apnea syndrome. *Respiration* **69**: 229–234.

Girard, P., Gerrest, F., Tommasi, M., *et al.* (1962). Ramollissement géant du pied de la protubérance. *Lyon Méd* **14**: 877–892.

Giubilei, F., Iannilli, M., Vitale, A., *et al.* (1992). Sleep patterns in acute ischemic stroke. *Acta Neurol Scand* **86**: 567–571.

Good, D. C., Henkle, J. Q., Gelber, D., Weösh, J., and Verhulst, S., (1996). Sleep-disordered breathing and poor functional outcome after stroke. *Stroke* **27**: 252–259

Gottselig, J.M, Bassetti, C. L., and Achermann, P. (2002). Power and coherence of sleep spindle frequency activity following hemispheric stroke. *Brain* **125**: 373–383.

Grade, C., Redford, B., Chrostowski, J., Tousaaint, L., and Blackwell, B. (1998). Methylphenidate in early post-stroke recovery: a double-blind, placebo controlled study. *Arch Phys Med Rehabil* **79**: 1047–1050.

Greenberg, R. (1966). Cerebral cortex lesions: the dream process and sleep spindles. *Cortex* **2**: 357–366.

Grünstein, A. M. (1924). Erforschung der Träume als eine Methode der topischen Diagnostik bei Grosshirnerkrankungen. *Zeitschr Ges Neurol Psychiatr* **93**: 416–420.

Guilleminault, C., Quera-Salva, M. A., and Goldberg, M. P. (1993). Pseudo-hypersomnia and pre-sleep behavior with bilateral paramedian thalamic lesions. *Brain* **116**: 1549–1563.

Hachinski, V., Mamelak, M., and Norris, J. W. (1978). *Prognostic Value of Sleep Morphology in Cerebral Infarction.* Amsterdam: Excerpta Medica.

(1990). Clinical recovery and sleep architecture degradation. *Can J Neurol Sci* **17**: 332–335.

Harbison, J., Ford, G. A., James, O. F. W., and Gibson, G. J. (2002). Sleep-disordered breathing following acute stroke. *Q J Med* **95**: 741–747.

Hermann, D. M. and Bassetti, C. L. (2003a). Sleep-disordered breathing and stroke. *Curr Opin Neurol* **16**: 87–90.

(2003b). Sleep apnea and other sleep–wake disorders in stroke. *Curr Treatm Opt Neurol* **5**: 241–249.

Hu, F. B., Willett, W. C., Colditz, G. A., *et al.* (1999). Prospective study of snoring and risk of hypertension in women. *Am J Epidemiol* **150**: 806–816.

Hu, F. B., Willett, W. C., and Manson, J. E. (2000). Snoring and risk of cardiovascular disease in women. *J Am Coll Cardiol* **35**: 308–313.

Hui, D. S. C., Choy, D. K. L., Wong, L. K. S., *et al.* (2002). Prevalence of sleep-disordered breathing and continuous positive airway pressure compliance: results in Chinese patients with first-ever ischemic stroke. *Chest* **122**: 852–860.

Ip, M. S., Lam, B., Chan, L. Y., *et al.* (2000). Circulating nitric oxide is suppressed in obstructive sleep apnea and is reversed by nasal continuous positive airway pressure. *Am J Respir Crit Care Med* **162**: 2166–2171.

Iranzo, A., Santamaria, J., Berenguer, J., Sanchez, M., and Chamorro, A. (2002). Prevalence and clinical importance of sleep apnea in the first night after cerebral infarction. *Neurology* **58**: 911–916.

Krachmann, S. L., D'Alonzo, G. E., and Criner, G. J. (1995). Sleep in the intensive care unit. *Chest* **107**: 1713–1720.

Lago, A., Geffner, D., Tembl, J., *et al.* (1998). Circadian variation in acute ischemic stroke: a hospital-based study. *Stroke* **29**: 1873–1875.

Laplane, D., Baulac, M., Widlöcher, D., and Dubois, B. (1984). Pure psychic akinesia with bilateral lesions of basal ganglia. *J Neurol Neurosurg Psychiatry* **47**: 377–385.

Lavie, P. (1991). The touch of Morpheus: pre-20th century accounts of sleepy patients. *Neurology* **41**: 1841–1844.

Lazar, R. M., Fitzsimmons, B. F., and Marshall, R. S. (2002). Reemergence of stroke deficits with midazolam challenge. *Stroke* **33**: 1456–1457.

Lee, M. C., Klassen, A. C., and Resch, J. A. (1974). Respiratory pattern disturbances in ischemic cerebral vascular disease. *Stroke* **5**: 612–616.

Lee, M. C., Klassen, A. C., Heaney, L. M., and Resch, J. A. (1976). Respiratory rate and pattern disturbances in acute brainstem infarction. *Stroke* **7**: 382–385.

Leppävuori, A., Pohjasvaara, T., Vataja, R., Kaste, M., and Erkinjuntti, T. (2002). Insomnia in ischemic stroke patients. *Cerebrovasc Dis* **14**: 90–97.

Levasseur, M., Baron, J. C., Sette, G., *et al.* (1992). Brain energy metabolism in bilateral paramedian thalamic infarcts. A PET study. *Brain* **115**: 795–807.

Lhermitte, M. J. (1922). Syndrome de la calotte du pédoncle cérébral. Les troubles psycho-sensoriels dans les lésions mésocéphaliques. *Rev Neurol* **29**: 1359–1365.

Markand, O. N. and Dyken, M. L. (1976). Sleep abnormalities in patients with brainstem lesions. *Neurology* **26**: 769–776.

Munschauer, F. E., Mador, J., Ahuja, A., and Jacobs, L. (1991). Selective paralysis of voluntary but not limbically influenced automatic respiration. *Arch Neurol* **48**: 1190–1192.

Müller, C., Achermann, P., Bischof, M., *et al.* (2002). Visual and spectral analysis of sleep EEG in acute hemispheric stroke. *Eur Neurol* **48**: 164–173.

Nachtmann, A., Siebler, M., Rose, G., Sitzer, M., and Steinmetz, H. (1995). Cheyne-Stokes respiration in ischemic stroke. *Neurology* **45**: 820–821.

Newsom-Davis, J. (1974). Autonomous breathing. *Arch Neurol* **30**: 480–483.

Obrador, S., Reinoso-Suarez, F., Carbonell, J., *et al.* (1975). Comatous state maintained during eight years following a vascular ponto-meencephalic lesion. *Electroencephalograph Clin Neurophysiol* **38**: 21–26.

Palomäki, H., Berg, A., Meririnne, E., *et al.* (2003). Complaints of post-stroke insomnia and its treatment with mianserin. *Cerebrovasc Dis* **15**: 56–62.

Parra, O., Arboix, A., Bechich, S., *et al.* (2000). Time course of sleep-related breathing disorders in first-ever stroke or transient ischemic attack. *Am J Respir Crit Care Med* **161**: 375–380.

Passouant, P., Cadilhac, J., and Baldy-Moulinier, M. (1967). Physio-pathologie des hypersomnies. *Rev Neurol* **116**: 585–629.

Peled, N., Abinader, E. G., Pillar, G., Sharif, D., and Lavie, P. (1999). Nocturnal ischemic events in patients with obstructive sleep apnea syndrome and ischemic heart disease: effects of continuous positive air pressure treatment. *J Am Coll Cardiol* **34**: 1744–1749.

Pepperell, J. C., Ramdassingh-Dow, S., Crosthwaite, N., *et al.* (2002). Ambulatory blood pressure after therapeutic and subtherapeutic nasal continuous positive airway pressure for obstructive sleep apnoea: a randomised parallel trial. *Lancet* **359**: 204–210.

Petitjean, F., Sakai, K., Blondaux, C., and Jouvet, M. (1975). Hypersomnie par lésion isthmique chez le chat. II. Etude neurophysiologique et pharmacologique. *Brain Res* **88**: 439–453.

Phillips, B. G., Narkiewicz, K., Pesek, C. A., *et al.* (1999). Effects of obstructive sleep apnea on endothelin-1 and blood pressure. *J Hypertens* **17**: 61–66.

Phillips, R. A., Sheinart, K. F., Godbold, J. H., Mahboob, R., and Tuhrim, S. (2000). The association of blunted nocturnal blood pressure dip and stroke in a multiethnic population. *Am J Hypertens* **13**: 1250–1255.

Plum, F. and Alvord, E. C. (1964). Apneustic breathing in man. *Arch Neurol* **10**: 101–112.

Plum, F. and Swanson, A. G. (1959). Central neurogenic hyperventilation in man. *Arch Neurol Psychiatry* **81**: 535–549.

Reinhart, W. H., Oswald, J., Walter, R., and Kuhn, M. (2002). Blood viscosity and platelet function in patients with obstructive sleep apnea syndrome treated with nasal continuous positive airway pressure. *Clin Hemorheol Microcirc* **27**; 201–207.

Rivera, V. M., Meyer, J. S., Hata, T., Ishikawa, Y., and Imai, A. (1986). Narcolepsy following cerebral hypoxic ischemia. *Ann Neurol* **19**: 505–508.

Robinson, R. W. and Zwillich, C. W. (2000). Medications, sleep, and breathing. In *Principles and Practice of Sleep Medicine*, 3rd edn, ed. M. H. Kryger, T. Roth, and W. C. Dement. Philadelphia: W. B. Saunders, pp. 797–812.

Rondot, P., Recondo, J., Davous, P., Bathien, N., and Coignet, A. (1986). Infarctus thalamique bilatéral avec mouvements abnormaux et amnésie durable. *Rev Neurol* **142**: 389–405.

Ropper, A. H. (1989). A preliminary MRI study of the geometry of brain displacement and level of consciousness with acute intracranial masses. *Neurology* **39**: 622–627.

Sandberg, O., Franklin, K. A., Bucht, G., and Gustafson, Y. (2001a). Sleep apnea, delirium, depressed mood, cognition, and ADL ability after stroke. *J Am Geriatr Soc* **49**: 391–397.

Sandberg, O., Franklin, K. A., Bucht, G., Eriksson, S., and Gustafson, Y. (2001b). Nasal continuous positive airway pressure in stroke patients with sleep apnoea: a randomized treatment study. *Eur Respir J* **18**: 630–634.

Sanner, B. M., Konermann, M., *et al.* (2000). Platelet function in patients with obstructive sleep apnoea syndrome. *Eur Respir J* **16**: 648–652.

Sastre, J. P., Buda, C., Kitahama, K., and Jouvet, M. (1996). Importance of the ventrolateral region of the periaqueductal gray and adjacent tegmentum in the control of paradoxical sleep as studied by uscinmol microinjections in the cat. *Neuroscience* **74**: 415–426.

Scammell, T. E., Nishino, S., Mignot, E., and Saper, C. B. (2001). Narcolepsy and low CSF orexin (hypocretin) concentration after a diencephalic stroke. *Neurology* **56**: 1751–1753.

Scheidtmann, K., Fries, W., Muller, F., and Koenig, E. (2001). Effect of levodopa in combination with physiotherapy on functional recovery after stroke: a prospective, randomized, double-blind study. *Lancet* **358**: 787–790.

Shahar, E., Whitney, C. W., Redline, S., *et al.* (2001). Sleep-disordered breathing and cardio-vascular disease: cross-sectional results of the Sleep Heart Health Study. *Am J Respir Crit Care Med* **163**: 19–25.

Shamsuzzaman, A. S., Winnicki, M., Lanfranchi, P., *et al.* (2002). Elevated C-reactive protein in patients with obstructive sleep apnea. *Circulation* **105**: 2462–2464.

Shamsuzzaman, A. S., Gersh, B. J., and Somers, V. K. (2003). Obstructive sleep apnea. *JAMA* **290**: 1906–1914.

Silvestrini, M., Rizzato, B., Placidi, F., *et al.* (2002). Carotid artery wall thickness in patients with obstructive sleep apnea syndrome. *Stroke* **33**: 1782–1785.

Solms, M. (1997). *The Neuropsychology of Dreams*. Mahwah, NJ: Lawrence Erlbaum Associates.

Stergiou, G. S., Vemmos, K. N., Pliarchopoulou, K. M., *et al.* (2002). Parallel morning and evening surge in stroke onset, blood pressure, and physical activity. *Stroke* **33**: 1480–1486.

Tamura, K., Karacan, I., Williams, R. L., and Meyer, J. S. (1983). Disturbances of the sleep–waking cycle in patients with vascular brain stem lesions. *Clin Electroencephalograph* **14**: 35–46.

Teschler, H., Döhrin, J., Wang, Y., and Berthon-Jones, M. (2001). Adaptive pressure support servo-ventilation. *Am J Respir Crit Care Med* **164**: 614–619.

Turkington, P. M., Bamford, J., Wanklyn, P., and Elliott, M. W. (2002). Prevalence and pre-dictors of upper airway obstruction in the first 24 hours after acute stroke. *Stroke* **33**: 2037–2042.

Valldeoriola, F., Santamaria, J., Graus, F., and Tolosa, E. (1993). Absence of REM sleep, altered NREM sleep and supranuclear horizontal gaze palsy caused by a lesion of the pontine tegmentum. *Sleep* **16**: 184–188.

van Bogaert, M. (1926). Syndrome de la calotte protubérentielle avec myoclonie localisée et troubles du sommeil. *Rev Neurol* (Paris) **45**: 977–988.

Villablanca, J. R., Marcus, R. J., and Olmstead, C. E. (1976). Effect of caudate nuclei or frontal cortex ablations in cats. II. Sleep-wakefulness, EEG, and motor activity. *Exp Neurol* **53**: 31–50.

Vock, J., Achermann, P., Bischof, M., *et al.* (2002). Evolution of sleep and sleep EEG after hemispheric stroke. *J Sleep Res* **11**: 331–338.

Wessendorf, T. E., Teschler, H., Wang, Y. M., Konietzko, N., and Thilmann, A. F. (2000a). Sleep-disordered breathing among patients with first-ever stroke. *J Neurol* **247**: 41–47.

Wessendorf, T. E., Thilmann, A. F., Wang, Y. M., *et al.* (2000b). Fibrinogen levels and obstruc-tive sleep apnea in ischemic stroke. *Am J Respir Crit Care Med* **162**: 2039–2042.

Wessendorf, T. E., Wang, Y. M., Thilmann, A. F., *et al.* (2001). Treatment of obstructive sleep apnea with nasal continuous positive airway pressure in stroke. *Eur Respir J* **18**: 619–622.

23

Technology for recovery after stroke

Neville Hogan

Massachusetts Institute of Technology, Cambridge, MA, USA

Hermano I. Krebs

Massachusetts Institute of Technology, Cambridge, MA and Cornell University, New York, USA

Brandon R. Rohrer

Sandia National Laboratories, Albuquerque, NM, USA

Susan E. Fasoli

Massachusetts Institute of Technology, Cambridge, MA, USA

Joel Stein

Spaulding Rehabilitation Hospital and Harvard Medical School, Boston, MA, USA

Bruce T. Volpe

Burke Medical Research Institute and Cornell University, New York, USA

Introduction

Stroke continues to be the leading cause of disability in the USA and elsewhere, despite the success of preventive strategies. In fact, recent studies have reported an increase in the incidence of stroke (Broderick *et al.*, 1998; Muntner *et al.*, 2002) with close to five million stroke survivors in the USA alone. This trend is likely to continue, driven by many factors, notably increasing life expectancy, aging of the "baby boom" generation, and improved medical treatment to increase stroke survivability. However, 90% of stroke survivors are left with significant impairment and require therapy.

While the number of patients is growing, pressure to contain and reduce the cost of healthcare has grown even faster, prompting a reduction of the time and resources available for post-stroke treatment. This generates a pressing need for new approaches to increase the effectiveness and efficiency of therapy, and one promising approach is to create innovative technology for rehabilitation. In principle, technology may be applied broadly across the entire spectrum of impairments that result

Recovery after Stroke, ed. Michael P. Barnes, Bruce H. Dobkin and Julien Bogousslavsky. Published by Cambridge University Press. © Cambridge University Press 2005.

from stroke: cognitive, affective, sensory, and motor. However, motor deficits persist chronically in about half of stroke survivors (Gresham *et al.*, 1979) and the following will focus on new technology for sensory–motor rehabilitation, in particular on robotic and information technologies.

Rehabilitation robots

In general, there are two broad classes of rehabilitation robot: those directed at recovery, attempting to reduce impairment and restore function, and those directed at compensation for disability. The latter is the older and more mature application. An excellent example is the wheelchair-mounted robot developed in the Netherlands (Verburg *et al.*, 1996). This is an elegant design that can fold unobtrusively when not in use and provides extended reach and limited manipulation to a seated patient.

Though both approaches arguably assist the patient, the term "assistive technology" is traditionally reserved for the direct use of technology to compensate for disability. More recently, attention has turned from such direct assistance to a more indirect role, helping clinicians to help patients recover. Though they present greater technical challenges (see below), robots to aid recovery have the potential for greater positive impact on patients' quality of life. They may be used throughout the process of recovery, beginning before a patient has regained voluntary movement, perhaps even at the bedside; in principle, they may minimize or eliminate the need for assistance.

Of course, the direct and indirect approaches are complementary. Robots may help a patient to recover as much function as possible, and robots may help to compensate for what cannot be recovered.

Robotic therapy

Robotic treatment may improve inpatient rehabilitation, where it can unburden the clinician of repetitive, time-consuming tasks and allow more time to focus on care delivery and individual patient needs. It may reduce cost by "leveraging" the know-how of clinical experts, allowing one to treat many simultaneously. Robots may also be an unprecedented vehicle to extend the reach of clinical expertise beyond the rehabilitation hospital, providing a means to deliver high-quality outpatient treatment in other venues that incur much lower fixed costs, including community care centers, skilled nursing facilities, assisted living facilities, and, ultimately, the patients' homes.

There are many ways in which robot technology might improve the quality and effectiveness of therapy. They provide better control of the delivery of movement therapy, allowing increased intensity or dosage, more timely correlation with sensory experience, and better responsiveness and adaptation to a patient's continually changing ability. They may provide alternative instruments for measurement and assessment that take less time to apply and yield reproducible, objective results. Through better measurement and control, they may ultimately improve our understanding of the process of recovery and how it might be accelerated and extended.

Of course, this optimistic vision does not yet match the present state of rehabilitation practice. That is likely to change rapidly as the development of neurorehabilitation technology is accelerating at a remarkable rate, but the key questions are pragmatic. Does robotic therapy work? How well? For which patients? By what mechanisms? How might it be improved? This chapter reviews our experience treating patients with a novel upper-extremity therapy robot, MIT-MANUS. (The name is derived from the motto of the Massachusetts Institute of Technology: *mens et manus*. The similarity to the name of the wheelchair-mounted assistive robot mentioned above (MANUS) is coincidental.) The chapter is by no means a comprehensive review (see Volpe *et al.*, 2001, 2002) as the work of many other groups is not reported but it represents a large body of experience (over 200 patients at the time of writing) and gives a practical sense of what may be expected of this new technology.

Robotic treatment of stroke

Initial pilot study

To test the benefits of robotic therapy, an initial pilot study was conducted with 20 hemiparetic patients (10 experimental, 10 control) at the Burke Rehabilitation Hospital in White Plains, New York State using a robot specifically designed to be safe and stable while capable of exerting large forces on a patient's upper limb (Hogan *et al.*, 1995; Krebs *et al.*, 1998). Robot therapy took the form of a highly simplified "game" in which patients were asked to move a handle on the end of the robot to move a cursor (a dot) on a computer display screen to whichever of eight target dots changed color (Fig. 23.1). In this way, the patient's action was visually evoked (by the target dot changing color) and could be visually guided (via the cursor motion on the screen).

The robot provided graded assistance: if the patient was unable to move, the robot moved the patient's hand to the target; if the patient moved inappropriately, the robot continually guided the patient's hand towards a nominal trajectory to the target. As the patient gained ability to control the limb, the robot provided less assistance. The continuously changing *interaction* between robot and patient was enabled by using robot impedance control (see below). With this highly interactive robot therapy, the target was always reached, providing at least some form of positive

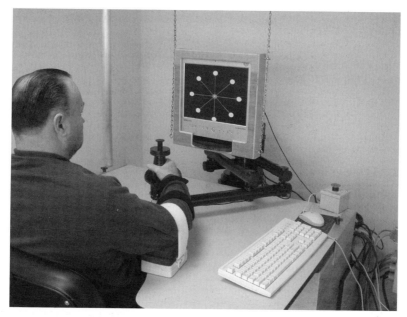

Fig. 23.1   Robotic therapy in the horizontal plane.

reinforcement on every trial. Further, because the robot kept the hand moving near the nominal trajectory, proprioceptive and kinesthetic feedback was well correlated with the appropriate movement.

All patients received a standard course of conventional physical and occupational therapy. In addition, the experimental group received a one-hour session of interactive robot therapy daily, four or five days a week for an average of four weeks, typically performing over 20 000 reaching movements in that period. A typical session consisted of five minutes to set up, 45 minutes of treatment, five minutes to disengage, and five minutes of slack time (e.g. for socializing). The control group was presented with the same robotic apparatus and visual display and also asked to move the handle of the robot to move the cursor to the target; the main difference was that the robot motors were not turned on. Without robotic assistance, patients had less success with the task. As a result (primarily to avoid discouraging them), the control group differed in that they had less exposure to the task, could assist the impaired limb with the unaffected limb, could use the unaffected limb alone, or a clinician could assist.

One important result of this study was clear, objective evidence that robot therapy matters. Clinical assessment by a blinded therapist using the Fugl–Meyer, Motor Power and Motor Status scores showed that, on average, all patients improved over the course of treatment. Most importantly, the robot-treated group out-performed the control group (Aisen *et al.*, 1997).

Replication study

The positive results of the pilot study prompted a second, larger clinical study to test the robustness of these findings and to improve our understanding of how robot therapy works. The replication study of 56 additional patients confirmed and extended the earlier results (Volpe *et al.*, 2000). Disability was assessed using the Functional Independence Measure (FIM). Although there was no significant difference in overall FIM scores, analysis of *motor* subsections of the FIM scores showed that the robot-treated group improved significantly more than the controls, whereas the *cognition* subsections of the FIM scores showed that both groups improved comparably. However encouraging this result may be, it must be interpreted cautiously since the FIM scores were not assessed with the restriction of using only the affected upper limb. In contrast, analysis of the impairment measures was unequivocal, showing first that interactive robot therapy significantly reduced motor impairment of the treated limbs and, second, that interactive robot therapy added to conventional therapy provided approximately *double* the impairment reduction. Robot therapy works.

Follow-up study

Another question was whether any benefits of robot therapy would outlast the treatment period. To test the long-term effects of robot therapy, patients from the first clinical study were reexamined; 12 of those 20 patients were recalled up to three years later (Volpe *et al.*, 1999). We found that all patients had improved after hospital discharge. Though we had no control over the experience of these patients between discharge and follow-up, this is an interesting observation in its own right, indicating that recovery is not complete at hospital discharge. More to the point, patients who received robot therapy sustained their improvement better than the control group. Subsequent follow-up studies reexamining the patients of the second (replication) study confirmed this finding. The benefits of robot therapy last.

Outpatient study

In the studies reviewed above, robot therapy was administered to stroke patients in the acute (inpatient) phase of recovery. Our observation that patients continued to improve after hospital discharge prompted an investigation of whether interactive robot therapy might benefit stroke patients in the chronic stable phase. In a study conducted at the Spaulding Rehabilitation Hospital in Boston, 20 community-dwelling stroke survivors were recruited who had suffered a single unilateral stroke one to five years previously. They were evaluated on three occasions at two-week intervals in the month prior to robot treatment, then received interactive robot therapy as outlined above, but three times a week for six weeks (without any regimen of conventional therapy), and evaluated again. The three pretreatment evaluations showed no significant change, verifying that these patients had, indeed, reached a plateau of performance prior to robot therapy. However, the post-treatment evaluation showed a significant improvement with robot therapy (Fasoli *et al.*, 2002, 2003). Robot therapy benefits chronic stroke.

How does robot therapy work?

We believe our studies provide unequivocal, objective evidence that therapy focused on physical activity has a positive effect on recovery from stroke. They also provide solid evidence that at least this form of robot therapy is beneficial. A natural question is how it works.

One possibility is that the benefits of robot therapy simply derive from the extra treatment that was provided. Though we cannot exclude this, two comments are appropriate. First, the robot provided movement coupled with sensory information from the periphery and a visual display that signaled when to move, showed the goal, the nominal path, the current hand position (and hence trajectory error), and provided knowledge of results. It is not clear that a human therapist could provide the same experience unaided. Second, even if the only benefit of robot therapy arose from the added movements, repetition is the forté of robotics; the number of movements provided by the robot (over 1000 moves in one session and more than 20 000 moves over the complete program) far exceeds any dosage that might reasonably be administered by a human therapist.

There remains the question why added movements help. Our clinical studies afford some insight into probable biological mechanisms.

Specificity versus generalization

Table 23.1 presents the composite results of two trials with 76 acute-phase inpatients (initial study with 20 patients, replication study with 56 patients).

All measures show a trend favoring the robot-treated group; it reaches statistical significance in the Motor Status score for shoulder and elbow and the Motor Power score but not in the Fugl–Meyer score and Motor Status score for wrist and fingers. Different results with different measures might be attributed to differences in their resolution (Krebs *et al.*, 2002) and in what they measure; for example, the Fugl–Meyer score measures motor behavior most sensitively from the acute injury to a point when the limb is developing tone and reflex changes and synergy but it may lose resolution thereafter. For that reason the Motor Status Scale was developed (Aisen *et al.*, 1995, 1996). Based on the Fugl–Meyer measures, it focuses motor

Table 23.1 Change during acute rehabilitation in patients treated with robot therapy or standard therapy

Group	Score change			
	F-M (out of 66)	MP (out of 20)	MS1 (out of 40)	MS2 (out of 42)
Robot therapy (*n* = 40)	9.25 ± 1.36	3.99 ± 0.43[*]	8.15 ± 0.79[*]	4.16 ± 1.16
Standard therapy (*n* = 36)	7.1 ± 1.20	2.0 ± 0.32	3.42 ± 0.62	2.64 ± 0.78

[a] From admission to rehabilitation hospital to discharge.
[*] Statistical signifigance for a one-way *t*-test that robot therapy score change is greater than that with standard therapy at $P < 0.05$.
F-M, Fugl–Meyer; MP, Motor Power score; MS1, Motor Status score for shoulder and elbow; MS2, Motor Status score for wrist and fingers.

analysis on the shoulder, elbow, wrist, and fingers. Recent work has confirmed the inter-rater reliability and criterion validity of this measure (Ferraro *et al.*, 2002).

The most telling and meaningful difference is between the two Motor Status scores. The statistical significance of the scores for shoulder and elbow demonstrates that (unlike the Fugl–Meyer score) this instrument is capable of detecting a significant advantage of robot therapy in these areas. Despite that fact, the same instrument applied to the wrist and fingers showed no significant difference between experimental and control groups. This difference in results was almost certainly a consequence of the initial experiments with robot therapy exercising the shoulder and elbow but not the wrist and fingers.

The benefits of sensory–motor training administered by robots (and perhaps by clinicians too) are specific to the muscle groups or limb segments exercised and do not generalize broadly. Because specificity is a distinctive characteristic of motor learning, these results are consistent with the proposal that recovery depends on an underlying neural plasticity, perhaps similar to motor learning in infants and adults.

Activity-dependent neural plasticity

The biology underlying recovery after stroke is not known. Candidate mechanisms include recovery of undamaged brain from functional inactivation caused by the damage, activation of undamaged regions of brain in the opposite hemisphere, and reorganization of synaptic connections. Recent results suggest that some recovery of function depends on the post-injury experience; plasticity or reorganizational potential is enhanced by activity. Several groups have described results from functional imaging of the brain in patients recovered from stroke (Cramer *et al.*, 2000, 2001; Miyai *et al.*, 2002). There was increased blood flow in areas around the lesion, in supplemental and premotor cortex, and in ipsilateral motor cortex. In patients recovering from stroke, other work tested the effect of enhanced treatment for the paralyzed arm using sequential positron emission tomography images performed while patients had their affected limb passively moved (Nelles *et al.*, 2001). Increased regional activation was also observed in a functional magnetic resonance imaging task in patients recovering from stroke (Marshall *et al.*, 2000).

Work with animal models has also indicated that training enhances recovery after central nervous system damage. Animals with focal cortical injury exposed to enriched or challenging sensory–motor environments registered greater anatomical responses. Other experiments in animals, in which highly practiced motor tasks were interrupted by specific focal brain injury, demonstrated that the motor-impaired animals exposed to early enhanced sensory–motor training had improved functional outcome (Nudo *et al.*, 1996; Schallert *et al.*, 1997; Plautz *et al.*, 2000).

The combination of clinical and animal studies indicates that repetitive exercise enhances or guides a neuroplastic recovery process after brain injury. If the process resembles motor learning, the most effective exercise will be a time-correlated sensory and motor stimulation of precisely the kind delivered by interactive robot therapy.

Influence of lesion anatomy

Another important practical consideration is which patients will benefit from robot therapy. Given the variability of brain lesions that result from stroke, we should expect a strong influence of lesion size and location.

Effect on recovery time course

We have studied whether differences in lesion anatomy affected response to therapy. We found a significant difference in the time course of recovery: patients with basal ganglia lesions improved much more slowly at first but subsequently their recovery accelerated (Krebs *et al.*, 2000) Figure 23.2 and Table 23.2 compare therapy outcomes for five patients with lesions confined to basal ganglia corpus striatum against six patients with much larger lesions that involved both the basal ganglia and cortical territories. Both groups of patients had comparable demographics and were evaluated by the same therapist on hospital admission (19 ± 2 days post-stroke), at discharge (33 ± 3 days later), and at follow-up (1002 ± 56 days after discharge). The patients with stroke confined to the basal ganglia had smaller lesion size than the basal ganglia plus cortical lesions ($13.3 \pm 3.9\,\mathrm{cm}^3$, $95.1 \pm 25.2\,\mathrm{cm}^3$, $P < 0.05$).

Patients with lesions including the cortex responded better to inpatient rehabilitation than patients with basal ganglia strokes even though the latter had smaller

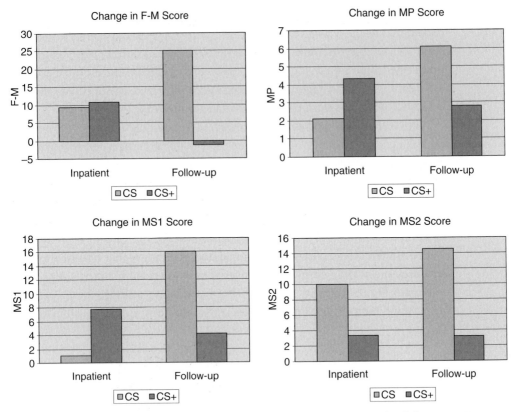

Fig. 23.2   Effect of lesion territory on change during acute rehabilitation and at follow-up. F-M,
Fugl–Meyer score; MP, Motor Power; MS1, Motor Status for shoulder and elbow; MS2, Motor
Status for wrist and fingers; CS, basal ganglia corpus striatum; CS+, basal ganglia plus cortex.

lesions ($\Delta 1$ in Table 23.2 and the left side of each part in Fig. 23.2). However, between
discharge and follow-up, the picture was reversed: patients with basal ganglia strokes
outperformed patients with strokes including the cortex ($\Delta 2$ in Table 23.2 and the
right side of each part in Fig. 23.2). In fact, comparing the total change from
admission to follow-up ($\Delta 3$ in Table 23.2), the patients with only basal ganglia
lesions exhibited greater overall improvement.

Effect on robot therapy benefits

An even more important question is whether lesion anatomy determines the
effectiveness of robot therapy. Figure 23.3 presents an analysis of the Motor
Power scores of 33 patients with middle cerebral artery strokes. In 14 of these
patients the lesions involved the pre-motor area; in 19 patients the pre-motor area
was spared. The top panel of Fig. 23.3 shows that patients with pre-motor
involvement fared more poorly overall, with lower scores at admission and at

Table 23.2 Effect of lesion territory on change during acute rehabilitation and at follow-up

Group	F-M (out of 66)[a]			MP (out of 20)[a]			MS1 (out of 40)[a]			MS2 (out of 42)[a]		
	Δ 1	Δ 2	Δ 3	Δ 1	Δ 2	Δ 3	Δ 1	Δ 2	Δ 3	Δ 1	Δ 2	Δ 3
Basal ganglia corpus stmatum ($n = 5$)	9.3	25.0*	34.3*	2.1	6.1	8.2	1.0	16.0*	17.0*	10.0	14.5*	24.5*
Basal ganglia and cortex ($n = 6$)	10.7	−1.3	9.4	4.3	2.8	7.1	7.7	4.2	11.9	3.3	3.2	6.5

[a] Score changes: Δ1, score change from rehabilitation hospital admission to discharge; Δ2, score change from discharge to follow-up; Δ3, score change from admission to follow-up.
* Statistically significant at $P < 0.05$ by one-way t-test for score with basal ganglia corpus striatum lesion only being greater than the score for the larger basal ganglia plus cortex lesions.

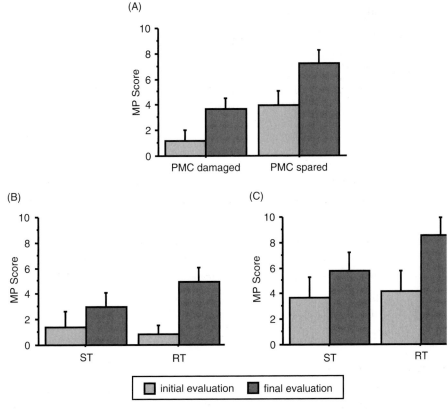

Fig. 23.3   Interaction of robot training with lesion type. Patients had middle cerebral artery strokes affecting the pre-motor area (PMC) or sparing it. The initial and final evaluations by the Motor Power (MP) scale are shown with standard CMOIS. (A) Overall performance for the two groups. (A) Comparison of standard treatment (ST) and robot therapy (RT) for the group with damage PMC. (C) Comparison of ST and RT for the group with PMC spared any damage.

discharge. However, further analysis to compare patients receiving robot therapy or standard therapy showed a clear trend: patients who received robot therapy improved more than those who did not, independent of the status of the pre-motor area.

Because of the modest sample size, these results should not be over-interpreted, but their implications are clear: as expected, lesion anatomy is a critical factor determining a patient's final outcome but it does not mitigate the advantages of robot therapy

Robotic measures

One of the most enticing promises of robotics for stroke recovery is that it allows high-precision measurements and information processing (at a minimum of that required for a computer to control the machine), which should provide objective, reliable, and possibly continual assessment of a patient's performance. The robots used in our studies are equipped to measure robot motions and also six independent forces and moments exerted by the patient (or applied to the patient); they typically sample these sensors hundreds to thousands of times per second. However, the technology challenge is not how to acquire data, but rather how to extract clinically useful knowledge from it.

Force

To obtain quantitative *robotic* measures of upper extremity impairment and recovery we measured the patient's ability to exert force in different directions at a fixed posture and to maintain a posture while the robot tried to move the arm (Krebs et al., 2002). These measures were combined into a single number as follows:

$$MP_{robot} = 8.313 + (6.866 \times \log_{10} Meanforce) - (158.882 \times holdradius)$$

where *Meanforce* is measured in newtons and is given by

$$\frac{1}{4} \left(\sum peakforce(Abduction + Adduction + Flexion + Extension) \right)$$

This is a measure of how well the patient can push in different directions.

Holdradius is measured in meters and is given by

$$\frac{1}{N} \sqrt{\sum_{i=1}^{N} (x_i^2 + y_i^2)}$$

where N is number of samples. Holdradius is a measure of how well the patient can hold a pose (x_i and y_i are displacements of the hand from a nominal pose in two directions).

This measure proved to be closely related to the widely used Motor Power scale. In a study of 48 patients, we found a correlation of almost 90% (Pearson's correlation coefficient $r = 0.895$) between the measures acquired by the clinician and by the robot. Procedures such as these take full advantage of the robot's unmatched objectivity, repeatability, and precision, yet they produce a simple number (MP_{robot}) that is meaningful to the clinician.

Note in passing that this interactive procedure – it may be visualized as a form of "arm-wrestling" between patient and robot – is a unique capability of the controllable-impedance robot designs that we advocate (see below). Using conventional high-impedance, motion-controlled robots, this would be difficult or impossible.

Motion

To take full advantage of robotic, measurement and computational technologies, it is important to study and understand the biology of movement control. Here, robotic tools may afford deeper insights. Our initial studies provided a detailed kinematic (time and motion) record of arm movements made by patients as they recover. Analysis of robot-acquired kinematic data revealed a striking feature of stroke patients' recovery: the earliest recovered movements are fragmented or broken, composed of a sequence of submovements. These submovements are remarkably stereotyped, exhibiting the same "signature" speed profile in all stroke patients (and one patient with myoclonus) for movement speeds ranging over two orders of magnitude: 0.02–1.0 m/s (Krebs et al., 1999). Further, as recovery progressed, these submovements became less obvious, more blended, and overlapped (Fig. 23.4).

We subsequently studied the arm movements of a further 31 stroke patients (12 acute and 19 chronic). We found that although movement smoothness generally improved with recovery, the interpretation of kinematic measures required considerable care; the best measure of smoothness showed a *decline* during inpatient treatment but *increased* during outpatient treatment (Rohrer et al., 2002a). This paradox was serendipitous; we were also able to show that this counter-intuitive result is a prediction of our theory that natural movements are produced as a string of submovements (like the composition of words into a sentence).

This suggests that a computer algorithm which could reliably identify and quantify submovements from continuous kinematic records would be a powerful tool to inform studies of recovery. However, this turned out to be extremely challenging, as the problem is "ill-posed" (in the mathematical sense that multiple spurious solutions exist). Nevertheless, we have recently developed a successful algorithm, verified its reliability, and used it to study how stroke patients recover (Rohrer et al., 2002a, b).

We analyzed the submovement characteristics of our 31 stroke patients. With changes considered significant at $P < 0.05$, we found that as recovery proceeds several changes occur.

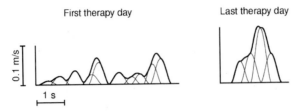

Fig. 23.4   Speed profiles of a single reaching movement made by a patient at the beginning and end of robot therapy. The heavy lines show observed speed; the light lines show underlying submovements.

1. The number of submovements used to reach declines. This implies greater reliability in producing movement and/or less need for corrections.
2. Individual submovements become larger. Both duration and speed increase; hence greater distance is traveled in each submovement. This indicates patients' growing confidence as well as movement vigor.
3. Submovements merge together and overlap in time. Later submovements begin while ongoing submovements are in progress. This implies improved coordination and convergence to normal function.
4. The inter-peak interval (time between adjacent submovement peaks) decreased for patients at the acute stage but not for chronic stages. This is consistent with a process of recovery that is made up of relearning two distinct maps, which has been postulated to underlie normal motor learning. It suggests that the forward map (which serves to predict movement consequences from sensory data) is refined earlier (Rohrer *et al.*, 2002b).

These observations – especially the last – add to the emerging picture that recovery is based on a biological substrate of activity-dependent neural plasticity and exhibits characteristics similar to motor learning.

Submovement analysis of robot-acquired movement data affords entirely new measures that may complement existing clinical instruments. In particular, the degree of blending of submovements promises to capture the important but hitherto intuitive sense of movement *quality* in a rigorous, quantitative manner

Technology challenges

Our experience to date (corroborated broadly by the work of many others not cited here) confirms the value of robot technology to assist recovery after stroke. However, it should be recognized that this robotic application is particularly challenging. To be effective, the robot should be capable of generating large forces; for example, the robot may be used to overcome abnormal muscle tone or spasticity. It should also be capable of moving about as fast as an unimpaired human (or faster). Together these dictate a capacity quite sufficient to cause injury. For example, industrial robots of similar capacity are typically turned off for safety reasons if a human is detected anywhere within the robot's reach.

Safety is, naturally, of paramount importance; the robot must not generate uncommanded forces or motions (or must turn off safely before that occurs), but this is not sufficient. For application to physiotherapy, the robot must operate in close physical contact with patients. As outlined below, physical interaction engenders its own unique problems for the robot controller; in addition, physiotherapy patients may be frail or elderly, with compromised sensory and neuromuscular function. Stroke patients may be especially vulnerable; joint pain and shoulder–hand syndrome are common after stroke and may be exacerbated if exercises are performed incorrectly. Therapy robots must be *gentle*.

It is also important for the robot not to suppress desirable movements made by a recovering patient. While in some stages of treatment it may be advantageous for the robot to offer resistance, in others the robot must be able to "get out of the way," to allow the patient to express appropriate motions, however weak they may be. The ability to get out of the way is *essential* for uncorrupted measurement of the patient's performance. Otherwise, movements made with the robot may give a distorted picture of the patient's ability and informative details may be masked. Therapy robots should have *low impedance*.

Impedance control

Our response to these technical challenges is to use impedance control (Hogan, 1980, 1985). Partly inspired by studies of biological motor control, the basic idea is straightforward: rather than design a robot's controller to regulate its motion or the force it exerts, design it to regulate and modulate the relation between force and motion. The relation between force and motion is rigorously defined by mechanical impedance (which may be considered a dynamic extension of stiffness) and determines what the robot feels like.

As with all controller design, this goal is an ideal; in practice, it can only be approximated to a degree that depends on a wealth of details: the robot's mechanical structure, actuators, sensors, controller bandwidth, control algorithm, modeling uncertainties, and so forth. Notwithstanding its inevitable imperfections, controlling impedance (or admittance, its inverse) has proven to be practical and effective, especially for tasks requiring physical contact and interaction. Example applications have been demonstrated in several industries: automotive (assembly of complex powertrain components; Newman *et al.*, 1999a,b), food packaging (fitting a delicate, compliant lid to a food container and sealing it; de Krijger *et al.*, 1997), construction (autonomous control of an excavator; Ha *et al.*, 2000), and more.

Contact stability

One of the surprising challenges is the problem of contact instability. Mechanical interaction between a robot and an object (both of which are stable and well behaved when not in contact) can induce pathological, unstable behavior that can be violent and destructive. One effective solution to this problem was identified by focusing on a property of the (controlled) robot that is invariant under contact with objects – that is, its impedance. The force exerted or motion achieved by a robot is fundamentally sensitive to object contact, but the robot's impedance properties are not; they describe the relation between force and motion that the robot presents to *any* object it encounters. Colgate & Hogan (1988) showed that constraining a robot's impedance to be *passive* provides robust stability properties.

With this condition, the stability of a robot is indifferent to contact with a large class of objects, even if their dynamic behavior is (almost) completely unknown. This substantially simplifies the problems of coordination between two or more robots, because each robot need not have a detailed model of the dynamics of the others. Schneider & Cannon (1992) have presented an elegant demonstration of impedance control as a platform for cooperative control.

Robot–human interaction

Once a robot is capable of stable interaction with another manipulator about which it has little knowledge, interaction with a human is a natural extension. Physical cooperation between impedance-controlled robots and humans has been demonstrated (Kosuge *et al.*, 1997, 2000). Robotic physiotherapy is another application that requires interaction and cooperation between robot and human; it is a natural application for impedance control. It enables the robot to cooperate with both the patient and a human therapist at the same time, should that be desirable.

The range of robot impedances can be chosen to approximate (however crudely) a human-like feeling. Most important, impedance control enables a *gentle* robot behavior. Throughout our clinical studies we have found no statistically significant difference in the incidence of common side-effects of therapy (joint pain and shoulder–hand syndrome) between patients who received robot therapy and those who did not (in fact, we consistently observed a trend to a *lower* incidence in the robot-treated patients); robot therapy evokes no more side-effects than conventional therapy. We believe this is because of the low impedance of our therapy robot, which makes the robot "gentle" in the sense that it yields easily when pushed – it can "get out of the way" as needed.

In consequence, because we have demonstrated an unequivocal positive benefit (however modest) with no increase in undesirable side-effects, robot treatment of stroke is now available as part of the treatment options for stroke patients at the Burke Rehabilitation Hospital.

Limitations of industrial robots

One important engineering subtlety is that a robot's mechanical design profoundly limits its achievable impedances. It might seem reasonable to reconfigure an industrial robot for application to therapy (and several groups have taken this approach), but most industrial robots are designed for motion control and are not "back-drivable": when pushed they yield poorly or not at all. To compensate and achieve the compliant (low-impedance) behavior appropriate for therapy, active-force feedback control may be used. Unfortunately, reducing impedance using active-force feedback is extremely vulnerable to contact instability. Over 20 years of experience with industrial robots has shown that non-back-drivable robots cannot practically achieve the low impedance appropriate to control interaction.

It is no coincidence that commercially available systems that interact physically with humans are low-impedance designs (e.g. the Phantom haptic interface from Sensable Technologies; the daVinci system for robotic endoscopic surgery from Intuitive Solutions). To work effectively with humans, robots should exhibit low, human-like impedance. While this can present a challenging engineering design problem, back drivability is critical to ensure robot stability, to allow uncorrupted measurements, and to facilitate interactive goal-directed therapy. It is a prominent feature of all the robot modules we have designed to assist recovery following stroke.

Summary

Experience to date warrants at least a cautious optimism about the future impact of technology (and robotics in particular) on recovery after stroke. There is unequivocal evidence that robotic therapy significantly enhances the return of voluntary motion; furthermore, the benefits last. While the effects reported above are modest (about a 10% impairment reduction for inpatients, 5% for outpatients), they are the result of a limited initial form of robot therapy focused on planar reaching motions that primarily involve the elbow and shoulder. It seems reasonable to expect that robot therapy focused on other limbs and functions will yield further improvements.

Equally important, an understanding of the biological basis of recovery has begun to emerge. Though as yet unproven, it offers a plausible account of how and why robot therapy works – by structuring sensory and motor stimuli so that a postulated neuroplastic process of recovery converges to functional patterns of motor behavior.

If structuring sensory and motor stimuli is important for recovery, there is plenty of room for improvement. The approaches taken in the work described above are rudimentary and give the merest hint of the vast potential of robotics and information technologies to assist and optimize recovery after stroke.

ACKNOWLEDGEMENTS

Work reported here was supported in part by the Burke Medical Research Institute, the National Institutes of Health under grants R01-HD37397, R01-HD36827, and F32-HD41795 (S. Fasoli), and a National Science Foundation fellowship (B. Rohrer).

REFERENCES

Aisen, M. L., Sevilla, D., Gibson, G., *et al.* (1995). 3,4-Diaminopyridine as a treatment for amyotrophic lateral sclerosis. *J Neurol Sci* **129**: 21–24

Aisen, M. L., Sevilla, D., Edelstein, L., and Blass, J. (1996). A double-blind placebo-controlled study of 3,4-diaminopyridine in amytrophic lateral sclerosis patients on a rehabilitation unit *J Neurol Sci* **138**: 93–96.

Aisen, M. L., Krebs, H. I., Hogan, N., McDowell, F., and Volpe, B. T. (1997). The effect of robot assisted therapy and rehabilitative training on motor recovery following stroke. *Arch Neurol* **54**: 443–446.

Broderick, J., Brott, T., Kothari, R., *et al.* (1998). The Greater Cincinnati/Northern Kentucky Stroke Study: preliminary first-ever and total incidence rates of stroke among blacks. *Stroke* **29**: 415–421.

Colgate, J. E. and Hogan, N. (1988). Robust control of dynamically interacting systems. *Int J Control* **48**: 65–88

Cramer, S. C., Moore, C. I., Finklestein, S. P., and Rosen, B. R. (2000). A pilot study of somatotopic mapping after cortical infarct. *Stroke* **31**: 668–671.

Cramer, S. C., Nelles, G., Schaechter, J. D., *et al.* (2001). A functional MRI study of three motor tasks in the evaluation of stroke recovery. *Neurorehabil Neural Repair* **15**: 1–8.

de Krijger, M. J., van Luenen, W. T. C., Pedersen, S. T., and Stramigioli, S. (1997). Reliable assembly of products using an impedance controlled manipulator. *In American Control Conference*, Albuquerque, New Mexico, pp. 2977–2981.

Fasoli, S. E., Krebs, H. I., Stein, J., *et al.* (2002). Effects of robotic therapy on upper limb motor impairments in chronic stroke. *Stroke* **33**: 350–351.

Fasoli, S. D., Krebs, H. I., Stein, J., Frontera, W. R., and Hogan, N. (2003). Effects of robotic therapy on motor impairment and recovery in chronic stroke. *Arch Phys Med Rehabil* **84**: 477–482.

Ferraro, M., Demaio, J. H., Krol, J., *et al.* (2002). Assessing the Motor Status score: a scale for the evaluation of upper limb motor outcomes in patients after stroke. *Neurorehabil Neural Repair* **16**: 301–307.

Gresham, G. E., Phillips, T. F., Wolf, P. A., *et al.* (1979). Epidemiologic profile of long term disability in stroke: the Framingham Study. *Arch Phys Med Rehab* **60**: 487–491.

Ha, Q. P., Nguyen, Q. H., Rye, D. C., and Durrant-Whyte, H. F. (2000). Impedance control of a hydraulically actuated robotic excavator. *Automation in Construction* **9**: 421–435.

Hogan, N. (1980). Mechanical impedance control in assistive devices and manipulators. *Proceedings of the 19th IEEE Joint Automatic Controls Conference,* San Francisco, vol. **1**, paper TA-10-B.

(1985). Impedance control: an approach to manipulation. *Am Soc Mech Eng J* **107**: 1–24.

Hogan, N., Krebs, H. I., Sharon, A., Charnnarong, J. (1995) Interactive robotic therapist. US Patent 5, 466, 213.

Kosuge, K., Oosumi, T., and Seki, H. (1997). Decentralized control of multiple manipulators handling an object in coordination based on impedance control of each arm. In *Proceedings of the IEEE/RSJ International Conference on Intelligent Robots and Systems,* Grenoble, pp. 17–22.

Kosuge, K., Sato, M., and Kazamura, N. (2000). Mobile robot helper. *In Proceedings of the IEEE International Conference on Robotics and Automation* San Francisco, pp. 583–588.

Krebs, H. I., Hogan, N., Aisen, M. L., and Volpe, B. T. (1998). Robot-aided neuro-rehabilitation, *IEEE Trans Rehabil Eng* **6**: 75–87.

Krebs, H. I., Hogan, N., Aisen, M. L., and Volpe, B. T. (1999) Quantization of continuous arm movement in humans with brain injury. *Proceedings of the National Academy of Sciences* **96**: 4645–4649.

Krebs, H. I., Volpe, B. T., Aisen, M. L., and Hogan, N. (2000). Increasing productivity and quality of care: robot-aided neurorehabilitation. *VA J Rehabil Res Dev* **37**: 639–652.

Krebs, H. I., Volpe, B. T., Ferraro, M., *et al.* (2002). Robot-aided neuro-rehabilitation: from evidence-based to science-based rehabilitation. *Top Stroke Rehabil* **8**: 54–70.

Marshall, R. S., Perera, G. M., Lazar, R. M., *et al.* (2000). Evolution of cortical activation during recovery from corticospinal tract infarction. *Stroke* **31**: 656–661.

Miyai, I., Suzuki, T., Mikami, A., Kubota, K., and Volpe, B. T. (2002). Functional MRI demonstrates persistent regional premotor cortex activation in patients with pure motor stroke and Wallerian degeneration. *J Stroke Cerebrovasc Dis*

Muntner, P., Garrett, E., Klag, M. J., and Coresh, J. (2002). Trends in stroke prevalence between 1973 and 1991 in the US population 25 to 74 years of age. *Stroke* **33**: 1209–1213.

Nelles, G., Jentzen, W., Jueptner, M., Muller, S., and Diener, H. C. (2001). Arm training induced brain plasticity in stroke studied with serial positron emission tomography. *Neuroimage* **13**: 1146–1154.

Newman, W. S., Branicky, M. S., Podgurski, H. A., *et al.* (1999a). Force-responsive robotic assembly of transmission components. In *Proceedings of the IEEE Internation Conference on Robotics and Automation,* San Francisco, **3**, pp. 2096–2102.

Newman, W. S., *et al.* (1999b). Impedance based assembly. In *Proceedings of the IEEE International on Robotics and Automation,* video proceedings.

Nudo, R. J., Milliken, G. W., Jenkins, W. M., and Merzenich, M. M. (1996). Use-dependent alterations of movement representations in primary motor cortex of adult squirrel monkeys. *J Neurosci* **16**: 785–807.

Plautz, E. J., Milliken, G. W., and Nudo, R. J. (2000). Effects of repetitive motor training on movement representations in adult squirrel monkeys: role of use versus learning. *Neurobiol Learn Mem* **74**: 27–55.

Rohrer, B. R., Fasoli, S., Krebs, H. I., *et al.* (2002a). Movement smoothness changes during stroke recovery. *J Neurosci* **22**: 8297–8304.

Rohrer, B. T., Krebs, H. I., Volpe, B., *et al.* (2002b). Patterns in stroke patient's submovements support a paired adaptive forward/inverse learning model. [Computational motor control symposium.] In *Society for Neuroscience Annual Meeting.*

Schallert, T., Kozlowski, D. A., Humm, J. L., and Cocke, R. R. (1997). Use-dependent structural events in recovery of function. *Adv Neurol* **73**: 229–238.

Schneider, S. A., and Cannon, R. H. (1992). Object impedance control for coordinated manipulation: theory and experiment. *IEEE Trans Robotics and Automation* **8**: 383–394.

Verburg, G., Kwee, H., Wisaksana, A., Cheetham, A., and van Woerden, J. (1996). Manus: the evolution of an assistive technology. *Tech Disabil* **5**: 217–228.

Volpe, B. T., Krebs, H. I., Hogan, N., *et al.* (1999). Robot training enhanced motor outcome in patients with stroke maintained over three years. *Neurology* **53**: 1874–1876.

(2000). A novel approach to stroke rehabilitation: robot-aided sensorimotor stimulation. *Neurology* **54**: 1938–1944.

(2001). Is robot aided sensori-motor training in stroke rehabilitation a realistic option? *Curr Opin Neurol* **14**: 745–752.

Volpe, B. T., Ferraro, M., Krebs, H. I., and Hogan, N. (2002). Robotics in the rehabilitation treatment of patients with stroke. In *Current Atherosclerosis Reports*, vol. 4, ed. A. M. Gotto, Jr., and J. P. Blass. Philadelphia, PA: Current Science, Inc.

24

Vocational rehabilitation

Ashish S. Macaden

Hunters Moor Regional Neurorehabilitation Centre, Newcastle upon Tyne, UK

Introduction

This chapter will discuss the principles, process, and practice of vocational rehabilitation in stroke. The definition of vocational rehabilitation is introduced
because this has implication on the width of its endeavour.

The word vocation is often used to specify a profession or trade. But vocation
also means choice of a life's career and a predisposition to a particular calling.
Vocational rehabilitation is, therefore, more than just getting a person back to
work. It is integrally woven into an attempt to bring back choices into a person's
life. It often is the person's way back to his or her calling and life work. It is a route
for a person with disability to gain back a right to give to society.

Vocational rehabilitation is defined as the attempt to maximize vocational
potential and function. Rehabilitation is an approach to maximize physical,
psychological, and social function of people with disability. There are three levels
at which rehabilitation attempts to maximize function: impairment, activity
(disability) and participation (handicap). Rehabilitation attempts to:

- alleviate impairment or actual loss of function
- improve activity that has been restricted by the impairment (i.e. it attempts to
  reduce disability)
- enable participation in a social role unfulfilled as a result of disability (i.e. it
  attempts to reduce handicap).

Vocational rehabilitation would need to address vocational needs at the three
levels of impairment, activity, and participation.

The discussion will draw on evidence from research on vocational rehabilitation
in traumatic brain injury as there is little published on stroke. There is a reasonable
amount of information available from similar, relevant research in traumatic
brain injury. It could be argued that brain injury following stroke is different
from brain injury following trauma. Comparatively, people with stroke might have
more focal and less-diffuse frontotemporal injury, resulting in fewer cognitive and

Recovery after Stroke, ed. Michael P. Barnes, Bruce H. Dobkin and Julien Bogousslavsky. Published by Cambridge University Press. © Cambridge University Press 2005.

more motor sequelae. In addition, people with stroke are generally older, closer to retirement, and would, therefore, face different expectations surrounding their return to work at full capacity. However, the causative factors and sequelae are similar in any brain injury and vocational rehabilitation programs talk about "acquired brain injury" and include both groups in their programs. Consequently, evidence will be drawn from research on vocational rehabilitation in traumatic brain injury.

Do those with stroke need vocational rehabilitation?

There is a small group of people with stroke who are affected during their vocational lives and need to maximize residual vocational potentials. In 1975, a Swedish study estimated the size of this group to be approximately 28 per 100 000. It also estimated that approximately 4–5 per 100 000 could be actively reemployed (Fugl-Meyer et al., 1975). Approximately 15–20% of all people with stroke are of working age; approximately 41% return to work and 21% try and fail to return to work (Heinemann et al., 1987; Vestling et al., 2003). Therefore, there is obviously a group of people with stroke who would need vocational rehabilitation. In addition, though the size of this group may be small, as the age of retirement increases, the numbers of people with stroke who are still working will obviously increase (Wozniak et al., 1999). Consequently, the numbers with stroke needing to return to their vocations is going to increase.

Principles of vocational rehabilitation

Basis in a partnership model

In a broad sense, the available models of rehabilitation are the medical and social models. The medical model of vocational rehabilitation focuses on addressing the difficulties in the person with disability while the social model focuses on addressing the social aspects creating difficulties for the person with disability. As in other areas of rehabilitation, the World Health Organization (WHO) suggest that both models will need to work together using a "biopsychosocial" approach in order to get people with stroke back to work (WHO, 2001). This has been called the partnership model (Barnes and Ward, 2000).

Requirement for personal empowerment

One of the principles of rehabilitation is empowerment. This means that the power and control of decisions are handed over to the person with disability. This is especially important in vocational rehabilitation as empowerment can positively influence motivation. When choosing life's career or deciding on a calling, the long-term results are always better when the individual has the freedom to choose from the options that the vocational rehabilitation program lays out (Brooke *et al.*, 2003).

Requirement for continuing support

Traditional vocational rehabilitation approaches have been limited to preplacement evaluations and interventions based on these evaluations. Both evaluation and interventions were provided in medical settings and their effects were expected to be transferred or generalized to real-life situations at work. These traditional services were generally provided by adult day centers, sheltered workshops, or segregated institutions (Fraser *et al.*, 1997). Not surprisingly, these approaches have reported disappointing results. Return to work was less than 40% in a day-care program (Haffey and Abrams, 1991) and averaged in the range 20–50% (Ip *et al.*, 1995; Greenspan *et al.*, 1996; Sander *et al.*, 1996; Cattelani *et al.*, 2002).

However, in the 1980s, two vocational program models evolved: the work reentry program (Haffey and Abrams, 1991) and the supported employment program (Wehman *et al.*, 1990). The basic principle of both was to provide continuing support. These programs, like their older counterparts, provided preplacement support and evaluation. However, in addition, they began to guide clients through specific job situations in actual work environments with the help of a "job coach." The programs continued follow-up and support, even after actual employment, through the job coaches. In addition the job coaches were involved in developing natural supports in the workplace; coworkers became mentors and technological supports were brought into the workplace to enable employment to be sustained. Both the work reentry program and the supported employment program are very similar in approach and results and, therefore, no attempt is made to differentiate between them. Not surprisingly, their results are superior to previous approaches. The supported employment approach has resulted in an encouraging return to work of 77% (Dean *et al.*, 2003). The work reentry program reports a 71% employment retention rate (Haffey and Abrams, 1991), resulting in increased governmental support. It has been felt that rehabilitation stopped too early. After stroke, people felt unprepared and wished for continued vocational rehabilitation support (Lock *et al.*, 2005).

Guiding values in vocational rehabilitation

The partnership model of vocational rehabilitation will need to address the needs of the individual as well as societal responses. This means that a common set of guiding values need to be identified that help in setting the goals of a vocational rehabilitation program.

The Department of Physical Medicine and Rehabilitation of the Medical School of the University of Virginia were instrumental in developing the supported

Table 24.1 Guiding values of a supported employment program

Value	Definition
Presumption of employment	Everyone, regardless of the level or the type of disability, has the capability and right to a job
Competitive employment	Employment occurs within the local labor market in regular community businesses
Control	When people with disabilities choose and regulate their own employment supports and services, career satisfaction will result
Commensurate wages and benefits	People with disabilities should earn wages and benefits equal to those of coworkers performing the same or similar jobs
Focus on capacity and capabilities	People with disabilities should be viewed in terms of their abilities, strengths, and interests rather than their disabilities
Importance of relationships	Community relationships both at and away from work lead to mutual respect and acceptance
Power of supports	People with disabilities need to determine their personal goals and receive assistance in assembling the supports necessary to achieve their ambitions
Systems change	Traditional systems must be changed to ensure customer control, which is vital to the integrity of supported employment
Importance of community	People need to be connected to the formal and informal networks of a community for acceptance, growth, and development

From the program of the Deptment of Physical Medicine and Rehabilitation, Medical School of the University of Virginia, USA (Brooke *et al.*, 2003).

employment program. They now are involved in training and have published an excellent manual that outlines the basics of the program in which they suggest a number of guiding values or principles (Brooke *et al.*, 2003; Table 24.1).

The process of vocational rehabilitation

The description here of the process of rehabilitation is divided into two major sections. The first section deals with the selection process, discussing the factors that are important in successful rehabilitation. The next section deals with the actual phases of a successful program.

Selection: which factors are associated with better return to work?

The list of factors associated with successful return to work is more important from the point of view of providing prognostic information to the client. The factors outlined should not be selection or exclusion criteria to a vocational rehabilitation program. Except for purposes of research, water-tight selection or exclusion criteria in a vocational rehabilitation program can often mislead the team and exclude potential successes.

It must be remembered that these criteria are based on relatively weak statistical evidence and can only shed light on the path; they cannot be the path itself. There have been no randomized control trials as attempts to form control groups have failed. Moreover, more than three quarters of failures in vocational rehabilitation occur for multiple reasons. Existing research reports a very wide variation: the percentage of people with stroke returning to work ranges from 21 to 73% (Wozniak *et al.,* 1999). There is a wide variation in results, probably because research in this field has yet to address the following methodological needs:

- sharper definition of temporal categories (acuteness of stroke)
- standardization of diagnostic categories of stroke
- standardization of vocational rehabilitation approaches
- long-term follow up data.

However weak the existing data, it is important for both the person with disability and the service provider to enter the process of vocational rehabilitation with clear sightedly. There are physical and psychosocial factors associated with success or failure in returning to work.

Physical factors

While most people with stroke returning to work will be younger than 65 years, the probability of returning to work decreases once the stroke survivor is past 55 years of age (Wozniak *et al.,* 1999). A corollary, however, is that individuals with brain injury in their late twenties are more difficult to place than those in their late thirties (Ponsford, 1995).

A higher level of function, as indicated by the Barthel Index, was also positively associated with return to work (Wozniak *et al.,* 1999).

Return to work does not seem to be affected by the extent of physical disability: aphasia level of consciousness and weakness at the time of the stroke, severity of stroke, race, sex, and pre-existing depression did not affect return to work significantly (Howard *et al.,* 1985; Wozniak *et al.,* 1999). There was no difference between right- and left-sided strokes. Neither was there any difference in return to work associated with race or with cortical, infratentorial, or lacunar strokes (Wozniak *et al.,* 1999) though fatigue was reported to be a problem (Lock *et al.,* 2005). However, the absence of either weakness or apraxia was identified as being predictive of return to work (Saeki *et al.,* 1995) as was preserved cognition and ability to walk (Vestling *et al.,* 2003).

Psychosocial factors

The case for psychosocial factors is much stronger than for physical factors.

Type of job
Return to work was shown to be better with white collar jobs rather than blue collar jobs (Howard *et al.,* 1985; Saeki *et al.,* 1995; Vestling *et al.,* 2003). A strong pre-injury work history was a strong predictor of return to work (Heinemann *et al.,* 1987). However, a client returning to a highly skilled job or work reentry at a lower level than the premorbid job are associated with poor outcomes (Heinemann *et al.,* 1987).

Economic disincentives
An income of more that US$30 000 annually was a positive predictor of return to work (Wozniak *et al.,* 1999). The time at which return to work seemed to peak appeared to be associated with the period allowed by social security: around 18 months in a Japanese study (Saeki *et al.,* 1995). It was also noticed that the reason why 6 of 25 clients with brain injury did not return to work was because the disability or compensation incomes were in excess of the potential earned income (Haffey and Abrams, 1991).

Substance abuse
Substance abuse is a strongly negative factor that emerges in almost every study at some point (Abrams *et al.,* 1991; Sale *et al.,* 1991; Ponsford, 1995). In around a third of clients who could not keep their jobs, substance abuse or criminal activity contributed to job separation (Sale *et al.,* 1991). This factor is so important that many vocational programs now exclude those with continuing problems with substance abuse.

Attitude to injury
Clients with a sense of responsibility did much better than those with a sense of victimization regarding the injury (Abrams *et al.,* 1991).

Interpersonal relationships
Factors relating to interpersonal relationships were reported to be responsible for around half of the job separations, including misinterpretation of social cues, interpersonal conflict, and inappropriate verbalization (Sale *et al.,* 1991).

Work-related skills

Skills such as initiating a task without prompting or direction, responding to non-verbal cues, observing safety requirements and using compensatory strategies consistently are important. Their absence makes it difficult for a person to return to work (Fraser *et al.,* 1997).

Family support

Strong family support is a useful predictor of successful return to work (Abrams *et al.,* 1991).

Phases of a supported employment program

The supported employment model would take a client through three phases: initial assessment, job placement, and long-term support and follow-up

Initial assessment

The first phase is the assessment and planning, which is focused on individual work-based skills and environmental opportunities and responses. The neuropsychological, medical, and social abilities of the client are perceived from this viewpoint. While test batteries and specialist scales are useful, none comprehensively discover all the needs or identify all the vocational potentials of a client (Tyerman, 1999a).

The individual's abilities in areas of functional independence, mobility, transfers, transportation, cognition, executive function, behavior, stress management, and safety cannot be assumed but must be tested and observed. Neurobehavioral aspects will be of special importance as motivation, behavior, and interpersonal relationships play an important role in maintaining employment. Abilities will need to be matched with felt needs. After abilities and felt needs are matched, the individual and the team sit down together to agree on goals and time frames. Progress along the agreed pathway will need follow-up and modification depending on the evolving situation.

Once the individual's ability and work-based skills are known, assessments for environmental opportunities will need to be carried out. This includes assessing skills required for the job development processes, for example preparing a resume, business interview skills, and phone conversations, including "cold calls" to employers.

The process of exploring environmental responses will need assessment. This includes identifying potential employers with whom the individual could undertake a placement. The pre-existing organizational marketing infrastructure and community networks of the rehabilitation service provider will come into play here. The employer or organization identified will need a SWOT (strength, weakness, opportunities, threats) analysis specific to the individual whose placement is planned. The rehabilitation service provider markets the individual and the individual's skills to employers within the network. It is often the case that employers actually benefit from the experience as they have work done in an environment of evaluation and support and have the opportunity to continue or stop the experience at the end of six weeks without any financial or legal implications. Assessment of environmental responses will also involve assessment and development of work-related family support.

This process can last for 6 to 12 weeks.

Job placement

The next phase is the placement and training. The job coach plays a central role from this point. Appropriate options are chosen in the light of the assessment and performance and evaluated. This process continues till a satisfactory result is obtained.

There are several models of placement, such as the traditional job clubs or job call lines, selective placement by the agency acting as a broker, the more active agency-generated job site support, and the proactive natural support in the workplace (training a coworker to be a mentor) (Fraser *et al.*, 1997).

During job placement, the assessment continues with job duty analysis both by the individual and by the employer. Assessment and development of natural supports in the work place might need to be supplemented with natural cues or extra cues that (a cue being a feature that would indicate to the individual what to do next). If cues are insufficient, verbal or gestural prompts may need to be introduced. Once cues are successfully instituted, fading of cues or prompts will need assessment. Other compensatory aids like imagery, mnemonics, a reminder notebook or whiteboard, and rehearsals might need to be instituted.

Again this could last anywhere from six weeks to six months.

Job support and long-term follow-up

The final phase is job seeking and continued support. The issue of job stability in brain injury is addressed by continued support at work and retraining when necessary. This support is usually offered for five years, though it might basically be a lifelong process.

Once back at work, persons with brain injury are challenged with being able to sustain a job. With the traditional approaches, 30–50% of those who returned to work could not sustain their jobs (Ip *et al.*, 1995; Greenspan *et al.*, 1996; Sander *et al.*, 1996; Cattelani *et al.*, 2002). Though a significantly larger percentage of people with stroke return to work with the supported employment approach, job stability seems to remain a problem with almost the same proportion of people (around 26%) requiring a second placement (Wehman *et al.*, 1995). Approximately 69% of those with job separations lose their jobs in the first six months (Sale *et al.*, 1991). This is such a common feature on vocational rehabilitation that it has been coined the "return loop syndrome" (Parenté *et al.*, 1991).

The return loop syndrome is characterized by successfully coached clients returning to the vocational program within a five-year period having either left or lost their jobs. The usual reasons for this are multiple and, apart from the factors mentioned above, include:

- upward mobility: after successful return to work and improved self-esteem, the client feels confident of taking up jobs with either increasing demands or poorly matching with their abilities; in addition, they do not put compensatory strategies into place
- change in job duties: a client who is able to stay with a job starts to experience change in environment, demands, managers, or coworkers; these changes cause stress and challenge coping abilities
- loss of support system: as the client becomes more engrossed in the vocational environment and the job coaching contact is slowly withdrawn by the program, contact and support of the peer interaction, therapy sessions, and feedback is lost.

There have been several approaches to prevent the return loop syndrome. The sense of loss of support could be countered by keeping follow-up open ended. The follow-up team could be more flexible and offer more intervention based on appropriate follow-up. This would mean that job coaches would need to be trained in trouble-shooting and crisis management skills (Parenté *et al.*, 1991). Employee assistance programs will need to be developed. Peer interaction sessions could be continued and hopefully these would address more than just vocational needs. Natural supports will need to be developed at the work place. This might include training, supporting, and advising, coworkers or employers to act in a mentors' role to improve job stability.

Putting principles and processes into practice

This section briefly describes some of the approaches used to deliver vocational rehabilitation services.

Provision of internal and external supports

There are various ways of supporting the values of supported employment and these can be broadly classified into internal supports (processes that people with disability train to use themselves) and external supports processes instituted in or on the surrounding environment (Table 24.2; Brooke *et al.*, 2003).

Table 24.2 Provision of internal and external support

Area of need	Internal supports	External supports
Capacity and capabilities	Physical enablement; cognitive enablement (e.g. initiation, dyspraxia, insight); behavioral enablement (e.g. coping skills for anger, stubbornness, consistency)	Education; control of substance abuse
Presumption of employment, competitive employment, control, commensurate wages and benefits	Develop self-image; develop motivation; education on rights, privileges and opportunities	Financial aid; modify level of responsibilities; adapt job environment
Power of supports and systems change		Specific vocational training; compensation; assistive technology; networking
Importance of relationships and importance of community	Positive family support: interdependent rather than dependent or undependable	Social, peer, and employer support; coworker (twinning) support

Customer-driven approach to supported employment

The Virginia University Manual suggests a customer-driven practice to enable the program to remain faithful to its principles (Brooke *et al.*, 2003).

1. Choice: the "customer–client" makes the informed choice, not the service provider.
2. Control: the "customer–employee" is the coordinator of the job with the employer, not the rehabilitation professional.
3. Careers: career development is built into the job and it cannot be assumed that the job obtained will be a dead end.
4. Full inclusion: there should be no discrimination, positive or negative, at the work place.
5. Long-term support: coworkers as much as job coaches can help to sustain employment.

6. Community and business supports: networking.
7. Total quality management: interaction and feedback from the client can improve the rehabilitation program.
8. Assistive technology: environmental engineering (ergonomic placement of commonly used articles, color-coded documents, cue cards at appropriate places), prosthetic memory aids (tele-memo watches, diaries, phones with number memories, dictaphones), and cognitive orthotic devices (spell check or word-finding software) (Parenté *et al.,* 1991).
9. Person-centered planning.

The job coach

The key to putting these principles and processes into practice is the job coach, who is the primary service provider in this approach. The Virginia University group have a fairly broad definition of the job coach, who has alternatively been called trainer advocate, job trainer, supported employment training specialist or employment specialist.

It is obvious that the job coach will need a host of skills deriving from various walks of life: psychology, counselling, education, marketing, and business (Brooke *et al.,* 2003). It might not be possible to find or train one person to fulfill all these functions and, therefore, several roles have been identified that could be fulfilled by one person or by various members of a vocational rehabilitation team. There are five distinct roles that job coaches perform.

1. Planner role: assess the client (customer profiling), assessing various job sites to match them with the client (resource matching), and training the client for interviews (resumes, cards, handling phones) using the person-centered planning approach.
2. Consultant role: provide recommendations to the client to get and keep a job.
3. Head hunter role: organizational marketing (building and maintaining a network of job providers), market and employer surveys, and matching client and job provider using a market-based planning approach.
4. Technician role: provide rehabilitation solutions for problems with transfers, cognitive dysfunction, and other disabilities at the work site. Suggest assistive technologies and develop natural supports at the work site.
5. Community resource role: networking and creative linking; fading from the job site neither too slowly (creates dependence) nor too fast (results in job losses).

Therefore, the function of the job coach would be customer profiling, career development, employment matching, job-site training and support, and provision of long-term support and extended follow-up.

Are vocational rehabilitation models beneficial?

Evaluating the efficacy of the supported employment and work reentry programs with a randomized double–blind control trial has not been possible, primarily because of the ethical difficulties of withholding vocational services to a control group.

However, the viability of modern vocational programs has been supported by cost–benefit analysis studies returned to the government funding agencies. This was done using comparison rather than control groups for 4000 clients in one state in the USA, comparing longitudinal incomes and service costs. The results were encouraging. The economic viability of the supported employment approach has been similarly demonstrated with qualitative and economic variables in small groups (Ponsford, 1995; Dean *et al.*, 2003). One recent 14-year longitudunal study reporting individual earnings of US$175 15 more than the costs associated with the individual's supported employment placement (Wehman *et al.*, 2003). A UK vocational rehabilitation project reported that, if savings in benefits and tax revenues as a result of return to work were calculated, the pay-back period to cover vocational rehabilitation costs was 21.6 months. They reported that, in their project, net savings to the exchequer were accumulating over three years at a rate of £300 per month (Tyerman, 1999b).

The improved percentages of those returning to work with supported employment or work reentry programs are the other soft evidence that vocational rehabilitation programs are beneficial, but there is a need for further, more robust research in this area.

Summary

Vocational rehabilitation would benefit around 15% of those who survive stroke beyond a year. The factors that influence return to work are more psychosocial than physical and, therefore, approaches need to include both medical and social aspects (partnership model). To empower the person with disability, the vocational rehabilitation program needs to be customer driven.

The supported employment and work reentry programs have reported more successful outcomes than previous approaches, probably because they provide continued support. They not only provide initial evaluation and counselling but also continue with ongoing evaluation and advice at job placements and follow-up and support through employment. The role of the job coach is the key to a successful supported employment program. However, people with disability continue to have problems with maintaining stable employment (return loop syndrome). The same factors that affect return to work continue to play a role in poor job stability.

Results are encouraging, with around 70% of clients in supported employment and work reentry programs returning to work, but there are methodological difficulties in obtaining controls for further research. Though largely reported for acquired brain injury in general, rather than stroke in particular, cost–benefit analyses of vocational rehabilitation projects are encouraging and evidenced by further governmental involvement in these programs.

REFERENCES

Abrams, D., Barker, L., Almandsmith, S., and Raffe, S. (1991). Enhancing employment success for individuals with traumatic brain injury. In *Report to Social Security Administration*. San Diego, CA: Sharp Rehabilitation Center, pp. 5–38.

Barnes, M. P. and Ward, A. B., ed. (2000). *Textbook of Rehabilitation Medicine*. Oxford: University Press.

Brooke, V., Inge, K., Armstrong, A., and Wehman, P. (2003). *Supported Employment: A Customer-driven Approach for Persons with Significant Disabilities*. Richmond, VA: Rehabilitation Research and Training Centre, Virginia Commonwealth University.

Cattelani, R., Tanzi, F., Lombardi, F., and Mazzucchi, A. (2002). Competitive reemployment after severe traumatic brain injury. *Brain Injury* **16**: 51–64.

Dean, D. H., Dolan, R. C., and Schmidt, R. M. (2003). A paradigm for evaluation of the Federal–State Vocational Rehabilitation program. *Disability Research Digest*, **vol. 3.** http://www.worksupport.com/main/downloads/dean/paradigmchap1.pdf.

Fraser, R. T., Cook, R., Clemmons, D. C., and Curl, R. H. (1997). Work access in traumatic brain injury rehabilitation. *Phys Med Rehabil Clin N Am*: **8**: 371–387.

Fugl-Meyer, A. R., Jaasko, L., and Norlin, V. (1975). The post stroke hemiplegic patient. II. Incidence, mortality and vocational return in Goteburg, Sweden with a review of literature. *Scand J Rehabil Med* **7**: 73–83.

Greenspan, A. I., Wrigley, J. M., Kresnow, M., Branche-Dorsey, C. M., and Fine, P. R. (1996). Factors influencing failure to return to work due to traumatic brain injury. *Brain Injury* **10**: 207–218.

Haffey, W. J. and Abrams, D. L. (1991). Employment outcomes for participants in a brain injury work reentry program: Preliminary findings. *J Head Trauma Rehabil* **6**: 24–34.

Heinemann, A. W., Roth, E. J., Cichowski, K., and Betts, H. B. (1987). Multivariate analysis of improvement and outcome following stoke rehabilitation. *Arch Neurol* **24**: 1478–1483.

Howard, G., Till, J. S., Matthews, C., Toole, J. F., and Truscott, B. L. (1985). Factors influencing return to work following cerebral infarction. *J Am Med Assoc* **253**: 226–32.

Ip, R. Y., Dornan, J., and Schentag, C. (1995). Traumatic brain injury: factors predicting return to work or school. *Brain Inj* **9**: 517–532.

Lock, S., Jordan, L., Bryan, K., and Maxim, J. (2005). Work after stroke: focusing on barriers and enablers. *Disabil Soc* **20**: 33–47.

Parenté, R., Stapleton, M. C., and Wheatley, C. J. (1991). Practical strategies for vocational reentry after traumatic brain injury. *J Head Trauma Rehabil* **6**: 35–45.

Ponsford, J. (1995). *Traumatic Brain Injury: Rehabilitation for Everyday Adaptive Living*. London: Psychology Press.

Saeki, S., Ogata, H., Okubo, T., Takahash, K., and Hoshuyama, T. (1995). Return to work after stroke: a follow-up study. *Stroke* **26**: 399–401.

Sale, P., West, M., Sherron, P., and Wehman, P. H. (1991). Exploratory analysis of job separations from supported employment for persons with traumatic brain injury. *J Head Trauma Rehabil* **6** : 1–11.

Sander, A. M., Kreutzer, J. S., Rosenthal, M., Delmonica, R., and Young, M. E. (1996). A multicenter longitudinal investigation of return to work and community integration following traumatic brain injury. *J Head Trauma Rehabil* **11**: 70–84.

Tyerman, A. D. (1999a). Outcome measures in a community head injury service. *Neuropsychol Rehabil* **9**: 481–491.

(1999b). *Working Out* [A joint report by the Department of Health and Employment Service Traumatic Brain Injury Vocational Rehabilitation Project and the Community Head Injury Service. Aylesbury.] Aylesbury, UK: Vale of Aylesbury Community Head Injury Service.

Vestling, M., Tufvesson, B., and Iwarsson, S. (2003). Indicators for return to work after stroke and the importance of work for subjective well-being and life satisfaction. *J Rehabil Med* **35**: 127–131.

Wehman, P. H., West, M. D., Kregel, J., Sherron, P. and Kreutzer, J. S. (1995). Return to work for persons with severe traumatic brain injury: a data based approach to program development. *J Head Trauma Rehabil* **10**: 27–39.

Wehman, P. H., Kreutzer, J. S., and West, M. D. (1990). Return to work for persons with traumatic brain injury: a supported employment approach. *Arch Phys Med Rehabil* **71**: 1047–1052.

Wehman, P. H., Kregel, J., Keyser-Marcus, L., *et al.* (2003). Supported employment for persons with traumatic brain injury: a preliminary investigation of long-term follow-up costs and program efficiency. *Arch Phys Med Rehabil* **84**: 192–196.

WHO (2001). *International Classification of Functioning, Disability and Health*. Resolution 54.21 Geneva: World Health Organization.

Wozniak, M. A., Kittner, S. J., Price, T. R., *et al.* (1999). Stroke location is not associated with return to work after first ischemic stroke. *Stroke* **30**: 2568–2573.

25

A patient's perspective

Donal O'Kelly

Different Strokes, Milton Keynes, UK

Introduction

Stroke is commonly seen as an affliction of old age, but it happens to younger people as well. It frequently strikes people in the prime of life, often for no known reason. Not only is it a big killer, along with heart disease, cancer, and respiratory illness, but also it is the largest single cause of severe disability. It happened to me in my early forties and completely changed my life.

Personal story

In June 1993, I was the defending barrister in a burglary case in North London. I was cross-examining a police sergeant about the vigorous arrest he had made of my "entirely innocent client." He'd seen my "entirely innocent client" backing out of someone else's bathroom window and had jumped to the wrong conclusion, as policemen sometimes do. Mid cross-examination I suddenly felt a slight pain in the back of my neck. I paused for a moment, wondering what was happening . . . and then the lights went out! I awoke a few minutes later, horizontal, unable to move and unable to speak. Although I had no idea what was going on, I realized that it must be serious as a para-medic was kneeling beside me trying to reassure me that it wasn't. I was stretchered into an ambulance and taken off to the nearest hospital, an old Victorian workhouse of a place that should have been pulled down years ago. I was borne into casualty still wearing full battle dress – my barrister's outfit, the wig and gown etc. – but I was totally incoherent. My words were slurred and were just not coming out right. I was thus unable to explain the eccentricities of court dress and the hospital staff just assumed that I was a drunken actor. Or maybe a brief on a bender. In any event, I was left in a corner to sleep it off. Soon I felt that slight pain in the back of my neck again and I was suddenly unable to breathe. My limbs were seizing up. The medics gave me some oxygen, which eased my situation, but they took it away after a short while. I passed out again and this time was gone for days.

Recovery after Stroke, ed. Michael P. Barnes, Bruce H. Dobkin and Julien Bogousslavsky. Published by Cambridge University Press. © Cambridge University Press 2005.

I woke later in the week in intensive care. I tried to get out of bed but could not. I was paralyzed on both sides, though feeling returned to my right side within the first few days. I still could not speak and my vision was blurred. Slowly I realized that the doctors who had deprived me of oxygen were trying to kill me. Not only that, but they had murdered most of my family and friends and were planning to finish me off at the earliest opportunity! When I actually saw my family and friends (all alive and well), I realized that I had got it wrong somehow. It was not till much later that I read that paranoia was a frequent symptom following stroke. At the time, however, I remembered the old saying, "Just because you're paranoid, doesn't mean they're not out to get you"; I determined to be vigilant just in case. I was very tired and very confused. It was as though my brain had closed down so that I couldn't take on the enormity of what had happened. Everything was such an effort, but I did not realize how serious my situation was. Later, in the third week, getting from the bed to the wheelchair was difficult, but adventurous and fun; never at that stage did I realize or understand that I might be a wheelchair user for the rest of my life. Even when the physiotherapist solemnly warned my friends that I might never walk again something in my head prevented me from really believing that.

My swallowing mechanism had been badly affected and, after I had nearly choked myself to death, I was tubed up to a drip-feed. In a particularly painful and disgusting procedure, a length of plastic with a bore no wider than a small rocket-launcher was fed up my nose and down into my stomach. Predigested peach gunk of supposedly high nutritional value was slowly leaked into my system. In the following days, when well-wishers arrived bearing grapes and flowers, I would grimace, twitch and inevitably sneeze up the tube. I went though eight tube insertions before hayfever was diagnosed and flowers were banned.

Nobody knew why this had happened to me, and I'm still not clear. I was 43 years old; I was fit, not overweight, a vegetarian; I'd given up smoking and drinking six years previously. My blood pressure was normal and I got plenty of rest and relaxation, and played a bit of sport. The consultant neurologist said that I was not the textbook candidate for a stroke but that an angiogram might provide the answer or at least some clues. The nearest available angiogram machine was in Central London, and if I was willing to pay for the procedure it could be done immediately. I was naive enough to believe that we still had a free health service, so I took my turn and waited six weeks before I could be properly diagnosed. It didn't really matter because as the neurologist said I wasn't going anywhere in a hurry.

Time passed slowly. Three weeks into my recovery, I was wheeled to the gym for physiotherapy. Although you may think that early intensive therapy is essential after a stroke, I was assigned just one session per week initially. It wasn't until a close friend got angry enough to demand more attention that my allocation was bumped up to four times a week. At this stage, I was still emotionally labile – more often laughing uncontrollably, but sometimes weeping inconsolably – and being curtained off because I may have been upsetting the other patients. There wasn't a dedicated stroke unit at the hospital. I was on an old-fashioned general medical ward with over 20 beds and most of the time we kept our spirits up with a mixture of camaraderie and graveyard humor. Much more disturbing than my occasional tears was the man opposite, who would begin to chant his daily prayers at 5 a.m. before even God had a chance to get up! The staff told me that I must not attempt to walk unassisted; one of the nurses would help me. However, the ward was always so pressed for staff that there was never any time to supervise me on walkies. One time I had a phone call. The student nurse who answered it, unthinkingly called out to me to come and get the phone, and for the first time I traversed the length of the ward unaided. None of the staff noticed until the rest of the patients burst into applause as I tottered to the phone.

Whilst the first hospital was solicitous for my welfare and probably over protective, when I got transferred for the angiogram it was a different story. My notes had been lost in transit and staff at the second hospital were not sure what I had been left to do on my own. "The lot" – I assured them – "bath, shower, toilet – leave it to me" and they did. I was able to exploit my new found freedom and before long was staggering about like an old drunk, unsteady, unbalanced, incontinent, but moving and improving. The angiogram eventually got done (despite my sabotaging it on several occasions by having a laughing fit at the critical moment), but I'm still not clear as to the cause of my stroke.

I was discharged from hospital after two months and re-entered the world without having any idea what to expect. As for the physiotherapy that I so obviously needed, I was to visit the local hospital as an outpatient once a week. The Barristers Benevolent Association (a charity run by and for the legal profession) offered to fund a private physiotherapist for me. When I mentioned this to the hospital physiotherapist she went ballistic! She insisted that she be the only one or she would withdraw and I would get no further help from the Health Service. This placed me in something of a dilemma as I knew it was important to get as much skilled assistance as was available, and yet I didn't want to exclude myself from the Health Service. I consulted family and friends as to what I should do – they were unanimous – *lie*! Tell the hospital physiotherapist she was the only one in the world but take advantage of the Barristers Benevolent Association's offer and get as much physiotherapy as I could. In fact, the outpatients department discharged me after three months, content that I could push a supermarket trolley without falling over, while the private physiotherapist continued to work on me for a whole year.

The same with speech therapy. My voice had completely gone and as a barrister I felt this more acutely than most. The hospital voice therapist discharged me when

I could just about croak and make myself understood. However, I sought further assistance privately at the Communications Department of University College London. There I worked with a sympathetic voice trainer for a further 12 months, singing and shouting like a lunatic. Although the hospital staff were very kind, they didn't feel it was necessary or essential for me to walk or talk as I had before. Their low expectation was oppressive. Their goal was a very limited recovery. If I wanted a full recovery, I could do it in my own time and at my own expense.

And expensive it was! I soon exhausted my own savings and had to rely on the charity of the Barrister's Benevolent Association to help me through. Family and friends helped out but essentially I was on my own. The advice and assistance I got from the professional carers was helpful but limited. For instance, nobody wanted to discuss sex or sexual dysfunction. My sexual appetite did not return immediately after the stroke and this caused a few problems. My partner and I eventually found out about an organization that deals specifically with this sort of difficulty and we were able to get some assistance with it. For a long while it was a topic I was encouraged to ignore; apparently I should be grateful to be alive and not be fussing about the finer details! I was only able to get help with this problem because both my partner and I were willing and able to spend the necessary time and money in researching what assistance was available.

I got back into office work five months after the stroke and I was back into court after nine months. I remember being terrified the first time I tried to shuffle down to the court. Everybody was walking so fast and confidently I felt sure I was going to be knocked over. I ended up clinging to a lamppost. It would be another two years before I would feel safe on the streets. I was still emotionally labile and often prone to inappropriate and excessive laughter. One time I was representing the wife in divorce proceedings. I weigh in at just over six foot (2.9 m). Mi'learned friend for the husband was 6′ 8″(3.2 m). Judge Williams, who was to hear the case, is a very pleasant and gentle man and a very good family lawyer, but sadly is vertically challenged. He is about five foot tall (2.4 m). As the judge came into court, my extremely large opponent leaned down to me and whispered, "These little things are sent to try us." I could not stop laughing and eventually had to be led away by the usher!

As a lawyer, I was finding work more difficult than before. My ability to concentrate seemed to have declined, I was still occasionally tripping over my words and I was running out of steam in the afternoons. I'd also lost confidence, having been out of court for over nine months. Eventually I found the stress and responsibility too much. I just wasn't enjoying it as I had in the past. I didn't want to do it anymore. I kept going for about 12 months when, after much soul searching, I decided to give up the law and look for something else; it has not been easy.

My recovery has not been without its low points. The problems associated with having a stroke are enormous; the problems a younger stroke patient has are even greater. One moment you're in charge – suddenly you lose all control, even over bodily functions. "Stroke shatters lives" says the advertising. My life has been shattered. It has been changed, changed utterly. Yet I have been lucky, very lucky. I am at the better end of the spectrum. I know that the studies done in this area estimate a prevalence of depression in 20–50% of stroke patients. I am sure it is much higher, if not 100%. Of the members who use the *Different Strokes* helpline (see below), at least 80% admit to having been through some sort of depression at some stage of their recovery; the other 20% are in denial!

The hidden side of stroke

Stroke is a traumatic and devastating experience. We are somewhere in the course of our daily life when it strikes: at work, on holiday, relaxing at home, socializing with friends, or even just defending entirely innocent clients. Wherever we are or whatever we are doing, our lives are brought to a complete standstill. Because many of us have had no previous experience of severe illness, the devastating effects of stroke are even more difficult to deal with. Stroke is about loss. The sudden loss of a fully functioning body and mind, which we have always taken for granted. Now instead we have paralyzed arms and legs, an inability to speak or be understood, incontinence, lack of concentration, poor vision, no short-term memory, uncontrollable laughter or tears, or any combination of the above and more. We find it very hard to relate to ourselves as "ill" people, let alone disabled in some way.

Possibly, we have never been in hospital before but almost certainly we will now experience hospitalization and/or rehabilitation units, usually for weeks or even months. We are removed from life, work, relationships, friends, and leisure time and become institutionalized as we begin the long, slow, and difficult process of rehabilitation. Anyone who has had a stroke will know about the huge changes that it brings. The loss of the freedom to "get on with life" while the rest of the world goes by. We are not allowed to function as before but are left feeling vulnerable, helpless, without dignity, frightened, and isolated.

This is the invisible side of stroke. No one can *see* those feelings, or those thoughts. Others can only see the sudden functional loss of parts of our body and, of course, it is vital that we work as hard as possible to regain as much as we can of what we have physically lost. However, it is equally vital that we allow ourselves to consider the "invisible side of stroke." It is not only our bodies that have been damaged, but our thoughts and feelings too. It is totally impossible to have a stroke and not experience extremes of emotion, fear, and anxiety about life, work, family, and close relationships, but most of all emotions about our relationship with, and perception of, ourselves. Everything changes after a stroke and everyone's recovery is individual. The most vital thing for our well-being is that we give ourselves the very best chance of getting better.

It is not easy to ignore the physical changes that a stroke causes, but it is easy to ignore the "invisible" ones. Acknowledging them and facing them can give a fuller, more rounded recovery.

The helpline hot list

When I was discharged from hospital, I found that such care services as were available were geared to the elderly. Bingo and basket-weaving were not the sort of therapies I was drawn to, but they seemed to be all that were on offer. A number of us "younger" patients thought about what sort of active rehabilitation would really help recovery and gradually the idea of a self-help support group grew. Although *Different Strokes* (Box 25.1) is active only in the UK at the moment, its findings and observations on stroke recovery are applicable around the world. In the first five years of its existence, the telephone helpline received calls on certain topics that would arise again and again. The most frequently used word was "dumped" – patients felt that after discharge there was nothing "out there"

Box 25.1 Different Strokes

Different Strokes is a UK charity run by stroke sufferers for stroke sufferers. It recognizes the need for a wider choice of services for younger patients to help them to return to a full life and an active role in their community. Stroke survivors have to learn everything from new, slowly moving and improving one day to the next: learning to talk, walk and live again. *Different Strokes* provides throughout the UK:

- a regional network of exercise classes and swimming sessions (over 30 classes are up and running)
- practical information packs to survivors
- access to counselling services
- benefits and rights information
- advice and info on education, special training information, and work opportunities
- a quarterly newsletter to keep members in touch with each other
- an interactive website
- a telephone helpline staffed by those who have had a stroke

---

to assist them. The points raised in this section draw directly on *Different Strokes'* experiences of working with younger stroke survivors, who frequently complain that help currently available has been designed primarily to meet the requirements of older people. *Different Strokes* advocates a need for a wider choice of services designed for younger stroke survivors to help them to return to a full life and active role in their community.

While in no way wishing to minimize the impact of stroke on older people and their families, *Different Strokes* suggests that the needs of a 20-year-old stroke survivor will be quite different to those of someone aged 80, not least because the 20 year old is faced not just by years but, hopefully, by decades over which to recover from stroke and cope with its impact on family, education, work, and social relationships. Rehabilitation, therefore, must be planned carefully and appropriately to maximize the potential of younger stroke survivors to return to independent living. *Different Strokes* believes that addressing the following issues would facilitate this process and at the same time contribute to reducing long-term dependence on health and social services.

The anecdotal nature of some of these issues is acknowledged but, in the absence of formal research evidence on younger stroke patients, it is hoped that listing them may generate discussion on the needs of this important but often ignored group of patients.

1. At the first onset of stroke, we want to be believed. We have often heard examples of people being treated by health professionals who appear not to understand that stroke can affect young people, with symptoms ascribed to other conditions, from migraine to being drunk.

2. We want to be looked after by staff who understand our specific needs. Specialized stroke nurses on dedicated stroke units would be a good start.

3. Younger adults with stroke often report distress at being admitted to and cared for on elderly care wards. Greater consideration needs to be given to the appropriate setting and location for the care and early rehabilitation of younger stroke patients while in hospital.

4. We want staff to be aware of and address not only the physical effects of stroke but also its emotional, social, and psychological impact. Consideration should be given to providing/improving access to counselling to help younger stroke survivors to come to terms and deal with the short-terms effect of stroke and also to adjust to its long-term implications for housing, personal finances, education, and employment.

5. At discharge from hospital, we do not want to be "written off" as disabled. We want a long-term plan of care which recognizes that we are embarking on a slow but gradual recovery.

6. Existing discharge advice and information is designed to meet the needs of older people. Information on long-term care or nursing homes, for example, is

usually not relevant to the needs of younger stroke survivors, who want discharge advice tailored to their own specific short- and longer-term needs and circumstances. The bingo and basket-weaving currently available at the local day center is not always appropriate!

7. The goals of most younger stroke survivors include achieving, as far as possible, a gradual return to independent living, to employment and to integration into family and social life. Those who design and provide services need to recognize that these goals may differ from those of older people and tailor rehabilitation services accordingly. Emphasis needs to be on treating us as individuals, taking age and personal factors into account.

8. After discharge, the transitional nature of recovery from stroke means that we should have an open-ended commitment to *ongoing* monitoring and assessment of our recovery so that rehabilitation services meet our needs appropriately as they change over time. Ensuring that as patients we have details of a specific person who can be contacted to organize re-assessment of our needs as we progress in our recovery could facilitate this.

9. In meeting the goals of younger stroke survivors, rehabilitation services need to address the specific issues of re-education, retraining, and re-employment.

10. Recognizing that existing health and social services cannot meet the full range of ongoing and long-term rehabilitation needs of younger stroke survivors, consideration should be given to developing innovative ways of meeting some of these needs. Models such as family doctor schemes for prescribing exercise, opportunities for using leisure centers etc. merit further investigation.

11. Younger stroke survivors have a range of information needs, including general advice on disability and help in getting aids and gadgets; information on benefits, social services and patients rights; applying to charities for individual grants; coping with the psychological impact of stroke and people's attitudes to stroke; advice on sex and relationships. (Notes on these topics are produced by *Different Strokes*.) Healthcare purchasers and providers should ensure that younger stroke survivors have timely access to these or comparable leaflets.

12. A number of organizations can provide advice on the specific issue of helping people with disabilities back to work. Health professionals in primary, community, and secondary care need to be aware of the different organizations that can help younger stroke survivors *and* need to convey this information to younger stroke survivors in systematic and timely ways.

13. Carers of people with stroke have their own support, advice, and information needs. Special consideration needs to be given to address the needs of carers of younger stroke survivors, taking into account both the possible long-term nature of this caring role and its transitional and variable nature over time.

Those getting over a stroke need all the help they can get. There is help, but the healthcare professionals who deal with the patient initially need to keep themselves informed of what is available in their area once the hospital treatment ceases. Every little thing you can do can help. Remember: "Nobody made a greater mistake than he who did nothing because he thought he could only do a little."

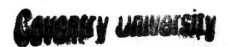

Index